Meyler's Side Effects of Drugs Used in Anesthesia

Meyler's Side Effects of Drugs Used in Anesthesia

Editor

J K Aronson, MA, DPhil, MBChB, FRCP, FBPharmacolS, FFPM (Hon)
Oxford, United Kingdom

ELSEVIER

AMSTERDAM • BOSTON • HEIDELBERG • LONDON • NEW YORK • OXFORD
PARIS • SAN DIEGO • SAN FRANCISCO • SINGAPORE • SYDNEY • TOKYO

Elsevier
Radarweg 29, PO Box 211, 1000 AE Amsterdam, The Netherlands
The Boulevard, Langford Lane, Kidlington, Oxford OX5 1GB, UK
525 B Street, Suite 1900, San Diego, CA 92101-4495, USA

Notice
No responsibility is assumed by the publisher for any injury and/or damage to persons
or property as a matter of products liability, negligence or otherwise, or from any use or operation
of any methods, products, instructions or ideas contained in the material herein. Because of rapid
advances in the medical sciences, in particular, independent verification of diagnoses and drug
dosages should be made

Medicine is an ever-changing field. Standard safety precautions must be followed, but as new
research and clinical experience broaden our knowledge, changes in treatment and drug therapy
may become necessary or appropriate. Readers are advised to check the most current product
information provided by the manufacturer of each drug to be administered to verify the
recommended dose, the method and duration of administrations, and contraindications. It is the
responsibility of the treating physician, relying on experience and knowledge of the patient, to
determine dosages and the best treatment for each individual patient. Neither the publisher nor the
authors assume any liability for any injury and/or damage to persons or property arising from this
publication.

British Library Cataloguing in Publication Data
A catalogue record for this book is available from the British Library

Library of Congress Catalog Number: 2008933969

ISBN: 978-044-453270-1

For information on all Elsevier publications
visit our web site at http://www.elsevierdirect.com

Printed and bound by CPI Group (UK) Ltd, Croydon, CR0 4YY

Transferred to Digital Print 2011

Working together to grow
libraries in developing countries

www.elsevier.com | www.bookaid.org | www.sabre.org

ELSEVIER   BOOK AID
International   Sabre Foundation

Contents

Preface

This volume covers the adverse effects of medicines used in anesthesia. The material has been collected from *Meyler's Side Effects of Drugs: The International Encyclopedia of Adverse Drug Reactions and Interactions* (15th edition, 2006, in six volumes), which was itself based on previous editions of *Meyler's Side Effects of Drugs*, and from the *Side Effects of Drugs Annuals* (SEDA) 28, 29, and 30. The main contributors of this material were JK Aronson, Z Baudoin, HMD Cardwell, P Flisberg, SA Jackson, I Kurowski, T Ledowski, M Leuwer, DJ O'Connor, A Raajkumar, SA Schug, ID Welters, Y Young, and O Zuzan.

A brief history of the Meyler series

Leopold Meyler was a physician who was treated for tuberculosis after the end of the Nazi occupation of The Netherlands. According to Professor Wim Lammers, writing a tribute in Volume VIII (1975), Meyler got a fever from para-aminosalicylic acid, but elsewhere Graham Dukes has written, based on information from Meyler's widow, that it was deafness from dihydrostreptomycin; perhaps it was both. Meyler discovered that there was no single text to which medical practitioners could look for information about unwanted effects of drug therapy; Louis Lewin's text "Die Nebenwirkungen der Arzneimittel" ("The Untoward Effects of Drugs") of 1881 had long been out of print (SEDA-27, xxv-xxix). Meyler therefore determined to make such information available and persuaded the Netherlands publishing firm of Van Gorcum to publish a book, in Dutch, entirely devoted to descriptions of the adverse effects that drugs could cause. He went on to agree with the Elsevier Publishing Company, as it was then called, to prepare and issue an English translation. The first edition of 192 pages (*Schadelijke Nevenwerkingen van Geneesmiddelen*) appeared in 1951 and the English version (*Side Effects of Drugs*) a year later.

The book was a great success, and a few years later Meyler started to publish what he called surveys of unwanted effects of drugs. Each survey covered a period of two to four years. They were labelled as volumes rather than editions, and after Volume IV had been published Meyler could no longer handle the task alone. For subsequent volumes he recruited collaborators, such as Andrew Herxheimer. In September 1973 Meyler died unexpectedly, and Elsevier invited Graham Dukes to take over the editing of Volume VIII.

Dukes persuaded Elsevier that the published literature was too large to be comfortably encompassed in a four-yearly cycle, and he suggested that the volumes should be produced annually instead. The four-yearly volume could then concentrate on providing a complementary critical encyclopaedic survey of the entire field. The first *Side Effects of Drugs Annual* was published in 1977. The first encyclopaedic edition of *Meyler's Side Effects of Drugs*, which appeared in 1980, was labelled the ninth edition, and since then a new encyclopaedic edition has appeared every four years. The 15th edition was published in 2006, in both hard and electronic versions.

Monograph structure

This volume is in three sections:

- general anesthetics—a general introduction to their adverse effects, followed by monographs on individual inhalational and intravenous anesthetics;
- local anesthetics—a general introduction to their adverse effects, including the adverse effects of different routes of administration, followed by monographs on individual local anesthetics;
- neuromuscular blocking agents and muscle relaxants—a general introduction to their adverse effects, followed by monographs on individual agents.

In each monograph in the Meyler series the information is organized into sections as shown on the next page (although not all the sections are covered in each monograph).

Drug names

Drugs have usually been designated by their recommended or proposed International Non-proprietary Names (rINN or pINN); when these are not available, chemical names have been used. In some cases brand names have been used.

Spelling

For indexing purposes, American spelling has been used, e.g. anemia, estrogen rather than anaemia, oestrogen.

Cross-references

The various editions of *Meyler's Side Effects of Drugs* are cited in the text as SED-13, SED-14, etc; the *Side Effects of Drugs Annuals* are cited as SEDA-1, SEDA-2, etc.

J K Aronson
Oxford, June 2008

Organization of material in monographs in the Meyler series (not all sections are included in each monograph)

General information
Drug studies
Observational studies
Comparative studies
Drug-combination studies
Placebo-controlled studies
Systematic reviews
Organs and systems
Cardiovascular
Respiratory
Ear, nose, throat
Nervous system
Neuromuscular function
Sensory systems
Psychological
Psychiatric
Endocrine
Metabolism
Nutrition
Electrolyte balance
Mineral balance
Metal metabolism
Acid-base balance
Fluid balance
Hematologic
Mouth
Teeth
Salivary glands
Gastrointestinal
Liver
Biliary tract
Pancreas
Urinary tract
Skin
Hair
Nails
Sweat glands
Serosae
Musculoskeletal
Sexual function
Reproductive system
Breasts
Immunologic
Autacoids
Infection risk

Body temperature
Multiorgan failure
Trauma
Death
Long-term effects
Drug abuse
Drug misuse
Drug tolerance
Drug resistance
Drug dependence
Drug withdrawal
Genotoxicity
Cytotoxicity
Mutagenicity
Tumorigenicity
Second-generation effects
Fertility
Pregnancy
Teratogenicity
Fetotoxicity
Lactation
Breast feeding
Susceptibility factors
Genetic factors
Age
Sex
Physiological factors
Disease
Other features of the patient
Drug administration
Drug formulations
Drug additives
Drug contamination and adulteration
Drug dosage regimens
Drug administration route
Drug overdose
Interactions
Drug-drug interactions
Food-drug interactions
Drug-device interactions
Smoking
Other environmental interactions
Interference with diagnostic tests
Diagnosis of adverse drug reactions
Management of adverse drug reactions
Monitoring therapy
References

GENERAL ANESTHETICS

General Information

The inhalational and injectable agents that are covered in separate monographs are listed in the table below.

The inhalational agents in common use share similar adverse effects, albeit with differing incidences. Initial hopes that new agents will be less problematic generally fade as their use increases and familiarity with their adverse effects grows. Although some untoward reactions related to inhalational anesthetics are unpredictable, it is important for the anesthetist/anesthesiologist to determine which patients are primarily at risk, so that safer use of anesthetic agents and better supervision of surgical patients can be achieved.

Inhalational	Injectable
Halogenated	*Barbiturates*
Chloroform	Methohexital
Desflurane	Thiamylal
Enflurane	Thiopental
Halothane	*Others*
Isoflurane	Alfadolone/alfaxolone
Methoxyflurane	Etomidate
Sevoflurane	Ketamine
Trichloroethylene	Propanidid
Others	Propofol
Anesthetic ether	
Cyclopropane	
Nitrous oxide	
Xenon	

Anesthetic combinations

The importance of multiple anesthetics should not be overlooked. For example, patients in whom halothane anesthesia is given twice, at an interval of less than 6 weeks, are at major risk of developing jaundice. Some anesthetists avoid any second exposure to this agent. However, there are several reasons why single agents are often insufficient in anesthesia: different problems require separate treatments; the severity of the adverse effects of individual drugs can sometimes be reduced by the use of combinations; and repeated administration of a single agent can lead to cumulative effects. Drug interactions in anesthesia are therefore potentially common and have been reviewed, both systematically (1) and as uncritical listings (2,3). Many of the interactions are beneficial, the concurrent use of two or more different agents improving the quality of anesthesia. Several reviews of this have appeared (4–6). Disadvantages of combinations include unpredictability of synergistic actions or toxicity, mutual alterations in pharmacokinetics, increased likelihood of errors in drug administration, and difficulties in planning drug therapy when adverse effects occur and are not attributable to a particular drug.

Dental anesthesia

Adverse effects of dental anesthesia represent a special problem, about which reliable data are hard to obtain. Several studies of the safety of dental anesthesia have been performed in the USA (SEDA-18, 113); unfortunately, all have weaknesses. More informative is an American survey in which 47 oral and maxillofacial surgeons were approached directly, and all responded (7). Among the 74 871 patients to whom they had given general anesthesia, there were 250 cases of laryngospasm, 51 of phlebitis, 30 of dysrhythmias sufficiently severe to require therapy, 17 of hypotension requiring drug therapy, and 13 of bronchospasm. A few patients had allergic reactions requiring drug therapy ($n = 4$), convulsions ($n = 4$), hypertension ($n = 2$), myocardial infarction ($n = 2$), or vomiting with aspiration ($n = 2$); in one case an injection was inadvertently given into an artery.

Sedation for endoscopy

Gastrointestinal endoscopy is one of the most commonly performed invasive procedures in clinical practice (for example about 500 000 procedures per annum in Australasia). Propofol is a short-acting intravenous anesthetic with a rapid onset of action and a short half-life, making it eminently suitable for day procedures. However, the use of propofol by non-anesthetists has been controversial because of the perceived risks of its low therapeutic ratio. In many jurisdictions, package inserts insist that it is only for use by anesthetists.

In a review of nurse-administered endoscopy sedation regimens that primarily used propofol the incidence of adverse events was examined (8). Respiratory depression, presenting as apnea and hypoxemia, is the most serious adverse event. The authors of this review have suggested that individuals administering propofol must be able to support ventilation. Respiratory depression appears to be more common after upper gastrointestinal endoscopy. Hypotension is also common, particularly in elderly people or in those with impaired left ventricular function. Most of the studies reviewed only examined American Society of Anesthesiology (ASA) Class 1 and 2 patients (i.e. they did not include patients with significant co-morbidity). The reviewers suggested that registered nurse-administered endoscopy sedation with propofol is safe, provided that the nurse is appropriately trained, that there is appropriate monitoring (probably including capnography), and that the nurse must attend solely to the patient and have no other functions to perform simultaneously in the endoscopy suite (for example assisting the endoscopist).

A contrary view has been taken in a prospective study of propofol sedation in 500 ASA 1 and ASA 2 patients undergoing upper gastrointestinal endoscopic ultrasound in a Canadian center (9). Propofol sedation (bolus plus infusion) was administered by the endoscopist and not a dedicated nurse. Patients were monitored by clinical observation, pulse oximetry, and automated sphygmomanometry. All received supplementary oxygen 2 l/minute during the procedures. There was oxygen desaturation (defined as an oxygen saturation below 95%) in 16 patients (3%). There was hypoxemia (saturation below 90%) in four patients (0.8%). Increasing the supplementary oxygen to 4 l/minute was all that was required in nine patients. Increasing the supplementary oxygen and jaw lift was needed in one patient. Increasing the supplementary oxygen, jaw lift, and stopping the propofol infusion was necessary in the other six patients. Assisted ventilation was not required. There were no cases of hypotension, bradycardia, or tachycardia. The authors concluded that propofol may be safely administered by endoscopists who are familiar with its pharmacological properties and uses, and that there was a high level of satisfaction for both patient and anesthetist. However, they went on to say that in fact they found using propofol without a dedicated administrator and observer rather stressful, and that most of the endoscopists had returned to using intermittent bolus midazolam + pethidine (meperidine).

The authors of a third prospective randomized study took a different approach, by comparing patient-controlled propofol with patient-controlled remifentanil (an ultra-short acting opioid) in 77 patients undergoing gastrointestinal endoscopy (10). Patient satisfaction was high in both groups. There were significantly more awake and oriented patients among those who received remifentanil (46 versus 24%). Unfortunately, nausea was also more common (29 versus 0%). There were two cases of oxygen desaturation (<92%) in the remifentanil group and none in the propofol group. Monitoring did not include capnography.

The incidence of adverse events related to an endoscopy sedation regimen that included propofol (in addition to midazolam and fentanyl), delivered by specially trained general practitioners, has been examined in a prospective audit (11); 28 472 procedures were performed over 5 years. There were 185 sedation-related adverse events, 107 with airway or ventilation problems; 123 interventions were necessary to maintain ventilation. No patients required tracheal intubation and there were no deaths. The authors concluded that appropriately trained general practitioners encountered a low incidence of adverse events and could safely use propofol for sedation during endoscopy. It should be noted that all the general practitioners had some experience in anesthesia or intensive care and were individually trained by the Director of Anesthesia.

Sedation for surgery under regional anesthesia

Sedation during prolonged surgical procedures under regional anesthesia can be quite challenging. The beta$_2$ adrenoceptor agonist dexmedetomidine has potent sedative and analgesic-sparing properties. In therapeutic doses it does not cause respiratory depression, making it attractive for infusion sedation. However, it causes reduced sympathetic outflow, which might cause untoward hemodynamic upset during intraoperative sedation. Dexmedetomidine has been compared with propofol in a prospective randomized trial in 40 patients (12). Dexmedetomidine provided slightly slower onset and offset of sedation, higher intraoperative blood pressure, and better postoperative analgesia.

Remifentanil is a highly selective OP$_3$ (μ, MOR) opioid receptor agonist with an extremely short onset and offset of action, allowing rapid and accurate titration of infusion rate to drug effect with rapid down-titration in case of

respiratory adverse effects. This makes it attractive for sedation. The efficacy and adverse effects profiles of remifentanil and propofol have been compared in a randomized, single-blind trial in 125 patients undergoing surgery with regional anesthesia (13). In those given remifentanil, nausea and vomiting were more frequent (27 versus 2%) and there was significantly more respiratory depression (46 versus 19%).

Sedation in intensive care

It has been proposed that a combination of propofol and midazolam may have advantages over either drug alone, reducing adverse effects while preserving the potential benefits ("co-sedation"). Propofol combined with a constant low dose of midazolam (1.0 mg/hour) has been compared with propofol alone for postoperative sedation in a randomized, placebo-controlled, double-blind trial in 60 patients undergoing coronary artery surgery under high-dose fentanyl anesthesia (14). Target sedation was achieved more readily with co-sedation (91 versus 79%) but at the expense of prolonged weaning from mechanical ventilation (432 versus 319 minutes). However, it is not clear whether this slightly prolonged time on the ventilator affected length of stay in the ICU.

It remains a source of much concern that those working in operating theaters spend their time in such a polluted environment, in spite of attempts to introduce scavenging of waste anesthetic gases (15). This is not without its effects. There is, for example, a relation between asthma and occupational exposure to various respiratory hazards, including anesthetic gases (16).

The α$_2$-adrenoceptor agonist dexmedetomidine has potent sedative and analgesia-sparing properties. In therapeutic doses it does not cause respiratory depression, making it attractive for infusion sedation. However, it causes reduced sympathetic outflow, which might cause untoward hemodynamic upset but might also have beneficial β-adrenoceptor antagonist-like value in patients undergoing cardiovascular surgery. Its use in pediatrics has been anecdotal. Dexmedetomidine has been compared with midazolam in a prospective randomized trial in 30 infants and children undergoing mechanical ventilation (17). Dexmedetomidine 0.5 micrograms/kg/hour provided more effective sedation, reduced supplementary morphine requirements, and reduced the number of patients with inadequate sedation. There was no difference in blood pressure, but heart rates were significantly lower in the children who received dexmedetomidine. One infant who received dexmedetomidine and concurrent digoxin developed bradycardia, but this resolved within an hour of withdrawing the dexmedetomidine.

Comparative studies

Halothane versus propofol

A randomized prospective trial in 60 children undergoing outpatient anesthesia showed a 30% shorter time from discontinuation of anesthesia to eye opening and return to full wakefulness in patients receiving propofol alone compared with halothane + nitrous oxide anesthesia (18). Propofol was associated with a 17% incidence of emesis compared with 58 and 53% for halothane + nitrous oxide and propofol + nitrous oxide anesthesia respectively.

Isoflurane + nitrous oxide versus propofol

The risk of postoperative nausea and vomiting has been studied in a randomized, controlled trial of total intravenous anesthesia with propofol versus inhalational anesthesia with isoflurane and nitrous oxide in 2010 patients (19). It was accompanied by an economic analysis. Propofol total intravenous anesthesia reduced the absolute risk of postoperative nausea and vomiting up to 72 hours postoperatively from 61 to 46%, in inpatients (NNT = 6) and from 46 to 28% in outpatients (NNT = 5). Both anesthetic techniques were otherwise similar. Anesthesia drug costs were more than three times higher for propofol total intravenous anesthesia (as propofol is substantially more expensive than isoflurane + nitrous oxide). However, the patients preferred propofol.

Isoflurane versus sevoflurane

A study of single vital-capacity breath inhalational induction using either isoflurane or sevoflurane combined with 67% nitrous oxide in 67 adults showed that isoflurane was unsuitable for this technique (20). There was an 87% incidence of induction complications with isoflurane, including involuntary movements, cough, laryngospasm, and failure of induction.

In 75 patients of ASA grades 1 or 2, recovery from anesthesia after maintenance with isoflurane + nitrous oxide was significantly slower than with sevoflurane + nitrous oxide (21).

Isoflurane and sevoflurane have been compared in a randomized study in 180 patients undergoing knee arthroscopy (22). In those given sevoflurane there were significantly more respiratory and cardiovascular complications and increased nausea and vomiting.

In a comparison of sevoflurane and isoflurane anesthesia in 2008 patients there was a 3–4 minute reduction in time to recovery end-points with sevoflurane (23). These differences became larger in anesthetics lasting over 3 hours and were trivial in cases less than 1 hour. Patients aged over 65 years had a 5-minute increase in recovery times after receiving isoflurane. There was no significant difference in the incidence of nausea or vomiting between isoflurane, sevoflurane, and propofol.

Propofol versus sevoflurane

Sevoflurane is pleasant to breathe and has a rapid onset and offset of action. It is challenging the tradition of intravenous anesthetic induction in adult patients. In a meta-analysis of 12 studies in 1102 adult patients, intravenous bolus doses of sevoflurane 7–8% and propofol for anesthetic induction were compared (24). Anesthesia maintenance included nitrous oxide 50–70% and either propofol infusion or sevoflurane inhalation, and spontaneous ventilation via a laryngeal mask. Patients in the sevoflurane group were significantly more likely to have postoperative nausea and vomiting (odds ratios 4.2 and 3.2). There were non-significant trends toward greater patient dissatisfaction and a longer induction time in the

sevoflurane group, and more frequent apnea in the propofol group. There were no significant complications in either group. Both agents are suitable for anesthetic induction, but propofol retains a small advantage in having better recovery characteristics.

Single-agent induction and maintenance of anesthesia has been compared in a randomized study of 44 patients undergoing elective spinal surgery (25). Patients received either propofol 4–6 µg/ml via a target-controlled infusion or sevoflurane 8% for induction, and sevoflurane 3.5% + 67% nitrous oxide for maintenance plus alfentanil as required. Patients in the propofol group required a significantly larger dose of opiate during the procedure (2.2 mg versus 0.3 mg). Two patients who received propofol complained of pain on injection. There was no significant breath-holding or laryngospasm in either group. Heart rate was significantly lower in the sevoflurane group compared with propofol both before and after incision. The numbers of adjustments to the patient's depth of anesthesia were similar in both groups. The authors concluded that either technique was suitable for spinal surgery. The inclusion of nitrous oxide in the sevoflurane group accounted for the differences in opioid requirements.

The effects of hypercapnia on cerebral autoregulation during sevoflurane or propofol anesthesia have been studied in a randomized, crossover study in eight healthy patients (26). Hypercapnia began to inhibit cerebral autoregulation, as measured by transcranial Doppler at a mean value of 56 mmHg P_aCO_2 with sevoflurane 1.0–1.1% and at 61 mmHg P_aCO_2 with propofol 140 µg/kg/minute. Patients also received remifentanil for analgesia, a drug with no known effects on cerebral autoregulation. The study is important, because one advantage of both propofol anesthesia and sevoflurane anesthesia is the lack of inhibition of cerebral autoregulation at standard doses. Clearly, careful control of ventilation is required for this to be true.

The effects of isoflurane, sevoflurane, and propofol on jugular venous oxygen saturation (S_jO_2) in patients undergoing coronary artery bypass surgery have been studied (27). S_jO_2 values were significantly lower in the propofol group 1 hour after bypass, suggesting an imbalance of oxygen supply and demand with propofol. Because anesthetic agents also reduce the cerebral metabolic rate, the implications of this finding are uncertain. However, low S_jO_2 values have previously been associated with postoperative neuropsychiatric dysfunction after cardiopulmonary bypass.

Vital capacity inhalational induction of anesthesia with sevoflurane has been compared with intravenous induction using propofol in 56 adults undergoing ambulatory anesthesia (28). The patients were randomized to either sevoflurane 8% + nitrous oxide 75% mixture at 8 l/minute ($n = 32$), or propofol 2 mg/kg bolus ($n = 24$), without any premedication. Induction time was significantly shorter with sevoflurane (average 51 seconds) than propofol (average 81 seconds). Adverse effects were different in the two groups: sevoflurane caused cough and hiccups, while propofol caused a fall in blood pressure and reduced movements. The overall incidence of adverse effects was similar. Postoperatively, there was mild nausea in 78% of the patients who received sevoflurane compared with 50%

for propofol. However, no antiemetics were needed and discharge times were not delayed.

The characteristics of sevoflurane anesthesia have been compared with those of target-controlled infusion of propofol in 61 day-case adults undergoing surgery (29). All received nitrous oxide 50% and fentanyl 1 µg/kg. After insertion of a laryngeal mask airway the propofol target concentration was reduced from 8 to 4 µg/ml and the inspired concentration of sevoflurane was reduced from 8 to 3% and subsequently titrated to clinical effects. Mean times to loss of consciousness and laryngeal mask airway insertion were significantly longer after sevoflurane (73 and 146 seconds respectively) than with propofol (50 and 116 seconds respectively). Sevoflurane was associated with a lower incidence of intraoperative movements (10 versus 55%), necessitating less adjustment to the dose. The incidence of movement in the propofol group was comparable to other studies. Emergence was faster after sevoflurane (5.3 versus 7.1 minutes) but sevoflurane was associated with more postoperative nausea (30 versus 17%) and vomiting (3 versus 0%), resulting in delayed discharge times (258 versus 193 minutes) and a higher total cost. The finding of significantly earlier discharge times after propofol anesthesia was unusual.

Propofol + alfentanil + nitrous oxide anesthesia has been compared with sevoflurane + nitrous oxide anesthesia in 44 patients undergoing dilatation and evacuation of the uterus (30). There was significantly less intraoperative uterine bleeding, as estimated by the gynecologist, with propofol. Above-average bleeding occurred in 5% of the patients with propofol anesthesia and 27% of patients with sevoflurane. This result was not surprising, given that sevoflurane reduces uterine tone, while propofol has no effect.

In a prospective randomized study of 120 day-surgery patients, desflurane and sevoflurane were associated with shorter times to awakening, extubation, and orientation than propofol infusion (31). Average times to awakening at the end of anesthesia were 5, 5, and 8 minutes respectively. There were no significant differences in time-to-home readiness or actual discharge times. A review of 436 patients undergoing either sevoflurane or propofol-based anesthesia showed no difference in similar recovery end-points (23).

There has been a prospective randomized comparison of 185 patients who received propofol 6–8 mg/kg/hour and sevoflurane 1.5% for maintenance of anesthesia (29). The patients were ventilated via a laryngeal mask and no muscle relaxants were given. Both agents were suitable for this technique. Emergence was significantly faster after sevoflurane but associated with more excitatory phenomena and tachycardia.

Sevoflurane versus thiopental
Sevoflurane 8% plus nitrous oxide 66% has been compared with thiopental 4 mg/kg for induction of anesthesia in brief outpatient procedures (30). Sevoflurane was safer, more efficacious, and better accepted by 78 unpremedicated adults with laryngeal cancer undergoing direct laryngoscopy for staging and biopsy. All received suxamethonium 50 mg on loss of the eyelash reflex and the surgeon then performed the laryngoscopy. Hemodynamic

stability was greater and immediate recovery was faster after sevoflurane (9.7 versus 11.4 minutes). The incidence of dysrhythmias was also higher with thiopental (19 versus 12 patients). The dysrhythmias were predominantly ventricular extra beats with sevoflurane and ventricular bigemini with thiopental. The high incidence of dysrhythmias was partly due to the lack of opioid medication as part of the anesthetic.

Organs and Systems

Cardiovascular

Volatile anesthetic agents depress cardiac output, especially in the elderly. A study of 80 patients aged over 60 years compared the effects of halothane and isoflurane with and without nitrous oxide 50% (34). Doses were carefully adjusted to be equipotent in all four groups. Isoflurane caused a 30% reduction in systolic and diastolic arterial pressures compared with a 17% reduction with halothane. The reductions in cardiac index were similar with the two agents, about 17%. The addition of nitrous oxide attenuated the reductions in arterial pressure. In the case of the combination of isoflurane with nitrous oxide, there was a small increase in cardiac index and a small reduction in the halothane/nitrous oxide group. Systemic vascular resistance was reduced by a greater extent with isoflurane compared with halothane and little altered by the addition of nitrous oxide. The result suggests that nitrous oxide supplementation may be advantageous in the elderly, but interpretation is limited by the fact that it does not include the effects of surgery on these important cardiac parameters.

The long QT syndrome is associated with potentially fatal ventricular dysrhythmias under anesthesia. The effect of halothane and isoflurane on the QT interval was studied in 51 healthy children (35). Isoflurane 2.3–3.0% increased the average QT interval from 425 to 475 milliseconds at the time of induction. Halothane reduced the average QT interval from 428 to 407 milliseconds. The result suggested that halothane may be the more desirable agent in children with a prolonged QT interval.

The frequencies of cardiac dysrhythmias during halothane and sevoflurane inhalation have been compared in 150 children aged 3–15 years undergoing outpatient general anesthesia for dental extraction (36). They were randomized into three groups and received either halothane or sevoflurane in 66% nitrous oxide whilst breathing spontaneously. One group received 0.75% increments of halothane every two to three breaths to a maximum of 3.0% for induction, and then 1.5% for maintenance of anesthesia. One group received sevoflurane in 2% increments to a maximum of 8% and then a maintenance dose of 4%. The final group received 8% sevoflurane for induction and then a maintenance dose of 4%. The children who received halothane had a 48% incidence of dysrhythmias, significantly higher than the 16% incidence in the sevoflurane group and 8% in the incremental sevoflurane group. The halothane-associated dysrhythmias mainly occurred during dental extraction or emergence from anesthesia, and were usually ventricular.

Six children in the halothane group had ventricular tachycardia. The longest run of ventricular tachycardia lasted 5.5 seconds, and one child had 13 separate episodes. Sevoflurane-associated dysrhythmias were mainly single supraventricular extra beats, and did not differ between the two administration methods. Although there was insufficient evidence to suggest that transient dysrhythmias associated with halothane in dental anesthesia can lead to cardiac arrest, sustained ectopic ventricular activity, including ventricular tachycardia, even if self-limiting, results in reduced cardiac output and cannot be ignored. These results imply that sevoflurane may be the preferable agent in this setting.

The hemodynamic responses to induction and maintenance of anesthesia with halothane have been compared with those of sevoflurane in 68 unpremedicated children aged 1–3 years undergoing adenoidectomy (37). The children received either sevoflurane 8% or halothane 5% + nitrous oxide 66% for induction of anesthesia and tracheal intubation, without neuromuscular blocking drugs. Anesthesia was maintained by adjusting the inspired concentration of the volatile anesthetic to maintain arterial blood pressure within 20% of baseline values, and the electrocardiogram was continuously recorded. The incidence of cardiac dysrhythmias was 23% with halothane and 6% with sevoflurane. Most of the dysrhythmias were short-lasting/self-limiting supraventricular extra beats or ventricular extra beats. Although the overall incidence of dysrhythmias was low in both groups, the result again shows that sevoflurane causes fewer dysrhythmias in children and may be the preferable agent.

QT dispersion, defined as the difference between QT_{max} and QT_{min} in the 12-lead electrocardiogram, is a measure of regional variation in ventricular repolarization (38). It is greater in patients with dysrhythmias. The effects of halothane and isoflurane on QT dispersion have been studied in 46 adult patients undergoing general anesthesia. QT dispersion was increased in both groups both with and without correction for heart rate. The increase was significantly greater with halothane than with isoflurane. The clinical significance of this finding is not known. In isolation, QT dispersion reflects an abnormality in ventricular repolarization and correlates with dysrhythmic events. Although there were no overt dysrhythmias in this study, the effect suggests a reason for the variable results of past studies of the QT interval: most studies showed prolongation of the QT interval, but some showed no change, or shortening. Larger studies are needed to elaborate on the possible clinical importance of this phenomenon, but it may be a significant cause of dysrhythmias with volatile anesthetics.

Respiratory

The incidence of perioperative respiratory complications has been studied prospectively in 602 children aged 1 month to 12 years undergoing elective surgery using a halothane-based anesthetic (39). Exposure to environmental smoke was assessed using the history of exposure to cigarette smoke and measurement of urinary cotinine concentrations, and the respiratory complications of laryngospasm, bronchospasm, stridor, breath holding, coughing, and excessive mucus production were recorded. The incidence of respiratory concentrations in patients with a urinary cotinine concentration over 40 ng/ml was 42%, dropping to 24% in patients with a urinary cotinine concentration less than 10 ng/ml. Female sex and lower socioeconomic status of the mother increased the incidence of respiratory complications. The study showed the importance of factors other than the anesthetic drugs and techniques used in determining complications precipitated by anesthesia.

The respiratory effects of sevoflurane and halothane have been investigated in 30 infants aged 6–24 months (40). Respiratory depression was greater in the sevoflurane group, with a mean minute ventilation of 4.5 compared with 5.4 l/minute/m^2 and respiratory rate was lower at 38 compared with 47 breaths/minute. There was a lower incidence of thoracoabdominal asynchrony with sevoflurane, but no difference in respiratory drive, as evidenced by the flow pressure generated during 100 milliseconds of occlusion of the airway.

The effects of desflurane and sevoflurane on bronchial smooth muscle reactivity have been compared in a randomized study of 40 patients (41). Anesthesia was induced with thiopental, followed by muscle relaxation and ventilation. Airway pressures were recorded during administration of desflurane or sevoflurane at one minimal alveolar concentration (MAC). Airway resistance increased by 5% in the desflurane group and fell by 15% in the sevoflurane group. The increase in airways resistance was greater in smokers and with desflurane, but did not differ with sevoflurane. The result was a surprise, given that desflurane stimulates the sympathetic nervous system. Thiopental also increased airways resistance by 10%. The result is important, because induction of anesthesia can cause bronchospasm and desflurane can exacerbate this.

Nervous system

The effects of sevoflurane and isoflurane anesthesia on interictal spike activity have been studied in 12 patients with refractory epilepsy (42). The patients were undergoing insertion of subdural electrodes and were also given fentanyl during surgery. Electroencephalogram spike frequency increased significantly in all patients during 1.5 MAC sevoflurane anesthesia compared with awake recordings; hypocapnia did not change this increased spike activity. The electrocorticographic interictal spike frequency was also significantly higher in all patients during 1.5 MAC sevoflurane anesthesia and in eight of 10 patients during 1.5 MAC isoflurane anesthesia, compared with 0.3 MAC isoflurane anesthesia. In susceptible individuals, both sevoflurane and isoflurane can provoke interictal spike activity. This effect is only well described for enflurane, but it is a dose-dependent feature of most volatile agents.

Convulsions during anesthesia are of concern because with the use of muscle relaxants they may go unrecognized. The epileptogenic properties of isoflurane and sevoflurane have been compared under a range of different ventilatory conditions in 24 ASA I or II mentally handicapped patients undergoing dental operations (43). Half had a history of epilepsy and half did not. Each patient was ventilated with 100% oxygen (end-tidal carbon dioxide = 40 mmHg; A), then 50% oxygen 50% nitrous oxide (end-tidal carbon dioxide = 40 mmHg; B), and then 100% oxygen (end-tidal carbon dioxide = 20 mmHg; C). With each different mode of ventilation, isoflurane was given at 1 MAC then at 1.5 and 2.0 MAC. The process was repeated 3 months later with sevoflurane. The electroencephalogram was concurrently recorded. The spike and wave index increased significantly from 2.0% during 1.0 MAC sevoflurane to 6.1% during 2.0 MAC in group A in those with epilepsy, while no spike activity was seen in those without epilepsy. Only a few spikes were observed in the isoflurane group in A, with none in B or C. Supplementation with nitrous oxide or hyperventilation suppressed the occurrence of spikes. The authors concluded that sevoflurane has stronger epileptogenic properties than isoflurane, but that this can be counteracted by nitrous oxide or hyperventilation.

There has been an impressive French study of the risks of occupational exposure of hospital personnel to anesthetics among the staff of 18 Paris hospitals (excluding doctors) over 12 years (44). Among 557 staff who had been exposed to anesthetics and 566 workers who had been less exposed, neuropsychological and neurological symptoms (tiredness, nausea, headaches, memory impairment, reduced reaction time, tingling, numbness, cramps) were reported some three times more commonly by workers in theaters that had been less often scavenged than by controls; no difference was found between workers from well-scavenging theaters and controls. Neuropsychological symptoms were reported in several earlier papers (45).

Neuromuscular function

Both desflurane and sevoflurane significantly increase the neuromuscular blocking effects of rocuronium compared with isoflurane or propofol (46,47). The effective doses of rocuronium for 50% depression of single twitch height were 95, 120, 130, and 150 µg/kg for desflurane, sevoflurane, isoflurane, and propofol respectively. There were no differences in recovery profiles between the four drugs using equieffective doses. Desflurane, sevoflurane, and to a lesser extent isoflurane, also potentiated the neuromuscular blocking effect of cisatracurium by 30% compared with propofol (48,49).

Hematologic

Hemostasis can be impaired by both surgery and general anesthetics (50). Fentanyl, halothane, and enflurane enhance fibrinolytic activity significantly (51). In addition, there was a raised plasma beta-thromboglobulin concentration (a good indicator of platelet activation) in 61 patients after the use of nitrous oxide, oxygen, and halothane compared with controls (52).

In an in vitro study of the inhibitory effects of thiopental, midazolam, and ketamine on human neutrophil function, thiopental and midazolam inhibited chemotaxis, phagocytosis, and reactive oxygen species production at clinically relevant concentrations (53). Ketamine only impaired chemotaxis. These results may be relevant in guiding anesthetic drug therapy in septic patients.

Gastrointestinal

About 2 million day-case anesthetics are administered annually in England. Most ophthalmic surgical procedures are carried out in the elderly as day-case procedures. Anesthetic practice varies widely in this context, because of a large and contradictory evidence base for optimal anesthetic in day surgery. In a prospective randomized controlled study in 96 elderly adults undergoing ophthalmic surgery (54) sevoflurane, when used for induction and maintenance, was more costly, less well tolerated, and associated with higher rates of postoperative nausea and vomiting than anesthetic regimens using propofol for induction of anesthesia.

In a prospective study of 556 adults using isoflurane-, halothane-, or enflurane-based anesthesia for ear, nose, throat, and eye procedures, the incidences of emesis in the various groups over the ensuing 24 hours were 36, 41, and 46% respectively (55). Other drugs given during anesthesia included midazolam, thiopental, morphine, and nitrous oxide. Antiemetic requirements were also less with isoflurane: 12% of patients required an antiemetic compared with 23% with halothane and enflurane. There were no differences in the overall incidences of headache or analgesic requirements in the three groups.

In another prospective study of nausea and vomiting in 50 patients undergoing arthroscopy, sevoflurane was compared with desflurane (56). Other drugs given during anesthesia included propofol and alfentanil. There was no difference in the incidence of nausea, 8 and 16% respectively, and no vomiting in either group. The desflurane group had a significantly higher incidence of sore throat (32 versus 8%). These studies have confirmed that the newer volatile anesthetics isoflurane, sevoflurane, and desflurane cause less nausea and vomiting than halothane or enflurane.

Because population measures of anesthetic dosages do not consider the individual's anesthetic needs, anesthetists often err on the side of relative overdosage during balanced anesthesia, in order to prevent the devastating consequences of unintentional awareness during surgery. This excessive depth of anesthesia contributes to delayed recovery and more adverse effects, which is particularly important in ambulatory surgery. Monitoring of the bispectral index-processed electroencephalogram has enabled anesthetists to monitor the depth of anesthesia and has brought greater precision to the administration of intravenous and inhaled anesthetics and opioids. The hypothesis that titration of the maintenance dose of sevoflurane during outpatient gynecological surgery using bispectral index monitoring reduces postoperative vomiting and improves recovery has been tested in a randomized, controlled study in 22 patients (57). The monitored patients had significantly less vomiting than the controls (16 versus 40%).

Several small clinical trials have suggested that total intravenous anesthesia with propofol reduces the incidence of postoperative nausea and vomiting and results in shorter emergence times. However, a systematic review (58) and a meta-analysis (59) have shown that most studies were small, did not have follow-up for more than 6 hours postoperatively, and were sponsored by industry.

The results were difficult to combine, owing to heterogeneous definitions of postoperative nausea and vomiting.

A simplified risk score for predicting postoperative nausea and vomiting in adult patients undergoing general anesthesia has been developed. In a study of 520 adults from Finland and 2202 patients from Germany who had received anesthesia that included benzodiazepine premedication, thiopental, fentanyl or alfentanil, isoflurane, enflurane or sevoflurane, and non-steroidal or opioid drugs for postoperative analgesia no antiemetic prophylaxis was given (60). The final derived score consisted of four predictors: female sex, a history of motion sickness or postoperative nausea and vomiting, non-smoking, and the use of postoperative opioids. The incidence of postoperative nausea and vomiting was 10% when there were no risk factors, 21% (one risk factor), 39% (two risk factors), 61% (three risk factors), and 79% (four risk factors). Only one of the four risk factors related to the drugs used.

Postoperative nausea and vomiting in children has been reviewed in detail, including multimodal strategies for management and prevention (61).

Urinary tract

Methoxyflurane, enflurane, isoflurane, and sevoflurane all release inorganic fluoride ions as a result of hepatic metabolism. Fluoride is nephrotoxic.

Renal function and fluoride ion release after anesthesia using not more than 2.4% sevoflurane or 1.9% isoflurane have been studied in 50 patients of ASA grades 1–3 undergoing operations lasting at least 1 hour (62). Serum fluoride ion concentrations were significantly increased in both groups, peaking at 28 μmol/l after sevoflurane and 5 μmol/l after isoflurane, both at 1 hour. Of more concern, three of the patients in the sevoflurane group had peak fluoride ion concentrations above 50 μmol/l; two of them had increases in serum blood urea nitrogen and creatinine at 24 hours after surgery. The half-life of fluoride ion was 22 hours.

Nephrotoxicity has been found with methoxyflurane when serum fluoride ion concentrations exceeded 50 μmol/l (SEDA-20, 106). Although this safety threshold has been applied to other volatile anesthetics as well, renal toxicity has not been reported for the other three anesthetics, even though the threshold can be exceeded during prolonged anesthesia.

Volatile agents do not cause nephrotoxicity in adults with normal renal function (63). However, using sensitive urinary markers, both sevoflurane and isoflurane caused mild transient glomerular and tubular functional impairment in 13 patients aged 70 years or over undergoing gastrectomy. The patients received epidural analgesia combined with inhalation anesthesia using 5 l/minute fresh gas flow. The mean dose of sevoflurane was 5.1 MAC-hours and of isoflurane 3.7 MAC-hours. The mean urinary albumin excretion increased from 65 to 148 mg/g creatinine in the sevoflurane group and from 44 to 197 mg/g creatinine in the isoflurane group, and returned to preoperative values on the first postoperative day. The mean urinary β_1 and β_2 microglobulin concentrations also increased markedly in both groups, from 9.3 and 0.8 mg/g to 31 and 6.2 mg/g with sevoflurane and from 7.4 and 0.7 mg/g to 44 and 11 mg/g with isoflurane.

These values had returned to normal by day 7 postoperatively. The mean urinary N-acetyl-β-D-glucosaminidase concentration also increased significantly. These changes suggest transient renal tubular injury in both groups. There has not been any agreement on how these results should be interpreted, and larger studies are warranted.

Musculoskeletal

A spectrum of muscle reactions to all inhalational agents has been described. Masseteric muscle spasm can occur as an isolated phenomenon or can progress either to rhabdomyolysis with renal insufficiency or to malignant hyperpyrexia (64–67).

Generalized muscle rigidity and hypercapnia, followed by raised creatine kinase activity, have been reported in a child undergoing general anesthesia (68).

- A 2-year-old girl with a past history of asthma, developmental delay, short neck, and lumbar lordosis, but no known genetic defect or syndrome underwent anesthesia with midazolam and paracetamol premedication, halothane and nitrous oxide induction, and isoflurane plus nitrous oxide for maintenance of anesthesia. Difficulty with mouth opening was noted and endotracheal intubation was difficult. Limb rigidity developed rapidly. Thiopental and cisatracurium were given and the muscle rigidity abated over the next 10 minutes. The procedure was continued with a propofol infusion. No treatment for malignant hyperpyrexia was undertaken and no other markers for malignant hyperpyrexia were observed. She made a normal recovery from anesthesia. Creatine kinase activities were raised at 2370 U/l intraoperatively and 18 046 U/l at 20 hours postoperatively.

The case is interesting in that although episodes of masseter spasm, rigidity, rhabdomyolysis, and malignant hyperpyrexia are well known after the use of halothane and suxamethonium, they have only rarely been reported when suxamethonium was not used.

Immunologic

The issue of hypersensitivity reactions during general anesthesia is a matter of concern. However, despite considerable work on the subject, there is divergence in interpretation (69). In patients with no pre-anesthetic immunological anomaly, general anesthesia is unlikely to affect immune status significantly (70).

Widespread erythema and edema, the most dangerous form of which affects the glottis, occur in some cases of hypersensitivity. Hypotension is also seen, together with compensatory tachycardia. Bronchospasm is a common respiratory finding (71).

There were significant immunological changes in the peripheral blood film of personnel working in unscavenged operating theaters in Croatia (72). Some of the effects persisted beyond a 4-week period away from that environment.

In a review of 23 444 anesthetics given during 12 months, one patient in 630 had generalized erythema and edema and one in 1230 had erythema and hypotension (73). One patient died of shock. Female patients aged 15–25 with a history of allergy, subjects with excessive anxiety, and those who had previously undergone general anesthesia had a statistically significant higher risk of developing non-allergic anaphylactic reactions. The incidence of allergic anaphylactic reactions (with IgE antibodies) is said to be one in 4500–20 000 general anesthetics per year (74). However, the diagnosis is often missed (75).

The patient's history is hardly helpful; neither the presence nor the absence of a previous reaction gives guidance as to the likelihood of its occurring on future exposure. The mechanisms underlying such reactions may or may not involve histamine release, but the distinction between allergic anaphylactic and non-allergic anaphylactic (anaphylactoid) reactions is often unclear, for lack of definitive and easily available investigations. Furthermore, because anesthetic drugs are often given rapidly and in combination, it can be impossible to decide which was responsible for the reaction. Intradermal injection of a test dose is of limited predictive value (76); false-positive and false-negative results are often obtained, particularly with opiates, tubocurarine, and atracurium. What is more, the test is dose-dependent and can itself precipitate a hypersensitivity reaction (77). It has been suggested that leukocyte histamine release on exposure to drugs can be used in combination with paper radioallergosorbent testing for IgE antibodies, to detect the precise cause of any anaphylactic reaction: these techniques point to neuromuscular blocking drugs as being most commonly implicated in anaphylaxis (76).

In a French study, 1585 patients underwent diagnostic investigations after anaphylactic shock during anesthesia; 813 of them had a reaction of immunological origin. The drugs involved were muscle relaxants (70%), latex (13%), anesthetic drugs (5.6%), opioids (1.7%), colloids (4.7%), and antibiotics (2.6%) (78). Among the 45 patients in whom anesthetics were involved, the agents implicated were thiopental ($n = 18$), propofol ($n = 10$), ketamine ($n = 1$), midazolam ($n = 7$), diazepam ($n = 5$), and flunitrazepam ($n = 4$). These data did not differ from those reported in a UK study (79). In both studies there was a high proportion of cases in which muscular relaxants were used alongside anesthetics, resulting in a two-fold risk of hypersensitivity.

Body temperature

Malignant hyperthermia

Malignant hyperpyrexia is a life-threatening condition that involves sustained muscle contraction, muscle damage, and the production of vast quantities of metabolic heat, carbon dioxide, and potassium. Although it is a rare complication of general anesthesia, it remains a topic of considerable interest (80).

The incidence is difficult to determine, but it is currently estimated at one in every 10 000–20 000 anesthetics.

Diagnosis

Generalized muscle rigidity (found in 70% of the patients involved) and a progressive rise in body temperature (sometimes beyond 43°C) are the main clinical features, often associated with tachycardia, hypoxia, metabolic acidosis, cardiac dysrhythmias and, less often, disseminated intravascular coagulation, cerebral edema, and acute renal insufficiency. Diagnosis relies on the clinical signs, that is muscle rigidity and hyperpyrexia, and on raised serum activities of skeletal and cardiac muscle enzymes, for example aldolase and creatine kinase.

Genetic markers for malignant hyperpyrexia may soon make identification of risk groups simpler than the currently used muscle biopsy technique (81).

Susceptibility factors and prophylaxis

Although malignant hyperthermia is usually associated with the muscle relaxant suxamethonium, all inhalational anesthetics have been implicated and will be unsafe if risk factors for this condition are present, for example a family history or one of the congenital muscle disorders (82). This must be considered in patients at risk, as there are readily acceptable alternatives, such as propofol (83) and midazolam (84).

Malignant hyperthermia is probably due to the inability of certain individuals to control calcium concentrations in the muscle fiber and may involve a generalized alteration in cellular or subcellular membrane permeability, as suggested from research on pigs. This anomaly is genetically determined, but pre-anesthetic evaluation of susceptibility to malignant hyperthermia is a matter of controversy: measurement of blood creatine kinase, ATP muscle depletion, or myophosphorylase A, histological examination of muscle fibers, and in vitro exposure to caffeine or halothane have all been proposed. However, if susceptible patients require general anesthesia, despite the risk, prophylactic use of intravenous dantrolene 2.4 mg/kg during induction of anesthesia has been recommended (85).

Treatment and prognosis

Around 1970, mortality was as high as 70%, but it is now less than 10%. This reduction in mortality has been due to the use of dantrolene, the only specific treatment available, and also to an increased understanding of the condition (80).

Treatment is by withdrawal of the anesthetic, hyperventilation with 100% oxygen, cooling, and dantrolene. Doses of dantrolene of 2.5–5 mg/kg are usually recommended, given as early as possible to ensure rapid and complete resolution of the hyperthermic response (86).

Death

Correct estimates of the incidence of anesthetic deaths are difficult to obtain, since many deaths are multifactorial. Mortality due to anesthetic drugs is one in 10 000–20 000 (81). The adverse effects of anesthetics have been reviewed (82). Dose-related reactions are common and carry a low mortality, while non-dose-related reactions are less common and carry a high mortality.

A national prospective survey of complications related to anesthesia was carried out in France from 1978 to 1982

(89,90). In 198 103 anesthetic procedures, only 63 deaths were recorded, of which only 15 were definitely attributed to anesthesia (91). The Confidential Enquiry into Perioperative Deaths, conducted a decade ago in three British Health Regions (92) and covering a total of 555 248 patients, showed that the incidence of death within 30 days of surgery and anesthesia was 0.73% (4034 cases). Only about 14 of these deaths were considered to be partly or totally attributable to the anesthesia, and indeed in most cases other factors were also involved, including the surgery itself, the presurgical condition, and intercurrent illnesses. In a review of 25 deaths during anesthesia in 1982–86, only six were considered to be drug-related; of these, two were due to overdose and two more were the result of adverse effects of non-anesthetic agents (93).

Finally, except for certain specific effects that have a clear relation to a particular agent (for example liver damage after halothane), it is difficult to designate one anesthetic as being more risky than another. It has been authoritatively concluded that "the current level of research effort cannot distinguish mortality and serious morbidity between the most common anesthetic agents, and the clear differences in hemodynamic patterns among these anesthetic agents have an unknown, perhaps non-existent, relationship with mortality and serious morbidity" (94).

Long-Term Effects

Mutagenicity

Genetic damage was demonstrated in 10 non-smoking veterinary surgeons exposed to isoflurane and nitrous oxide compared with 10 non-smoking, non-exposed veterinary physicians acting as controls (95). The surgeons were monitored for 1 week in a working environment comparable to that of pediatric anesthesia, with the use of uncuffed endotracheal tubes and open-circuit breathing systems during operations on small animals. The overall calculated 8-hour time-weighted average exposure of cases was 5.3 ppm for isoflurane and 13 ppm for nitrous oxide. The European exposure limits are 10 ppm and 100 ppm respectively, and the corresponding values recommended by USA-NIOSH are 2 ppm and 25 ppm respectively. These values therefore violated the USA-NIOSH limit for isoflurane. The mean frequency of sister chromatid exchanges in peripheral blood lymphocytes was significantly higher in exposed workers than in controls (10 versus 7.4) and the proportion of micronuclei was also significantly higher in exposed workers (8.7 versus 6.8 per 500 binucleated cells). These measures reflect the mutagenicity of isoflurane and nitrous oxide. The findings are comparable to smoking 11–20 cigarettes a day. However, this study did not distinguish between the potential genotoxic effects of isoflurane and nitrous oxide; nor did it show a dose-dependency of genotoxicity, owing to the small sample size.

Second-Generation Effects

Fertility

Nitrous oxide may be the most serious of anesthetic pollutants; female dental assistants exposed to large amounts of nitrous oxide (5 hours or more of exposure per week) are significantly less fertile than women who are not exposed or who are exposed to lower amounts (96).

Pregnancy

The pharmacology and adverse effects of anesthetic drugs used for cesarean section have been reviewed (97).

Teratogenicity

In an epidemiological study, anesthetists had significantly greater exposure and perhaps more adverse effects than other operating-room personnel (98). Among women, exposure certainly causes an increased risk of spontaneous abortions in the first trimester, although teratogenicity is less clear-cut (99).

Susceptibility Factors

Underlying disease

Underlying disease is probably one of the most complex risk factors. Although general anesthesia is potentially more hazardous in patients with underlying disease in general (100) or specifically suffering from intracardiac conduction disturbances (101), severe hypertension (102), hypothyroidism (103), or cancer (104), it is extremely difficult to provide clear-cut recommendations, because the relative severity of disease in a given patient and the patient's response to the pathological process needs to be taken into account: while, for instance, thiopental may precipitate cardiovascular collapse, both pre-existing cardiac status and the dose of the drug are relevant.

Critically ill patients

Drug metabolism is reduced in critically ill patients. When the serum from five critically ill patients was incubated with microsomes prepared from three different human livers, the activity of CYP3A4, assessed by metabolism of midazolam to 1-hydroxymidazolam, was significantly inhibited compared with serum from healthy volunteers (105). The authors pointed out that many other drugs are also metabolized by this enzyme, including alfentanil, ciclosporin, cortisol, erythromycin, lidocaine, and nifedipine. This observation accounts for past reports of very slow metabolism of midazolam in seriously ill patients, resulting in high blood concentrations and delayed awakening.

Pre-anesthetic drug therapy

The consequences of pre-anesthetic drug therapy as a risk factor are obviously closely related to those of the underlying disease. The problem has attracted considerable attention in recent years and has been extensively reviewed (106). Interactions of drugs with anesthesia are dealt with here primarily in monographs on the drugs concerned. Although many pharmacological interactions with general anesthesia are firmly established, others remain ill-explained or unpredictable. Individual factors are likely to play a major role. Moreover, pre-anesthetic drug withdrawal in itself can be more dangerous than continuation of therapy, as exemplified by the case of the antihypertensive drug clonidine (107) or beta-blockers (108).

Driving

The hazard of driving shortly after general anesthesia is still difficult to evaluate. Although abstention from driving has been recommended for 48 hours after general anesthesia (109), it is still difficult to draw clear-cut conclusions from the available data. The matter is also referred to under individual anesthetic drugs.

Amiodarone

It has been reported that there is an increased risk of adverse reactions to amiodarone in patients undergoing anesthesia (SEDA-15, 171). However, in a retrospective survey of 12 patients who underwent anesthesia for urgent thyroidectomy due to amiodarone there were no anesthetic complications or deaths (110).

There is an increased risk of some of the adverse effects of amiodarone (including dysfunction of the liver and lungs) in patients who have had or who are having surgery (111). In addition the perioperative mortality in these patients is higher than in controls (112). The factors that increase the risks of amiodarone-associated adverse cardiovascular effects during surgery (113) include pre-existing ventricular dysfunction, too rapid a rate of intravenous infusion, hypocalcemia, and an interaction between amiodarone and both the general anesthetics used and other drugs with negative inotropic or chronotropic effects. It has therefore been recommended (113) that serum concentrations of calcium, amiodarone, and digoxin should be within the reference or target ranges before operation, and that other drugs with negative inotropic or chronotropic effects should be withdrawn before surgery.

The use of amiodarone in the prevention of atrial fibrillation after cardiac surgery has been reviewed (114). When an intravenous loading dose of amiodarone was used, bradycardia was a common adverse effect but was rarely severe enough to warrant withdrawal. When only oral amiodarone was used there were no serious adverse reactions.

Fenfluramine

Following a report of death after an anesthetic in a 23-year-old woman who had been taking fenfluramine, a study was undertaken in rabbits to investigate the possibility of an interaction of fenfluramine with halothane. Electrocardiographic and phonocardiographic changes were recorded in rabbits given the combined treatment, and could not readily be reversed with beta-blockers and resuscitative drugs. It was recommended that fenfluramine be discontinued a week before anesthesia (SED-9, 13)

References

1. Hindle AT, Columb MO, Shah MV. Drug interactions and anaesthesia. Curr Anaesth Crit Care 1995;6:103–12.
2. McAuliffe MS, Hartshorn EA. Anesthetic drug interactions. CRNA 1995;6(2):103–7.
3. McAuliffe MS, Hartshorn EA. Anesthetic drug interactions. CRNA 1995;6(3):139–42.
4. Stoltzfus DP. Advantages and disadvantages of combining sedative agents. Crit Care Clin 1995;11(4):903–12.
5. Whitwam JG. Co-induction of anaesthesia: day-case surgery. Eur J Anaesthesiol Suppl 1995;12:25–34.
6. Amrein R, Hetzel W, Allen SR. Co-induction of anaesthesia: the rationale. Eur J Anaesthesiol Suppl 1995;12:5–11.
7. D'Eramo EM. Morbidity and mortality with outpatient anesthesia: the Massachusetts experience. J Oral Maxillofac Surg 1992;50(7):700–4.
8. Chen SC, Rex DK. Review article: registered nurse-administered propofol sedation for endoscopy. Aliment Pharmacol Ther 2004;19:147–55.
9. Yussoff IF, Raymond G, Sahai AV. Endoscopist administered propofol for upper-GI EUS is safe and effective: a prospective study in 500 patients. Gastrointestinal Endoscopy 2004;60:356–60.
10. Bouvet L, Allaouchiche B, Duflo F, Debon R, Chassard D, Boselli E. Remifentanil is an effective alternative to propofol for patient-controlled analgesia during digestive endoscopic procedures. Can J Anesth 2004;51:122–5.
11. Clarke AC, Chiragakis L, Hillman LC, Kaye GL. Sedation for endoscopy: the safe use of propofol by general practitioner sedationists. Med J Aust 2002;176(4):158–61.
12. Arain SR, Ebert TJ. The efficacy, side effects, and recovery characteristics of dexmedetomidine versus propofol when used for intraoperative sedation. Anesth Analg 2002;95(2):461–6.
13. Servin FS, Raeder JC, Merle JC, Wattwil M, Hanson AL, Lauwers MH, Aitkenhead A, Marty J, Reite K, Martisson S, Wostyn L. Remifentanil sedation compared with propofol during regional anaesthesia. Acta Anaesthesiol Scand 2002;46(3):309–15.
14. Walder B, Borgeat A, Suter PM, Romand JA. Propofol and midazolam versus propofol alone for sedation following coronary artery bypass grafting: a randomized, placebo-controlled trial Anaesth Intensive Care 2002;30(2):171–8.
15. Gray WM. Occupational exposure to nitrous oxide in four hospitals. Anaesthesia 1989;44(6):511–4.
16. Gold DR. Indoor air pollution. Clin Chest Med 1992;13(2):215–29.
17. Tobias JD, Berkenbosch JW. Sedation during mechanical ventilation in infants and children: dexmedetomidine versus midazolam. Southern Med J 2004;97:451–5.
18. Crawford MW, Lerman J, Sloan MH, Sikich N, Halpern L, Bissonnette B. Recovery characteristics of propofol anaesthesia, with and without nitrous oxide: a comparison with halothane/nitrous oxide anaesthesia in children. Paediatr Anaesth 1998;8(1):49–54.
19. Visser K, Hassink EA, Bonsel GJ, Moen J, Kalkman CJ. Randomized controlled trial of total intravenous anesthesia with propofol versus inhalation anesthesia with isoflurane–nitrous oxide: postoperative nausea with vomiting and economic analysis. Anesthesiology 2001;95(3):616–26.
20. Ti LK, Pua HL, Lee TL. Single vital capacity inhalational anaesthetic induction in adults—isoflurane vs sevoflurane. Can J Anaesth 1998;45(10):949–53.
21. Smith I, Ding Y, White PF. Comparison of induction, maintenance, and recovery characteristics of sevoflurane–N_2O and propofol–sevoflurane–N_2O with propofol–isoflurane–N_2O anesthesia. Anesth Analg 1992;74(2):253–9.

22. Elcock DH, Sweeney BP. Sevoflurane vs. isoflurane: a clinical comparison in day surgery. Anaesthesia 2002;57(1):52–6.

23. Ebert TJ, Robinson BJ, Uhrich TD, Mackenthun A, Pichotta PJ. Recovery from sevoflurane anesthesia: a comparison to isoflurane and propofol anesthesia. Anesthesiology 1998;89(6):1524–31.

24. Joo HS, Perks WJ. Sevoflurane versus propofol for anesthetic induction: a meta-analysis. Anesth Analg 2000;91(1):213–9.

25. Watson KR, Shah MV. Clinical comparison of "single agent" anaesthesia with sevoflurane versus target controlled infusion of propofol. Br J Anaesth 2000;85(4):541–6.

26. McCulloch TJ, Visco E, Lam AM. Graded hypercapnia and cerebral autoregulation during sevoflurane or propofol anesthesia. Anesthesiology 2000;93(5):1205–9.

27. Nandate K, Vuylsteke A, Ratsep I, Messahel S, Oduro-Dominah A, Menon DK, Matta BF. Effects of isoflurane, sevoflurane and propofol anaesthesia on jugular venous oxygen saturation in patients undergoing coronary artery bypass surgery. Br J Anaesth 2000;84(5):631–3.

28. Philip BK, Lombard LL, Roaf ER, Drager LR, Calalang I, Philip JH. Comparison of vital capacity induction with sevoflurane to intravenous induction with propofol for adult ambulatory anesthesia. Anesth Analg 1999;89(3):623–7.

29. Smith I, Thwaites AJ. Target-controlled propofol vs. sevoflurane: a double-blind, randomised comparison in day-case anaesthesia. Anaesthesia 1999;54(8):745–52.

30. Nelskyla K, Korttila K, Yli-Hankala A. Comparison of sevoflurane–nitrous oxide and propofol–alfentanil–nitrous oxide anaesthesia for minor gynaecological surgery. Br J Anaesth 1999;83(4):576–9.

31. Song D, Joshi GP, White PF. Fast-track eligibility after ambulatory anesthesia: a comparison of desflurane, sevoflurane, and propofol. Anesth Analg 1998;86(2):267–73.

32. Keller C, Sparr HJ, Brimacombe JR. Positive pressure ventilation with the laryngeal mask airway in non-paralysed patients: comparison of sevoflurane and propofol maintenance techniques. Br J Anaesth 1998;80(3):332–6.

33. Nishiyama T, Nakayama H, Hanaoka K. Sevoflurane or thiopental–isoflurane for induction and laryngeal mask insertion? Comparison by side effects, hemodynamics, and spectral analysis of heart rate variability. Anesth Resusc 1999;35:99–103.

34. Mckinney MS, Fee JP. Cardiovascular effects of 50% nitrous oxide in older adult patients anaesthetized with isoflurane or halothane. Br J Anaesth 1998;80(2):169–73.

35. Michaloudis D, Fraidakis O, Petrou A, Gigourtsi C, Parthenakis F. Anaesthesia and the QT interval. Effects of isoflurane and halothane in unpremedicated children. Anaesthesia 1998;53(5):435–9.

36. Blayney MR, Malins AF, Cooper GM. Cardiac arrhythmias in children during outpatient general anaesthesia for dentistry: a prospective randomised trial. Lancet 1999;354(9193):1864–6.

37. Viitanen H, Baer G, Koivu H, Annila P. The hemodynamic and Holter-electrocardiogram changes during halothane and sevoflurane anesthesia for adenoidectomy in children aged one to three years. Anesth Analg 1999;89(6):1423–5.

38. Guler N, Bilge M, Eryonucu B, Kati I, Demirel CB. The effects of halothane and sevoflurane on QT dispersion. Acta Cardiol 1999;54(6):311–5.

39. Skolnick ET, Vomvolakis MA, Buck KA, Mannino SF, Sun LS. Exposure to environmental tobacco smoke and the risk of adverse respiratory events in children receiving general anesthesia. Anesthesiology 1998;88(5):1144–53.

40. Brown K, Aun C, Stocks J, Jackson E, Mackersie A, Hatch D. A comparison of the respiratory effects of sevoflurane and halothane in infants and young children. Anesthesiology 1998;89(1):86–92.

41. Goff MJ, Arain SR, Ficke DJ, Uhrich TD, Ebert TJ. Absence of bronchodilation during desflurane anesthesia: a comparison to sevoflurane and thiopental. Anesthesiology 2000;93(2):404–8.

42. Watts AD, Herrick IA, McLachlan RS, Craen RA, Gelb AW. The effect of sevoflurane and isoflurane anesthesia on interictal spike activity among patients with refractory epilepsy. Anesth Analg 1999;89(5):1275–81.

43. Iijima T, Nakamura Z, Iwao Y, Sankawa H. The epileptogenic properties of the volatile anesthetics sevoflurane and isoflurane in patients with epilepsy. Anesth Analg 2000;91(4):989–95.

44. Saurel-Cubizolles MJ, Estryn-Behar M, Maillard MF, Mugnier N, Masson A, Monod G. Neuropsychological symptoms and occupational exposure to anaesthetics. Br J Ind Med 1992;49(4):276–81.

45. Vaisman AI. Usloviia truda v operatisionnykh i ikh vliianie na zdorov'e anesteziologov. [Working conditions in the operating room and their effect on the health of anesthetists.] Eksp Khir Anesteziol 1967;12(3):44–9.

46. Lowry DW, Mirakhur RK, Carrol MT. Time course of action of rocuronium during sevoflurane, isoflurane or i.v. anaesthesia Br J Anaesth 1998;80:544.

47. Wulf H, Ledowski T, Linstedt U, Proppe D, Sitzlack D. Neuromuscular blocking effects of rocuronium during desflurane, isoflurane, and sevoflurane anaesthesia. Can J Anaesth 1998;45(6):526–32.

48. Wulf H, Kahl M, Ledowski T. Augmentation of the neuromuscular blocking effects of cisatracurium during desflurane, isoflurane, and sevoflurane anaesthesia. Can J Anaesth 1998;45:526–32.

49. Tran TV, Fiset P, Varin F. Pharmacokinetics and pharmacodynamics of cisatracurium after a short infusion in patients under propofol anesthesia. Anesth Analg 1998;87(5):1158–63.

50. Sparacia A, Mangione S, Sansone A. Alterazioni dell'emostasi in relazione al farmaci anestetici ed all'emostasi ed all'intervento chirurgico. [Hemostatic changes related to anesthetic drugs and surgical intervention.] Minerva Anestesiol 1980;46(7):791–814.

51. Simpson PJ, Radford SG, Forster SJ, et al. The fibrinolytic effects of anesthesia. Anesth Analg 1982;60:319.

52. Zahavi J, Price AJ, Kakkar VV. Enhanced platelet release reaction associated with general anaesthesia. Lancet 1980;1(8178):1132–3.

53. Nishina K, Akamatsu H, Mikawa K, Shiga M, Maekawa N, Obara H, Niwa Y. The inhibitory effects of thiopental, midazolam, and ketamine on human neutrophil functions. Anesth Analg 1998;86(1):159–65.

54. Luntz SP, Janitz E, Motsch J, Bach E, Böttiger BW. Cost-effectiveness and high patient satisfaction in the elderly: sevoflurane versus propofol anaesthesia. Eur J Anaesthesiol 2004;21:115–22.

55. van den Berg AA, Honjol NM, Mphanza T, Rozario CJ, Joseph D. Vomiting, retching, headache and restlessness after halothane-, isoflurane- and enflurane-based anaesthesia. An analysis of pooled data following ear, nose, throat and eye surgery. Acta Anaesthesiol Scand 1998;42(6):658–63.

56. Naidu-Sjosvard K, Sjoberg F, Gupta A. Anaesthesia for videoarthroscopy of the knee. A comparison between desflurane and sevoflurane. Acta Anaesthesiol Scand 1998;42(4):464–71.

57. Nelskyla KA, Yli-Hankala AM, Puro PH, Korttila KT. Sevoflurane titration using bispectral index decreases postoperative vomiting in phase II recovery after ambulatory surgery. Anesth Analg 2001;93(5):1165–9.

58. Tramèr M, Moore A, McQuay H. Propofol anaesthesia and postoperative nausea and vomiting: quantitative systematic review of randomized controlled studies. Br J Anaesth 1997;78(3):247–55.

59. Sneyd JR, Carr A, Byrom WD, Bilski AJ. A meta-analysis of nausea and vomiting following maintenance of anaesthesia with propofol or inhalational agents. Eur J Anaesthesiol 1998;15(4):433–45.

60. Apfel CC, Laara E, Koivuranta M, Greim CA, Roewer N. A simplified risk score for predicting postoperative nausea and vomiting: conclusions from cross-validations between two centers. Anesthesiology 1999;91(3):693–700.

61. Rose JB, Watcha MF. Postoperative nausea and vomiting in paediatric patients. Br J Anaesth 1999;83(1):104–17.

62. Goldberg ME, Cantillo J, Larijani GE, Torjman M, Vekeman D, Schieren H. Sevoflurane versus isoflurane for maintenance of anesthesia: are serum inorganic fluoride ion concentrations of concern? Anesth Analg 1996;82(6):1268–72.

63. Hase K, Meguro K, Nakamura T. Assessment of renal effects of sevoflurane in elderly patients using urinary markers. Anesth Analg 1999;88(6):1426–7.

64. McGuire N, Easy WR. Malignant hyperthermia during isoflurane anaesthesia. Anaesthesia 1990;45(2):124–7.

65. Rubiano R, Chang JL, Carroll J, Sonbolian N, Larson CE. Acute rhabdomyolysis following halothane anesthesia without succinylcholine. Anesthesiology 1987;67(5):856–7.

66. Littleford JA, Patel LR, Bose D, Cameron CB, McKillop C. Masseter muscle spasm in children: implications of continuing the triggering anesthetic. Anesth Analg 1991;72(2):151–60.

67. Lee SC, Abe T, Sato T. Rhabdomyolysis and acute renal failure following use of succinylcholine and enflurane: report of a case. J Oral Maxillofac Surg 1987;45(9):789–92.

68. Medina KA, Mayhew JF. Generalized muscle rigidity and hypercarbia with halothane and isoflurane. Anesth Analg 1998;86(2):297–8.

69. Walton B. Anaesthesia, surgery and immunology. Anaesthesia 1978;33(4):322–48.

70. Ryhanen P. Effects of anaesthesia and operative surgery on the immune response of patients of different ages. Ann Clin Res 1977;19(Suppl):9.

71. Clarke RS. The clinical presentation of anaphylactoid reactions in anesthesia. Int Anesthesiol Clin 1985;23(3):1–16.

72. Peric M, Vranes Z, Marusic M. Immunological disturbances in anaesthetic personnel chronically exposed to high occupational concentrations of nitrous oxide and halothane. Anaesthesia 1991;46(7):531–7.

73. Laxenaire MC, Manel J, Borgo J, Moneret-Vautrin DA. Facteurs de risque d'histamino-libération: étude prospective dans une population anestésie. [Risk factors in histamine liberation: a prospective study in an anesthetized population.] Ann Fr Anesth Reanim 1985;4(2):158–66.

74. Watkins J. Investigation of allergic and hypersensitivity reactions to anaesthetic agents. Br J Anaesth 1987;59(1):104–11.

75. Youngman PR, Taylor KM, Wilson JD. Anaphylactoid reactions to neuromuscular blocking agents: a commonly undiagnosed condition? Lancet 1983;2(8350):597–9.

76. Assem ES. Anaphylactic anaesthetic reactions. The value of paper radioallergosorbent tests for IgE antibodies to muscle relaxants and thiopentone. Anaesthesia 1990;45(12):1032–8.

77. Assem ES, Symons IE. Anaphylaxis due to suxamethonium in a 7-year-old child: a 14-year follow-up with allergy testing. Anaesthesia 1989;44(2):121–4.

78. Laxenaire MC, Moneret-Vautrin DA, Guéant JL, et al. Drugs and other agents involved in anaphylactic shock occurring during anaesthesia. A French multicenter epidemiological inquiry. Ann Fr Anesth Reanim 1993;12(2):91–6.

79. Clarke RS, Watkins J. Drugs responsible for anaphylactoid reactions in anaesthesia in the United Kingdom. Ann Fr Anesth Reanim 1993;12(2):105–8.

80. Halsall PJ, Ellis FR. Malignant hyperthermia. Bailliere's Clin Anaesthesiol 1993;7:343–56.

81. MacKenzie AE, Allen G, Lahey D, Crossan ML, Nolan K, Mettler G, Worton RG, MacLennan DH, Korneluk R. A comparison of the caffeine halothane muscle contracture test with the molecular genetic diagnosis of malignant hyperthermia. Anesthesiology 1991;75(1):4–8.

82. Chalkiadis GA, Branch KG. Cardiac arrest after isoflurane anaesthesia in a patient with Duchenne's muscular dystrophy. Anaesthesia 1990;45(1):22–5.

83. Gallen JS. Propofol does not trigger malignant hyperthermia. Anesth Analg 1991;72(3):413–4.

84. Brooks JH. Midazolam in a malignant hyperthermia-susceptible patient. Anesthesiology 1989;70(1):167–8.

85. Flewellen EH, Nelson TE, Jones WP, Arens JF, Wagner DL. Dantrolene dose response in awake man: implications for management of malignant hyperthermia. Anesthesiology 1983;59(4):275–80.

86. Harrison GG. Malignant hyperthermia. Dantrolene—dynamics and kinetics. Br J Anaesth 1988;60(3):279–86.

87. Derrington MC, Smith G. A review of studies of anaesthetic risk, morbidity and mortality. Br J Anaesth 1987;59(7):815–33.

88. Berthoud MC, Reilly CS. Adverse effects of general anaesthetics. Drug Saf 1992;7(6):434–59.

89. Harrison GG. Death attributable to anaesthesia. A 10-year survey (1967–1976). Br J Anaesth 1978;50(10):1041–6.

90. Saarnivaara L. Comparison of halothane and enflurane anaesthesia for tonsillectomy in adults. Acta Anaesthesiol Scand 1984;28(3):319–24.

91. Vourc'h G, Hatton F, Tiret L, Desmonts JM. Étude épidemiologique sur les complications de l'anesthésie en France. [Epidemiologic study of anesthesia complications in France.] Bull Acad Natl Med 1983;167(8):939–45.

92. Buck N, Devlin HB, Lunn JN. The Report of a Confidential Enquiry into Perioperative Deaths. London: Nuffield Provincial Hospitals Trust and The King's Fund;. 1987.

93. Gannon K. Mortality associated with anaesthesia. A case review study. Anaesthesia 1991;46(11):962–6.

94. Pace NL. Adverse outcomes and the multicenter study of general anesthesia: II. Anesthesiology 1992;77(2):394–6.

95. Hoerauf K, Lierz M, Wiesner G, Schroegendorfer K, Lierz P, Spacek A, Brunnberg L, Nusse M. Genetic damage in operating room personnel exposed to isoflurane and nitrous oxide. Occup Environ Med 1999;56(7):433–7.

96. Rowland AS, Baird DD, Weinberg CR, Shore DL, Shy CM, Wilcox AJ. Reduced fertility among women employed as dental assistants exposed to high levels of nitrous oxide. N Engl J Med 1992;327(14):993–7.

97. D'Alessio JG, Ramanathan J. Effects of maternal anesthesia in the neonate. Semin Perinatol 1998;22(5):350–62.

98. Sass-Kortsak AM, Purdham JT, Bozek PR, Murphy JH. Exposure of hospital operating room personnel to potentially harmful environmental agents. Am Ind Hyg Assoc J 1992;53(3):203–9.

99. In: Eger EI, editor. Nitrous Oxide. New York: Edward Arnold, 1985:43.

100. Train M, Lepage JY, Le Forestier K, Dixneuf B, Duveau D. Incidents et accidents observés lors de l'anesthésie-réanimation en chirurgie coronaire. [Accidents and

complications seen during anesthesia and postoperative recovery in coronary surgery.] Ann Anesthesiol Fr 1979;20(5):431–4.

101. Tachoires D, Poisot D, Erny P, Mourot F, Bergeron JL. Les troubles de la conduction intra-cardiaque en anesthésie-réanimation. [Disorders of intracardiac conduction in anesthesia-resuscitation.] Ann Anesthesiol Fr 1979;20(4):357–69.

102. Rodriguez PR, Mangans DT. Anesthesia and hypertension. Semin Anaesthesiol 1982;1:226.

103. Murkin JM. Anesthesia and hypothyroidism: a review of thyroxine physiology, pharmacology, and anesthetic implications. Anesth Analg 1982;61(4):371–83.

104. Chung F. Cancer, chemotherapy and anaesthesia. Can Anaesth Soc J 1982;29(4):364–71.

105. Park GR, Miller E, Navapurkar V. What changes drug metabolism in critically ill patients?—II Serum inhibits the metabolism of midazolam in human microsomes Anaesthesia 1996;51(1):11–5.

106. Craig DB, Bose D. Drug interactions in anaesthesia: chroic antihypertensive therapy. Can Anaesth Soc J 1984;31(5):580–9.

107. Stevens JE. Rebound hypertension during anaesthesia. Anaesthesia 1980;35(5):490–1.

108. Ponten J, Biber B, Bjuro T, Henriksson BA, Hjalmarson A. Beta-receptor blocker withdrawal. A preoperative problem in general surgery? Acta Anaesthesiol Scand Suppl 1982;76:32–7.

109. Havard J. In: Medical Aspects of Fitness to Drive. 3rd ed. London: A Rapple, 1976:43.

110. Sutherland J, Robinson B, Delbridge L. Anaesthesia for amiodarone-induced thyrotoxicosis: a case review. Anaesth Intensive Care 2001;29(1):24–9.

111. Kupferschmid JP, Rosengart TK, McIntosh CL, Leon MB, Clark RE. Amiodarone-induced complications after cardiac operation for obstructive hypertrophic cardiomyopathy. Ann Thorac Surg 1989;48(3):359–64.

112. Andersen HR, Bjorn-Hansen LS, Kimose HH, et al. Amiodaronebehandling og arytmikirurgi. Ugeskr Laeger 1989;151:2264.

113. Perkins MW, Dasta JF, Reilley TE, Halpern P. Intraoperative complications in patients receiving amiodarone: characteristics and risk factors. DICP 1989; 23(10):757–63.

114. Morady F. Prevention of atrial fibrillation in the postoperative cardiac patient: significance of oral class III antiarrhythmic agents. Am J Cardiol 1999; 84(9A):R156–60.

INHALATIONAL ANESTHETICS—HALOGENATED

Chloroform

General Information

Chloroform (SED-8, 250) should no longer be used, because of its toxic effects on the heart, liver, and kidneys, although the exact nature and extent of these complications has been debated (1). The very serious adverse effects of chloroform anesthesia when poorly administered have been briefly reviewed (2).

References

1. Payne JP. Chloroform in clinical anaesthesia. Br J Anaesth 1981;53(Suppl 1):S11–5.
2. Defalque RJ, Wright AJ. An anesthetic curiosity in New York (1875–1900): a noted surgeon returns to "open drop" chloroform. Anesthesiology 1998;88(2):549–51.

Desflurane

General Information

Desflurane is identical in structure to isoflurane, except that it is halogenated completely with fluorine instead of fluorine and chlorine. Desflurane is a volatile anesthetic that combines low blood gas solubility with moderate potency and high volatility. Its pharmacology has been reviewed (1,2).

Compared with volatile anesthetics in current use, desflurane has the advantages of being practically inert and of having a low blood-gas partition coefficient (0.4), making its onset and offset of action rapid. Its disadvantages include its low boiling point (close to room temperature) and the fact that it requires a specially heated vaporizer for delivery. It is also irritating to airways, precluding its use for induction of anesthesia and making the safety of mask anesthesia questionable. It also has excitatory effects on the sympathetic nervous system, causing tachycardia and mydriasis, which can make it difficult to judge the adequacy of anesthetic depth.

When desflurane is used with the proper equipment, alveolar concentrations can be adjusted more rapidly and precisely during administration, and recovery is quicker in both the short and long term than with other agents (3).

In a prospective, randomized study of 120 patients undergoing day-surgery, desflurane and sevoflurane were associated with shorter times to awakening, extubation, and orientation than propofol by infusion (4).

Average times to awakening at the end of anesthesia were 5, 5, and 8 minutes respectively.

Comparative studies

In a systematic review of 25 published, randomized controlled comparisons of sevoflurane (746 patients) and desflurane (752 patients) there was no significant difference in the rates of postoperative nausea and vomiting (5).

Organs and Systems

Cardiovascular

Desflurane increases the heart rate and reduces both mean arterial pressure and systemic vascular resistance while maintaining cardiac output (6,7). In high concentrations it can cause transient activation of the sympathetic nervous system, predisposing to hypertension and dysrhythmias (8).

Despite some coronary vasodilatation in dogs, there is no evidence of coronary steal in man. Desflurane may benefit elderly patients by allowing more rapid recovery from anesthesia (9).

Cardiac arrest due to desflurane toxicity has been attributed to accidental delivery of a high concentration of desflurane due to vaporizer malfunction (10).

- A healthy 36-year-old woman underwent anesthesia maintained with desflurane, which was delivered at 3.5% using a Tec 6 Plus Vaporizer (Datex Ohmeda, Steeton, England) via a partially closed circuit with a low flow of fresh gases (1 l/minute). Five minutes after induction, she developed hypoxia and bradycardia, rapidly followed by cardiac arrest with asystole. She was resuscitated and a chest x-ray showed pulmonary edema.

Examination of the memory of the halogenated anesthetic monitor (Viridia 24 C; Hewlett Packard, Boeblingen, Germany) showed a progressive increase in end-expiratory desflurane concentration up to 23%. There was an internal crack in the control dial, which normally regulates the control valve, but the damage did not limit the rotation of the control valve, which remained uncontrolled. The authors thought that this defect had been responsible for massive administration of desflurane in the inhalation circuit. Cardiac arrest was probably due to the negative inotropic effect of desflurane.

Duchenne's muscular dystrophy can be associated with cardiac arrest during anesthesia, and this has been reported in a 16-year-old boy who was anesthetized with desflurane (11).

Respiratory

Desflurane is a mild respiratory irritant (7). Moderate to severe laryngospasm and moderate to severe coughing occurred often (50% of cases) during induction of anesthesia with desflurane in 206 children aged 1 month to 12 years; the authors concluded that the high incidence of these airway complications during induction limit the use of desflurane in children, but that anesthesia could be safely maintained with desflurane after induction with another anesthetic (12).

The effects of 6% or 12% desflurane and 1.8% or 3.6% sevoflurane, which have markedly different pungencies, on airway reactivity have been tested in 60 patients breathing equivalent concentrations through a laryngeal mask airway (13). Compared with sevoflurane, desflurane titration to 12% increased heart rate, increased mean arterial blood pressure, and initiated frequent coughing (53% versus 0%) and body movements (47% versus 0%). During emergence, there was a two-fold greater incidence of coughing and a five-fold increase in breath holding with desflurane.

Nervous system

Increasing doses of desflurane caused no demonstrable fall in cerebral blood flow. Consequently, it can be advocated for patients undergoing neurosurgical procedures (14).

Neuromuscular function

Depression of neuromuscular function occurred 10 minutes after the introduction of desflurane 1.3% in a 32-year-old man who had previously received midazolam, fentanyl, and thiopental for induction. On withdrawal his neuromuscular function returned to baseline (15).

Liver

Poorly metabolized gases are generally safer than those that undergo extensive metabolism. Desflurane is poorly metabolized, and appeared to have no toxic effects on the liver and kidneys in 13 young men (16).

However, a case of severe hepatotoxicity after desflurane anesthesia has been reported (17).

- An obese 37-year-old woman with a past history of allergy to penicillin, nickel, and cobalt, and unexplained mild hepatitis 6 weeks after halothane anesthesia 9 years before, was given an anesthetic including etomidate, alcuronium, metamizole, piritramizide, fentanyl, nitrous oxide, and desflurane. Ten days later she developed the symptoms and signs of hepatitis, an eosinophilia, and raised hepatic enzymes, including alanine transaminase 1776 IU/l, aspartate transaminase 1258 IU/l, gamma-glutamyl transpeptidase 48 IU/l, and bilirubin 503 μmol/l. After exclusion of common causes of hepatitis, a liver biopsy confirmed acute hepatitis. There were increased titers of antitrifluoroacetylated IgG antibodies, which peaked at 0.159 on day 25 postoperatively. She eventually recovered.

This patient had multiple risk factors for anesthesia-induced hepatitis, including obesity, middle age, female sex, a history of drug allergies, and multiple exposures to fluorinated anesthetic agents. Desflurane has a very low

rate of hepatic oxidative metabolism (0.02 versus 20% for halothane), and is considered to be one of the safest volatile agents as far as hepatotoxicity is concerned. Nevertheless, this case shows that it can cause severe hepatotoxicity.

Acute liver damage has also been reported in an 81-year-old woman after general anesthesia with desflurane (18).

Urinary tract

The effects of sevoflurane, isoflurane, and desflurane on macroscopic renal structure have been studied in 24 patients undergoing nephrectomy (19). All the anesthetics were administered using a fresh gas flow of 1 l/minute and a sodium hydroxide absorber and had an average duration of 3 hours. No injury to nephrons was observed by pathologists blinded to which anesthetic agent had been used. Postoperative creatinine concentrations and urine volumes did not differ significantly between the groups.

Body temperature

Malignant hyperthermia has been reported with desflurane (20).

- Malignant hyperthermia has been described in a 10-year-old boy who received thiopental and suxamethonium for induction of anesthesia, followed by desflurane for maintenance of anesthesia (21).

The role of suxamethonium must also be considered in this case.

Long-term effects

Genotoxicity

The effects of desflurane on the frequency of sister chromatid exchange has been studied in the peripheral blood lymphocytes of 15 women during and after anesthesia maintained with desflurane 5–6% in an oxygen/air mixture (22). The numbers of sister chromatid exchanges per cell at 60 and 120 minutes were significantly higher than the numbers before anesthesia. In addition, the numbers of sister chromatid exchange per cell on the 1st, 3rd, and 7th postoperative days were significantly higher than preoperatively, but there was no difference by the 12th postoperative day. The authors concluded that desflurane may be capable of causing genetic damage. This view has been supported by the results of an in vitro study of the effect of desflurane on peripheral blood lymphocytes, in which both halothane and desflurane increased DNA migration in a concentration-related manner (23).

Susceptibility Factors

Age

In old people, the MAC of desflurane, with or without nitrous oxide, was less than that in patients aged 18–65 years. Doses of desflurane must therefore be reduced in older people, as with all other inhalation agents (24).

Drug–Drug Interactions

Adrenaline

Adrenaline used during anesthesia can cause ventricular dysrhythmias. The threshold dose of adrenaline for dysrhythmias is reduced by halothane, but not by desflurane; the dose of adrenaline required to produce dysrhythmias in 50% of patients was three times that needed when anesthesia was with halothane (25).

Fentanyl

The MAC of desflurane was significantly reduced 25 minutes after a single dose of fentanyl (26).

Propofol

Desflurane-based anesthesia, with and without prophylactic ondansetron, to reduce the incidence of postoperative nausea and vomiting, has been compared with a propofol infusion in 90 women of ASA grades 1 and 2 undergoing outpatient gynecological laparoscopic surgery (27). The incidence of postoperative nausea and vomiting was 80% with desflurane alone, 40% with desflurane plus ondansetron, and 20% with propofol. Postoperative antiemetic requirements were larger and times-to-home readiness longer with desflurane alone, but sedation and analgesic requirements were similar. The high incidence of postoperative nausea and vomiting suggests that routine antiemetic prophylaxis should be considered in outpatients receiving desflurane-based anesthesia.

Rocuronium

Both desflurane and sevoflurane significantly increase the neuromuscular blocking effects of rocuronium compared with isoflurane or propofol (28,29).

References

1. Westrin P. Intravenous and inhalational anaesthetic agents. Baillière's Clin Anaesthesiol 1996;10:687–715.
2. Anonymous. Sevoflurane and desflurane: comparison with older inhalational anaesthetics. Drugs Ther Perspect 1996;7:1–5.
3. Eger EI 2nd. Desflurane animal and human pharmacology: aspects of kinetics, safety, and MAC. Anesth Analg 1992;75(Suppl 4):S3–9.
4. Song D, Joshi GP, White PF. Fast-track eligibility after ambulatory anesthesia: a comparison of desflurane, sevoflurane, and propofol. Anesth Analg 1998;86(2):267–73.
5. Macario A, Dexter F, Lubarsky D. Meta-analysis of trials comparing postoperative recovery after anesthesia with sevoflurane or desflurane. Am J Health Syst Pharm 2005;62(1):63–8.
6. Rodig G, Wild K, Behr R, Hobbhahn J. Effects of desflurane and isoflurane on systemic vascular resistance during hypothermic cardiopulmonary bypass. J Cardiothorac Vasc Anesth 1997;11(1):54–7.
7. Warltier DC, Pagel PS. Cardiovascular and respiratory actions of desflurane: is desflurane different from isoflurane? Anesth Analg 1992;75(Suppl 4):S17–31.
8. Bunting HE, Kelly MC, Milligan KR. Effect of nebulized lignocaine on airway irritation and haemodynamic changes during induction of anaesthesia with desflurane. Br J Anaesth 1995;75(5):631–3.
9. Bennett JA, Lingaraju N, Horrow JC, McElrath T, Keykhah MM. Elderly patients recover more rapidly from desflurane than from isoflurane anesthesia. J Clin Anesth 1992;4(5):378–81.
10. Geffroy JC, Gentili ME, Le Pollés R, Triclot P. Massive inhalation of desflurane due to vaporizer dysfunction. Anesthesiology 2005;103(5):1096–8.
11. Smelt WL. Cardiac arrest during desflurane anaesthesia in a patient with Duchenne's muscular dystrophy. Acta Anaesthesiol Scand 2005;49(2):267–9.
12. Zwass MS, Fisher DM, Welborn LG, Cote CJ, Davis PJ, Dinner M, Hannallah RS, Liu LM, Sarner J, McGill WA, et al. Induction and maintenance characteristics of anesthesia with desflurane and nitrous oxide in infants and children. Anesthesiology 1992;76(3):373–8.
13. Arain SR, Shankar H, Ebert TJ. Desflurane enhances reactivity during the use of the laryngeal mask airway. Anesthesiology. 2005;103(3):495–9.
14. Ornstein E, Young WL, Fleischer LH, Ostapkovich N. Desflurane and isoflurane have similar effects on cerebral blood flow in patients with intracranial mass lesions. Anesthesiology 1993;79(3):498–502.
15. Kelly RE, Lien CA, Savarese JJ, Belmont MR, Hartman GS, Russo JR, Hollmann C. Depression of neuromuscular function in a patient during desflurane anesthesia. Anesth Analg 1993;76(4):868–71.
16. Weiskopf RB, Eger EI 2nd, Ionescu P, Yasuda N, Cahalan MK, Freire B, Peterson N, Lockhart SH, Rampil IJ, Laster M. Desflurane does not produce hepatic or renal injury in human volunteers. Anesth Analg 1992;74(4):570–4.
17. Berghaus TM, Baron A, Geier A, Lamerz R, Paumgartner G, Conzen P. Hepatotoxicity following desflurane anesthesia. Hepatology 1999;29(2):613–4.
18. Tung D, Yoshida EM, Wang CS, Steinbrecher UP. Severe desflurane hepatotoxicity after colon surgery in an elderly patient. Can J Anaesth 2005;52(2):133–6.
19. Annila P, Rorarius M, Reinikainen P, Oikkonen M, Baer G. Effect of pre-treatment with intravenous atropine or glycopyrrolate on cardiac arrhythmias during halothane anaesthesia for adenoidectomy in children. Br J Anaesth 1998;80(6):756–60.
20. Uskova AA, Matusic BP, Brandom BW. Desflurane, malignant hyperthermia, and release of compartment syndrome. Anesth Analg 2005;100(5):1357–60.
21. Fu ES, Scharf JE, Mangar D, Miller WD. Malignant hyperthermia involving the administration of desflurane. Can J Anaesth 1996;43(7):687–90.
22. Akin A, Ugur F, Ozkul Y, Esmaoglu A, Gunes I, Ergul H. Desflurane anaesthesia increases sister chromatid exchanges in human lymphocytes. Acta Anaesthesiol Scand 2005;49(10):1559–61.
23. Karpiński TM, Kostrzewska-Poczekaj M, Stachecki I, Mikstacki A, Szyfter K. Genotoxicity of the volatile anaesthetic desflurane in human lymphocytes in vitro, established by comet assay. J Appl Genet 2005;46(3):319–24.

24. Gold MI, Abello D, Herrington C. Minimum alveolar concentration of desflurane in patients older than 65 yr. Anesthesiology 1993;79(4):710–4.
25. Moore MA, Weiskopf RB, Eger EI 2nd, Wilson C, Lu G. Arrhythmogenic doses of epinephrine are similar during desflurane or isoflurane nesthesia in humans. Anesthesiology 1993;79(5):943–7.
26. Sebel PS, Glass PS, Fletcher JE, Murphy MR, Gallagher C, Quill T. Reduction of the MAC of desflurane with fentanyl. Anesthesiology 1992;76(1):52–9.
27. Eriksson H, Korttila K. Recovery profile after desflurane with or without ondansetron compared with propofol in patients undergoing outpatient gynecological laparoscopy. Anesth Analg 1996;82(3):533–8.
28. Lowry DW, Mirakhur RK, Carrol MT. Time course of action of rocuronium during sevoflurane, isoflurane or i.v. anaesthesia Br J Anaesth 1998;80:544.
29. Wulf H, Ledowski T, Linstedt U, Proppe D, Sitzlack D. Neuromuscular blocking effects of rocuronium during desflurane, isoflurane, and sevoflurane anaesthesia. Can J Anaesth 1998;45(6):526–32.

Enflurane

General Information

Enflurane is a non-explosive halogenated volatile anesthetic that was first marketed in 1966. It was developed in the search for agents safer than halothane and methoxyflurane (1). However, the list of its halothane-like adverse effects has continued to grow.

Organs and Systems

Cardiovascular

Despite conflicting results, enflurane is generally considered to have little effect on the cardiovascular system. Cardiac output was mildly influenced in healthy men and the negative inotropic effects of enflurane (2) were more pronounced in patients with congestive heart failure (3). Myocardial damage was suggested to be an unlikely complication of enflurane anesthesia, even in patients with ischemic heart disease (4).

Cardiac dysrhythmias are generally considered to be less frequent, or at least less severe, with enflurane than with halothane (5,6). However, caution in the use of adrenaline is advisable, especially in patients with cardiac disease or hyperthyroidism. Isorhythmic atrioventricular dissociation was seen in 16 of 105 patients after the use of 1.0–1.5% enflurane (7).

Respiratory

Enflurane is usually not irritant to the respiratory tract, although bronchospasm has been reported (8). However, it is generally considered to be a bronchodilator. It causes respiratory depression at concentrations over 2%.

Nervous system

Cerebral irritability is a potential consequence of enflurane anesthesia, as evidenced by electroencephalographic recordings and by reported cases of convulsions (SED-11, 208) (9). Enflurane should be used with care (although it is probably not absolutely contraindicated) in patients with epileptiform tendencies, especially if they are deeply anesthetized and hyperventilated. There are reports of delayed convulsions after light general anesthesia not involving hyperventilation. A patient had a convulsion in a car after being discharged from a day-care anesthetic involving enflurane (9).

Motor neuron disease has been attributed to enflurane (10). The authors proposed that enflurane-induced release of glutamate may have caused changes in the spinal cord motor neurons. It is not clear what role alcohol abuse had in this case.

Neuromuscular function

Enflurane increased the sensitivity of the neuromuscular junction to d-tubocurarine in man (11).

Psychological, psychiatric

There was a reduced capacity for learning and decision-making in healthy volunteers after exposure to subanesthetic concentrations of enflurane (12,13).

Endocrine

The endocrine effects of enflurane anesthesia are minimal and clinically insignificant (14).

Metabolism

The effect of enflurane on heme metabolism has been tested in mice (15); the authors suggested that enflurane be added to the list of drugs that can precipitate acute attacks of porphyria.

Liver

One of the main advantages of enflurane over halothane is a reduced rate of liver damage, although such damage can occur (about one in 800 000 exposures) (16,17). With increasing use since 1980 there has been an increasing number of reports of enflurane-induced hepatitis (SED-11, 209), some in patients previously affected by halothane (18), and with some evidence that the risk may be higher in obese middle-aged women (19); some deaths have occurred. All the same, its hepatotoxic potential, although not entirely defined, is probably low, as evidenced by prospective studies of liver function during repeated enflurane anesthesia (20). Indeed, in May 1982 the FDA decided against incorporating a warning of hepatotoxicity on the drug's American labelling, and this policy has been maintained since.

Two patients with hepatic failure after enflurane anesthesia were reported from a hepatic transplant unit in France; both died while waiting for a liver transplant (21). In common with halothane, hepatic failure after enflurane is thought to be caused by the metabolite trifluoroacetic acid.

Urinary tract

Nephrotoxicity leading to renal insufficiency, particularly after prolonged anesthesia, is a potential consequence of general anesthesia with enflurane (22). Several cases of renal insufficiency have been described (SED-11, 209) (23,24), and the mechanism studied. On experimental grounds, it has been suspected that the inorganic fluoride ions to which enflurane is transformed may play a role. Despite evidence that enflurane can cause a significant reduction in maximum urinary osmolarity (tested using vasopressin administration) and in creatinine clearance in healthy volunteers (25), further investigations are warranted. Superimposition of nephrotoxic factors, for example drugs or underlying disease, should be avoided (1).

Musculoskeletal

Myoglobinuria, developing immediately after enflurane anesthesia, has been reported (26).

Second-Generation Effects

Teratogenicity

Experimental evidence is against a teratogenic role of enflurane (1).

Susceptibility Factors

Renal disease

It has been thought that patients with chronically impaired renal function might be at increased risk of nephrotoxicity due to enflurane, because of an increased fluoride load due to reduced excretion. However, this was not confirmed in 41 patients undergoing elective surgery with a stable increased preoperative serum creatinine concentration who were randomly allocated to receive sevoflurane ($n = 21$) or enflurane ($n = 20$) at a fresh gas inflow rate of 4 l/minute for maintenance of anesthesia (27). Peak serum inorganic fluoride concentrations were significantly higher after sevoflurane than after enflurane anesthesia. Laboratory measures of renal function remained stable throughout the postoperative period in both groups. No patient had permanent deterioration of pre-existing renal insufficiency and none required dialysis.

Drug–Drug Interactions

Amitriptyline

Amitriptyline may potentiate enflurane-induced cerebral irritability (19).

References

1. Black GW. Enflurane. Br J Anaesth 1979;51(7):627–40.
2. Shimosato S, Iwatsuki N, Carter JG. Cardio-circulatory effects of enflurane anesthesia in health and disease. Acta Anaesthesiol Scand Suppl 1979;71:69–70.
3. Rifat K. Effets cardiovasculaires de l'enflurane. Med Hyg 1979;37:3602.
4. Reves JG, Samuelson PN, Lell WA, McDaniel HG, Kouchoukos NT, Rogers WJ, Smith LR, Carter MR. Myocardial damage in coronary artery bypass surgical patients anaesthetized with two anaesthetic techniques: a random comparison of halothane and enflurane. Can Anaesth Soc J 1980;27(3):238–45.
5. Saarnivaara L. Comparison of halothane and enflurane anaesthesia for tonsillectomy in adults. Acta Anaesthesiol Scand 1984;28(3):319–24.
6. Willatts DG, Harrison AR, Groom JF, Crowther A. Cardiac arrhythmias during outpatient dental anaesthesia: comparison of halothane with enflurane. Br J Anaesth 1983;55(5):399–403.
7. Chander S. Isorhythmic atrioventricular dissociation during enflurane anesthesia. South Med J 1982;75(8):945–50.
8. Lowry CJ, Fielden BP. Bronchospasm associated with enflurane exposure—three case reports. Anaesth Intensive Care 1976;4(3):254–8.
9. Fahy LT. Delayed convulsions after day case anaesthesia with enflurane. Anaesthesia 1987;42(12):1327–8.
10. Schnorf H, Landis T. Motor neuron disease after enflurane/ propofol anaesthesia in patient with alcohol abuse. Lancet 1995;346(8978):850–1.
11. Stanski DR, Ham J, Miller RD, Sheiner LB. Time-dependent increase in sensitivity to d-tubocurarine during enflurane anesthesia in man. Anesthesiology 1980;52(6):483–7.
12. Bentin S, Collins GI, Adam N. Decision-making behaviour during inhalation of subanaesthetic concentrations of enflurane. Br J Anaesth 1978;50(12):1173–8.
13. Bentin S, Collins GI, Adam N. Effects of low concentrations of enflurane on probability learning. Br J Anaesth 1978;50(12):1179–83.
14. Oyama T, Taniguchi K, Ishihara H, Matsuki A, Maeda A, Murakawa T, Kudo T. Effects of enflurane anaesthesia and surgery on endocrine function in man. Br J Anaesth 1979;51(2):141–8.
15. Buzaleh AM, Enriquez de Salamanca R, Batlle AM. Porphyrinogenic properties of the anesthetic enflurane. Gen Pharmacol 1992;23(4):665–9.
16. Holt C, Csete M, Martin P. Hepatotoxicity of anesthetics and other central nervous system drugs. Gastroenterol Clin North Am 1995;24(4):853–74.
17. Kenna JG, Jones RM. The organ toxicity of inhaled anesthetics. Anesth Analg 1995;81(Suppl 6):S51–66.
18. Sigurdsson J, Hreidarsson AB, Thjodleifsson B. Enflurane hepatitis. A report of a case with a previous history of halothane hepatitis. Acta Anaesthesiol Scand 1985;29(5):495–6.
19. Paull JD, Fortune DW. Hepatotoxicity and death following two enflurane anaesthetics. Anaesthesia 1987;42(11):1191–6.
20. Fee JP, Black GW, Dundee JW, McIlroy PD, Johnston HM, Johnston SB, Black IH, McNeill HG, Neill DW, Doggart JR, Merrett JD, McDonald JR, Bradley DS, Haire M, McMillan SA. A prospective study of liver enzyme and other changes following repeat administration of halothane and enflurane. Br J Anaesth 1979;51(12):1133–41.
21. Lo SK, Wendon J, Mieli-Vergani G, Williams R. Halothane-induced acute liver failure: continuing occurrence and use of liver transplantation. Eur J Gastroenterol Hepatol 1998;10(8):635–9.
22. Motuz DJ, Watson WA, Barlow JC, Velasquez NV, Schentag JJ. The increase in urinary alanine aminopeptidase excretion associated with enflurane anesthesia is increased further by aminoglycosides. Anesth Analg 1988;67(8):770–4.

23. Eichhorn JH, Hedley-Whyte J, Steinman TI, Kaufmann JM, Laasbert LH. Renal failure following enflurane anesthesia. Anesthesiology 1976;45(5):557–60.

24. Delhumeau A, Cocaud J, Bourganneau MC, Cavellat M. La toxicité rénale de l'enflurane: hypothése ou certitude? Anesth Analg Reanim 1981;38:549.

25. Mazze RI, Calverley RK, Smith NT. Inorganic fluoride nephrotoxicity: prolonged enflurane and halothane anesthesia in volunteers. Anesthesiology 1977;46(4):265–71.

26. Miyagishima T, Takagi N, Oka N, et al. Myoglobinuria associated with enflurane anesthesia. Hiroshima J Anesth 1981;16:122.

27. Conzen PF, Nuscheler M, Melotte A, Verhaegen M, Leupolt T, Van Aken H, Peter K. Renal function and serum fluoride concentrations in patients with stable renal insufficiency after anesthesia with sevoflurane or enflurane. Anesth Analg 1995;81(3):569–75.

Halothane

General Information

Halothane is a non-inflammable hydrocarbon that induces anesthesia, with little tendency to excitement. Contrary to earlier assumptions, halothane is metabolized, the consequences of which are discussed below (1,2).

Organs and Systems

Cardiovascular

Halothane, isoflurane, and sevoflurane are potent coronary vasodilators, able to produce some degree of coronary steal in ischemic regions. Despite this, halothane may preferentially dilate large coronary arteries and/or interfere with platelet aggregation. If these experimental effects are confirmed, halothane may be the anesthetic of choice in the non-failing ischemic heart (3).

Halothane has a mild depressive effect on cardiac performance (4). In human ventricular myocardium, halothane interacted with L-type calcium channels by interfering with the dihydropyridine binding site; this may, at least in part, explain its negative inotropic effect (5).

Halothane depressed cardiovascular function significantly more than isoflurane in younger adults, but the falls in systolic and diastolic blood pressures in elderly patients were significantly greater with isoflurane (6).

Cardiac dysrhythmias

Halothane produces bradycardia, but dysrhythmias, most often ventricular in origin, also occur during maintenance of anesthesia. They were noted in 53% of 679 patients (7). Concomitant administration of catecholamines increases the risk of dysrhythmias.

Bundle branch block and aberrant conduction were noted in children during halothane anesthesia (8).

In a double-blind, randomized, controlled study of 77 children undergoing halothane anesthesia for adenoidectomy, the effects of atropine 0.02 mg/kg, glycopyrrolate 0.04 mg/kg, and physiological saline were compared (9). There was no difference in the incidence of ventricular dysrhythmias. Atropine prevented bradycardia but was associated with sinus tachycardia in most patients. The bradycardias that occurred in the groups that received glycopyrrolate or placebo were short-lived and resolved spontaneously.

Pulsus alternans in association with hypercapnia occurred in a study of 120 patients who breathed spontaneously during halothane anesthesia (10). End-tidal carbon dioxide concentration was allowed to rise freely until pulsus alternans or other cardiac dysrhythmias occurred. Ten of the patients developed pulsus alternans, which was promptly relieved on institution of positive pressure ventilation and the return of end-tidal carbon dioxide concentration to normal. The mechanism and the significance of this phenomenon are not well understood.

Respiratory

Halothane is not irritant to the respiratory tract. Respiratory depression is a consequence only of high concentrations of halothane. A certain degree of bronchodilatation is observed, and may explain the fact that a beneficial effect of halothane was described in a 17-year-old woman with acute severe asthma who did not respond to conventional treatment (11).

Preterm infants can become apneic during the immediate postoperative period, even if the ventilatory response to CO_2 is not depressed after halothane anesthesia (12). In a prospective study in 167 preterm infants after inguinal herniorrhaphy with halothane/nitrous oxide anesthesia, only one had an episode of apnea up to 2 days postoperatively; however, the authors recommended careful monitoring until complete recovery from anesthesia has occurred (13).

Nervous system

In contrast to enflurane, cerebral irritability is very rare with halothane (14).

Halothane can cause an increase in intracranial pressure (15), as can other inhalational anesthetics, which can constitute a particular risk if the pressure is already raised before anesthesia. In neonates, the intracranial pressure may fall (16).

A child who underwent induction of anesthesia with halothane developed hiccups associated with pulmonary edema (17).

- An 8-year-old girl with a history of seizures and cerebral ischemic strokes secondary to moyamoya disease underwent anesthetic induction with halothane and 70% nitrous oxide. She had had three previous uneventful anesthetics. Hiccups started within seconds of induction of anesthesia and did not cease until 20 minutes later, when she was paralysed, intubated, and ventilated. During the next 20 minutes a period of hemodynamic instability ensued, with increasing oxygen requirements. The procedure was stopped and pulmonary edema was confirmed on chest X-ray. The child was transferred to the intensive care unit and ventilated overnight. Further recovery was uneventful.

Hiccups during anesthesia are often thought to be benign. Negative pressure pulmonary edema is usually associated with an obstructed airway, as occurs with laryngospasm, or other causes of upper airway obstruction, but was presumably the cause in this child.

The effect of increasing and decreasing concentrations of halothane on the cerebral circulation in 11 young children (aged 4 months to 3.5 years) undergoing minor urological surgery under general relaxant and caudal anesthesia has been studied (18). Cerebral blood flow velocity was measured in the middle cerebral artery using transcranial Doppler ultrasound. There was significantly increased cerebral blood flow velocity when the dose was increased from 0.5 to 1.0 minimum alveolar concentration (MAC) and from 0.5 to 1.5 MAC, but not when it was increased from 1.0 to 1.5 MAC. When the halothane concentration was reduced from 1.5 to 1.0 MAC, cerebral blood flow velocity fell significantly, whereas there was no effect when the concentration was reduced from 1.0 to 0.5 MAC. These results suggest that there is cerebrovascular hysteresis in response to increasing and decreasing concentrations of halothane.

Psychological, psychiatric

Slight depression of mood, lasting up to 30 days, along with a non-specific slowing of the electroencephalogram for 1–2 weeks, was observed after halothane. In 16 healthy young men, halothane anesthesia had negative effects on postoperative mood and intellectual function, the changes being greatest 2 days after anesthesia, with restoration of function after 8 days (19). In seven subjects, serial electroencephalography, serum bromide determinations, and psychological tests before and after halothane anesthesia showed that there was significant psychological impairment 2 days after anesthesia (20).

The effect of a single preoperative dose of the opioid oxycodone on emergence behavior has been studied in a randomized trial in 130 children (21). Oxycodone prophylaxis, compared with no premedication, significantly reduced the incidence of post-halothane agitation.

Mineral balance

Halothane can cause an increase in circulating concentrations of bromide and fluoride (20), which can be associated with impaired urine-concentrating ability in response to antidiuretic hormone (22).

Hematologic

Halothane produced inhibition of in vitro platelet aggregation and an increase in bleeding time (23).

Gastrointestinal

Postoperative nausea and vomiting can occur after halothane anesthesia (24). In one series, postoperative vomiting occurred in 13 of 29 patients who had received halothane for induction, but when dyxirazine was added during anesthesia the incidence of postoperative vomiting was significantly reduced (three of 29 patients) (25).

Liver

The greatest disadvantage of halothane is its ability to cause liver damage (26).

Incidence

The death rate due to halothane-induced liver damage was estimated in 1993 at one in 35 000 anesthetics (27), three times greater than the one in 110 000 incidence reported in 1976 (28). Both immune function and the metabolism of halothane play important roles in the pathophysiology of liver damage (29). Human hepatic microsomal carboxylesterase is a target antigen in halothane hepatitis, protein disulfide isomerase is an important factor in the mechanism of liver impairment, and an associated immune response may be involved (SEDA-18, 116). So-called halothane-induced liver antigens are novel antigens found in the livers of some individuals who have been exposed to halothane, but not in the livers of unexposed individuals (30).

A retrospective review of the case-notes of 44 patients with drug-induced hepatotoxicity diagnosed in 1978–96 found only one case attributable to halothane (31). Antibiotics, non-steroidal anti-inflammatory drugs, and psychotropic drugs accounted for 73% of the cases.

Mechanisms

The mechanisms by which halothane causes hepatic toxicity have been reviewed (32). Oxidative metabolism of halothane to trifluoroacetate occurs in the liver, probably via CYP2E1. In rats, trifluoroacetylated CYP2E1 has been identified after exposure to halothane, as has antibody formation to this antigen (33). Covalent binding of halothane (34), after its activation to the trifluoroacetyl halide, to proteins in human liver microsomes has also been shown (35). It has been suggested that some genetic factor determines the risk of developing halothane hepatitis (36). A report of halothane hepatitis in three pairs of closely related women (37) raised the possibility of a pharmacogenetic defect in these patients, with increased production of hepatotoxic metabolites.

Most recorded cases of liver disorders occurred after either repeated exposure (38) or prolonged exposure (39) to halothane. In one case, hepatitis developed 3 weeks after a single halothane anesthetic in a 37-year-old renal transplant recipient who had previously been exposed to isoflurane (40); this report suggests that previous exposure to isoflurane may predispose to subsequent halothane toxicity.

Halothane also reduces liver blood flow during anesthesia, and this could increase the release of potentially hepatotoxic halothane metabolites. The role of reduced halothane metabolites and inorganic fluoride, which may covalently link to liver macromolecules, has been stressed; in keeping with this hypothesis is the observation of halothane hepatitis in patients who simultaneously take enzyme-inducing agents, for example barbiturates (41) or rifampicin (42).

It is therefore tempting to suggest that patients with one or several predisposing factors, for example a pharmacogenetic trait, hepatic hypoxia, or enzyme induction, are likely to produce large amounts of hepatotoxic halothane metabolites that covalently bind to liver macromolecules, rendering them immunogenic. The finding that repeated administration increases the risk of halothane jaundice (43,44) supports this hypothesis.

Presentation

Two patterns of liver damage associated with halothane have been observed (45). One pattern is a mild derangement of liver enzymes, which occurs in about one in four anesthetics. The other pattern is rare but is associated with severe hepatitis, often resulting in fulminant liver failure. This severe form occurs more often in middle-aged, obese women, usually after multiple anesthetics, and is known as halothane hepatitis. It is defined as unexplained severe liver damage occurring within 28 days of halothane exposure in a person with a previously normal liver, and it occurs in 1:35 000 halothane exposures. With repeated exposure to halothane within 1 month, the frequency of acute liver failure increases to 1:3700. The overall incidence of halothane hepatitis is falling, owing to reduced use of halothane. Survival after liver transplantation in patients with fulminant hepatic failure is lower than that after liver transplantation for other reasons.

A case of halothane hepatitis has been reported in a child (46).

- A 6-year-old boy sustained pelvic injuries and a femoral fracture. The first anesthetic he received consisted of thiopental, suxamethonium, isoflurane, and nitrous oxide. He also received two units of blood. He subsequently underwent four halothane anesthetics over 6 weeks for dilatation of a urethral stricture. Two days after the last anesthetic he was noted to be jaundiced. He had a negative viral screen but was positive for antitrifluoroacetyl IgG antibodies. He developed fulminant hepatic failure with grade 2 hepatic encephalopathy and underwent an auxiliary liver transplantation 24 days after his last exposure to halothane. He died of septicemia 18 days later. Both at autopsy and on a previous hepatobiliary scan he was noted to have had extensive native liver regeneration.

Halothane hepatitis in children is rare, and occurs in 1:82 000 to 1:200 000 exposures. Children as young as 11 months are not exempt from the risk, contrary to what was once thought and there is a growing number of reports of halothane hepatitis in children (47). It has been noted that sevoflurane is not metabolized to trifluoroacetic acid and may prove to be a better alternative for repeated anesthesia in children (48).

A retrospective review of the case-notes of 44 patients with drug-induced hepatotoxicity diagnosed in 1978–96 found only one case attributable to halothane (31). Antibiotics, non-steroidal anti-inflammatory drugs, and psychotropic drugs accounted for 73% of the cases.

Urinary tract

Renal blood flow, glomerular filtration rate, and urinary volume are sometimes mildly and reversibly reduced. In contrast, repeated massive polyuria has been reported in a 46-year-old man after two anesthetics with halothane (49). Acute renal insufficiency has been described (50) but is rare.

Skin

A young nurse complained of a skin rash with edema of the eyelids after repeated professional exposure to halothane (51).

Immunologic

Halothane can suppress host defence mechanisms; the clinical consequences are unclear (SED-11, 210) (SEDA-3, 101) (SEDA-4, 77) (SEDA-5, 121) (SEDA-11, 109).

Body temperature

Halothane reduces body temperature and can cause shivering, although active thermoregulation does not occur until the core temperature is reduced by 2.5°C (52). The shivering can be attenuated by flumazenil, despite a lower core temperature (53).

Halothane in association with suxamethonium is the most frequent cause of malignant hyperthermia attributed to general anesthesia (54). Standard in vitro caffeine-halothane contracture testing was performed on 32 patients with a past history of malignant hyperthermia diagnosed on clinical grounds; they were compared with a matched control group of 120 subjects who were considered clinically to be at low risk of malignant hyperthermia (55). The sensitivity of the test was 97% and the specificity 78%.

Second-Generation Effects

Pregnancy

Halothane strongly reduces uterine contractility during labor (56).

Fetotoxicity

Halothane can be used as an anesthetic by maternal inhalation for fetal surgery and improves surgical exposure by relaxing the uterus. However, the effects of halothane on fetal cardiovascular homeostasis have been evaluated, and the authors concluded that halothane had a significant negative effect on the fetal heart and peripheral vasculature; it was therefore considered a poor anesthetic for this purpose (57).

Lactation

Halothane is readily excreted into breast milk (58).

Drug Administration

Drug administration route

In a randomized, double-blind, placebo-controlled comparison of intranasal and intramuscular atropine in 80 children, the intranasal route was equally effective at preventing halothane-induced bradycardia (59).

Drug overdose

Suicide attempts with halothane have sometimes succeeded, but in patients who recovered there was no residual damage. A 4-year-old boy was accidentally given halothane intravenously; he recovered fully within a few hours (60). Accidental intravenous injection and illicit inhalation have both caused pulmonary edema (61).

Drug–Drug Interactions

Atracurium dibesilate

From animal experiments (65) it seems likely that drug interactions with atracurium will be similar to those for other non-depolarizing neuromuscular blocking agents. Laudanosine has been reported to increase the MAC for halothane in animals (66).

In man, potentiation and prolongation of the action of atracurium by halothane (67–69) have been reported, as has potentiation after 30 minutes of isoflurane anesthesia (70). Whether the dose of atracurium should be reduced from that used during balanced anesthesia by 20, 30, or 50% when patients are anesthetized with inhalational anesthetics can only be decided in the case of an individual patient if neuromuscular monitoring is available, since many other variables, such as the tissue concentrations of the volatile anesthetic and the response of the individual patient to the neuromuscular blocking drug, will influence the overall blocking effect.

Disulfiram

Disulfiram is an inhibitor of CYP2E1. In 20 patients undergoing halothane-based maintenance of anesthesia at an end-tidal concentration of 1% for an average of 3 hours, disulfiram 500 mg taken the night before substantially attenuated trifluoroacetate production, as judged by its urinary excretion (62). It was suggested that a single dose of disulfiram may provide effective prophylaxis against halothane hepatitis.

Ephedrine

Halothane and some other anesthetics sensitize patients to the risk of ephedrine-induced ventricular dysrhythmias and acute pulmonary edema, especially if hypoxia is present (71).

Midazolam

Midazolam produced marked reduction of the MAC of halothane in humans at lower serum concentrations than required to cause sleep (64).

Nitrous oxide

The addition of nitrous oxide to halothane in coronary patients produced hypotension, with a subsequent risk of myocardial damage (72).

Non-depolarizing muscle relaxants

Halothane potentiates the effects of non-depolarizing muscular relaxants (SED-11, 210) (63).

References

1. Weis KH, Engelhardt W. Is halothane obsolete? Two standards of judgement. Anaesthesia 1989;44(2):97–100.
2. Pedersen T, Johansen SH. Serious morbidity attributable to anaesthesia. Considerations for prevention. Anaesthesia 1989;44(6):504–8.
3. Merin RG. Physiology, pathophysiology and pharmacology of the coronary circulation with particular emphasis on anesthetics. Anaesthesiol Reanim 1992;17(1):5–26.
4. Maze M, Mason DM. Aetiology and treatment of halothane-induced arrhythmias. Clin Anaesthesiol 1983;1:301.
5. Schmidt U, Schwinger RH, Bohm S, Uberfuhr P, Kreuzer E, Reichart B, Meyer L, Erdmann E, Bohm M. Evidence for an interaction of halothane with the L-type Ca^{2+} channel in human myocardium. Anesthesiology 1993;79(2):332–9.
6. McKinney MS, Fee JP, Clarke RS. Cardiovascular effects of isoflurane and halothane in young and elderly adult patients. Br J Anaesth 1993;71(5):696–701.
7. Yokoyama K. Arrhythmias due to halothane anesthesia. Jpn J Anesthesiol 1978;27:64.
8. Lindgren L. E.C.G changes during halothane and enflurane anaesthesia for E.N.T. surgery in children Br J Anaesth 1981;53(6):653–62.
9. Reinoso-Barbero F, Gutierrez-Marquez M, Diez-Labajo A. Prevention of halothane-induced bradycardia: is intranasal premedication indicated? Paediatr Anaesth 1998;8(3):195–9.
10. Saghaei M, Mortazavian M. Pulsus alternans during general anesthesia with halothane: effects of permissive hypercapnia. Anesthesiology 2000;93(1):91–4.
11. Obata T, Masaki T, Nezu T, Iikura Y. Treatment of status asthmaticus with halothane: a case report. Iryo 1992;46:204–10.
12. Palmisano BW, Setlock MA, Doyle MK, Rosner DR, Hoffman GM, Eckert JE. Ventilatory response to carbon dioxide in term infants after halothane and nitrous oxide anesthesia. Anesth Analg 1993;76(6):1234–7.
13. Haga S, Shima T, Momose K, Andoh K, Hoshi K, Hashimoto Y. [Postoperative apnea in preterm infants after inguinal herniorrhaphy.]Masui 1993;42(1):120–2.
14. Smith PA, Macdonald TR, Jones CS. Convulsions associated with halothane anaesthesia. Two case reports. Anaesthesia 1966;21(2):229–33.
15. Cunitz G, Danhauser I, Gruss P. Die Wirkung von Enflurane (Ethrane) im Vergleich zu Halothan auf den intracraniellen Druck. [Effect of enflurane (Ethrane) on intracranial pressure in comparison with halothane.] Anaesthesist 1976;25(7):323–30.
16. Friesen RH, Thieme RE, Honda AT, Morrison JE Jr. Changes in anterior fontanel pressure in preterm neonates receiving isoflurane, halothane, fentanyl, or ketamine. Anesth Analg 1987;66(5):431–4.
17. Stuth EA, Stucke AG, Berens RJ. Negative-pressure pulmonary edema in a child with hiccups during induction. Anesthesiology 2000;93(1):282–4.
18. Paut O, Bissonnette B. Effect of halothane on the cerebral circulation in young children: a hysteresis phenomenon. Anaesthesia 2001;56(4):360–5.
19. Davison LA, Steinhelber JC, Eger EI 2nd, Stevens WC. Psychological effects of halothane and isoflurane anesthesia. Anesthesiology 1975;43(3):313–24.

20. Bruchiel KJ, Stockard JJ, Calverley RK, Smith NT, Scholl ML, Mazze RI. Electroencephalographic abnormalities following halothane anesthesia. Anesth Analg 1978; 57(2):244–51.
21. Neunteufl T, Berger R, Pacher R. Endothelin receptor antagonists in cardiology clinical trials. Expert Opin Investig Drugs 2002;11(3):431–43.
22. Mazze RI, Calverley RK, Smith NT. Inorganic fluoride nephrotoxicity: prolonged enflurane and halothane anesthesia in volunteers. Anesthesiology 1977;46(4):265–71.
23. Dalsgaard-Nielsen J, Risbo A, Simmelkjaer P, Gormsen J. Impaired platelet aggregation and increased bleeding time during general anaesthesia with halothane. Br J Anaesth 1981;53(10):1039–42.
24. Kenny GN. Risk factors for postoperative nausea and vomiting. Anaesthesia 1994;49(Suppl):6–10.
25. Karlsson E, Larsson LE, Nilsson K. The effects of prophylactic dixyrazine on postoperative vomiting after two different anaesthetic methods for squint surgery in children. Acta Anaesthesiol Scand 1993;37(1):45–8.
26. Feher J, Vasarhelyi B, Blazovics A. A halotan hepatitis. [Halothane hepatitis.] Orv Hetil 1993;134(33):1795–8.
27. Elliott RH, Strunin L. Hepatotoxicity of volatile anaesthetics. Br J Anaesth 1993;70(3):339–48.
28. Bottiger LE, Dalen E, Hallen B. Halothane-induced liver damage: an analysis of the material reported to the Swedish Adverse Drug Reaction Committee, 1966–1973. Acta Anaesthesiol Scand 1976;20(1):40–6.
29. Smith GC, Kenna JG, Harrison DJ, Tew D, Wolf CR. Autoantibodies to hepatic microsomal carboxylesterase in halothane hepatitis. Lancet 1993;342(8877):963–4.
30. Kenna JG, Knight TL, van Pelt FN. Immunity to halothane metabolite-modified proteins in halothane hepatitis. Ann NY Acad Sci 1993;685:646–61.
31. Aithal PG, Day CP. The natural history of histologically proved drug induced liver disease. Gut 1999;44(5):731–5.
32. Pumford NR, Halmes NC, Hinson JA. Covalent binding of xenobiotics to specific proteins in the liver. Drug Metab Rev 1997;29(1–2):39–57.
33. Eliasson E, Kenna JG. Cytochrome P450 2E1 is a cell surface autoantigen in halothane hepatitis. Mol Pharmacol 1996;50(3):573–82.
34. Nuscheler M, Conzen P, Schwender D, Peter K. Fluoridinduzierte Nephrotoxizität: Fakt oder Fiktion?. [Fluoride-induced nephrotoxicity: factor fiction?.] Anaesthesist 1996;45(Suppl 1):S32–40.
35. Madan A, Parkinson A. Characterization of the NADPH-dependent covalent binding of [^{14}C]halothane to human liver microsomes: a role for cytochrome P450 2E1 at low substrate concentrations. Drug Metab Dispos 1996;24(12):1307–13.
36. Ranek L, Dalhoff K, Poulsen HE, Brosen K, Flachs H, Loft S, Wantzin P. Drug metabolism and genetic polymorphism in subjects with previous halothane hepatitis. Scand J Gastroenterol 1993;28(8):677–80.
37. Hoft RH, Bunker JP, Goodman HI, Gregory PB. Halothane hepatitis in three pairs of closely related women. N Engl J Med 1981;304(17):1023–4.
38. Dahmash NS, Ayoola EA, Al-Nozha M. Halothane induced hepatotoxicity in a Saudi male. Ann Saudi Med 1993;13:314–6.
39. Shimizu H, Namba H, Ishima T. Liver dysfunction after halothane therapy in two cases with life threatening asthma. KoKyu 1993;12:229–32.
40. Slayter KL, Sketris IS, Gulanikar A. Halothane hepatitis in a renal transplant patient previously exposed to isoflurane. Ann Pharmacother 1993;27(1):101.
41. Bidard JM, Casio N, Gerolami A, et al. Deux observations d'hépatite toxique par association d'halothane—un inducteur enzymatique. Nouv Presse Méd 1980;9:883.
42. Steiner F, Pottecher T, Bellocq JP. Ictère grave post opératoire: rôle de l'halothane et des tuberculostatiques. Cah Anesthesiol 1980;23:1019.
43. Fee JP, Black GW, Dundee JW, McIlroy PD, Johnston HM, Johnston SB, Black IH, McNeill HG, Neill DW, Doggart JR, Merrett JD, McDonald JR, Bradley DS, Haire M, McMillan SA. A prospective study of liver enzyme and other changes following repeat administration of halothane and enflurane. Br J Anaesth 1979;51(12):1133–41.
44. Schlippert W, Anuras S. Recurrent hepatitis following halothane exposures. Am J Med 1978;65(1):25–30.
45. Neuberger J. Halothane hepatitis. Eur J Gastroenterol Hepatol 1998;10(8):631–3.
46. Munro HM, Snider SJ, Magee JC. Halothane-associated hepatitis in a 6-year-old boy: evidence for native liver regeneration following failed treatment with auxiliary liver transplantation. Anesthesiology 1998;89(2):524–7.
47. Kenna JG, Neuberger J, Mieli-Vergani G, Mowat AP, Williams R. Halothane hepatitis in children. BMJ (Clin Res Ed) 1987;294(6581):1209–11.
48. Murat I. There is no longer a place for halothane in paediatric anaesthesia. Paediatr Anaesth 1998;8(2):184.
49. Dallera F, Caccialanza E, Segalini A, et al. Un caso di poliuria probabilmente da fluotano. Acta Anaesthesiol Ital 1983;34:83.
50. Gelman ML, Lichtenstein NS. Halothane-induced nephrotoxicity. Urology 1981;17(4):323–7.
51. Bodman R. Skin sensitivity to halothane vapour. Br J Anaesth 1979;51(11):1092.
52. Sessler DI, Olofsson CI, Rubinstein EH, Beebe JJ. The thermoregulatory threshold in humans during halothane anesthesia. Anesthesiology 1988;68(6):836–42.
53. Weinbroum AA, Geller E. Flumazenil improves cognitive and neuromotor emergence and attenuates shivering after halothane-, enflurane- and isoflurane-based anesthesia. Can J Anaesth 2001;48(10):963–72.
54. Drury PM, Gilbertson AA. Malignant hyperpyrexia and anaesthesia. Two case reports. Br J Anaesth 1970;42(11):1021–3.
55. Allen GC, Larach MG, Kunselman AR. The sensitivity and specificity of the caffeine-halothane contracture test: a report from the North American Malignant Hyperthermia Registry. The North American Malignant Hyperthermia Registry of MHAUS. Anesthesiology 1998;88(3):579–88.
56. Neumark J, Faller T. Halothan, Enfluran und ihr Einfluss auf die Uterusaktivität am Geburts-Termin. [The effects of halothane and enflurane on uterine activity during childbirth.] Prakt Anaesth 1978;13(1):7–12.
57. Sabik JF, Assad RS, Hanley FL. Halothane as an anesthetic for fetal surgery. J Pediatr Surg 1993;28(4):542–6.
58. Cote CJ, Kenepp NB, Reed SB, Strobel GE. Trace concentrations of halothane in human breast milk. Br J Anaesth 1976;48(6):541–3.
59. Annila P, Rorarius M, Reinikainen P, Oikkonen M, Baer G. Effect of pre-treatment with intravenous atropine or glycopyrrolate on cardiac arrhythmias during halothane anaesthesia for adenoidectomy in children. Br J Anaesth 1998;80(6):756–60.
60. Trombini Garcia R, Salomao JB, Benincasa SC, et al. Instilagaio acidental de halotano em una crianca de quatro anos. J Pediatr 1984;56:323.
61. Martindale. The Extra Pharmacopoeia. London: Pharmaceutical Press;. 1977.

62. Kharasch ED, Hankins D, Mautz D, Thummel KE. Identification of the enzyme responsible for oxidative halothane metabolism: implications for prevention of halothane hepatitis. Lancet 1996;347(9012):1367–71.

63. Hughes R, Payne JP. Interaction of halothane with nondepolarizing neuromuscular blocking drugs in man. BMJ 1979;2:1425.

64. Inagaki Y, Sumikawa K, Yoshiya I. Anesthetic interaction between midazolam and halothane in humans. Anesth Analg 1993;76(3):613–7.

65. Chapple DJ, Clark JS, Hughes R. Interaction between atracurium and drugs used in anaesthesia. Br J Anaesth 1983;55(Suppl 1):S17–22.

66. Shi WZ, Fahey MR, Fisher DM, Miller RD, Canfell C, Eger EI 2nd. Laudanosine (a metabolite of atracurium) increases the minimum alveolar concentration of halothane in rabbits. Anesthesiology 1985;63(6):584–8.

67. Payne JP, Hughes R. Evaluation of atracurium in anaesthetized man. Br J Anaesth 1981;53(1):45–54.

68. Katz RL, Stirt J, Murray AL, Lee C. Neuromuscular effects of atracurium in man. Anesth Analg 1982;61(9):730–4.

69. Stirt JA, Murray AL, Katz RL, Schehl DL, Lee C. Atracurium during halothane anesthesia in humans. Anesth Analg 1983;62(2):207–10.

70. Rupp SM, Fahey MR, Miller RD. Neuromuscular and cardiovascular effects of atracurium during nitrous oxide-fentanyl and nitrous oxide–isoflurane anaesthesia. Br J Anaesth 1983;55(Suppl 1):S67–70.

71. Haller CA, Benowitz NL. Dietary supplements containing Ephedra alkaloids. New Engl J Med 2001;344:1096–7.

72. Moffitt EA, Sethna DH, Gary RJ, Raymond MJ, Matloff JM, Bussell JA. Nitrous oxide added to halothane reduces coronary flow and myocardial oxygen consumption in patients with coronary disease. Can Anaesth Soc J 1983;30(1):5–9.

Isoflurane

General Information

Isoflurane is a potent inhalation anesthetic. An isomer of enflurane, it has many of the same adverse effects. It is hardly metabolized (about 0.2%), which has encouraged its prolonged use as a sedative agent or bronchodilator in patients with acute severe asthma. However, it may not be as inert in all patients.

Organs and Systems

Cardiovascular

Although atrial dysrhythmias have been reported in 3.9% of patients and ventricular dysrhythmias in 2.5% (1), the dysrhythmogenicity of isoflurane is less pronounced than that of halothane (2). Indeed, the incidence of dysrhythmias due to catecholamines in cardiovascular anesthesia and during oral surgery is reduced by using isoflurane rather than the other agents.

The most controversial adverse effect of isoflurane is its potential to cause coronary steal in patients with critical stenosis in the coronary circulation. Most recent work suggests that the risk of myocardial ischemia is not increased, as long as the hemodynamics, especially heart rate, are well controlled (3). However, there are still isolated reports, suggesting that the issue is not settled. In some cases isoflurane has caused a specific coronary steal even with good hemodynamic control (4).

Isoflurane can cause marked hypertension during induction of anesthesia. Of 26 patients who were anesthetized with 0.5% isoflurane in oxygen, increased to 4% in 2 minutes, nine had increases in systolic blood pressure by more than 10 mmHg (mean 26) (5). Tracheal intubation markedly increased the blood pressure in all patients, but there was a negative correlation between the isoflurane-induced increase and that induced by intubation. Tracheal intubation produced a larger increase in blood pressure in the isoflurane-induced hypertensive patients.

Respiratory

Marked respiratory depression has been documented in children (6) and coughing associated with nausea and vomiting occurs in about 10% of subjects (1).

Like halothane, isoflurane is useful in cases of life-threatening acute severe asthma refractory to drug therapy.

- An 11-year-old girl with acute asthma, severe CO_2 narcosis, and ventricular fibrillation induced by hypoxemia was successfully treated with isoflurane in oxygen for 14 hours. Her recovery may have been due to bronchodilatation and the treatment that was possible because of the low dysrhythmogenic effect of isoflurane (7).

Nervous system

Seizures are uncommon with isoflurane, but reports continue to appear.

The neuromuscular blocking effects of vecuronium bromide can be enhanced by inhalation anesthetics.

- Symptoms suggestive of severe sensorimotor neuropathy developed in a 40-year-old woman 15 days after admission for a severe exacerbation of asthma (8). During this time she was given isoflurane 0.5–3% in oxygen, vecuronium bromide 4–6 mg/hour, and fentanyl 100 micrograms/hour. The neuropathy resolved spontaneously over the next 3 months.

In this case, isoflurane may have been the trigger.

- A fine tremor occurred when isoflurane was used in the management of a 3-year-old boy with pneumonia and underlying congenital myasthenia gravis (9).

Psychological

Memory function and its relation to depth of hypnotic state has been prospectively evaluated in anesthetized and non-anesthetized subjects, using the Bispectral Index during general anesthesia and an auditory word stem completion test and process dissociation procedure after anesthesia (10). Isoflurane was used in 47 patients and propofol in one. There was evidence of memory for words presented during light anesthesia (Bispectral Index score 61–80) and adequate anesthesia (score 41–60) but not during deep anesthesia (score 21–40). The process dissociation procedure showed a significant implicit memory contribution but not reliable explicit memory contribution. Memory performance was better in non-anesthetized subjects than in anesthetized patients, with a higher contribution from explicit memory and a comparable contribution from implicit memory. The authors concluded that during general anesthesia for elective surgery, implicit memory persists, even in adequate hypnotic states, to a comparable degree as in non-anesthetized subjects.

Endocrine

The effects of anesthesia for more than 10 hours with either isoflurane or sevoflurane on hormone secretion have been studied in 20 patients (11). Adrenaline and noradrenaline concentrations increased continuously during and after surgery in the isoflurane group whereas they increased only after surgery in the sevoflurane group; both concentrations were higher in the isoflurane group during anesthesia. Cortisol increased continuously but adrenocorticotropic hormone increased only during surgery. Antidiuretic hormone increased during surgery and the isoflurane group had significantly higher values than the sevoflurane group. Glucose increased both during and after surgery but insulin increased only after surgery; glucagon fell during surgery in both groups.

Metabolism

The effects of anesthesia with sevoflurane (0.5, 1.0, and 1.5 MAC) and isoflurane (0.5, 1.0, and 1.5 MAC) on glucose tolerance have been studied in a randomized study in 30 patients (12). The insulinogenic index (change in concentration of immunoreactive insulin/change in glucose concentration), the acute insulin response, and the rates of glucose disappearance were significantly lower in all anesthesia groups than in the control group. However, there were no differences among the six anesthesia groups.

Liver

Hepatic damage related to isoflurane anesthesia has very occasionally been described (13,14), including one report of hepatic necrosis and death (15). Hepatitis or hepatocellular injury has been described with all current volatile anesthetics. Among these, halothane-associated hepatitis has been best characterized and is probably caused by an immune reaction induced by hepatocyte proteins that have been covalently trifluoroacetylated by the trifluoroacetyl metabolite of halothane. The reactive acyl-halide metabolite of trifluoroacetic acid can trifluoroacetylate liver proteins, resulting in immune-mediated hepatic necrosis (16). However, isoflurane biotransformation to trifluoroacetate is less than 0.2%, compared with 15–20% for halothane.

In an interesting case report, clinical, histochemical, and immunohistochemical evidence supporting the role of trifluoroacetyl-modified proteins has been presented in a patient with hepatitis associated with isoflurane (17).

The role of CYP2E1 as the predominant route of metabolism of isoflurane to trifluoroacetic acid and inorganic fluoride ions has been confirmed using the enzyme inhibitor disulfiram as a metabolic probe in 22 adults randomized to either disulfiram 500 mg the evening before surgery or placebo. Anesthesia with 1.5% isoflurane lasted for an average of 8 hours. Postoperative plasma concentrations were increased and urinary excretion of trifluoroacetic acid was inhibited by 80–90% in the disulfiram group. Whether the use of disulfiram would reduce the incidence of hepatitis is unknown. Patients with increased activity of CYP2E1 or CYP2A6 appear to be at higher risk of isoflurane hepatotoxicity.

Acute hepatotoxicity has been reported with isoflurane (18). The authors hypothesized that induction of cytochrome P-450 by phenytoin had caused enhanced transformation of isoflurane to trifluoroacetic acid. They suggested that caution should be taken in the use of halogenated anesthetics in patients taking drugs that induce cytochrome P-450 isozymes.

- An obese 35-year-old diabetic woman developed isoflurane-induced hepatotoxicity (19). She had had four previous halothane anesthetics, the last two of which were associated with jaundice. She made a full recovery and during a subsequent anesthetic received an infusion of propofol. Unfortunately, trifluoroacetic acid antibody titers were not performed. Liver function does not appear to have been severely affected: peak alanine transaminase activity was 1410 IU/l.

Fatal hepatotoxicity associated with isoflurane has been reported (20).

- A 76-year-old woman with previous exposure to isoflurane 3 years earlier underwent an above-knee amputation for a liposarcoma using isoflurane anesthesia. On day 3 postoperatively she became febrile and confused. Bacterial cultures later showed *Staphylococcus aureus* in the sputum and *Escherichia coli* in the urine. Associated hypotension for 2 hours resolved with inotropic support and here renal function remained normal. On day 6 she became jaundiced and developed further hypotension. Despite intensive care treatment she died on day 7. An autopsy showed centrilobular necrosis consistent with drug-induced hepatitis. All liver serology was negative.

The clinical details in this case were similar to those seen in halothane hepatitis. The authors concluded that although there was no direct evidence that isoflurane was the causative agent, it was likely to have caused this type of hepatitis. Unfortunately, trifluoroacetic acid antibodies titers were not measured, because this test, if positive, would have confirmed the diagnosis.

Urinary tract

High concentrations of fluorine ions, potentially damaging to the kidney, can be found after prolonged use (21).

Four patients with renal dysfunction in an intensive care unit received isoflurane inhalation for sedation for 8–26 days. The concentrations of isoflurane used were 20–50% of the minimum alveolar concentration. Only small increases in fluoride ion concentration, the highest being

25 μmol/l, were recorded, well below the 50 μmol/l threshold associated with adverse effects on renal function (22).

Immunologic

Anaphylaxis has been reported in a patient who received isoflurane (23).

Body temperature

Malignant hyperthermia is a possible complication of isoflurane anesthesia (24).

Shivering after an anesthetic develops in as many as a half of patients recovering from isoflurane anesthesia. Most postoperative shivering appears to be thermoregulatory, although volatile anesthetics can themselves facilitate muscular activity. In 60 adult patients the incidence of postoperative shivering was 40% in a control group, 7% after physostigmine 0.04 mg/kg, zero after meperidine 0.5 mg/kg, and zero after clonidine 1.5 micrograms/kg (25). The centrally acting adrenoceptor agonist phenylpropylamine methylphenidate, the 5-hydroxytryptamine antagonist ketanserin, magnesium sulfate, doxapram, and hypercapnia also reduce the incidence of postoperative shivering.

Drug–Drug Interactions

Alfentanil and esmolol

The effects of alfentanil and esmolol on isoflurane requirements for anesthesia have been studied in a randomized trial in 100 patients (26). Alfentanil infusion to a targeted effect site concentration of 50 ng/ml, but not esmolol, reduced the minimum alveolar concentration of isoflurane required to suppress movement to surgical pain by 25%. The combination of esmolol and alfentanil caused a 74% reduction in isoflurane requirements. This study is interesting, because the beta-blocker esmolol had a profound effect on the isoflurane-sparing effects of alfentanil, while having little effect on its own.

Atracurium dibesilate

A synergistic interaction between isoflurane and atracurium (high doses) has been incriminated in the causation of an increased incidence of generalized tonic-clonic seizures after neurosurgical operations (SEDA-15, 125) (27).

Clonidine

In a randomized, double-blind, controlled trial in 61 patients, oral clonidine 5 micrograms/kg was given 90 minutes before surgery to reduce the concentration of isoflurane at which patients wake at the end of surgery by 8% (28). There was a 6–7 minute delay in waking in the clonidine group compared with the control group. Clonidine 2.5 micrograms/kg had no significant effect.

Midazolam

The effects of the combination of midazolam and isoflurane on memory were studied in a randomized, double-blind study in 28 volunteers (29). Midazolam 0.03 mg/kg or 0.06 mg/kg combined with isoflurane 0.2% almost completely abolished explicit and implicit memory, but there were more variable effects on the level of sedation. The duration of the deficit averaged 45 minutes. The study was remarkable for the very low doses required to abolish memory, owing to synergy of the combination of midazolam and isoflurane and abolition of memory at subhypnotic doses with this combination. However, the subjects did not undergo surgery, so caution must be exercised in extrapolating the result to surgical patients, because painful stimuli increase the dosage required to abolish memory.

Rocuronium

The infusion requirements of rocuronium necessary to maintain twitch depression were reduced by 40% during anesthesia involving isoflurane (30). In another study in 60 patients undergoing maintenance anesthesia, isoflurane plus nitrous oxide anesthesia reduced the dosage requirement of rocuronium by 35–40% (31).

Suxamethonium

Isoflurane in nitrous oxide inhibited suxamethonium-induced muscle fasciculation in children (32).

References

1. Levy WJ. Clinical anaesthesia with isoflurane. A review of the multicentre study. Br J Anaesth 1984;56(Suppl 1):S101–12.
2. Rodrigo MR, Moles TM, Lee PK. Comparison of the incidence and nature of cardiac arrhythmias occurring during isoflurane or halothane anaesthesia. Studies during dental surgery. Br J Anaesth 1986;58(4):394–400.
3. Slogoff S, Keats AS. Randomized trial of primary anesthetic agents on outcome of coronary artery bypass operations. Anesthesiology 1989;70(2):179–88.
4. Inoue K, Reichelt W, el-Banayosy A, Minami K, Dallmann G, Hartmann N, Windeler J. Does isoflurane lead to a higher incidence of myocardial infarction and perioperative death than enflurane in coronary artery surgery? A clinical study of 1178 patients. Anesth Analg 1990;71(5):469–74.
5. Kobayashi Y. [Pressor responses to inhalation of isoflurane during induction of anesthesia and subsequent tracheal intubation.] Masui 2005;54(8):869–74.
6. Murat I, Beydon L, Chaussain M, Levy J, Saint-Maurice JP. Ventilatory changes during nitrous oxide isoflurane anaesthesia in children. Eur J Anaesthesiol 1986;3(5):403–11.
7. Shibata Y, Kukita I, Baba T, Goto T, Yoshinaga T. [A critical patient relieved from status asthmaticus with isoflurane inhalation therapy.]Masui 1993;42(1):116–9.
8. du Peloux Menage H, Duffy S, Yates DW, Hughes JA. Reversible sensorimotor impairment following prolonged ventilation with isoflurane and vecuronium for acute severe asthma. Thorax 1992;47(12):1078–9.
9. McBeth C, Watkins TG. Isoflurane for sedation in a case of congenital myasthenia gravis. Br J Anaesth 1996;77(5):672–4.
10. Iselin-Chaves IA, Willems SJ, Jermann FC, Forster A, Adam SR, Van der Linden M. Investigation of implicit memory during isoflurane anaesthesia for elective surgery using the process dissociation procedure. Anesthesiology 2005;103(5):925–33.
11. Nishiyama T, Yamashita K, Yokoyama T. Stress hormone changes in general anesthesia of long duration:

isoflurane-nitrous oxide vs sevoflurane-nitrous oxide anesthesia. J Clin Anesth 2005;17(8):586–91.

12. Tanaka T, Nabatame H, Tanifuji Y. Insulin secretion and glucose utilization are impaired under general anesthesia with sevoflurane as well as isoflurane in a concentration-independent manner. J Anesth 2005;19(4):277–81.

13. Gregoire S, Kennedy A, Smiley RK. Acute hepatitis in a patient with mild factor IX deficiency after anesthesia with isoflurane. CMAJ 1986;135(6):645–6.

14. Scheider DM, Klygis LM, Tsang TK, Caughron MC. Hepatic dysfunction after repeated isoflurane administration. J Clin Gastroenterol 1993;17(2):168–70.

15. Carrigan TW, Straughen WJ. A report of hepatic necrosis and death following isoflurane anesthesia. Anesthesiology 1987;67(4):581–3.

16. Kharasch ED, Hankins DC, Cox K. Clinical isoflurane metabolism by cytochrome P450 2E1. Anesthesiology 1999;90(3):766–71.

17. Njoku DB, Shrestha S, Soloway R, Duray PR, Tsokos M, Abu-Asab MS, Pohl LR, West AB. Subcellular localization of trifluoroacetylated liver proteins in association with hepatitis following isoflurane. Anesthesiology 2002; 96(3):757–61.

18. Sinha A, Clatch RJ, Stuck G, Blumenthal SA, Patel SA. Isoflurane hepatotoxicity: a case report and review of the literature. Am J Gastroenterol 1996;91(11):2406–9.

19. Hasan F. Isoflurane hepatotoxicity in a patient with a previous history of halothane-induced hepatitis. Hepatogastroenterology 1998;45(20):518–22.

20. Turner GB, O'Rourke D, Scott GO, Beringer TR. Fatal hepatotoxicity after re-exposure to isoflurane: a case report and review of the literature. Eur J Gastroenterol Hepatol 2000;12(8):955–9.

21. Truog RD, Rice SA. Inorganic fluoride and prolonged isoflurane anesthesia in the intensive care unit. Anesth Analg 1989;69(6):843–5.

22. Fujino Y, Nishimura M, Nishimura S, Taenaka N, Yoshiya I. Prolonged administration of isoflurane to patients with severe renal dysfunction. Anesth Analg 1998;86(2):440–1.

23. Slegers-Karsmakers S, Stricker BH. Anaphylactic reaction to isoflurane. Anaesthesia 1988;43(6):506–7.

24. Boheler J, Hamrick JC Jr, McKnight RL, Eger EI 2nd. Isoflurane and malignant hyperthermia. Anesth Analg 1982;61(8):712–3.

25. Horn EP, Standl T, Sessler DI, von Knobelsdorff G, Buchs C, Schulte am Esch J. Physostigmine prevents postanesthetic shivering as does meperidine or clonidine. Anesthesiology 1998;88(1):108–13.

26. Johansen JW, Schneider G, Windsor AM, Sebel PS. Esmolol potentiates reduction of minimum alveolar isoflurane concentration by alfentanil. Anesth Analg 1998;87(3):671–6.

27. Beemer GH, Dawson PJ, Bjorksten AR, Edwards NE. Early postoperative seizures in neurosurgical patients administered atracurium and isoflurane. Anaesth Intensive Care 1989;17(4):504–9.

28. Goyagi T, Tanaka M, Nishikawa T. Oral clonidine premedication reduces the awakening concentration of isoflurane. Anesth Analg 1998;86(2):410–3.

29. Ghoneim MM, Block RI, Dhanaraj VJ. Interaction of a subanaesthetic concentration of isoflurane with midazolam: effects on responsiveness, learning and memory. Br J Anaesth 1998;80(5):581–7.

30. Shanks CA, Fragen RJ, Ling D. Continuous intravenous infusion of rocuronium (ORG 9426) in patients receiving balanced, enflurane, or isoflurane anesthesia. Anesthesiology 1993;78(4):649–51.

31. Olkkola KT, Tammisto T. Quantifying the interaction of rocuronium (Org 9426) with etomidate, fentanyl, midazolam, propofol, thiopental, and isoflurane using closed-loop feedback control of rocuronium infusion. Anesth Analg 1994;78(4):691–6.

32. Randell T, Yli-Hankala A, Lindgren L. Isoflurane inhibits muscle fasciculations caused by succinylcholine in children. Acta Anaesthesiol Scand 1993;37(3):262–4.

Methoxyflurane

General Information

Methoxyflurane is a volatile halogenated anesthetic.

Organs and Systems

Liver

Hepatitis has been reported (1), with possible cross-allergy between halothane and methoxyflurane.

Urinary tract

The nephrotoxicity of methoxyflurane is well established (2).

References

1. Ansuategui Sanchez M, Gonzalez Miranda F, Rodriguez-Hernandez JL. Icteria y metoxiflurano. [Jaundice and methoxyflurane.] Rev Esp Anestesiol Reanim 1980;27(6):481–6.

2. Desmond JW. Methoxyflurane nephrotoxicity. Can Anaesth Soc J 1974;21(3):294–307.

Sevoflurane

General Information

Sevoflurane is an isoflurane-related anesthetic, which is pleasant to breathe and has a rapid onset and offset of action. It can be used for both the induction and maintenance of anesthesia.

It has become popular in day surgery, despite little evidence of clear advantages over current alternatives.

Inhalational induction of anesthesia is common in children, and sevoflurane is challenging the tradition of halothane induction in children. Deep anesthesia with sevoflurane can be obtained rapidly, and recovery is also faster than with halothane.

Compound A

Compound A is a haloalkene degradation product of sevoflurane metabolism by carbon dioxide absorbers, and it has been suggested that prolonged low-flow closed-circuit anesthesia with sevoflurane may maximize exposure to the degradation product. Compound A can cause convulsions and neural damage in rats (1). It also causes nephrotoxicity and hepatotoxicity in rats, particularly if barium hydroxide lime is used (2).

Observational studies

In 640 infants aged 1 day to 12 months, who were given sevoflurane in high concentrations for sedation during MRI examination, the only adverse events were one case of vomiting, eight of minor hypoxia, and two of severe hypoxia (3).

Organs and Systems

Cardiovascular

In 28 subjects given either sevoflurane + nitrous oxide or enflurane + nitrous oxide anesthesia, sevoflurane caused fewer cardiodepressant effects than enflurane (4). Nevertheless, in 10 healthy subjects atrial contraction and left ventricular diastolic function, including active relaxation, passive compliance, and elastic recoil were impaired by sevoflurane (1 MAC) (5).

Sevoflurane has a similar effect on regional blood flow to other halogenated anesthetics, although it is perhaps slightly less of a coronary artery vasodilator than isoflurane. It reduces myocardial contractility and does not potentiate adrenaline-induced cardiac dysrhythmias (6). It also reduces baroreflex function, and in that respect is similar to other halogenated anesthetics. Coronary artery disease is not a risk factor for the use of these agents (7).

In contrast to isoflurane and desflurane, sevoflurane tends not to increase the heart rate, and is usually well tolerated for induction of anesthesia in young children. However, profound bradycardia was reported in four unpremedicated children aged 6 months to 2 years during anesthesia induction with sevoflurane 8% and nitrous oxide 66% (8). The episodes were not associated with loss of airway or ventilation. In three of the children there was spontaneous recovery of heart rate when the sevoflurane concentration was reduced; the other child received atropine because of evidence of significantly reduced cardiac output. In a previous study of sevoflurane induction of anesthesia in children with atropine premedication there was also a low incidence of this complication (9), which is probably due to excessive sevoflurane concentrations.

Sudden death in infants is associated with prolongation of the QT_c interval to 440ms or longer, and sevoflurane prolongs the QT_c in adults. In a prospective randomized trial the QT_c interval was measured in pre-, peri-, and post-operative electrocardiograms in 36 infants aged 1-6 months scheduled for inguinal or umbilical hernia repair (10). Anesthesia was by either sevoflurane or halothane. There was prolongation of the QT_c interval during sevoflurane anesthesia (mean 473 ms) and 60 minutes after emerging from anesthesia (433 ms) compared with infants who received halothane. The JT_c interval was analogously

affected. The authors suggested that despite sevoflurane's shorter half-life, electrocardiographic monitoring until the QT_c interval has returned to preanesthetic values may increase safety after sevoflurane anesthesia.

The effects of sevoflurane on cardiac conduction have been studied in 60 healthy unpremedicated infants (11). They received sevoflurane either as a continuous concentration of 8% from a primed circuit or in incrementally increasing doses. Nodal rhythm occurred in 12 cases. The mean duration of the nodal rhythm was 62 seconds in the incremental group and 90 seconds in the 8% group. All of the dysrhythmias were self-limiting and there were no ventricular or supraventricular dysrhythmias. No adverse events occurred as a result of the dysrhythmias. This study highlights the importance of using electrocardiographic monitoring when inducing anesthesia with volatile agents.

- Complete atrioventricular block occurred in a 10-year-old child with a history of hypertension, severe renal dysfunction, incomplete right bundle branch block, and a ventricular septal defect that had been repaired at birth (12). After slow induction with sevoflurane and nitrous oxide 66%, complete atrioventricular block occurred when the inspired sevoflurane concentration was 3% and reverted to sinus rhythm after withdrawal of the sevoflurane. The dysrhythmia recurred at the end of the procedure, possibly caused by lidocaine, which had infiltrated into the abdominal wound, and again at 24 hours in association with congestive cardiac failure following absorption of peritoneal dialysis fluid.

Congenital or acquired forms of the long QT syndrome can result in polymorphous ventricular tachycardia (torsade de pointes). Many drugs, including inhalational anesthetics, alter the QT interval, and sevoflurane prolongs the rate-corrected QT interval (QT_c). In a randomized study of whether sevoflurane-associated QT_c prolongation was rapidly reversed when propofol was used instead, 32 patients were randomly allocated to one of two groups (13). All received sevoflurane induction and maintenance for the first 15 minutes. In one group, sevoflurane was then withdrawn, and anesthesia was maintained with propofol for another 15 minutes; the other group continued to receive sevoflurane for 30 minutes. Sevoflurane-associated QT_c prolongation was fully reversed within 15 minutes when propofol was substituted.

The effects of sevoflurane on QT dispersion have been compared with those of halothane in 50 children aged 5-15 years in a blind randomized study (14). Neither sevoflurane nor halothane caused a significant increase in QT dispersion compared with baseline.

The effects of propofol and sevoflurane on the corrected QT (QT_c) and transmural dispersion of repolarization have been investigated in 50 unpremedicated children aged 1–16 years (15). Sevoflurane significantly prolonged the preoperative QT_c; propofol did not. Neither anesthetic had any significant effect on the preoperative transmural dispersion of repolarization.

Life-threatening dysrhythmias during anesthesia have been reported in patients with increased QT dispersion

(QT_d), the difference between the longest and shortest QT intervals in any of the 12 leads of the electrocardiogram. Sevoflurane prolongs the QT_c and QT_d. In a prospective randomized study of the QT interval, the QT_c, the QT_d, and the QT_{cd} in preoperative, perioperative, and postoperative electrocardiograms in 90 adults undergoing non-cardiac surgery under general anesthesia, sevoflurane, desflurane, and isoflurane all prolonged QT_c, QT_d, and QT_{cd}, but there were no significant intergroup differences (16).

The effects of single-breath vital capacity rapid inhalation with sevoflurane 5% on QT_c has been assessed in comparison with propofol in 44 adults undergoing laparoscopic surgery in a blind, randomized study (17). Sevoflurane significantly prolonged the QT_c and seven patients developed ventricular dysrhythmias.

A case of torsade de pointes has been attributed to sevoflurane anesthesia (18).

- A 65-year-old woman, who had had normal preoperative serum electrolytes and a normal QT interval with sinus rhythm, received hydroxyzine and atropine premedication followed by thiopental and vecuronium for anesthetic induction. Endotracheal intubation was difficult and precipitated atrial fibrillation, which was refractory to disopyramide 100 mg. Anesthesia was then maintained with sevoflurane 2% and nitrous oxide 50%. Ten minutes later ventricular tachycardia ensued, refractory to intravenous lidocaine, disopyramide, and magnesium. DC cardioversion resulted in a change to a supraventricular tachycardia, which then deteriorated to torsade de pointes. External cardiac massage and further DC cardioversion were initially unsuccessful, but the cardiac rhythm reverted to atrial fibrillation 10 minutes after the sevoflurane was switched off. Two weeks later she had her operation under combined epidural and general anesthesia, with no changes in cardiac rhythm.

In this case the role of excessive sympathetic drive as a result of the difficult intubation and the lack of opioid use during induction must be considered, even if sevoflurane played a role in precipitating the dysrhythmia.

Severe bradycardia has been described after sevoflurane induction for adeno-tonsillectomy in three children aged 42, 26, and 5 months with trisomy 21 (19). Two had normal electrocardiography and echocardiography. The third had had a complete AV canal repaired early in life, and had first degree heart block but normal echocardiography. Severe bradycardia (40-44/minute from a baseline of 110-130) and hypotension occurred on induction of anesthesia. Two children responded to atropine and glycopyrrolate, but the third required adrenaline for resuscitation. The authors suggested that children with trisomy 21 should be premedicated with an anticholinergic agent either orally or intramuscularly.

Respiratory

In a randomized study of the respiratory effects of high concentrations of halothane and sevoflurane in 21 healthy boys undergoing inguinal or penile surgery, there was similar respiratory depression with each agent (20). Minute ventilation fell by about 50% as a result of a reduction in tidal volume, despite an increase in respiratory rate.

The incidence and duration of apnea during sevoflurane anesthesia has been studied in 131 women who were given increasing concentrations of sevoflurane from 1% to 8% (n = 42), decremental–incremental concentrations from 8% to 4% and then from 4% to 8% (n = 36), or fixed concentrations of 8% (n = 53) (21). Although apnea occurred in all groups, it was more frequent and more pronounced in the fixed-dose group.

Nervous system

Despite a fall in mean arterial pressure, with a consequent reduction in cerebral perfusion pressure, sevoflurane should be a suitable agent for neuroanesthesia (22). Even in patients with ischemic cerebrovascular diseases, both the CO_2 response and cerebral autoregulation were well maintained during sevoflurane anesthesia (0.88 MAC) (23).

A case of acute dystonia has been reported during induction of anesthesia with sevoflurane (24).

- A 19-year-old man with schizophrenia, who was taking cyamemazine (a phenothiazine) 75 mg/day, and dihydroergotamine 180 mg/day to avoid neuroleptic drug-induced hypotension, had no history of involuntary movements, and neurological examination was normal preoperatively. Anesthesia was induced with midazolam 5 mg oral premedication and an inhalational induction using 4–5 maximum breaths of sevoflurane 8% and nitrous oxide 50% in oxygen. One minute after loss of consciousness, he developed a torticollic posture and stiffness, rapidly extending to the left trapezius and scalene muscles. There was severe rotation of the head accompanied by trismus and opisthotonos. An intravenous injection of the muscle relaxant atracurium 30 mg resolved the muscle spasms. Subsequent anesthesia was uneventful.

Dystonia after inhalational anesthesia is rare and is presumably due to an alteration in the dynamic relation between dopaminergic and other receptors in the brain.

Seizwes

Sevoflurane can cause epileptiform activity on the electroencephalogram, especially during emergence from anesthesia. It has also been associated with epileptiform discharges in volunteer studies, but clinical convulsions appear to very be rare. Two cases of epileptiform activity during sevoflurane anesthesia have been reported in healthy volunteers (25). They were taking part in a study of the effects of sevoflurane on regional cerebral blood flow and received twice the minimum alveolar concentration (MAC) of sevoflurane (4.4%). The only other drug administered was rocuronium, a muscle relaxant. Sevoflurane was used at up to twice its MAC, to induce burst suppression of the electroencephalogram. One of the subjects had partial motor seizure activity in the form of slight clonic movements in the right and then later in the left leg. There was an associated increase in heart rate (from 65 to 79 beats/minute) and systolic blood pressure (from 85 to 106 mmHg) and rhythmic epileptiform discharges on the electroencephalogram. The second subject had epileptiform activity on his electroencephalogram, consisting of partial and secondarily generalized discharges lasting for 2 and 3 minutes respectively. There were no clinical signs of an epileptic seizure. Burst suppression appeared on the electroencephalogram in both subjects before the seizure activity, and the Bispectral Index increased dramatically during the epileptiform discharge to maximum values of 44 and 73 respectively. As expected, regional cerebral blood flow and regional metabolism of the epileptic focus fell interictally and increased ictally. Although the concentrations of sevoflurane used in this study were high compared with usual anesthetic practice, further human studies are warranted, because prolonged epileptiform discharge is known to be harmful.

In another case, epileptiform activity was reported during sevoflurane anesthesia, but not with propofol in the same individual (26).

- A 62-year-old woman with no personal or family history of seizures had general relaxant anesthesia for plastic surgery using a total intravenous anesthetic technique with propofol, remifentanil, and cisatracurium, after benzodiazepine premedication. Routine electroencephalographic monitoring showed continuous slowing followed by burst suppression (consistent with very deep anesthesia), but no epileptiform activity. At a second procedure, and following identical benzodiazepine premedication and induction with propofol, anesthesia was maintained with sevoflurane (plus remifentanil for analgesia and cisatracurium for neuromuscular blockade). During the procedure, sevoflurane was increased from 2% to 8%. After 5 minutes, at an end-tidal concentration of 5.9%, there was epileptiform activity on the electroencephalogram. There were no hemodynamic changes.

Epileptiform activity on the electroencephalogram in association with sevoflurane induction has also been reported in a prospective study of 20 non-premedicated healthy children in whom electroencephalographic monitoring was started before sevoflurane induction (27). At 2 MAC there was epileptiform activity in two boys, with spontaneously resolving myoclonic movements.

Epileptiform activity on the electroencephalogram in association with sevoflurane has also been reported in two children aged 3 and 5 years in a center in which electroencephalographic monitoring is routine (28). In both cases the activity occurred after several minutes of anesthesia, when the sevoflurane concentrations were increased to 7–8%. The epileptiform activity resolved after a reduction in sevoflurane concentrations. No seizure activity was noted.

In a prospective, observational study in 30 children undergoing adenoidectomy anesthesia was induced with midazolam and thiopental (both potent anticonvulsants) and maintained with sevoflurane; no electroencephalographic epileptiform activity was observed (29).

Two types of tonic–clonic movement disorders during sevoflurane anesthesia have been described (30):

- agitation during early induction shortly after the loss of the eyelash reflex, characterized by discoordinate movements of the arms and legs, often followed by hypertonia and respiratory obstruction, both of which resolve with deepening of anesthesia;
- localized or generalized tonic–clonic movements during deep anesthesia at the end of induction and persisting at that level of anesthesia.

During sevoflurane anesthesia electroencephalography shows a brief increase in beta activity, which occurs at around the time when the eyelash reflex is lost (30–60 seconds after beginning induction); this is rapidly followed by sudden slowing to <2 Hz delta activity maximal at the end of the second minute of induction, and then acceleration to delta predominance (2–4 Hz) until the pupils are constricted and central. The bispectral index monitor also shows a higher index number at concentric pupils than during the middle of induction, when slowing down is maximal. Some subjects have episodes of burst suppression with deeper anesthesia (higher end-tidal sevoflurane and longer duration of anesthesia). Epileptiform activity also occurs. Spikes occur first, usually during delta oscillations (spike-wave). They may be simple or complex or periodic, leading to periods of epileptiform discharges or frank seizures. Generally, major discharges or frank seizure activity occur during deep anesthesia and are occasionally accompanied by tonic–clonic movements. Susceptibility factors include pre-existing epilepsy, febrile convulsions, and intracranial pathology.

The authors of this review made the following recommendations:

- benzodiazepine premedication, such as midazolam in children, might be useful;
- nitrous oxide might have a minimal protective effect;
- narcotic analgesics might be useful, but their protective qualities have not yet been documented.
- A 3-year-old child had tonic convulsions after inhaling 3.9% sevoflurane for 45 minutes associated with moderate hyperventilation; he was later discovered to have epileptiform activity on electroencephalography (31).
- A 5-day-old girl was underwent excision of an axillary lymphangioma (32). Induction of anesthesia was with sevoflurane and nitrous oxide, and maintenance with sevoflurane. No other sedative or analgesic drugs were given. Surgery took 4.5 hours, and there was rhythmic myoclonic movement of all four limbs immediately after tracheal extubation and twice more in the intensive care unit. Each episode lasted about 5 minutes and was terminated with diazepam and phenytoin. Further investigations showed no underlying cause.
- Generalized tonic–clonic seizure-like movements lasting 40 seconds occurred in a healthy 32-year-old man after emergence from sevoflurane-based anesthesia (33).
- A 19-year-old man with a history of metamfetamine abuse 3 weeks earlier, but no personal or family history of seizure activity had anesthesia induced with

midazolam 1 mg, nitrous oxide 50%, and sevoflurane 8% (34). The sevoflurane was subsequently reduced to 2%. After radical orchidectomy the sevoflurane and nitrous oxide were withdrawn and oxygen 100% was given and 2 minutes later rhythmic jerking movements began in the legs and quickly spread to the rest of the body. The movements were accompanied by an arched back and a stiff neck. Arterial oxygen saturation dropped to 50% and ventilation was controlled, again using sevoflurane 8%. The duration of the seizure was about 4 minutes. The sevoflurane was again withdrawn 3 minutes later, and a similar seizure occurred. This time it was controlled with midazolam 1 mg and propofol 30 mg. Recovery was marked only by mild disorientation. Postoperative computerized tomography showed a ganglioneuroma in the posterior cortex. The electroencephalogram was normal.

These reports show that clinicians need to be aware of the possibility of generalized seizures, especially in patients who are predisposed to seizures.

Postanesthetic agitation

The use of sevoflurane in children is complicated by a high incidence of postanesthetic agitation, probably due to residual sevoflurane during washout.

Rapid emergence and postoperative pain have been proposed as possible mechanisms. This has been assessed in a randomized, prospective study in 80 infants and children undergoing inguinal hernia repair, all of whom received sevoflurane or halothane as the sole anesthetic for induction and maintenance (35). All received preoperative oral midazolam. For analgesia a caudal epidural block was performed with a mixture of 0.25% bupivacaine and 1% lidocaine before surgery. The time to recovery was similar in the two groups, but emergence agitation was significantly more common with sevoflurane group than with halothane (27% versus 5%) 5 minutes after arrival in the Post Anesthetic Care Unit.

In another study postanesthetic agitation was not related to the speed of emergence (36).

Rapid emergence has also been assessed in a randomized, prospective study in 53 infants and children, all of whom received sevoflurane as the sole anesthetic for induction and then either sevoflurane or propofol for maintenance (37). A caudal epidural block was performed before surgery for analgesia with 0.25% bupivacaine or intravenous fentanyl 2 micrograms/kg was used. The times to extubation and recovery were similar between the two groups, but emergence agitation was significantly more common with sevoflurane than with propofol (23% versus 3.7%). There was no relation between analgesic technique and agitation.

The effect of clonidine 2 micrograms/kg on the risk of sevoflurane-induced postanesthetic agitation has been quantified in 169 children (38). Clonidine significantly reduced pain and discomfort scores, reduced the incidence of agitation by 57%, and reduced the incidence of severe agitation by 67%. The relative risks of agitation and severe agitation were 0.43 (95% CI = 0.24, 0.78) and 0.32 (0.09, 1.17) respectively.

In a randomized prospective study of the effect of a single dose of dexmedetomidine on emergence agitation in 90 children undergoing superficial lower abdominal and genital surgery no premedication was used (39). After induction of anesthesia with 8% sevoflurane in 50% nitrous oxide and oxygen, the patients received either saline (group 1), dexmedetomidine 0.15 micrograms/kg (group 2), or dexmedetomidine 0.3 micrograms/kg (group 3). All received a caudal epidural block with 0.25% bupivacaine. The time to eye opening was similar in all the groups. The incidences of agitation (95% CI) were 37% (20–54%) in group 1, 17% (4–30%) in group 2, and 10% (0–21%) in group 3. Paired comparisons between groups showed a significant difference between groups 1 and 3.

Nitrous oxide has been used to mitigate postanesthetic agitation in 20 children, by continued administration after the end of sevoflurane anesthesia (40). The end-tidal concentrations of sevoflurane at awakening were significantly lower in those who had been given nitrous oxide than in the control group and postanesthetic agitation was significantly less.

Peripheral neuropathy

Peripheral neuropathy has been reported in two healthy men anesthetized with 1.25 MAC sevoflurane at 2 l/minute fresh gas flow for 8 hours. Their average concentrations of compound A were 45 and 28 ppm. Both had had previous minor injuries in the regions in which the neuropathies were reported. The authors suggested that compound A, or other factors associated with sevoflurane anesthesia, may predispose patients to peripheral neuropathy. Both men were volunteers for earlier published studies comparing the nephrotoxic properties of sevoflurane and desflurane, sponsored by Baxter PPD, New Jersey, the manufacturer of desflurane, a rival inhalational anesthetic agent; these reports need to be regarded with caution.

Neuromuscular function

Prolongation of rapacuronium-induced neuromuscular blockade by sevoflurane has been studied in a randomized, placebo-controlled comparison with suxamethonium in 40 children (41). Patients received sevoflurane and nitrous oxide anesthesia followed by rapacuronium 2 mg/kg. The study was stopped after only seven patients had been recruited, because the mean time to return of twitch height to 25% of baseline was 26 minutes. This time represents a stage at which neuromuscular blockade can be reversed and in this case it was twice as long as predicted from experience in adult patients. The authors suggested that the prolonged neuromuscular relaxation was due to the interaction of sevoflurane with rapacuronium, because such prolongation has not been observed using other inhalation agents.

Sensory systems

Visual pathway abnormalities have been described in a prospective study of 10 patients undergoing sevoflurane anesthesia (42). Postoperative electroretinographic abnormalities and associated reductions in contrast sensitivity were consistently present in patients who underwent sevoflurane anesthesia and these persisted beyond the time standard clinical discharge criteria were met. As ambulatory surgery now comprises more than 60–70% of all surgery, this finding is important.

Psychological, psychiatric

Delirium during emergence from sevoflurane anesthesia has often been documented. Four patients, an adult and three children aged 3–8 years, who were able to recount the experience, have been reported (43). They had full recall of postoperative events, were terrified, agitated, and distressed, and hence presented with acute organic mental state dysfunction which was short-lived. Two were disoriented and had paranoid ideation. They were not in any pain or were not distressed by pain if it was present. The authors hypothesized that misperception of environmental stimuli associated with sevoflurane's particular mode of action may have been the underlying cause of this phenomenon. Anxiolytic premedication and effective analgesia did not necessarily prevent the problem.

The effect of intravenous clonidine 2 micrograms/kg on the incidence and severity of postoperative agitation has been assessed in a double-blind, randomized, placebo-controlled trial in 40 boys who had anesthetic induction with sevoflurane after oral midazolam premedication (44). There was agitation in 16 of those who received placebo and two of those who received clonidine; the agitation was severe in six of those given placebo and none of those given clonidine.

The effects of intravenous and caudal epidural clonidine on the incidence and severity of postoperative agitation have been assessed in a randomized, double-blind study in 80 children, all of whom received sevoflurane as the sole general anesthetic for induction and maintenance (45). A caudal epidural block was performed before surgery for analgesia with 0.175% bupivacaine 1 ml/kg. The children were assigned randomly to four groups: (I) clonidine 1 microgram/kg added to the caudal bupivacaine; (II) clonidine 3 micrograms/kg added to the caudal bupivacaine; (III) clonidine 3 micrograms/kg intravenously; and (IV) no clonidine. The incidences of agitation were 22, 0, 5, and 39% in the four groups respectively. Thus, clonidine 3 micrograms/kg effectively prevented agitation after sevoflurane anesthesia independent of the route of administration.

The effect of a single preoperative dose of the opioid oxycodone on emergence behavior has been studied in a randomized trial in 130 children (46). Oxycodone prophylaxis had no effect on post-sevoflurane delirium.

The effect of a single bolus dose of midazolam before the end of sevoflurane anesthesia has been investigated in a double-blind, randomized, placebo-controlled trial in 40 children aged 2–7 years (47). Midazolam significantly reduced the incidence of delirium after anesthesia. However, when it was used for severe agitation midazolam only reduced the severity without abolishing agitation. The authors concluded that midazolam attenuates, but does not abolish, agitation after sevoflurane anesthesia.

Gastrointestinal

About 2 million day-case anesthetics are given annually in England, and anesthetic practice varies widely, because of a large and contradictory evidence base for the optimal anesthetic in day surgery. In a randomized controlled trial in 1063 adults and 322 children sevoflurane, when used for induction and maintenance, was more costly and associated with higher rates of postoperative nausea and vomiting than anesthetic regimens using propofol for induction of anesthesia (48).

Liver

Sevoflurane can be used to induce hypotension during neurosurgery. Hypotensive anesthesia has little effect on postoperative liver function (49).

• A 3-day-old boy underwent inguinal herniorrhaphy under sevoflurane anesthesia, and 2 days later developed vomiting, anorexia, and fever (50). His aspartate transaminase, alanine transaminase, and lactate dehydrogenase activities were increased and peaked 12–16 days after the operation. Viral markers were negative, as was a lymphocyte stimulation test with sevoflurane. Toxic (not allergic) liver damage due to exposure to sevoflurane was considered to be the most probable diagnosis.

In a randomized study of the renal and hepatic effects of prolonged low-flow anesthesia with sevoflurane or isoflurane in patients undergoing prolonged operations (over 8 hours), using a technique that maximized compound A production, there were no differences in markers of hepatocellular injury at 24 or 72 hours (51).

The effect of minimal-flow (as opposed to low-flow) anesthesia with sevoflurane and isoflurane has been examined in a randomized trial in 76 patients (52). There were no significant differences between the groups in blood chemistry markers of hepatic function, despite high exposure to Compound A in the patients who received sevoflurane.

Plasma activity of alpha-glutathione S-transferase activity (αGT) is a more sensitive and specific marker of hepatocellular injury than transaminase activity and it correlates better with hepatic histology. Anesthesia with halothane leads to transiently raised αGT activity, but propofol and isoflurane do not. In a randomized study of plasma αGT activity during and after low-flow anesthesia with sevoflurane or isoflurane, there were no significant differences in αGT activities between the two groups during or after anesthesia (53).

Thus, the evidence suggests that sevoflurane is as safe as isoflurane in low-flow anesthesia with respect to liver dysfunction.

Hepatitis after sevoflurane exposure has been described in an infant with primary hyperoxaluria type 1 undergoing urological surgery (54).

- An 11-month-old infant developed hepatomegaly 2 days postoperatively associated with marked increases in serum transaminases (alanine transaminase 543 IU/l, aspartate transaminase 683 IU/l). No data on synthetic function were given. Viral serology was negative. The transaminases resolved after 11 days, and the child went on to have another urological procedure after a further 4 days, avoiding volatile agents completely. There was no subsequent liver dysfunction.

Severe hepatotoxicity occurred after anesthesia with sevoflurane in a child with pre-existing mild renal dysfunction (55).

Urinary tract

The effects of sevoflurane, isoflurane, and desflurane on macroscopic renal structure have been studied in 24 patients undergoing nephrectomy (56). All anesthetics were administered using a fresh gas flow of 1 l/minute and a sodium hydroxide absorber and had an average duration of 3 hours. No injury to nephrons was observed by pathologists blinded to which anesthetic agent had been used. Postoperative creatinine concentrations and urine volumes did not differ significantly between the groups.

- Transient renal tubular dysfunction has been reported in a patient with asthma requiring mechanical ventilation who received sevoflurane for 9 days (57). Soda lime was not used, and the cumulative dose was 298 MAC-hours. Serum and urinary inorganic fluoride concentrations reached maximum concentrations of 71 and 2047 µmol/l respectively. Markers of renal tubular injury were also greatly raised (urinary N-acetyl-beta-D-glucosaminidase and beta$_2$-microglobulin). However, urine volume, creatinine clearance, and serum creatinine and urea concentrations were unaffected.

There has been a meta-analysis of 22 controlled trials in 3436 patients (82% ASA I or II, 16% ASA III, and 2% ASA IV) (58). The trials had compared sevoflurane for anesthesia maintenance with isoflurane, propofol, or enflurane. Serum creatinine and blood urea nitrogen were used to assess preoperative and postoperative renal function. The duration of anesthesia was 0.5–11 hours. Most patients (97%) were exposed to less than 4 MAC-hours of volatile agent. Falls in the serum creatinine and blood urea nitrogen were significantly smaller with isoflurane than with sevoflurane. In patients who received concurrent aminoglycosides, sevoflurane was associated with a small increase in serum creatinine. The following factors had no effect on renal function: the type of anesthetic circuit, the choice of carbon dioxide absorber, the inorganic fluoride ion concentration, the duration of anesthesia, the use of nitrous oxide, or how sick patients were. When all patients were considered, the incidences of clinically significant increases in serum creatinine were the same between agents. In patients with baseline creatinine values greater than 132 µmol/l (1.5 mg/dl), the incidence of clinically important increases in serum creatinine was significantly higher in both treatment groups compared with baseline. This meta-analysis has provided strong evidence that sevoflurane does not contribute to clinically significant renal insufficiency.

Renal impairment often follows cardiac surgery, but in a randomized trial in elective coronary artery surgery in 354 patients, sevoflurane did not produce greater increases in serum creatinine concentrations than isoflurane or propofol (59).

The role of compound A
Sevoflurane is metabolized to compound A by carbon dioxide absorbers. It is nephrotoxic in rats, but nephrotoxicity in humans has not been proven. The accumulation of compound A is greatest with low fresh gas flows and barium hydroxide absorbers, both of which cause higher temperatures in the absorber. Current anesthetic practice is to use sodium hydroxide for carbon dioxide absorption, because it produces less compound A than barium hydroxide.

There has been controversy over whether compound A causes significant renal damage in humans. The potential for renal damage using sevoflurane was investigated in 42 patients without renal disease scheduled for surgery lasting more than 4 hours (60). The patients were given low-flow sevoflurane or isoflurane (fresh gas flow 1 l/minute/m^2) or high-flow sevoflurane (6 l/minute/m^2). None of these increased blood urea nitrogen concentrations, creatinine concentrations, or creatinine clearance. There were no significant differences in beta$_2$-microglobulin, a marker of tubular function, or urinary glucose concentrations. However, there was an increase in the 24-hour urinary excretion of N-acetyl-beta-glucosaminidase, a marker of proximal tubular necrosis, with both doses of sevoflurane but not with isoflurane. There were no significant differences in the serum and urinary fluoride concentrations between the two sevoflurane groups, despite the higher concentration of compound A (29 versus 3.9 ppm) in the expired gases of those who received low-flow sevoflurane. The maximum 24-hour protein excretion was higher with low-flow sevoflurane compared with the other two groups.

The effect of the nephrotoxic aminoglycoside antibiotic amikacin on renal function during low-flow sevoflurane anesthesia has been studied in a randomized study in 37 men undergoing orthopedic surgery (61). Markers of renal tubular injury (urinary N-acetyl-beta-D-glucosaminidase and beta$_2$-microglobulin) were not abnormally raised, and urine volume, creatinine clearance, and serum creatinine and urea concentrations were unaffected. The duration of anesthesia and compound A concentrations were similar in the two groups.

In a randomized study of the renal and hepatic effects of prolonged low-flow anesthesia with sevoflurane or isoflurane in patients undergoing prolonged operations (over 8 hours), using a technique that maximized compound A production, there were no significant differences between the groups in serum creatinine or urea concentrations, creatinine clearance, or urinary protein or glucose excretion at 24 or 72 hours (51). Proteinuria and glycosuria were common in both groups. There was no correlation between exposure to compound A and any measure of renal function. There were no differences in markers of hepatocellular injury. There was no evidence of nephrotoxicity of sevoflurane even at high degrees of exposure to compound A for as long as 17 hours.

The effect on renal function of minimal-flow (as opposed to low-flow) anesthesia with sevoflurane and isoflurane has been examined in a randomized trial in 76 patients (52). There were no significant differences between the groups in blood chemistry markers of renal or hepatic function or in urinary markers of tubular injury, despite high exposure to compound A in the patients who received sevoflurane.

In a randomized prospective study of the effects of prolonged (>10 hour) low-flow sevoflurane, high-flow sevoflurane, and low-flow isoflurane anesthesia on renal function in 25 patients undergoing orthopedic surgery the AUC compound A was higher in the low-flow than the high-flow sevoflurane group (mean 360 ppm versus 61 ppm) (62). However, there were no differences between the groups in markers of renal function, renal tubular damage, or hepatic transaminases. Prolonged anesthesia with low flow sevoflurane appears to be safe.

These studies have confirmed earlier findings that although there is biochemical evidence of renal damage after sevoflurane anesthesia, there are no clinically significant effects.

The role of fluoride
Serum and urinary inorganic fluoride concentrations can rise after inhalation of sevoflurane, because of hepatic metabolism (63). The authors concluded that lengthy sevoflurane anesthesia could alter renal function, although there was no other evidence of nephrotoxicity. Although patients with normal renal function are probably not at risk during normal anesthesia with sevoflurane, those with pre-existing renal impairment may be at risk.

A randomized, open study in 26 patients with renal dysfunction who received either isoflurane or sevoflurane for operations lasting up to 6 hours showed no significant differences in postoperative creatinine clearances. However, there was a significant increase in the plasma fluoride ion concentration with sevoflurane (64). In 10 adults who were given repeat high-flow sevoflurane anesthesia there was no evidence of renal or hepatic injury and no increases in serum or urine fluoride concentrations that would indicate an increase in sevoflurane metabolism with repeated use (65).

Renal function has been assessed after low fresh gas flow anesthesia (1 l/minute or less) with either sevoflurane or isoflurane in a multicenter study of 254 patients (66). The mean duration of anesthesia was 3.0 MAC-hours in both groups. Peak serum fluoride concentrations were significantly higher (40 μmol/l) after sevoflurane compared with isoflurane (3 μmol/l), and 26 patients had peak fluoride concentrations over 50 μmol/l, a concentration that is associated with renal dysfunction after methoxyflurane anesthesia. There were no significant differences in the renal function of the two groups, as measured by serum creatinine, urea, glycosuria, proteinuria, urine pH, or specific gravity. Absence of renal dysfunction, despite high

serum fluoride concentrations after sevoflurane anesthesia, was consistent with previous reports. It appears that low fresh gas flow anesthesia with sevoflurane is not associated with clinically significant renal damage.

The role of aquaporins
Aquaporin-2 is a protein involved in regulation of water permeability in the kidneys. The effects of sevoflurane- and propofol-based anesthesia on urine concentrating ability and aquaporin-2 concentrations have been compared in 30 patients undergoing major surgical procedures given sevoflurane + nitrous oxide or propofol + nitrous oxide (67). Sevoflurane caused a transient 25% fall in aquaporin-2 concentrations 90 minutes after surgery, rather than the usual 40% increase, which occurred in the propofol group. By 3 hours after surgery the aquaporin concentrations in the sevoflurane group had increased and were similar to those in the propofol group. There was a 40% fall in urine osmolarity in the sevoflurane group, but recovery occurred by 3 hours postoperatively. This effect is the likely cause of the occasional cases of polyuria reported in association with sevoflurane anesthesia, rather than nephrotoxicity caused by fluoride ion or compound A.

Musculoskeletal

There have been reports of rhabdomyolysis after anesthesia with halothane, enflurane, and isoflurane in patients with muscular dystrophy, in whom suxamethonium was not used. Rhabdomyolysis has also been reported after sevoflurane anesthesia (68).

- An 11-year-old boy with Duchenne's muscular dystrophy underwent strabismus repair. He also had asthma, for which he was taking prednisone 25 mg/day and theophylline. He underwent inhalational induction with sevoflurane 4% and nitrous oxide 64%; tracheal intubation was then performed without the use of a muscle relaxant. Anesthesia was maintained using sevoflurane 1.5–3.0% and nitrous oxide 64%. He also received hydrocortisone 100 mg and diclofenac 25 mg. The operation lasted 51 minutes and anesthesia was uneventful. He suffered heel pain during the first few hours postoperatively, and 3 hours postoperatively passed 300 ml of dark red urine, containing large amounts of myoglobin. His serum enzymes increased from preoperative values, serum aspartate transaminase from 76 to 458 IU/l, alanine transaminase from 136 to 254 IU/l, and creatine kinase from 4430 to 55 700 IU/l. He was treated with dantrolene 1 mg/kg and recovered over the next day.

The history and finding in this case are strongly diagnostic of rhabdomyolysis. The most likely cause of rhabdomyolysis in this patient was thought to be inhalation of sevoflurane.

Rhabdomyolysis triggered by sevoflurane in a child with Duchenne muscular dystrophy has been reported in one case (69).

Body temperature

Malignant hyperthermia has occurred in people treated with sevoflurane.

- In the case of a 4-year-old girl, dantrolene was effective; susceptibility to malignant hyperthermia was later confirmed by muscle biopsy (70).
- A 28-year-old man, who developed malignant hyperthermia after anesthesia induced with isoflurane and maintained with sevoflurane, died 4 days later, despite cooling and intravenous dantrolene (71).

Other cases of malignant hyperthermia have been reported in patients who received sevoflurane (72,73). Although it is highly likely that sevoflurane caused malignant hyperpyrexia in these cases, suxamethonium was also given and was also a suspect.

Of two other cases (74,75), the second was remarkable, in that the specific-treatment dantrolene was not available, and yet the patient survived with aggressive active cooling and general supportive measures, including sodium bicarbonate.

In more than 3000 cases in Japan, there were two cases of malignant hyperthermia, one fatal (50). In this case isoflurane had been used early in anesthesia, and could have been at least in part responsible. There was some reason to consider that the patient, a 12-year-old girl, had a family propensity to malignant hyperthermia, as indicated by higher resting Pi/Pcr values. However, sevoflurane itself can trigger malignant hyperthermia in swine (76).

Long-term effects

Genogenicity

Sevoflurane can cause toxicity (for example nephrotoxicity) from either inorganic fluoride ions or the haloalkene degradation product Compound A. Fluoride ions are produced by metabolism of sevoflurane and can reach high concentrations after prolonged anesthesia. Compound A is produced in carbon dioxide absorbers (soda lime and barium hydroxide lime in particular) and is nephrotoxic in rats but not in humans. Compound A induces sister chromatid exchanges in Chinese hamster ovary cells in vitro as a marker for possible genotoxicity. The formation of sister chromatid exchanges in mitogen-stimulated T lymphocytes of 40 children undergoing sevoflurane anesthesia for minor operations has been investigated (77) Anesthesia was induced and maintained with sevoflurane in oxygen and nitrous oxide at a fresh gas flow rate of 3l/minute in a circle system, using soda lime as the carbon dioxide absorbent. Blood samples were drawn immediately before induction and after the end of anesthesia. The average duration of anesthesia was 50 minutes. There was no difference in sister chromatid exchanges rate after sevoflurane anesthesia and so no evidence of a genotoxic effect.

Susceptibility Factors

Renal disease

It has been thought that patients with chronically impaired renal function might be at increased risk of nephrotoxicity due to sevoflurane, because of an increased fluoride load due to reduced excretion. However, this was not confirmed in 41 patients undergoing elective surgery, with a stable increased preoperative serum creatinine concentration, who were randomly allocated to receive sevoflurane ($n = 21$) or enflurane ($n = 20$) at a fresh gas inflow rate of 4 l/minute for maintenance of anesthesia (78). Peak serum inorganic fluoride concentrations were significantly higher after sevoflurane than after enflurane anesthesia. Laboratory measures of renal function remained stable throughout the postoperative period in both groups. No patient had permanent deterioration of pre-existing renal insufficiency and none required dialysis.

Other features of the patient

Insulinoma

- A 56-year-old woman with insulinoma, operated under sevoflurane anesthesia, had an uneventful perioperative course, and the authors suggested that sevoflurane suppressed the spontaneous release of insulin (79).

Sevoflurane may therefore be useful for anesthesia in patients with insulinoma.

Transplantation

- A 29-year-old man was anesthetized after renal transplantation with sevoflurane + nitrous oxide + oxygen for replacement of the head of the left femur (80). His serum fluoride concentration was always below 40 µmol/l and sevoflurane had little effect on the transplanted kidney.

It seems therefore that sevoflurane might be suitable for patients with renal transplants.

Drug–Drug Interactions

Aloeaceae

Massive intraoperative bleeding in a 35-year-old woman has been attributed to an interaction of preoperative *Aloe vera* tablets and sevoflurane, since both may inhibit platelet function (81).

Dexmedetomidine

In 45 adult patients undergoing elective surgery, the α_2-adrenoceptor agonist dexmedetomidine in a concentration of 0.7 ng/ml reduced the minimum alveolar concentration of sevoflurane required to suppress movement to skin incision by 17%, but a plasma concentration of 0.39 ng/ml had no effect (82). The larger reductions in isoflurane requirements found in earlier studies of dexmedetomidine were probably due to the use of potent opioids and intravenous induction as part of the anesthetic.

Fentanyl

The minimum alveolar concentrations of sevoflurane required to suppress movements and adrenergic responses to surgery in the presence of the potent opioid fentanyl have been quantified in 226 adults (83). Fentanyl 3 ng/ml and 6 ng/ml reduced sevoflurane requirements to suppress movement to pain by 61% and 74%, respectively, and requirements to suppress the adrenergic responses to pain by 83% and 91%, respectively. There was no further reduction in sevoflurane requirements at concentrations of fentanyl above 6 ng/ml. The degree of interaction was similar to that seen in previous studies of other volatile anesthetic + opioid combinations.

Ketorolac

Ketorolac, which can cause renal vasoconstriction by inhibiting cyclo-oxygenase, is often given to patients anesthetized with sevoflurane, which is also potentially nephrotoxic. The effect of ketorolac has been assessed in a placebo-controlled, randomized study in 30 women undergoing breast surgery with sevoflurane anesthesia (84). There were no differences in several markers of renal injury in those who did or did not receive ketorolac.

Mexiletine

- A 79-year-old woman was given mexiletine 125 mg intravenously over 10 minutes during anesthesia after having been given lidocaine 100 mg intravenously, and had a marked drop in blood pressure 1 hour later (85). The blood pressure rose when sevoflurane was withdrawn.

The authors proposed that the effect had been brought about by the combination of mexiletine and sevoflurane, although it is more likely that the effect was due to the combination of mexiletine with lidocaine.

Probenecid

The effect of the uricosuric agent probenecid in prolonged sevoflurane anesthesia has been examined in 64 patients randomized to receive high-flow or low-flow anesthesia with sevoflurane with or without preoperative oral probenecid (86). There were no differences in urea, creatinine, or creatinine clearance among the treatments. However, patients who received low-flow sevoflurane had some evidence of renal tubular injury (raised urinary markers) compared with those who received either high-flow anesthesia or probenecid.

References

1. Goldberg ME, Larijani GE, Eger EI 2nd. Peripheral neuropathy in healthy men volunteers anesthetized with 1.25 MAC sevoflurane for 8 hours Pharmacotherapy 1999;19(10):1173–6.
2. Kharasch ED. Compound A: Toxikologie und klinische Relevanz. [Compound A: toxicology and clinical relevance.] Anaesthesist 1998;47(Suppl 1):S7–S10.
3. De Sanctis Briggs V. Magnetic resonance imaging under sedation in newborns and infants: a study of 640 cases using sevoflurane. Paediatr Anaesth 2005;15(1):9–15.
4. Kikura M, Ikeda K. Comparison of effects of sevoflurane/nitrous oxide and enflurane/nitrous oxide on myocardial contractility in humans. Load-independent and noninvasive assessment with transesophageal echocardiography. Anesthesiology 1993;79(2):235–43.
5. Kitahata H, Tanaka K, Kimura H, Saito T. [Effects of sevoflurane on left ventricular diastolic function using transesophageal echocardiography.]Masui 1993;42(3):358–64.
6. Ebert TJ, Harkin CP, Muzi M. Cardiovascular responses to sevoflurane: a review. Anesth Analg 1995;81(Suppl 6): S11–22.
7. Malan TP Jr, DiNardo JA, Isner RJ, Frink EJ Jr, Goldberg M, Fenster PE, Brown EA, Depa R, Hammond LC, Mata H. Cardiovascular effects of sevoflurane compared with those of isoflurane in volunteers. Anesthesiology 1995;83(5):918–28.
8. Townsend P, Stokes MA. Bradycardia during rapid inhalation induction with sevoflurane in children. Br J Anaesth 1998;80(3):410.
9. Sigston PE, Jenkins AM, Jackson EA, Sury MR, Mackersie AM, Hatch DJ. Rapid inhalation induction in children: 8% sevoflurane compared with 5% halothane. Br J Anaesth 1997;78(4):362–5.
10. Loeckinger A, Kleinsasser A, Maier S, Furtner B, Keller C, Kuehbacher G, Lindner KH. Sustained prolongation of the QTc interval after anesthesia with sevoflurane in infants during the first 6 months of life. Anesthesiology 2003;98:639–42.
11. Green DH, Townsend P, Bagshaw O, Stokes MA. Nodal rhythm and bradycardia during inhalation induction with sevoflurane in infants: a comparison of incremental and high-concentration techniques. Br J Anaesth 2000;85(3):368–70.
12. Maruyama K, Agata H, Ono K, Hiroki K, Fujihara T. Slow induction with sevoflurane was associated with complete atrioventricular block in a child with hypertension, renal dysfunction, and impaired cardiac conduction. Paediatr Anaesth 1998;8(1):73–8.
13. Kleinsasser A, Loeckinger A, Lindner KH, Keller C, Boehler M, Puehringer F. Reversing sevoflurane-associated Q-Tc prolongation by changing to propofol. Anaesthesia 2001;56(3):248–50.
14. Gurkan Y, Canatay H, Agacdiken A, Ural E, Toker K. Effects of halothane and sevoflurane on QT dispersion in paediatric patients. Paediatr Anaesth 2003;13:223–7.
15. Whyte SD, Booker PD, Buckley DG. The effects of propofol and sevoflurane on the QT interval and transmural dispersion of repolarization in children. Anesth Analg 2005;100(1):71–7.
16. Yildrim H, Adanir T, Atay A, Kataricioglu K, Savaci S. The effects of sevoflurane, isoflurane and desflurane on QT interval of the ECG. Eur J Anaesthesiol 2004;21:566–70.
17. Sen S, Ozmert G, Boran N, Turan H, Caliskan E. Comparison of the effects of single-breath vital capacity rapid inhalation with sevoflurane 5% and propofol induction on QT interval and haemodynamics for laparoscopic surgery. Eur J Anaesthesiol 2004;21:543–6.
18. Abe K, Takada K, Yoshiya I. Intraoperative torsade de pointes ventricular tachycardia and ventricular fibrillation during sevoflurane anesthesia. Anesth Analg 1998;86(4):701–2.
19. Roodman S, Bothwell M, Tobias JD. Bradycardia with sevoflurane induction with patients with trisomy 21. Paediatr Anaesth 2003;13:538–40.
20. Walpole R, Olday J, Haetzman M, Drummond GB, Doyle E. A comparison of the respiratory effects of high concentrations of halothane and sevoflurane. Paediatr Anaesth 2001;11(2):157–60.
21. Pancaro C, Giovannoni S, Toscano A, Peduto VA. Apnea during induction of anesthesia with sevoflurane is related to its mode of administration. Can J Anaesth 2005;52(6):591–4.

22. Takahashi H, Murata K, Ikeda K. Sevoflurane does not increase intracranial pressure in hyperventilated dogs. Br J Anaesth 1993;71(4):551–5.

23. Kitaguchi K, Ohsumi H, Kuro M, Nakajima T, Hayashi Y. Effects of sevoflurane on cerebral circulation and metabolism in patients with ischemic cerebrovascular disease. Anesthesiology 1993;79(4):704–9.

24. Bernard JM, Le Roux D, Pereon Y. Acute dystonia during sevoflurane induction. Anesthesiology 1999;90(4):1215–6.

25. Kaisti KK, Jaaskelainen SK, Rinne JO, Metsahonkala L, Scheinin H. Epileptiform discharges during 2 MAC sevoflurane anesthesia in two healthy volunteers. Anesthesiology 1999;91(6):1952–5.

26. Schultz B, Schultz A, Grouven U, Korsch G. Epilepsietypische EEG-Aktivitat: Auftreten bei Sevofluran-anflutung und nicht unter Propofolapplikation. [Epileptoform EEG activity: occurrence under sevoflurane and not during propofol application.] Anaesthesist 2001;50(1):43–5.

27. Conreux F, Best O, Preckel MP, Lhopitault C, Beydon L, Pouplard F, Granry JC. Effects electroencephalrahiques du sevoflurane a l'induction chez le jeune enfant: etude prospective sur 20 cas. [Electroencephalographic effects of sevoflurane in pediatric anesthesia: a prospective study of 20 cases.] Ann Fr Anesth Reanim 2001;20(5):438–445.

28. Schultz A, Schultz B, Grouven U, Korsch G. Epileptiform activity in the EEGs of two nonepileptic children under sevoflurane anaesthesia. Anaesth Intensive Care 2000;28(2):205–7.

29. Ohkoshi N, Shoji S. Reversible ageusia induced by losartan: a case report. Eur J Neurol 2002;9(3):315.

30. Constant I, Seeman R, Murat I. Sevoflurane and epileptiform EEG changes. Paediatr Anaesth 2005;15(4):266–74.

31. Boutin F, Bonnet A, Cros AM. Survenue d'une crise pileptiforme avec le s voflurane chez un enfant. Ann Fr Anesth Reanim 2005;24(5):559–60.

32. Hsieh S-W, Lan K-M, Luk H-N, Jawan B. Postoperative seizures after sevoflurane anesthesia in a neonate. Acta Anaesthesiol Scand 2004;48:663.

33. Terasako K, Ishii S. Postoperative seizure-like activity following sevoflurane anesthesia. Acta Anaesthesiol Scand 1996;40(8 Pt 1):953–4.

34. Hilty CA, Drummond JC. Seizure-like activity on emergence from sevoflurane anesthesia. Anesthesiology 2000;93(5):1357–9.

35. Weldon BC, Bell M, Craddock T. The effect of caudal analgesia on emergence agitation in children after sevoflurane versus halothane anesthesia. Anesth Analg 2004;98:321–6.

36. Oh AY, Seo KS, Kim SD, Kim CS, Kim HS. Delayed emergence process does not result in a lower incidence of emergence agitation after sevoflurane anesthesia in children. Acta Anaesthesiol Scand 2005;49(3):297–9.

37. Cohen IT, Finkel JC, Hannallah RS, Hummer KC, Patel KM. Rapid emergence does not explain agitation following sevoflurane anaesthesia in infants and children a comparision with propofol. Paediatr Anaesth 2003;13:63–7.

38. Tesoro S, Mezzetti D, Marchesini L, Peduto VA. Clonidine treatment for agitation in children after sevoflurane anesthesia. Anesth Analg 2005;101(6):1619–22.

39. Ibacache ME, Munoz HR, Brandes V, Morales AL. Single-dose dexmedetomidine reduces agitation after sevoflurane anesthesia in children. Anesth Analg 2004;98:360–3.

40. Shibata S, Shigeomi S, Sato W, Enzan K. Nitrous oxide administration during washout of sevoflurane improves postanesthetic agitation in children. J Anesth 2005;19(2):160–3.

41. Cara DM, Armory P, Mahajan RP. Prolonged duration of neuromuscular block with rapacuronium in the presence of sevoflurane. Anesth Analg 2000;91(6):1392–3.

42. Iohom G, Gardiner C, Whyte A, O'Connor G, Shorten G. Abnormalities of contrast sensitivity and electroretinogram following sevoflurane anaesthesia. Eur J Anaesthesiol 2004;21:646–52.

43. Wells LT, Rasch DK. Emergence "delirium" after sevoflurane anesthesia: a paranoid delusion? Anesth Analg 1999;88(6):1308–10.

44. Kulka PJ, Bressem M, Tryba M. Clonidine prevents sevoflurane-induced agitation in children. Anesth Analg 2001;93(2):335–8.

45. Tabak F, Mert A, Ozaras R, Biyikli M, Ozturk R, Ozbay G, Senturk H, Aktuglu Y. Losartan-induced hepatic injury. J Clin Gastroenterol 2002;34(5):585–6.

46. Neunteufl T, Berger R, Pacher R. Endothelin receptor antagonists in cardiology clinical trials. Expert Opin Investig Drugs 2002;11(3):431–43.

47. Kulka PJ, Bressem M, Wiebalck A, Tryba M. Prophylaxe des "Postsevoflurandelirs" mit Midazolam. [Prevention of "post-sevoflurane delirium" with midazolam.] Anaesthesist 2001;50(6):401–5.

48. Elliott RA, Payne K, Moore JK, Harper NJN, St Leger AS, Moore EW, Thoms GM, Pollard BJ, McHugh GA, Bennett J, Lawrence G, Kerr J, Davies LM. Clinical and economic choices in anaesthesia for day surgery: a prospective randomised controlled trial. Anaesthesia 2003;58:412–21.

49. Hasegawa J, Mitsuhata H, Matsumoto S, Komatsu H, Mizunuma T. [The effects of induced hypotension with sevoflurane and PGE$_1$ on liver functions during neurosurgery.]Masui 1992;41(5):772–8.

50. Watanabe K, Hatakenaka S, Ikemune K, Chigyo Y, Kubozono T, Arai T. [A case of suspected liver dysfunction induced by sevoflurane anesthesia.]Masui 1993;42(6):902–5.

51. Kharasch ED, Frink EJ Jr, Artru A, Michalowski P, Rooke GA, Nogami W. Long-duration low-flow sevoflurane and isoflurane effects on postoperative renal and hepatic function. Anesth Analg 2001;93(6):1511–20.

52. Goeters C, Reinhardt C, Gronau E, Wusten R, Prien T, Baum J, Vrana S, Van Aken H. Minimal flow sevoflurane and isoflurane anaesthesia and impact on renal function. Eur J Anaesthesiol 2001;18(1):43–50.

53. Higuchi H, Adachi Y, Wada H, Kanno M, Satoh T. Comparison of plasma alpha glutathione S-transferase concentrations during and after low-flow sevoflurane or isoflurane anaesthesia. Acta Anaesthesiol Scand 2001;45(10):1226–9.

54. Reich A, Everding AS, Bulla M, Brinkmann OA, Van Aken H. Hepatitis after sevoflurane exposure in an infant suffering from primary hyperoxaluria type 1. Anesth Analg 2004;99:370–2.

55. Jang Y, Kim I. Severe hepatotoxicity after sevoflurane anesthesia in a child with mild renal dysfunction. Paediatr Anaesth 2005;15(12):1140–4.

56. Pertek JP, Le Chaffotec L, Cormier L, Champigneulle J, Omar-Amrani M, Meistelman C. Effects of sevoflurane and isoflurane or desflurane on kidney structure and function in

patients undergoing nephrectomy. Cah Anesthesiol 1999;47:365–70.

57. Ishikawa M, Miyazaki M, Ohta Y. Transient renal tubular dysfunction in a patient with severe asthmatic attack treated with sevoflurane. J Anesth 2001;15(1):49–52.

58. Mazze RI, Callan CM, Galvez ST, Delgado-Herrera L, Mayer DB. The effects of sevoflurane on serum creatinine and blood urea nitrogen concentrations: a retrospective, twenty-two-center, comparative evaluation of renal function in adult surgical patients. Anesth Analg 2000;90(3):683–8.

59. Story DA, Poustie S, Liu G, McNicol PL. Changes in plasma creatinine concentration after cardiac anesthesia with isoflurane, propofol, or sevoflurane: a randomized clinical trial. Anesthesiology 2001;95(4):842–8.

60. Higuchi H, Sumita S, Wada H, Ura T, Ikemoto T, Nakai T, Kanno M, Satoh T. Effects of sevoflurane and isoflurane on renal function and on possible markers of nephrotoxicity. Anesthesiology 1998;89(2):307–22.

61. Higuchi H, Adachi Y. Renal function in surgical patients after administration of low-flow sevoflurane and amikacin. J Anesth 2002;16(1):17–22.

62. Fukuda H, Kawamoto M, Yuge O, Fuji K. A comparison of the effects of prolonged (>10 hour) low-flow sevoflurane, high-flow sevoflurane and low-flow isoflurane anesthesia on hepatorenal function in orthopaedic patients. Anesth Intensive Care 2004;32:210–18.

63. Kobayashi Y, Ochiai R, Takeda J, Sekiguchi H, Fukushima K. Serum and urinary inorganic fluoride concentrations after prolonged inhalation of sevoflurane in humans. Anesth Analg 1992;74(5):753–7.

64. McGrath BJ, Hodgins LR, DeBree A, Frink EJ Jr, Nossaman BD, Bikhazi GB. A multicenter study evaluating the effects of sevoflurane on renal function in patients with renal insufficiency. J Cardiovasc Pharmacol Ther 1998;3(3):229–34.

65. Nishiyama T, Hanaoka K. Inorganic fluoride kinetics and renal and hepatic function after repeated sevoflurane anesthesia. Anesth Analg 1998;87(2):468–73.

66. Groudine SB, Fragen RJ, Kharasch ED, Eisenman TS, Frink EJ, McConnell S, Ebert TJ, Muzi M, Hannon V, Jellish WS, Johnson JO, Jones RM, Sebel PS, Vinik HR, Boyd G. Comparison of renal function following anesthesia with low-flow sevoflurane and isoflurane. J Clin Anesth 1999;11(3):201–7.

67. Morita K, Otsuka F, Ogura T, Takeuchi M, Mizobuchi S, Yamauchi T, Makino H, Hirakawa M. Sevoflurane anaesthesia causes a transient decrease in aquaporin-2 and impairment of urine concentration. Br J Anaesth 1999;83(5):734–9.

68. Obata R, Yasumi Y, Suzuki A, Nakajima Y, Sato S. Rhabdomyolysis in association with Duchenne's muscular dystrophy. Can J Anaesth 1999;46(6):564–6.

69. Takahashi H, Shimokawa M, Sha K, Sakamoto T, Kawaguchi M, Kitaguchi K, Furuya H. [Sevoflurane can induce rhabdomyolysis in Duchenne's muscular dystrophy.]Masui 2002;51(2):190–2.

70. Otsuka H, Komura Y, Mayumi T, Yamamura T, Kemmotsu O, Mukaida K. Malignant hyperthermia during sevoflurane anesthesia in a child with central core disease. Anesthesiology 1991;75(4):699–701.

71. Ochiai R, Toyoda Y, Nishio I, Takeda J, Sekiguchi H, Fukushima K, Kohda E. Possible association of malignant hyperthermia with sevoflurane anesthesia. Anesth Analg 1992;74(4):616–8.

72. Hoshino K, Yamashiro Y, Nitta K, Kawaguchi H, Fukui H, Ikeda M, Ooshima Y. A case of postoperative malignant

hyperthermia after 15 hours induced anesthesia. Hiroshima J Anesth 1996;32:15–8.

73. Yamamoto Y, Tanaka H, Ikeda K. A case in which it was difficult to differentiate between malignant hyperthermia and thyroid storm. Anesth Resusc 1996;32S:85–9.

74. Massaro F, De Klerk DYJ, Snoeck MMJ. A case of malignant hyperthermia during use of sevoflurane. Ned Tijdschr Anesthesiol 2001;14:71–3.

75. Baris S, Karakaya D, Guldogus F, Sarihasan B, Tekat A. A case of malignant hyperthermia during sevoflurane anesthesia. Turk J Med Sci 2001;31:171–3.

76. Shulman M, Braverman B, Ivankovich AD, Gronert G. Sevoflurane triggers malignant hyperthermia in swine. Anesthesiology 1981;54(3):259–60.

77. Krause T, Scholz J, Jansen L, Boettcher H, Koch C, Wappler F, Schulte am Esch J. Sevoflurane anaesthesia does not induce the formation of sister chromatid exchanges in peripheral blood lymphocytes of children. Br J Anaesth 2003;90:233–5.

78. Conzen PF, Nuscheler M, Melotte A, Verhaegen M, Leupolt T, Van Aken H, Peter K. Renal function and serum fluoride concentrations in patients with stable renal insufficiency after anesthesia with sevoflurane or enflurane. Anesth Analg 1995;81(3):569–75.

79. Matsumoto M, Sakai H. [Sevoflurane anesthesia for a patient with insulinoma.]Masui 1992;41(3):446–9.

80. Saitoh K, Hirabayashi Y, Fukuda H, Shimizu R. [Sevoflurane anesthesia in a patient following renal transplantation.]Masui 1993;42(5):746–9.

81 Lee A, Chui PT, Aun CS, Gin T, Lau AS. Possible interaction between sevoflurane and Aloe vera. Ann Pharmacother 2004;38(10):1651–4.

82. Fragen RJ, Fitzgerald PC. Effect of dexmedetomidine on the minimum alveolar concentration (MAC) of sevoflurane in adults age 55 to 70 years. J Clin Anesth 1999;11(6): 466–70.

83. Katoh T, Kobayashi S, Suzuki A, Iwamoto T, Bito H, Ikeda K. The effect of fentanyl on sevoflurane requirements for somatic and sympathetic responses to surgical incision. Anesthesiology 1999;90(2):398–405.

84. Laisalmi M, Eriksson H, Koivusalo AM, Pere P, Rosenberg P, Lindgren L. Ketorolac is not nephrotoxic in connection with sevoflurane anesthesia in patients undergoing breast surgery. Anesth Analg 2001;92(4):1058–63.

85 Kudo M, Ohke H, Kawai T, Kato M, Kokubu M, Shinya N. Geriatric patient who suffered transitory cardiovascular collapse under sevoflurane anesthesia due to continuous medication with mexiletine hydrochloride. J Jpn Dent Soc Anesthesiol 1999;27:614–8.

86. Higuchi H, Wada H, Usui Y, Goto K, Kanno M, Satoh T. Effects of probenecid on renal function in surgical patients anesthetized with low-flow sevoflurane. Anesthesiology 2001;94(1):21–31.

Trichloroethylene

General Information

Trichloroethylene is a volatile halogenated anesthetic with weak anesthetic properties compared with other halogenated anesthetics and poor muscle relaxant activity.Trichloroethylene is not used as an inhalational anesthetic, but still has industrial uses, including dry cleaning, metal degreasing, and as a solvent for oils and resins.

Organs and Systems

Nervous system

A population-based study of 143 people who had been exposed to long-term low concentrations of trichloroethylene because of a contaminated water supply showed significant neurobehavioral deficits (1).

Liver

Hepatitis and acute liver failure (associated with skin and mucosal lesions similar to Stevens–Johnson syndrome) has been described in two young Thai women who used trichloroethylene to clean metal watch straps (2). One 23-year-old woman died from acute liver failure within a fortnight of occupational exposure. The other woman, aged 24 years, recovered spontaneously.

Immunologic

In 35 workers who had been exposed to environmental trichloroethylene there were significant increases in serum interleukin-2 and interferon-gamma concentrations and a reduction in interleukin-4 concentrations compared with 30 control workers (3).

Long-Term Effects

Tumorigenicity

The incidence of cancer among 803 Danish workers exposed to trichloroethylene has been evaluated (4). There was no overall increase. However, the standardized incidence ratio was significantly higher in men with non-Hodgkin's lymphoma or esophageal cancer and in women with cervical cancer.

In a consecutive case-control study of 134 renal cell cancer cases and 401 controls (5) median urinary α_1-microglobulin excretion was significantly higher in patients with renal cell cancer who had been exposed to trichloroethylene than in non-exposed cases. A significant excess risk of renal cell cancer was associated with occupational exposure to trichloroethylene (for example for metal degreasers, OR=5.57, 95%CI=2.33, 13.32).

The carcinogenicity of trichloroethylene has been evaluated in a consecutive case-control study in 134 patients with renal cell cancers and 401 controls (6). There was a significant excess risk with occupational exposure to trichloroethylene (for example, for metal degreasing OR=5.57; 95%CI=2.33, 13.32).

Second-Generation Effects

Teratogenicity

Reviewers of the industrial uses of trichloroethylene have concluded that there is no evidence that it is teratogenic (7) (8).

Previous studies have suggested that trichloroethylene is a selective cardiac teratogen. In a case-control study of 4025 infants born between 1997 and 1999 in Milwaukee the risk of congenital heart disease was more than three-fold greater in older trichloroethylene exposed mothers than in non-exposed mothers (9).

Drug Administration

Drug overdose

Overdosage with trichloroethylene has been reported (10).

A man in his 40s drank an unknown amount of trichloroethylene in a suicide attempt. He became comatose, with acute respiratory failure, hypotension, sinus tachycardia, and severe diarrhea. He was mechanically ventilated and on day 4 developed ventricular bigeminy. His serum creatine kinase and lactate dehydrogenase activities were persistently raised. He died with complete heart block after 24 days.

A muscle biopsy in this case showed evidence of muscle damage, with large lipid droplets compressed the myofilaments, degenerating mitochondria, and markedly reduced succinate and NAD cytochrome c reductase activities.

References

1. Reif JS, Burch JB, Nuckols JR, Metzger L, Ellington D, Anger WK. Neurobehavioral effects of exposure to trichloroethylene through a municipal water supply. Environ Res 2003;93:248–58.
2. Pantucharoensri S, Boontee P, Likithsan P, Padungtod C, Prasartsansoui S. Generalized eruption accompanied by hepatitis in two Thai metal cleaners exposed to trichloroethylene. Industrial Health 2004;42:385–8.
3. Iavicoli I, Marinaccio A, Carelli G. Effects of occupational trichloroethylene exposure on cytokine levels in workers. J Occup Environ Med 2005;47(5):453–7.
4. Hansen J, Raaschou-Nielsen O, Christensen JM, Johansen I, McLaughlin JK, Lipworth L, Blot WJ, Olsen JH. Cancer incidence among Danish workers exposed to trichloroethylene. J Occup Environ Med 2001;43(2):133–9.
5. Bolt HM, Lammert M, Selinski S, Bruning T. Urinary ?1-microglobulin as biomarker of renal toxicity in trichloroethylene-exposed persons Int Arch Occup Environ Health 2004;77:186–90.
6. Bruning T, Pesch B, Wiesenhutter B, Rabstein S, Lammert M, Baumuller A, Bolt HM. Renal cell cancer risk and occupational exposure to trichloroethylene: results of a consecutive case-control study in Arnsberg, Germany. Am J Ind Med 2003;43:274–85.

7. Hardin BD, Kelman BJ, Brent RL. Trichloroethylene and dichloroethylene: a critical review of teratogenicity. Birth Defects Res A Clin Mol Teratol 2005;73(12):931–55.

8. Watson RE, Jacobson CF, Williams AL, Howard WB, DeSesso JM. Trichloroethylene-contaminated drinking water and congenital heart defects: a critical analysis of the literature. Reprod Toxicol 2006;21(2):117–47.

9. Yauck JS, Malloy ME, Blair K, Simpsin P, McCarver DG. Proximity of residence to trichloroethylene-emitting sites and increased risk of offspring congenital heart defects among older women. Birth Defects Res (Part A) 2004;70:808–14.

10. Vattemi G, Tonin P, Filosto M, Rizzuto N, Tomelleri G, Perbellini L, Iacovelli W, Petrucci N. Human skeletal muscle as a target organ of trichloroethylene toxicity. JAMA 2005;294(5):554–6.

INHALATIONAL ANESTHETICS—NON-HALOGENATED

Anesthetic ether

General Information

Diethyl ether (SED-9, 172) is obsolete as a general anesthetic (1). It is highly inflammable and therefore incompatible with modern surgical and anesthetic techniques. It has an unpleasant smell and irritates mucous membranes; this can cause coughing, straining, laryngeal spasm, and hypersalivation. Recovery is slow and accompanied by nausea and vomiting in up to 85% of patients. Liver damage is as frequent as with halothane. Ether raises intracranial pressure and can cause convulsions. It can cause impaired immune responsiveness and contact dermatitis has been reported, together with a systemic allergic reaction (SEDA-5, 120).

Reference

4. Whaten FX, Bacon DR, Smith HM. Inhaled anesthetics: an historical overview. Best Pract Res Clin Anaesthesiol 2005;19(3):323–30.

Cyclopropane

General Information

Cyclopropane is an inhalational anesthetic gas. Its minimum alveolar concentration (MAC) is 9.2%. Because of the risk of explosion, it is usually administered by closed circuit (1).

Organs and Systems

Cardiovascular

Cardiac dysrhythmias, which can be ventricular, can complicate the use of cyclopropane (2), and the risk is increased in patients who have also been given catecholamines (3).

Nervous system

Delirium can occur in patients given cyclopropane (4).

Gastrointestinal

Nausea and vomiting are fairly frequent after recovery from cyclopropane anesthesia (5,6).

Liver

Liver dysfunction due to cyclopropane, as judged by effects on indocyanine green clearance, has been reported (7).

Urinary tract

Cyclopropane has an antidiuretic effect that is partly reversed by alcohol (8).

Body temperature

There has been a report of malignant hyperthermia in a patient who was given cyclopropane during cesarean section (9), consistent with the in vitro effect of cyclopropane on caffeine-induced muscle contraction (10).

References

1. Jansen U, Moller-Petersen J, Pedersen S. Eksplosionsdod fald under cyklopropan–anaestesi. [A fatal case after explosion during cyclopropane anesthesia.] Ugeskr Laeger 1979;141(49):3375.
2. Hansen DD, Fernandes A, Skovsted P, Berry P. Cyclopropane anaesthesia for renal transplantation. Report of 100 cases. Br J Anaesth 1972;44(6):584–9.
3. Wong KC. Sympathomimetic drugs. In: Smith NT, Miller RD, Corbascio AN, editors. Drug Interactions in Anesthesia. Philadelphia: Lea & Febiger, 1981:66.
4. Denson JS. Cyclopropane. Int Anesthesiol Clin 1963;21:1005–32.
5. Gold MI. Postanesthetic vomiting in the recovery room. Br J Anaesth 1969;41(2):143–9.
6. Kenny GN. Risk factors for postoperative nausea and vomiting. Anaesthesia 1994;49(Suppl):6–10.
7. Abdel Salam AR, Drummond GB, Bauld HW, Scott DB. Clearance of indocyanine green as an index of liver function during cyclopropane anaesthesia and induced hypotension. Br J Anaesth 1976;48(3):231–8.
8. Deutsch S, Pierce EC Jr, Vandam LD. Cyclopropane effects on renal function in normal man. Anesthesiology 1967;28(3):547–58.
9. Lips FJ, Newland M, Dutton G. Malignant hyperthermia triggered by cyclopropane during cesarean section. Anesthesiology 1982;56(2):144–6.
10. Reed SB, Strobel GE Jr. An in-vitro model of malignant hyperthermia: differential effects of inhalation anesthetics on caffeine-induced muscle contractures. Anesthesiology 1978;48(4):254–9.

Nitrous oxide

General Information

Nitrous oxide is a relatively potent analgesic but a weak anesthetic, in use since 1842. At body temperature, its blood/gas partition ratio is only 0.47. It is excreted unchanged via the lungs. Because of the large mass of gas delivered to the patient, important physicochemical problems arise. Its ability to diffuse into and expand any air-filled cavity continues to produce new reports. Nitrous oxide is occasionally abused (1).

The continued use of nitrous oxide in anesthetic practice has been questioned on the basis of its serious adverse effects and the availability of potentially safer short-acting potent analgesic drugs, such as xenon and remifentanil (2).

Organs and Systems

Cardiovascular

Although myocardial depression has been described in healthy volunteers after the use of 40 or 50% nitrous oxide in oxygen, it is usually mild. It is likely that nitrous oxide can worsen myocardial ischemia in patients with critical coronary stenosis, although this may not be of clinical significance (3,4).

Homocysteine concentrations
Nitrous oxide inhibits methionine synthase, thereby preventing the conversion of homocysteine to methionine. A high homocysteine concentration has also been identified as an independent risk factor for coronary artery and cerebrovascular disease.

The effect of nitrous oxide on homocysteine concentrations and perioperative myocardial ischemia/infarction has been extensively reviewed (5). Nitrous oxide causes acute rises in postoperative homocysteine concentrations temporally associated with postoperative myocardial ischemia. Preoperative oral folate and vitamins B_6 and B_{12} blunt nitrous oxide-induced postoperative increases in plasma homocysteine (6).

The effect of nitrous oxide on homocysteine concentrations and myocardial ischemia has been studied in a randomized controlled study in 90 patients, ASA grades 1–3, who received a standardized anesthetic consisting of propofol induction, an opioid, and either inhalational isoflurane or isoflurane + 50% nitrous oxide (7). They underwent carotid endarterectomy (average operation duration 3.3 hours). Electrocardiographic monitoring consisted of a three-channel Holter monitor (leads II, V2, and V5), which was later examined for periods of ischemia by a physician blinded to treatment group. Myocardial enzyme activities were not measured. Baseline homocysteine concentrations (12.7 µmol/l) were significantly increased in the recovery room and at 48 hours to 15.5 and 18.8 µmol/l respectively. The concentrations did not increase in those given nitrous oxide. Periods of preoperative and intraoperative ischemia did not differ. Postoperatively the nitrous oxide group had more patients with ischemia (19 versus 11), longer ischemic events in the first 24 hours (54 minutes versus 17 minutes), and more episodes of ischemia lasting more than 30 minutes (23 versus 14). The authors concluded that nitrous oxide is associated with increased myocardial ischemia. However, they conceded that they had not shown causality. Previous studies have not shown this outcome, but were less sensitive, using only two-channel or once-daily 12-lead electrocardiography, or not

monitoring patients postoperatively. The subject warrants a major study before a firm conclusion can be drawn.

Respiratory

Although airway conductance may be reduced by nitrous oxide, respiratory depression is unlikely after short-term exposure (8). The respiratory safety of nitrous oxide inhalation in children has been confirmed (9).

The effects of intraoperative air or nitrous oxide on postoperative oxygen saturation (S_aO_2) in blood have been compared in 40 patients of ASA classes 1 and 2 undergoing elective open cholecystectomy. The incidence of hypoxemia was significantly higher in those treated with nitrous oxide than in those given air 48 hours postoperatively (10). Hypoxemia may also have some mechanical origins. Nitrous oxide diffuses into the endotracheal tube cuff, overexpanding it, and can thus provoke upper airway obstruction, hypoxemia, and trauma in intubated patients during general anesthesia (11).

The poor solubility of nitrous oxide may be dangerous for patients with pneumothorax, pneumoperitoneum, ileus, or air embolism.

Nervous system

Nitrous oxide inactivates the enzyme methionine synthetase, and caution is urged in giving nitrous oxide to patients who may be deficient in vitamin B_{12}. Low serum vitamin B_{12} concentrations have previously been reported in patients with sickle cell disease, but the reason for this is uncertain. Three cases of peripheral neuropathy have been reported in patients with sickle cell disease who received nitrous oxide (12–14). All three had a history of frequent painful sickle crises, for which they received nitrous oxide for prolonged periods. Serum vitamin B_{12} concentrations were slightly reduced in two patients and very low in the third. The patients all presented with difficulty in walking and paresthesia. Peripheral sensorimotor neuropathy was confirmed by nerve conduction studies. The patients all responded well to vitamin B_{12} injections and avoiding further exposure to nitrous oxide. Caution is therefore recommended when using nitrous oxide in patients with sickle cell disease or who are suspected of vitamin B_{12} deficiency. Two cases of polyneuropathy have also been reported after the use of nitrous oxide for 80 minutes and 3 hours in patients who were subsequently found to have pernicious anemia. They both responded well to hydroxocobalamin.

Nitrous oxide has a potential for abuse (15), one of the major complications of which is myeloneuropathy. Altered vitamin B_{12} metabolism has been suggested as a mechanism (16), and in some cases the patients concerned have been found to have pre-existing subclinical B_{12} deficiency (17). Nitrous oxide interferes with vitamin B_{12} formation by causing irreversible oxidation of cobalt in an essential co-enzyme. Three cases of myeloneuropathy after nitrous oxide anesthesia have been reported in patients with subclinical vitamin B_{12} deficiency (18,19). In 12 patients who were heavily exposed to nitrous oxide either deliberately or professionally for periods ranging from 3 months to several years, numbness in the hands or legs developed initially, followed by Lhermitte's sign, gait ataxia, impotence, and sphincter disturbances (20). Several similar cases have been reported by others (SEDA-11, 110). Numbness and/or muscle weakness were found four times more often among exposed than non-exposed dental personnel (21).

Since nitrous oxide has some effects on the nervous system, it is not entirely surprising to note a further report that under experimental conditions it can affect memory. That memory changes can occur has been known for a long time, but the pattern of the effects now appears to be distinctly odd.

Myelopathy associated with nitric oxide anesthesia typically occurs in individuals who have been discovered postoperatively to be B_{12} deficient, and another case has been reported in a 24-year-old man who used nitric oxide for recreational purposes (22).

Myelopathy associated with nitrous oxide abuse has also been reported (23).

- A 23-year-old man presented with a 5-day history of gait disturbance and incoordination. He had severe loss of proprioception in his legs and could not walk. He was hypomanic. Severe posterior column myelopathy was diagnosed using MRI scanning. His nitrous oxide use had consisted of 40–60 whipped cream bulbs per day for 6 months. He also admitted to intermittent diamorphine abuse, but not for the 3 weeks before admission. He was treated with hydroxocobalamin and methionine, but still had minor abnormalities 3 months later.

The authors noted that although the evidence is scant, treatment should consist of both vitamin B_{12} and methionine.

Two cases of polyneuropathy and myelopathy associated with chronic nitrous oxide abuse have been reported (24,25).

Inhalation of 50 or 70% nitrous oxide in oxygen for 15 minutes impaired driving skill (26). Patients who receive nitrous oxide should be informed that its after-effects can alter their functioning without their being conscious of the fact (27).

Nitrous oxide can diffuse into any cavity that has air inserted or left in situ. Intraoperative subdural tension pneumocephalus arising during neurosurgery has been described (28). Air injected into the epidural space can cause symptomatic pressure effects if nitrous oxide diffuses into the air pocket.

A mixture of nitrous oxide and oxygen in equal proportions ("Entonox") can cause damage to the spinal cord, mimicking subacute combined degeneration (29).

- A 21-year-old man had a series of major operations for inflammatory bowel disease over 4 years—colectomy, ileostomy, and laparotomy, with the formation of an ileoanal pouch. He developed pelvic sepsis and an extensive perineal abscess had to be laid open. Postoperative analgesia proved difficult during daily changes of packs to the cavity. He was given regular paracetamol, diclofenac, and opioids. A 50:50 mixture of nitrous oxide and oxygen was used to manage acute pain. The hospital gave him a 300-liter cylinder of the

mixture as a short-term arrangement over Christmas and issued increasing amounts over the next 4 months, resulting in weekly consumption of 1280 liters of the nitrous oxide mixture. He then developed progressive difficulty in walking over 6 weeks. He had severe pseudoathetosis of the fingers and arms, brisk reflexes, and normal bilateral flexor plantar responses. There was severe loss of joint position sense in the hands and feet and loss of vibration sense in all four limbs, with no spinothalamic sensory loss or truncal sensory level. There was a long lesion in the dorsal column, typical of subacute combined degeneration, on an MRI scan. Although his serum B_{12} concentration was normal, he was given hydroxocobalamin and at follow-up at 3 months he had no gait ataxia and normal hand function and was independent in all activities of daily living.

A patient who developed a diffuse myelopathy after receiving nitrous oxide on two occasions within 8 weeks had hyperhomocysteinemia and low concentrations of vitamin B_{12}, and had a polymorphism in the 5,10-methylenetetrahydrofolate reductase (MTHFR) gene associated with the thermolabile isoform of the enzyme (30). The authors suggested that this explained the myelopathy. Treatment with folic acid and vitamin B_{12} caused the neurological symptoms to improve.

Subacute combined degeneration of the cord occurred 4 weeks after prolonged exposure to nitrous oxide in a man with diabetes who had hyperhomocysteinemia and vitamin B_{12} deficiency (31).

Sensory systems

Eyes

Nitrous oxide is 34 times more soluble than nitrogen in enclosed body cavity gas spaces and it enters such spaces rapidly, causing expansion and a rise in pressure. Vitreoretinal surgery often uses intraocular gases to replace vitreous humor, in order to internally tamponade the neuroretina to the retinal pigment epithelium. Various long-acting inert gases, such as sulfur hexafluoride(SF_6) or perfluoropropane, can be used as intraocular tamponading agents. Several cases of blindness and severe visual loss associated with nitrous oxide in people with intraocular gas bubbles have been reported (32–34). It has been suggested that all such patients should have warning bracelets detailing the presence of intraocular gas and that nitrous oxide be avoided until it has been shown that the gas bubble has been absorbed.

- A 71-year-old man with glaucoma developed a left retinal detachment which was yreated with vitrectomy and retinal cryotherapy (35). He subsequently underwent general anesthesia with oxygen in nitrous oxide for 2 hours, and had intense pain and complete loss of vision in the left eye while recovering from the anaesthetic. He had no light perception in the left eye, the pupil was mid-dilated and non-reactive, and the intraocular pressure was 31 mmHg. The vitreous cavity was 50% full of gas and the retinal vasculature was attenuated. Three months later he still had no light perception and the optic disc was pale.

- A 66-year-old man had a vitrectomy and peeling of an epiretinal membrane in the right eye (36). Perioperatively, the eye was filled with 20% sulfur hexafluoride gas to tamponade retinal breaks. Five days later he underwent prostatectomy under general anesthesia using nitrous oxide. Postoperatively the eye had no light perception as a result of ischemic retinopathy.

Another case of blindness associated with nitrous oxide in a patient with an intraocular gas bubble has been reported, this time 37 days after vitreoretinal surgery (37). The author's institution now insists that all such patients should have warning bracelets detailing the presence of intraocular gas, and that nitrous oxide be avoided until it has been demonstrated by an ophthalmologist that the gas bubble has been absorbed.

Ears

- Rupture of the tympanic membrane was attributed to nitrous oxide in a 28-year-old woman with a history of tonsillectomy and a recent respiratory tract infection who underwent dilatation and curettage during laparoscopy (38).

Hematologic

The effect of nitrous oxide on vitamin B_{12} and folate metabolism can cause megaloblastic bone marrow changes, the period required depending on the patient's nutritional status (39).

Dyshemopoiesis after exposure to nitrous oxide may be mediated through a direct inhibitory effect (40). Although clinical sequelae have not been reported, the use of nitrous oxide in bone marrow transplantation needs to be evaluated further and cannot currently be recommended (41).

Gastrointestinal

Nausea and vomiting seldom occur. Nitrous oxide had no effect on recovery from laparoscopic cholecystectomy (42).

Liver

Jaundice after general anesthesia in which nitrous oxide was the only anesthetic has been described (43). However, contamination with halothane was not definitely ruled out.

Urinary tract

Renal blood flow is moderately reduced by nitrous oxide (44). Disturbances of kidney function have been described (45).

Body temperature

Malignant hyperthermia is very rare; the possible role of nitrous oxide as a triggering agent has not been confirmed in pigs (46).

Second-Generation Effects

Pregnancy

Nitrous oxide has been widely used in pregnancy and is generally regarded as being safe (47).

Teratogenicity

Some experimental data have suggested a possible teratogenic potential of nitrous oxide, the clinical relevance of which is unclear (48). The interaction with vitamin B_{12} causes changes in DNA synthesis that could be important in the first trimester of pregnancy. Nitrous oxide is the only inhalational anesthetic that has definitely been shown to be teratogenic in experimental animals, but epidemiological studies have suggested that it is not teratogenic in human (49).

Drug–Drug Interactions

Halothane

The addition of nitrous oxide to halothane in coronary patients produced hypotension, with a subsequent risk of myocardial damage (49).

Midazolam

The combination of midazolam with nitrous oxide produced retrograde amnesia in 21 women undergoing elective cesarean section (51). All had spinal anesthesia. After delivery the patients received intravenous midazolam, average dose 94 µg/kg, and inhaled nitrous oxide 50%. At the end of surgery, flumazenil was given in 0.1 mg increments until the patient awoke. Another nine women were given only nitrous oxide inhalation after delivery. Of the women who received midazolam and nitrous oxide, 33% could not recall their baby's face, while all of the women not given midazolam could. The results suggest that midazolam plus nitrous oxide can produce retrograde amnesia not reversed by flumazenil.

Other inhalation agents

The uptake of any other inhalation agent, given at the same time as nitrous oxide, is accelerated by the rate of uptake of nitrous oxide. This is termed the "second gas effect" (52). Direct pharmacodynamic interactions do not occur.

Drug-Device Interactions

Nitrous oxide is 34 times more soluble than nitrogen in enclosed body cavity gas spaces, and it enters such spaces rapidly, causing expansion and a rise in pressure. It can therefore cause pneumothorax, air embolism, or pneumocephalus. Nitrous oxide also diffuses into the cuff of endotracheal tubes and can cause a marked increase in cuff pressure. In a 27-year-old woman with placenta percreta at 37 weeks gestation who required elective cesarean hysterectomy, internal iliac artery occlusion balloons ruptured during nitrous oxide anesthesia (53).

Interference with Diagnostic Tests

Oxygen dissociation

Nitrous oxide inhalation can give false PO_2 measurement results and shift the oxyhemoglobin curve to the left (54).

References

1. LiPuma JP, Wellman J, Stern HP. Nitrous oxide abuse: a new cause of pneumomediastinum. Radiology 1982;145(3):602.
2. Shaw AD, Morgan M. Nitrous oxide: time to stop laughing? Anaesthesia 1998;53(3):213–5.
3. Kozmary SV, Lampe GH, Benefiel D, Cahalan MK, Wauk LZ, Whitendale P, Schiller NB, Eger EI 2nd. No finding of increased myocardial ischemia during or after carotid endarterectomy under anesthesia with nitrous oxide. Anesth Analg 1990;71(6):591–6.
4. Lampe GH, Donegan JH, Rupp SM, Wauk LZ, Whitendale P, Fouts KE, Rose BM, Litt LL, Rampil IJ, Wilson CB, et al. Nitrous oxide and epinephrine-induced arrhythmias. Anesth Analg 1990;71(6):602–5.
5. Badner NH, Spence JD. Homocyst(e)ine, nitrous oxide and atherosclerosis. Balliere's Best Pract Res Clin Anesthesiol 2001;15:185–93.
6. Badner NH, Freeman D, Spence JD. Preoperative oral B vitamins prevent nitrous oxide-induced postoperative plasma homocysteine increases. Anesth Analg 2001;93(6):1507–10.
7. Badner NH, Beattie WS, Freeman D, Spence JD. Nitrous oxide-induced increased homocysteine concentrations are associated with increased postoperative myocardial ischemia in patients undergoing carotid endarterectomy. Anesth Analg 2000;91(5):1073–9.
8. Jin T, Ishihara H, Ohshiro Y, Murakawa T, Kogure M, Ookura I, Tsukamoto A, Sakaki T, Oyama T. [Effect of nitrous oxide on the circulatory and respiratory functions.]Masui 1980;29(5):458–61.
9. Litman RS, Berkowitz RJ, Ward DS. Levels of consciousness and ventilatory parameters in young children during sedation with oral midazolam and nitrous oxide. Arch Pediatr Adolesc Med 1996;150(7):671–5.
10. Maroof M, Khan RM, Siddique M. Ventilation with nitrous oxide during open cholecystectomy increases the incidence of postoperative hypoxemia. Anesth Analg 1993;76(5):1091–4.
11. Komatsu H, Mitsuhata H, Hasegawa J, Matsumoto S. [Decreased pressure of endotracheal tube cuff in general anesthesia without nitrous oxide.] Masui 1993;42(6):831–4.
12. Ogundipe O, Walker M, Pearson MW, Slater NG, Adepegba T, Westerdale N. Sickle cell disease and nitrous oxide-induced neuropathy. Clin Lab Haematol 1999;21(6):409–12.
13. Sesso RM, Iunes Y, Melo AC. Myeloneuropathy following nitrous oxide anesthaesia in a patient with macrocytic anaemia. Neuroradiology 1999;41(8):588–90.
14. Alarcia R, Ara JR, Serrano M, Garcia M, Latorre AM, Capablo JL. [Severe polyneuropathy after using nitrous oxide as an anesthetic. A preventable disease?] Rev Neurol 1999;29(1):36–8.

15. Atkinson RM, Moorozumi P, De Wayne-Green J, Kramer JC. Nitrous oxide intoxication: subjective effects in healthy young men. J Psychedelic Drugs 1977;6:317.
16. Nunn JF. Clinical aspects of the interaction between nitrous oxide and vitamin B_{12}. Br J Anaesth 1987;59(1):3–13.
17. Holloway KL, Alberico AM. Postoperative myeloneuropathy: a preventable complication in patients with B_{12} deficiency. J Neurosurg 1990;72(5):732–6.
18. Nestor PJ, Stark RJ. Vitamin B_{12} myeloneuropathy precipitated by nitrous oxide anaesthesia. Med J Aust 1996;165(3):174.
19. Takacs J. [N_2O-induced acute funicular myelosis in latent vitamin B_{12} deficiency.] Anasthesiol Intensivmed Notfallmed Schmerzther 1996;31(8):525–8.
20. Layzer RB. Myeloneuropathy after prolonged exposure to nitrous oxide. Lancet 1978;2(8102):1227–30.
21. Brodsky JB, Cohen EN, Brown BW Jr, Wu ML, Whitcher CE. Exposure to nitrous oxide and neurologic disease among dental professionals. Anesth Analg 1981;60(5):297–301.
22. Waters MF, Kang GA, Mazziotta JC, DeGiorgio CM. Nitrous oxide inhalation as a cause of cervical myelopathy. Acta Neurol Scand. 112(4):270–2.
23. Sur RL, Kane CJ. Sildenafil citrate-associated priapism. Urology 2000;55(6):950.
24. Iwata K, O'Keefe GB, Karanas A. Neurologic problems associated with chronic nitrous oxide abuse in a non-healthcare worker. Am J Med Sci 2001;322(3):173–4.
25. Eichhorn M, Watson M, Wurst F. Polyneuropathie und myelopathie bei N_2O-Abusus im Rahmeneiner Polytoxikomanie. [Polyneuropathy and myelopathy in N2O abuse within the scope of multiple drug abuse.] Psychiatr Prax 2001;28(4):204–5.
26. Moyes D, Cleaton-Jones P, Lelliot J. Evaluation of driving skills after brief exposure to nitrous oxide. S Afr Med J 1979;56(23):1000–2.
27. Ramsay DS, Leonesio RJ, Whitney CW, Jones BC, Samson HH, Weinstein P. Paradoxical effects of nitrous oxide on human memory. Psychopharmacology (Berl) 1992;106(3):370–4.
28. Goodie D, Traill R. Intraoperative subdural tension pneumocephalus arising after opening of the dura. Anesthesiology 1991;74(1):193–5.
29. Doran M, Rassam SS, Jones LM, Underhill S. Toxicity after intermittent inhalation of nitrous oxide for analgesia. BMJ 2004;328:1364–5.
30. Lacassie HJ, Nazar C, Yonish B, Sandoval P, Muir HA, Mellado P. Reversible nitrous oxide myelopathy and a polymorphism in the gene encoding 5,10-methylenetetrahydrofolate reductase. Br J Anaesth 2006;96(2):222–5.
31. Ahn SC, Brown AW. Cobalamin deficiency and subacute combined degeneration after nitrous oxide anesthesia: a case report. Arch Phys Med Rehabil 2005;86(1):150–3.
32. Yang YF, Herbert L, Ruschen H, Cooling RJ. Nitrous oxide anaesthesia in the presence of intraocular gas can cause irreversible blindness. BMJ 2002;325(7363):532–3.
33. Seaberg RR, Freeman WR, Goldbaum MH, Manecke GR Jr. Permanent postoperative vision loss associated with expansion of intraocular gas in the presence of a nitrous oxide-containing anesthetic. Anesthesiology 2002;97(5):1309–10.
34. Fu AD, McDonald HR, Eliott D, Fuller DG, Halperin LS, Ramsay RC, Johnson RN, Ai E. Complications of general anesthesia using nitrous oxide in eyes with pre-existing gas bubbles. Retina 2002;22(5):569–74.
35. Yang YF, Herbert L, Ruschen H, Cooling RJ. Nitrous oxide anaesthesia in the presence of intraocular gas can cause irreversible blindness. Br Med J 2002;325:532–3.

36. Astrom S, Kjellgren D, Monestam E, Backlund U. Nitrous oxide anaesthesia and intravitreal gas tamponade. Acta Anaesthesiol Scand 2003;47:361–2.

37. Lee EJK. Use of nitrous oxide causing severe visual loss 37 days after retinal surgery. Br J Anaesth 2004;93:464–6.

38. Ohryn M. Tympanic membrane rupture following general anesthesia with nitrous oxide: a case report. AANA J 1995;63(1):42–4.

39. Waldman FM, Koblin DD, Lampe GH, Wauk LZ, Eger EI 2nd. Hematologic effects of nitrous oxide in surgical patients. Anesth Analg 1990;71(6):618–24.

40. Warren DJ, Christensen B, Slordal L. Effect of nitrous oxide on haematopoiesis in vitro: biochemical and functional features. Pharmacol Toxicol 1993;72(1):69–72.

41. Carmel R, Rabinowitz AP, Mazumder A. Metabolic evidence of cobalamin deficiency in bone marrow cells harvested for transplantation from donors given nitrous oxide. Eur J Haematol 1993;50(4):228–33.

42. Jensen AG, Prevedoros H, Kullman E, Anderberg B, Lennmarken C. Peroperative nitrous oxide does not influence recovery after laparoscopic cholecystectomy. Acta Anaesthesiol Scand 1993;37(7):683–6.

43. Hart SM, Fitzgerald PG. Unexplained jaundice following non-halothane anaesthesia. A case report. Br J Anaesth 1975;47(12):1321–6.

44. Bethune DW. Organ damage after open-heart surgery. Lancet 1976;2(8000):1410–1.

45. Nuutinen LS. The effect of nitrous oxide on renal function in open heart surgery. Ann Chir Gynaecol 1976;65(3):200–6.

46. Gronert GA, Milde JH. Hyperbaric nitrous oxide and malignant hyperpyrexia. Br J Anaesth 1981;53(11):1238.

47. Crawford JS, Lewis M. Nitrous oxide in early human pregnancy. Anaesthesia 1986;41(9):900–5.

48. Fujinaga M. Teratogenicity of nitrous oxide. Ballière's Best Pract Res Clin Anaesthesiol 2001;15:363–75.

49. Nunn JF. Nitrous oxide and pregnancy. Anaesthesia 1987;42(4):427–8.

50. Moffitt EA, Sethna DH, Gary RJ, Raymond MJ, Matloff JM, Bussell JA. Nitrous oxide added to halothane reduces coronary flow and myocardial oxygen consumption in patients with coronary disease. Can Anaesth Soc J 1983;30(1):5–9.

51. Takano M, Takano Y, Sato I. [The effect of midazolam on the memory during cesarean section and the modulation by flumazenil.] Masui 1999;48(1):73–5.

52. Epstein RM, Rackow H, Salanitre E, Wolf GL. Influence of the concentration effect on the uptake of anesthetic mixtures: the second gas effect. Anesthesiology 1964;25:364–71.

53. Kuczkowski KM, Eisenmann UB. Nitrous oxide as a cause of internal iliac artery occlusion balloon rupture. Ann Fr Anesth Reanim 2005;24(5):564.

54. Fournier L, Major D. Nitrous oxide effects on PO_2 measurements in the operating room: shift of the oxyhaemoglobin curve. Can Anaesth Soc J 1982;29:498.

Xenon

General Information

Xenon is a heavy gas (symbol Xe; atomic no 54) that is normally present in the atmosphere. It has been used as an anesthetic and as a diagnostic tool in functional neuroimaging (1).

Xenon has many characteristics of the ideal anesthetic (2) and has analgesic properties. In addition to its lack of effects on the cardiovascular system (most other anesthetics are negative inotropes), xenon has low solubility, enabling faster induction of anesthesia and faster emergence. Although its high cost limits its use, the development of closed rebreathing systems has led to further interest. It has no effects on the cardiovascular system and has low solubility, enabling faster induction of and emergence from anesthesia.

Xenon-enhanced CT scanning in functional neuroimaging is based on the use of stable xenon gas, which is radiodense and lipid-soluble, as an inhaled contrast agent. The patient inhales a mixture of xenon, usually 26–33%, and oxygen for several minutes via a face mask. The inhaled xenon dissolves in the blood and passes into the brain parenchyma. CT scans can be acquired before, during, and after inhalation. Fast spiral CT has improved the capability of this technique.

Comparative studies

In a prospective randomized study in 21 patients following thoracic surgery xenon sedation (delivered via a closed circuit) was compared with a standard regimen of propofol plus alfentanil (3). Xenon sedation was very well tolerated and was not associated with any adverse physiological effects. In addition, there was extremely rapid recovery.

In a multicenter randomized study in 224 patients the hypothesis that xenon anesthesia would be associated with faster recovery than an established isoflurane based regimen, and be as effective and safe, was tested [4]. Patients who received xenon recovered much faster, and there were no more adverse effects than with the standard regimen.

The subjective, psychomotor, and physiological properties of subanesthetic concentrations of xenon have been studied in 10 volunteers (5). Xenon sedation was well tolerated and was not associated with any adverse physiological effects. In particular, there was no nausea or vomiting. It was preferred to sedation with nitrous oxide and was subjectively dissimilar (xenon was more pleasant).

Drug-Drug Interactions

In a prospective randomized study in 40 patients rocuronium neuromuscular block under xenon anesthesia (delivered via a closed circuit) was compared with a standard propofol regimen [6]. Xenon did not prolong neuromuscular block due to rocuronium.

References

1. Taber KH, Zimmerman JG, Yonas H, Hart W, Hurley RA. Applications of xenon CT in clinical practice: detection of hidden lesions. J Neuropsychiatry Clin Neurosci 1999;11(4):423–5.

2. Leclerc J, Nieuviarts R, Tavernier B, Vallet B, Scherpereel P. Anesthésie an xénon: du mythe à la réalité. [Xenon anesthesia: from myth to reality.] Ann Fr Anesth Reanim 2001; 20(1):70–6.

3. Bedi A, Murray JM, Dingley J, Stevenson MA, Fee JPH. Use of xenon as a sedative for patients requiring critical care. Crit Care Med 2003;31:2470–7.

4. Rossaint R, Reyle-Hahn M, Schulte am Esch J, Scholz J, Scherpereel P, Vallet B, Giunta F, Del Turco M, Erdmann W, Tenbrick R, Hammerle AF, Nagele P. Multicenter comparision of the efficacy and safety of xenon and isoflurane in patients undergoing elective surgery. Anesthesiology 2003;98:6–13.

5. Bedi A, McCarroll C, Murray JM, Stevenson MA, Fee JP. The effects of subanaesthetic concentrations of xenon volunteers. Anaesthesia 2002;57(3):233–41.

6. Kunitz O, Baumert J-H, Hecker K, Beeker T, Coburn M, Zuhlsdorff A, Rossaint R. Xenon does not prolong neuromuscular block of rocuronium. Anesth Analg 2004;99: 1398–401.

INJECTABLE ANESTHETICS–BARBITURATES

Methohexital

General Information

Methohexital is an ultrashort-acting barbiturate that is widely used in dental anesthesia because of its rapid onset and short duration of action.

Of 4379 dental patients who received methohexital, 6.7% experienced restlessness, 5.5% respiratory disorders (respiratory obstruction, hiccuping, laryngeal spasm, apnea, or sneezing), 1.1% venous complications, 1.0% delayed recovery, 0.5% excitation, 0.27% nausea and vomiting, and 0.2% other mild reactions (1). Pain at the site of injection occurs in up to 64% of patients; the addition of lidocaine 10 mg significantly reduced the incidence to 22% (2).

A selective inhibitor of neuronal nitric oxide synthase, 7-nitroindazole, prolonged the duration of methohexital-induced narcosis in rats (3). This finding is consistent with previous work showing potentiation of anesthetic agents by non-specific nitric oxide synthase inhibitors.

Organs and Systems

Cardiovascular

Vasodilatation and depressed myocardial contractility are possible hemodynamic consequences of high-dose methohexital anesthesia (4).

Respiratory

Rectal administration of methohexital, sometimes used for children with needle-phobia, can cause apnea, particularly if there are pre-existing nervous system abnormalities (SED-12, 242) (5).

Nervous system

Seizures are a possible but rare complication of methohexital (6); it is inadvisable to use it in a patient with a history of epilepsy.

References

1. McDonald D. Methohexitone in dentistry. Aust Dent J 1980;25(6):335–42.
2. Millar JM, Barr AM. The prevention of pain on injection. A study of the effect of intravenous lignocaine before methohexitone. Anaesthesia 1981;36(9):878–80.
3. Motzko D, Glade U, Tober C, Flohr H. 7-Nitro indazole enhances methohexital anesthesia. Brain Res 1998;788(1–2):353–5.
4. Todd MM, Drummond JC, Sang H. The hemodynamic consequences of high-dose methohexital anesthesia in humans. Anesthesiology 1984;61(5):495–501.
5. Yemen TA, Pullerits J, Stillman R, Hershey M. Rectal methohexital causing apnea in two patients with meningomyeloceles. Anesthesiology 1991;74(6):1139–41.
6. Rockoff MA, Goudsouzian NG. Seizures induced by methohexital. Anesthesiology 1981;54(4):333–5.

Thiamylal sodium

General Information

Thiamylal sodium is a short-acting intravenous barbiturate anesthetic.

Organs and Systems

Electrolyte balance

Severe hypokalemia occurred in a 14-year-old boy undergoing emergency aortic arch replacement under deep hypothermic cardiopulmonary bypass (1). He was treated with thiamylal by infusion, total dose 30 mg/kg, for persistent convulsive waves on his electroencephalogram. This caused his serum potassium concentration to fall to 1.6 mmol/l. The hypokalemia was resistant to potassium chloride infusion 80 mmol/hour, but responded to replacing the thiamylal infusion with midazolam. It was noted that there have also been reports of severe hypokalemia in brain-injured patients undergoing thiopental coma therapy.

Reference

1. Irita K, Kawasaki T, Uenotsuchi T, Sakaguchi Y, Takahashi S. Does barbiturate therapy cause severe hypokalemia? Anesth Analg 1998;86(1):214.

Thiopental sodium

General Information

Thiopental sodium, a barbiturate and one of the oldest anesthetics, still remains the first-choice induction drug for cesarean section (1).

Organs and Systems

Cardiovascular

Cardiovascular depression is a well-documented complication of thiopental. However, the plasma concentrations necessary to produce loss of corneal reflex and trapezius muscle tone were only minimally depressant to the heart (2). Problems can in any case be reduced or avoided by proper fluid administration before induction of anesthesia, as well as by cautious choice of dosage and administration in patients with uncompensated cardiac failure.

Surgery for cerebral artery aneurysms sometimes requires cardiopulmonary bypass and deep hypothermic circulatory arrest if they are to be operated on safely. During such bypass procedures patients with such aneurysms often receive large doses of thiopental, in the hope of providing additional cerebral protection. In 42 non-cardiac patients thiopental loading to the point of suppressing electroencephalographic bursts caused only negligible cardiac impairment and did not impede withdrawal of cardiopulmonary bypass; however, there were no data on patients with cardiac disease (3).

Sensory systems

Patients sometimes notice a taste of onions or garlic before they lose consciousness; the incidence of this sensation was 42% in 113 adult patients (4).

Endocrine

Thiopental given for cerebral protection after cardiac arrest to patients in intensive care caused altered thyroid function (5). Five patients received 5 mg/kg as a bolus followed by 3 mg/kg/hour for 48–72 hours. Free T3 concentrations fell dramatically in three of them and remained near normal in the other two. In those in whom T3 concentrations fell they returned to near normal on withdrawal of thiopental. Reverse T3 concentrations increased in these patients. Although the study was not controlled, the authors speculated that thiopental causes conversion of T3 to reverse T3, and that this can intensify the sick euthyroid syndrome that can occur after cardiac arrest.

Electrolyte balance

Life-threatening hyperkalemia after therapeutic barbiturate coma with thiopental has been described in three patients; it was fatal in one (6). All the episodes occurred after the withdrawal of thiopental. There have also been reports of severe hyperkalemia following hypokalemia related to prolonged thiopental coma [7].

- A 35-year-old woman with a history of tonic–clonic seizures gave birth to a healthy child at term, but 2 weeks later developed tonic–clonic seizures refractory to combined antiepileptic drug therapy [8]. She was mechanically ventilated and was sedated with midazolam, sufentanil, and thiopental (2–3 mg/kg/hour) for 84 hours, controlled by burst suppression on continuous electroencephalographic monitoring. After 2 days she developed symptoms of puerperal sepsis and underwent hysterectomy. During thiopental coma, she developed mild hypokalemia, which was treated with potassium 2–5 mmol/hour. The potassium infusion was stopped several hours before hysterectomy. Renal function was not compromised. A few hours later she developed a ventricular tachycardia, associated with a serum potassium concentration of 7.1 mmol/l. Despite treatment with insulin, glucose, calcium, and immediate hemofiltration, the hyperkalemia persisted, and she became asystolic and died.

It is unclear whether the rise in serum potassium in this case was related to rhabdomyolysis or some other effect. However, hypokalemia has previously been described after barbiturate coma, with hyperkalemia after withdrawal; hyperkalemia in such cases may therefore be a rebound effect. Clinicians may choose to manage asymptomatic barbiturate-induced hypokalemia expectantly in an attempt to avoid rebound hyperkalemia.

Hematologic

- Immune hemolytic anemia with acute renal insufficiency has been reported in a 55-year-old patient after induction of anesthesia with thiopental 450 mg; a specific thiopental antibody was detected; the patient recovered fully (9).

Gastrointestinal

Vomiting is common during many types of anesthesia (10). By reducing upper esophageal sphincter pressure during induction, thiopental can contribute to this complication (11).

Skin

Fixed drug eruptions after thiopental administration have been reported (12).

Immunologic

Anaphylaxis has been repeatedly reported after thiopental (SED-10, 190) (SED-11, 211), but is rare, with an estimated incidence of one in 30 000.

- An extreme example reported in 1993 involved a 55-year-old obese man with no history of allergy to penicillin, who had on earlier occasions received sodium thiopental without reaction; on this occasion he stopped breathing and had severe bronchial constriction and vascular collapse requiring prolonged resuscitation and mechanical ventilation (13).

Multiorgan failure

A syndrome with striking similarities to propofol infusion syndrome has been reported in association with thiopental [14].

- A 59-year-old man with a history of epileptic convulsions developed status epilepticus. Intravenous midazolam was ineffective and he was mechanically ventilated and given high-dose thiopental with continuous electroencephalographic monitoring. After 3 days he developed a fever, severe hemodynamic instability, and multiorgan dysfunction. He was given inotropic drugs in high doses, low-dose glucocorticoids, and renal replacement therapy. After 5 days, thiopental and midazolam were withdrawn. He died after 2 weeks with persistent cardiac failure, severe rhabdomyolysis, renal insufficiency, metabolic acidosis, and fulminant hepatic failure.

The clinical symptoms that led to this patient's death mimicked propofol infusion syndrome. The authors hypothesized that total suppression of cerebral activity by any sedative drug could lead to physiological compromise and development of a lethal syndrome resembling the propofol infusion syndrome. As observed in propofol infusion syndrome, which is usually associated with high-dose propofol infusion, very high dosages of thiopental were used as a sedative anticonvulsant regimen in this patient. Although rhabdomyolysis and renal insufficiency have been described as complications of status epilepticus (15), a toxic drug-related cellular effect in susceptible patients, possibly involving mitochondrial pathways, could provide an alternative explanation.

Second-Generation Effects

Fetotoxicity

A mother with eclampsia was unsuccessfully treated with diazepam, total dose 120 mg, and phenytoin 750 mg; she received thiopental and had an emergency cesarean section at 33 weeks gestation (16). The infant was unresponsive and floppy, requiring intubation and ventilation. At 10 hours after delivery a flumazenil infusion was begun; the baby responded with facial and limb movements within 30 seconds, resumed spontaneous ventilation, and was extubated 4 hours later. She was maintained on a slowly reducing flumazenil infusion over the next 4 days while the benzodiazepines were metabolized.

Susceptibility Factors

In one case, undetected congenital methemoglobinemia caused severe cyanosis during anesthesia with thiopental 500 mg and nitrous oxide 50% (17).

The use of thiopental or any other barbiturate is contraindicated in acute intermittent porphyria; a progressive neuropathy can occur and can be fatal.

Drug Administration

Drug administration route

Inadvertent injection into extravascular tissues causes pain, swelling, and possibly tissue necrosis. Pain on intravenous injection has been noted in 10% of patients (18). Intra-arterial injection causes vascular spasm and can cause gangrene of a distal extremity.

References

1. Celleno D, Capogna G, Emanuelli M, Varrassi G, Muratori F, Costantino P, Sebastiani M. Which induction drug for cesarean section? A comparison of thiopental sodium, propofol, and midazolam. J Clin Anesth 1993;5(4):284–8.
2. Becker KE Jr, Tonnesen AS. Cardiovascular effects of plasma levels of thiopental necessary for anesthesia. Anesthesiology 1978;49(3):197–200.
3. Stone JG, Young WL, Marans ZS, Khambatta HJ, Solomon RA, Smith CR, Ostapkovich N, Jamdar SC, Diaz J. Cardiac performance preserved despite thiopental loading. Anesthesiology 1993;79(1):36–41.
4. Nor NB, Fox MA, Metcalfe IR, Russell WJ. The taste of intravenous thiopentone. Anaesth Intensive Care 1996;24(4): 483–5.
5. Kotake Y, Matsumoto M, Takeda J. Thiopental intensifies the euthyroid sick syndrome after cardiopulmonary resuscitation. J Anesth 2000;14(1):38–41.
6. Cairns CJ, Thomas B, Fletcher S, Parr MJ, Finfer SR. Life-threatening hyperkalaemia following therapeutic barbiturate coma. Intensive Care Med 2002;28(9):1357–60.
7. Schaefer M, Link J, Hannemann L, Rudolph KH. Excessive hypokalemia and hyperkalemia following head injury. Intensive Care Med 1995;21:235–7.
8. Machata AM, Gonano C, Birsan T, Zimpfer M, Spiss CK. Rare but dangerous adverse effects of propofol and thiopental in intensive care. J Trauma 2005;58:643–5.
9. Habibi B, Basty R, Chodez S, Prunat A. Thiopental-related immune hemolytic anemia and renal failure. Specific involvement of red-cell antigen I. N Engl J Med 1985;312(6):353–5.
10. Vaughan GG, Grycko RJ, Montgomery MT. The prevention and treatment of aspiration of vomitus during pharmacosedation and general anesthesia. J Oral Maxillofac Surg 1992;50(8):874–9.
11. Vanner RG, Pryle BJ, O'Dwyer JP, Reynolds F. Upper oesophageal sphincter pressure and the intravenous induction of anaesthesia. Anaesthesia 1992;47(5):371–5.
12. Desmeules H. Nonpigmenting fixed drug eruption after anesthesia. Anesth Analg 1990;70(2):216–7.
13. Seymour DG. Anaphylactic reaction to thiopental. JAMA 1993;270:2503.
14. Enting D, Ligtenberg JJ, Aarts LP, Zijlstra JG. Total suppression of cerebral activity by thiopental mimicking propofol infusion syndrome: a fatal common pathway? Anesth Analg 2005;100:1864–5.
15. Guven M, Oymak O, Utas C, Emeklioglu S. Rhabdomyolysis and acute renal failure due to status epilepticus. Clin Nephrol 1998;50:204.
16. Dixon JC, Speidel BD, Dixon JJ. Neonatal flumazenil therapy reverses maternal diazepam. Acta Paediatr 1998;87(2):225–6.
17. Festimanni F, Orvieto A, Peduto VA. Metaemoglobinemia congenita come causi di cianosi durante l'anesthesia. Acta Anaesthesiol Ital 1980;31:601.
18. Kawar P, Dundee JW. Frequency of pain on injection and venous sequelae following the I.V. administration of certain anaesthetics and sedatives Br J Anaesth 1982;54(9):935–9.

INJECTABLE ANESTHETICS–NON-BARBITURATES

Alfadolone and alfaxolone

General Information

Alfadolone and alfaxolone are two steroid anesthetics that were used in combination, with the brand name Althesin. However, the mixture has been withdrawn because of safety considerations regarding the solvent used, polyethoxylated castor oil (Cremophor EL), which can cause non-IgE-mediated anaphylactic (anaphylactoid) reactions (SED-15, 1016) (1).

Reference

1. Anonymous. Glaxo discontinues Althesin. Scrip 1984;882:17.

Dexmedetomidine

General Information

The α_2-adrenoceptor agonist dexmedetomidine has potent sedative and analgesic-sparing properties. In therapeutic doses it does not cause respiratory depression, making it attractive for infusion sedation. However, it causes reduced sympathetic outflow, which might cause untoward hemodynamic upset but might also have beneficial β-adrenoceptor antagonist-like action in patients undergoing cardiovascular surgery.

Comparative studies

Dexmedetomidine has been compared with propofol in a prospective randomized open trial in 295 patients undergoing coronary artery surgery (1). Mean times to weaning and extubation were similar in the two groups, but fewer patients given dexmedetomidine remained on the ventilator beyond 8 hours postoperatively. Then use of morphine was significantly less in those who were given dexmedetomidine, only 28% of whom required morphine while being ventilated compared with 69% of propofol-treated patients (the latter also required four times the mean dose of morphine than the former). No patients who received dexmedetomidine had ventricular tachycardia, whereas 5% of propofol patients did. Significantly fewer patients who were given dexmedetomidine required β-adrenoceptor antagonists, antiemetics, non-steroidal anti-inflammatory drugs, adrenaline, and high-dose diuretics. Mean blood pressure fell by 3 mmHg relative to baseline in patients who were given dexmedetomidine and rose by 9 mmHg in those who were given propofol.

Reference

1. Herr DL, Sum-Ping STJ, England M. ICU sedation after coronary artery bypass graft surgery: dexmedetomidine-based versus propofol-based sedation regimens. J Cardiothorac Vasc Anesth 2003;17:576–84.

Etomidate

General Information

Etomidate, a non-barbiturate anesthetic, is considered to be safe, especially in patients with hemodynamic instability. The most common complications of using etomidate are venous sequelae, pain on injection (1), and involuntary muscle movements (SED-11, 211) (2).

Organs and Systems

Cardiovascular

The cardiorespiratory tolerance of etomidate is usually excellent (3), but cardiovascular instability has been described after a bolus dose (4).

Nervous system

In 104 patients, the frequency of pain on injection of etomidate was 32–53% and was severe in 5–20% of patients (5). The frequency of involuntary movements was 15–35%. The frequency of both pain and involuntary muscle movements was least when fentanyl 2.5 μg/kg was given before etomidate. There was no significant relation between pain and muscle movement. A medium-chain triglyceride and soya bean emulsion formulation has been used for anesthetic induction, in an attempt to reduce the unwanted adverse effects of pain on injection and thrombophlebitis (6).

Myoclonus has been noted, and can be dangerous in open eye surgery (7). Methods for preventing myoclonus have been assessed in two prospective placebo-controlled studies from the same group. In the first they assessed the effect of midazolam pre-treatment in 60 patients (8). Midazolam 0.15 mg/kg 90 seconds before induction of anesthesia with etomidate 0.3 mg/kg was significantly better than placebo in reducing the incidence of myoclonus. In the second study they assessed the effect of sufentanil 0.3 micrograms/kg pre-treatment in 40 patients; sufentanil abolished myoclonus completely (9).

Myoclonic movements and pain on injection are common during induction of anesthesia with etomidate. In a double-blind study in 100 patients in whom anesthesia was induced with etomidate, ketamine 0.2 mg/kg, ketamine 0.5 mg/kg, magnesium sulfate 2.48 mmol, or isotonic saline were used to prevent myoclonic muscle movements. Of the 25 patients who received magnesium sulfate, 19 did not have myoclonic movements after the administration of etomidate; ketamine did not reduce the incidence of myoclonic movements (10).

Etomidate produced activation of epileptiform activity, and electrographic seizures during craniotomy in epileptic patients (11). Generalized seizures were noted after etomidate induction in 20% of 30 patients without a history of epilepsy (12). Cerebral excitation can also occur after recovery from etomidate anesthesia, with potential respiratory disturbance (13,14). Caution should be exercised when giving etomidate to patients with a history of seizures (SEDA-18, 113).

When etomidate was given to 12 patients who had seizures of short duration during electroconvulsive therapy conducted previously under propofol anesthesia, mean seizure duration was significantly increased with etomidate anesthesia (15). However, there is no evidence that this observation is associated with an improved psychiatric outcome.

Endocrine

Etomidate inhibits adrenal function resulting in reduced steroidogenesis after administration of both single boluses and maintenance infusions (16). In a prospective cohort study of 62 critically ill patients who were mechanically ventilated for more than 24 hours, about half developed adrenal insufficiency on the day after intubation. Administration of a single intravenous dose of etomidate 0.2–0.4 mg/kg for intubation led to a 12-fold increased risk of adrenal insufficiency (17). Etomidate should therefore be avoided as an induction agent in critical illness, in particular in patients with septic shock, among whom the incidence of adrenal insufficiency is high (18,19,20).

Adrenocortical function has been assessed in a randomized trial after intravenous etomidate in 30 patients who required rapid-sequence induction and tracheal intubation (21). The controls received midazolam. Etomidate caused adrenocortical dysfunction, which resolved after 12 hours.

Cortisol and aldosterone concentrations were reduced by etomidate in adults (22,23), but the clinical relevance was minimal after a single bolus (24). A reduction in cortisol was reported 2 hours after delivery in 40 infants whose mothers received etomidate for cesarean section. There were also nine cases of severe to moderate hypoglycemia in this study, but the changes in blood glucose concentration were not significantly different from those in controls (25).

Hematologic

Hemolysis has been reported after the administration of etomidate (26). It may be related to the use of propylene glycol as a solvent (27,28).

Platelet hyperaggregability after general anesthesia has been reported in patients undergoing vascular surgery. The effect of etomidate and thiopental on platelet function has now been examined in 46 patients undergoing infrainguinal vascular surgery (29). Etomidate caused significant platelet inhibitory effects, whereas the effects of thiopental were minor. This may affect the choice of anesthetic in patients with compromised hemostasis.

Immunologic

Transient erythema has been described, but histamine release does not occur (30).

Etomidate is the induction agent of choice in atopic patients, in whom etomidate, fentanyl, and vecuronium comprise the safest combination of drugs for general anesthesia. However, non-allergic anaphylactic (anaphylactoid) reactions have been observed, even with this combination (31,32), and it can even be life-threatening; one patient also had a myocardial infarction (32).

Drug Administration

Drug formulations

An oral transmucosal formulation of etomidate, which is absorbed over 15 minutes, has been studied in 10 healthy adults at four doses: 12.5, 25, 50, and 100 mg (33). Dose-related drowsiness and light sleep occurred 10–20 minutes after administration. Peak serum concentrations and clinical effects were noted at about 20 minutes, with no clinical effect noticeable by 60 minutes. There was no vomiting and only four patients had transient nausea. Two patients had brief episodes of involuntary tremor with the 100 mg dose. Of note was the increasingly unpleasant taste with increasing dose and the apparent reduction in absorption with higher doses.

References

1. Kawar P, Dundee JW. Frequency of pain on injection and venous sequelae following the I.V. administration of certain anaesthetics and sedatives Br J Anaesth 1982;54(9):935–9.
2. Holdcroft A, Morgan M, Whitwam JG, Lumley J. Effect of dose and premedication on induction complications with etomidate. Br J Anaesth 1976;48(3):199–205.
3. Colvin MP, Savege TM, Newland PE, Weaver EJ, Waters AF, Brookes JM, Inniss R. Cardiorespiratory changes following induction of anaesthesia with etomidate in patients with cardiac disease. Br J Anaesth 1979; 51(6):551–6.
4. Price ML, Millar B, Grounds M, Cashman J. Changes in cardiac index and estimated systemic vascular resistance during induction of anaesthesia with thiopentone, methohexitone, propofol and etomidate. Br J Anaesth 1992; 69(2):172–6.
5. Korttila K, Tammisto T, Aromaa U. Comparison of etomidate in combination with fentanyl or diazepam, with thiopentone as an induction agent for general anaesthesia. Br J Anaesth 1979;51(12):1151–7.
6. Mayer M, Doenicke A, Nebauer AE, Hepting L. Propofol und Etomidat-Lipuro zur Einleitung einer Allgemeinanästhesie. Hämodynamik, Venenverträglichkeit, subjektives Empfinden und postoperative Übelkeit. [Propofol and etomidate-Lipuro for induction of general anesthesia. Hemodynamics, vascular compatibility, subjective findings and postoperative nausea.] Anaesthesist 1996;45(11):1082–4.

7. Berry JM, Merin RG. Etomidate myoclonus and the open globe. Anesth Analg 1989;69(2):256–9.

8. Schwarzkopf KRG, Hueter L, Simon M, Fritz HG. Midazolam pre-treatment reduces etomidate-induced myoclonic movements. Anaesth Intensive Care 2003; 31:18–20.

9. Hueter L, Schwarzkopf KRG, Simon M, Bredle D, Fritz HG. Pretreatment with sufentanil reduces myoclonus after etomidate. Acta Anaesthesiol Scand 2003;47:482–4.

10. Guler A, Satilmis T, Akinci SB, Celebioglu B, Kanbak M. Magnesium sulfate pretreatment reduces myoclonus after etomidate. Anesth Analg 2005;101(3):705–9.

11. Krieger W, Koerner M. Generalized grand mal seizure after recovery from uncomplicated fentanyl–etomidate anesthesia. Anesth Analg 1987;66(3):284–5.

12. Nickel B, Schmickaly R. Gesteigerte Anfallsbereitschaft unter Etomidatlangzeitinfusion beim Delirium tremens. [Increased tendency to seizures as affected by long-term infusions of etomidate in delirium tremens.] Anaesthesist 1985;34(9):462–9.

13. Parker CJ. Respiratory disturbance during recovery from etomidate anaesthesia. Anaesthesia 1988;43(1):16–7.

14. Hansen HC, Drenck NE. Generalised seizures after etomidate anaesthesia. Anaesthesia 1988;43(9):805–6.

15. Stadtland C, Erfurth A, Ruta U, Michael N. A switch from propofol to etomidate during an ECT course increases EEG and motor seizure duration. J ECT 2002;18(1):22–5.

16. Wagner RL, White PF, Kan PB, Rosenthal MH, Feldman D. Inhibition of adrenal steroidogenesis by the anesthetic etomidate. N Engl J Med 1984;310:1415–21.

17. Malerba G, Romano-Girard F, Cravoisy A, Dousset B, Nace L, Lvy B, Bollaert PE. Risk factors of relative adrenocortical deficiency in intensive care patients needing mechanical ventilation. Intensive Care Med 2005;31:388–92.

18. Jackson WL jr.. Should we use etomidate as an induction agent for endotracheal intubation in patients with septic shock? A critical appraisal. Chest 2005;127:1031–8.

19. Annane D. ICU physicians should abandon the use of etomidate!. Intensive Care Med 2005;31:325–6.

20. Morris C, McAllister C. Etomidate for emergency anaesthesia; mad, bad and dangerous to know? Anaesthesia 2005;60(8):737–40.

21. Schenarts CL, Burton JH, Riker RR. Adrenocortical dysfunction following etomidate induction in emergency department patients. Acad Emerg Med 2001;8(1):1–7.

22. Weber MM, Lang J, Abedinpour F, Zeilberger K, Adelmann B, Engelhardt D. Different inhibitory effect of etomidate and ketoconazole on the human adrenal steroid biosynthesis. Clin Investig 1993;71(11):933–8.

23. Varga I, Racz K, Kiss R, Futo L, Toth M, Sergev O, Glaz E. Direct inhibitory effect of etomidate on corticosteroid secretion in human pathologic adrenocortical cells. Steroids 1993;58(2):64–8.

24. Vanacker B, Wiebalck A, Van Aken H, Sermeus L, Bouillon R, Amery A. Induktionsqualität und Nebennierenrindenfunktion. Ein klinischer Vergleich von Etomidat-Lipuro und Hypnomidate. [Quality of induction and adrenocortical function. A clinical comparison of Etomidate-Lipuro and Hypnomidate.] Anaesthesist 1993;42(2):81–9.

25. Crozier TA, Flamm C, Speer CP, Rath W, Wuttke W, Kuhn W, Kettler D. Effects of etomidate on the adrenocortical and metabolic adaptation of the neonate. Br J Anaesth 1993;70(1):47–53.

26. Nebauer AE, Doenicke A, Hoernecke R, Angster R, Mayer M. Does etomidate cause haemolysis? Br J Anaesth 1992;69(1):58–60.

27. Wertz E. Does etomidate cause haemolysis? Br J Anaesth 1993;70(4):490–1.

28. Doenicke A, Nebauer AE, Hoernecke R, Angster R, Mayer M. Does etomidate cause haemolysis? In response. Br J Anaesth 1993;70:491.

29. Gries A, Weis S, Herr A, Graf BM, Seelos R, Martin E, Bohrer H. Etomidate and thiopental inhibit platelet function in patients undergoing infrainguinal vascular surgery. Acta Anaesthesiol Scand 2001;45(4):449–57.

30. Doenicke A, Hartel U, Buttner T, Kropp W. Anaesthesien für endoskopischdiagnostische Eingriffe unter besonderer Berücksightigung von Etomidate. In: Proceedings, 8th International Anaesthesia Postgraduate Course. Vienna: p.l. Egermann.

31. Fazackerley EJ, Martin AJ, Tolhurst-Cleaver CL, Watkins J. Anaphylactoid reaction following the use of etomidate. Anaesthesia 1988;43(11):953–4.

32. Moorthy SS, Laurent B, Pandya P, Fry V. Anaphylactoid reaction to etomidate: report of a case. J Clin Anesth 2001;13(8):582–4.

33. Streisand JB, Jaarsma RL, Gay MA, Badger MJ, Maland L, Nordbrock E, Stanley TH. Oral transmucosal etomidate in volunteers. Anesthesiology 1998;88(1):89–95.

Ketamine

General Information

Ketamine is a non-competitive antagonist at the phencyclidine site of the N-methyl-d-aspartate (NMDA) receptor for glutamate. However, its effects are also mediated by interactions with many others receptors. It is a short-acting anesthetic that has been widely used by emergency physicians (1) and can be given intravenously, intramuscularly, orally, and even nasally (2). Multiple ketamine anesthetics may be safe (3).

Ketamine was introduced as early as the 1960s, and is not generally used today as a general anesthetic, because of its adverse psychological effects, including delirium, disturbed dreaming, motor adverse effects, and emergence reactions in about 12% of patients. However, subanesthetic low-dose ketamine has been used for acute pain therapy, day-case surgery, and chronic pain management. Ketamine is available in chiral ($S+$ and $R-$) forms as well as the standard racemic form. S-ketamine has twice the analgesic potency of racemic ketamine and four times that of R-ketamine. Thus, low dose S-ketamine may avoid adverse effects while providing high-quality analgesia.

The pharmacology of ketamine, including its adverse effects, has been reviewed (4), as has the use and adverse effects of S-ketamine in the intensive care unit (5).

Ketamine relaxes smooth muscles in the airways and may therefore be a useful induction agent in children with asthma (6). If endotracheal intubation is required, lidocaine 1–2 mg/kg intravenously before intubation has been recommended, although the use of a laryngeal mask airway may be more appropriate. When used in combination with midazolam by infusion, ketamine provides analgesia and prevents and relieves bronchospasm (7).

Comparative studies

The addition of ketamine to bupivacaine for spinal anesthesia has been studied in 60 patients undergoing spinal anesthesia for insertion of intracavitary brachytherapy implants for cervical carcinoma (8). They were randomly assigned to receive either bupivacaine 10 mg or bupivacaine 7.5 mg plus ketamine 25 mg. Motor recovery was significantly quicker in the ketamine group. Blood pressure was significantly lower in the bupivacaine group 5 minutes after administration, and perioperative intravenous fluid requirements were significantly higher. Patients given ketamine reported more sedation and dizziness, both intraoperatively and postoperatively. There were no nightmares or dissociative features. Overall satisfaction was better with bupivacaine. The study was abandoned after 30 patients, because of the high rate of adverse effects with ketamine. Although ketamine had local anesthetic-sparing properties, its adverse effects made it unsuitable for intrathecal administration.

When added to standard doses of morphine and a nonsteroidal analgesic, S-ketamine 0.5 mg/kg had no additional benefit in a randomized, double-blind study in 30 patients undergoing anterior cruciate ligament repair (9).

Placebo-controlled studies

The effect of low-dose intravenous ketamine in combination with continuous femoral nerve block on postoperative pain and rehabilitation after total knee arthroplasty has been evaluated in a randomized placebo-controlled study (10). Those who received ketamine required significantly less morphine. No patients reported sedation, hallucinations, nightmares, or diplopia, and there were no differences in the incidence of nausea and vomiting between the two groups.

Systematic reviews

In a systematic review perioperative subanesthetic doses of ketamine reduced rescue analgesic requirements, pain intensity, or both in 27 of 37 clinical trials (2240 participants) (11–12). Ketamine reduced both 24-hour PCA morphine consumption and postoperative nausea and vomiting. Adverse effects were mild or absent.

Organs and Systems

Cardiovascular

Tachycardia and hypertension are common after anesthetic induction with ketamine, although the hypertension can be limited by the addition of diazepam (13). Nodal dysrhythmias can also occur (14). Because of possible reduced cardiac and pulmonary performance, ketamine should be avoided in critically ill patients (15). Pulmonary vasoconstriction and increased ventricular preload secondary to ketamine can be deleterious (16).

The effects of intramuscular premedication with either clonidine 2 micrograms/kg or midazolam 70 micrograms/kg on perioperative responses to ketamine anesthesia have been assessed in a placebo-controlled study in 30

patients (17). Clonidine significantly reduced intraoperative oxygen consumption, mean arterial pressure, and heart rate compared with midazolam and placebo. Thus, clonidine was as effective as midazolam, the standard drug used for this purpose, in reducing the undesirable sympathetic stimulation of ketamine.

Oral clonidine, 2.5 or 5.0 micrograms/kg, 90 minutes before ketamine 2 mg/kg has been compared with placebo in 39 patients (18). In those given clonidine 2.5 micrograms/kg, heart rate responses were reduced compared with placebo (maximum heart rate 97 versus 76 beats/minute). In those given clonidine 5 micrograms/kg, heart rate responses were less (maximum heart rate 97 versus 77 beats/minute) and mean arterial pressure was lower (121 versus 141 mmHg), and there were fewer nightmares and less drooling.

Angina pectoris has been reported with subanesthetic low-dose ketamine.

- Subcutaneous low-dose ketamine precipitated angina in an elderly man with metastatic bladder cancer and venous gangrene of a leg, in whom antianginal medication had been withdrawn (19).

Respiratory

Apnea occurred after the intramuscular injection of ketamine 4 mg/kg to sedate a healthy 4-year-old boy (20). This case illustrates the need for adequate monitoring and preparation for emergency airway management when using ketamine for sedation.

Nervous system

Ketamine causes a significant rise in cerebrospinal fluid pressure, increased electroencephalographic activity, and possibly epileptiform discharges (21). However, although ketamine has long been regarded as contraindicated in patients with, or at risk of, neurological damage, this view has been revised, with emphasis that there is evidence that ketamine does not increase intracranial pressure when used under conditions of controlled ventilation, co-administration of a gamma-aminobutyric acid (GABA) receptor agonist, and without nitrous oxide (22). Based on clinical, laboratory, and experimental results, ketamine may be safely used in patients with neurological damage. Ketamine may have neuroprotective effects, and S(+)-ketamine additional neuroregenerative effects, even when administered after the onset of a cerebral insult. Ketamine's hemodynamic effects may also improve cerebral perfusion and thereby influence outcome.

Delayed acute intracranial hypertension has been described after ketamine anesthesia (23).

Oral ketamine is an effective analgesic in patients with chronic pain. In 21 patients with central and peripheral chronic neuropathic pain treated with oral ketamine, the starting dose was ketamine 100 mg/day, titrated upward by 40 mg/day increments every 2 days until a satisfactory effect was achieved, or until adverse effects became limiting (24). Nine patients discontinued ketamine because of intolerable adverse effects, including psychotomimetic symptoms, such as "elevator" effect or dissociative feelings, somnolence or insomnia, and sensory changes such as taste disturbance and somatic sensations.

In a study of 21 outpatients with refractory neuropathic pain treated with oral ketamine, 17 reported adverse events (25). The most common were light-headedness, dizziness, tiredness, headache, a nervous floating feeling, and bad dreams. The adverse effects were sufficiently important to prevent ten patients from continuing with the trial.

Neurotoxicity due to focal lymphocytic vasculitis has been reported close to the catheter injection site in a patient who received intrathecal ketamine infusion for chronic cancer pain (26).

- A 72-year-old woman with abdominal pain due to peritoneal malignant mesothelioma was given patient-controlled analgesia with morphine and then a thoracic epidural infusion of bupivacaine 0.125% and morphine 0.04 mg/ml at a rate of 6–12 ml/hour, with minor success. A thoracic intrathecal catheter was inserted for infusion of bupivacaine 0.25% plus morphine 0.12 mg/ml at a rate of up to 3.5 ml/hour. The morphine concentration was increased to 0.3 mg/ml and then clonidine 3 micrograms/ml was added. Satisfactory pain relief was finally achieved by adding ketamine 1 mg/ml, containing benzethonium chloride as a preservative. The mean daily intrathecal dose of ketamine was 67 mg. After 7 days she had an acute psychotic reaction and the ketamine was withdrawn. There were no neurological deficits. She died 10 days later. There was focal lymphocytic vasculitis in the spinal medullary tissue, in the nerves, and in the leptomeninges of the thoracolumbar spinal cord.

This neurotoxicity could have been due to the preservative benzethonium chloride or the ketamine. However, several other agents, including bupivacaine, morphine, and clonidine, were also given intrathecally, so causality was not proven, even though the other agents have not been associated with this problem.

There have been several attempts to understand the pathophysiology of schizophrenia using subanesthetic doses of ketamine to probe glutaminergic function in healthy and schizophrenic volunteers; no long-term adverse consequences were attributable to ketamine (27).

Psychological, psychiatric

In a randomized, double-blind, crossover study of cognitive impairment in 24 volunteers who received S-ketamine 0.25 mg/kg, racemic ketamine 0.5 mg/kg, or R-ketamine 1.0 mg/kg, the ketamine isomers caused less tiredness and cognitive impairment than equianalgesic doses of racemic ketamine (28). In addition, S-ketamine caused less reduction in concentration capacity and primary memory.

A placebo-controlled study of low-dose ketamine infusion in ten volunteers showed formal thought disorder and impairments in working and semantic memory (29). The degree of thought disorder correlated with the impairment in working memory.

Subanesthetic low-dose ketamine is thought to cause delirium and disturbing dreaming. A systematic review of NMDA receptor antagonists in preventive analgesia has shown that only one of 20 studies documented adverse

psychotomimetic effects attributable to ketamine (30). In that study, ketamine was given by the epidural route in a relatively high dose.

The effects of ketamine 50 or 100 ng/ml on memory have been investigated in a double-blind, placebo-controlled, randomized, within-subject study in 12 healthy volunteers (31). Deleterious effects of ketamine on episodic memory were primarily attributable to its effects on encoding, rather than retrieval. The authors suggested that the effects they observed were similar to the memory deficits seen in schizophrenia and thus provide some support for the ketamine model of the disease.

Psychotomimetic effects

The psychotomimetic effects of ketamine, apart from encouraging illicit use, can lead to distressing psychic disturbances, particularly in children (16); there can be nightmares, delirium, and hallucinations (32). Oral ketamine is an effective analgesic in patients with chronic pain. In 21 patients with central and peripheral chronic neuropathic pain treated with oral ketamine, the starting dose was ketamine 100 mg/day, titrated upward by 40 mg/day increments every 2 days until a satisfactory effect was achieved, or until adverse effects became limiting (24). Nine patients discontinued ketamine because of intolerable adverse effects, including psychotomimetic symptoms, such as "elevator" effect or dissociative feelings, somnolence or insomnia, and sensory changes such as taste disturbance and somatic sensations.

The pharmacological effects of the R- and S-enantiomers of ketamine have been compared in 11 subjects who received R-ketamine 0.5 mg and then S-ketamine 0.15 mg, separated by 1 week (33). Before and after each drug administration they were subjected to a painful stimulus using a nerve stimulator applied to the right central incisor tooth. Pain suppression was equal with the two drugs. The subjects reported more unpleasant psychotomimetic effects with S-ketamine and more pleasant effects with R-ketamine. Seven of eleven subjects preferred R-ketamine, while none preferred S-ketamine. These results suggest that the neuropsychiatric effect of ketamine may be predominantly due to the S-enantiomer, and that R-ketamine may be a better alternative. This study is in direct distinction to earlier work suggesting that R-ketamine is responsible for most of the undesirable neuropsychiatric side effects of ketamine.

A placebo-controlled study in 10 healthy young men showed a linear relation between ketamine plasma concentrations of 50–200 ng/ml and the severity of psychotomimetic effects (34). The psychedelic effects were also similar to those observed in a previous study of dimethyltryptamine, an illicit LSD-25 type of drug, and were a function of plasma concentration rather than simply an emergence phenomenon. Clinically useful analgesia was obtained at plasma concentrations of 100–200 ng/ml. At plasma concentrations of 200 ng/ml, all subjects had lateral nystagmus. When ketamine is given in large doses, patients rapidly become unresponsive, and so the effects described in this study are usually only observed during the recovery phase.

There have been several attempts to understand the pathophysiology of schizophrenia using subanesthetic doses of ketamine to probe glutaminergic function in healthy and schizophrenic volunteers; no long-term adverse consequences were attributable to ketamine (27).

Prevention
There have been several attempts to attenuate the unpleasant psychological adverse effects that occur after sedation with ketamine.

Prior use of benzodiazepines or opiates limits the psychotomimetic effects of ketamine. There has been a double-blind, placebo-controlled study of the role of lorazepam in reducing these effects after subanesthetic doses of ketamine in 23 volunteers who received lorazepam 2 mg or placebo, 2 hours before either a bolus dose of ketamine 0.26 mg/kg followed by an infusion of 0.65 mg/kg/hour or a placebo infusion (35). The ability of lorazepam to block the undesirable effects of ketamine was limited to just some effects. It reduced the ketamine-associated emotional distress and perceptual alterations, but exacerbated the sedative, attention-impairing, and amnesic effects of ketamine. However, it failed to reduce many of the cognitive and behavioral effects of ketamine. There were no pharmacokinetic interactions between subanesthetic doses of ketamine and lorazepam.

The effect of intravenous midazolam 0.05 mg/kg on emergence phenomena after ketamine 1.5 mg/kg intravenously for painful procedures has been assessed in a randomized, double-blind, placebo-controlled study in 104 children (36). Midazolam was given 2 minutes after the ketamine. There was no significant difference between the two groups in levels of agitation. The overall rate of agitation was low, but probably high enough to detect any significant differences between the groups.

The neuropsychiatric effects of ketamine were modulated by lamotrigine, a glutamate release inhibitor, in 16 healthy volunteers (37). Lamotrigine 300 mg was given 2 hours before ketamine 0.26 and 0.65 mg/kg on two separate days. There were fewer ketamine-induced perceptual abnormalities, fewer schizophreniform symptoms, and less learning and memory impairments. Mood-elevating effects were increased with lamotrigine. The authors commented that the results were experimental and that further studies are needed to confirm the potential benefits in a larger group of patients.

The hypothesis that the unpleasant emergence phenomena that often accompany the use of ketamine, including odd behavior, vacant stare, and abnormal affect, would be reduced by the use of a selected recorded tape played during the perioperative period has been tested in 28 adults (38). The incidence of dreams was higher when the recorded tape was connected. This report emphasizes the current recommendations that a quiet room with minimal stimuli is best for reducing emergence phenomena after ketamine sedation.

Management
Benzodiazepines are often co-administered to attempt to manage emergence delirium and disturbing dreaming.

The optimal dose of diazepam to add to ketamine–fentanyl field anesthesia has been assessed in a randomized double-blind study in 400 patients from Vanuatu; the optimal dose was 0.1 mg/kg (39).

Endocrine

In a double-blind, randomized, placebo-controlled crossover comparison of the effects of ketamine and memantine in 15 male volunteers, ketamine increased serum prolactin and cortisol concentrations, whereas memantine and placebo did not (40).

Gastrointestinal

Ketamine is used as an oral premedication in many pediatric centers. Benzodiazepines are often co-administered. In an excellent randomized, double-blind study in 72 children from New Delhi the optimal dose of oral ketamine to add to midazolam in order to minimize adverse effects was assessed (41). The optimal regimen consisted of ketamine 3 mg/kg + midazolam 0.25 mg/kg. Excessive salivation was significantly more common in children who received the higher dose of 6 mg/kg.

Liver

Serum enzyme activities (alkaline phosphatase, aspartate transaminase, alanine transaminase, and gamma-glutamyl transpeptidase) were raised in 14 of 34 patients anesthetized with ketamine; the significance of this is unknown (42).

Long-Term Effects

Drug abuse

Media reports suggest that in some countries the nonmedical (illicit) use of ketamine has greatly increased (43,44). It is sold as a liquid or powder that can be injected, ingested, or added to materials for smoking. Its psychedelic effects usually dissipate within 1 hour, and repeated use is therefore common. Its acute pharmacological effects include tachycardia, increased blood pressure, impaired memory and cognitive function, and visual alterations. High doses can cause out-of-body or near-death experiences. Its toxic effects include hyperexcitability, severe agitation, and paranoid psychoses. Hyperthermia, seizures, rhabdomyolysis, and transient respiratory depression can occur. Physical dependence has not been reported.

Dopamine D_1 receptor availability has been assessed using positron emission tomography and the selective D_1 receptor radioligand $[^{11}]$-NNC 112 ((+)-5-(7-benzofuranyl)-8-chloro-7-hydroxy-3-methyl-2,3,4,5-tetrahydro-1H-3-benzazepine) in 14 chronic recreational users of ketamine and matched healthy subjects (45). Dorsolateral prefrontal cortex D_1 receptor availability was significantly up-regulated in chronic ketamine, confirming similar observations in animals. Prefrontal dopamine neurotransmission is important for working memory and executive functions.

Drug Administration

Drug administration route

The addition of ketamine to bupivacaine for spinal anesthesia has been studied in 60 patients undergoing spinal anesthesia for insertion of intracavitary brachytherapy implants for cervical carcinoma (8). They were randomly assigned to receive either bupivacaine 10 mg or bupivacaine 7.5 mg plus ketamine 25 mg. Motor recovery was significantly quicker in the ketamine group. Blood pressure was significantly lower in the bupivacaine group 5 minutes after administration, and perioperative intravenous fluid requirements were significantly higher. Patients given ketamine reported more sedation and dizziness, both intraoperatively and postoperatively. There were no nightmares or dissociative features. Overall satisfaction was better with bupivacaine. The study was abandoned after 30 patients, because of the high rate of adverse effects with ketamine. Although ketamine had local anesthetic-sparing properties, its adverse effects made it unsuitable for intrathecal administration.

Drug overdose

Chronic homicidal ketamine poisoning has been reported in a 34-year-old married woman with no previous medical history, who died in her own home (46). She had been chronically poisoned by her husband over about 1 year. There was cardiac muscle fibrosis and hyaline degeneration of the small cardiac arteries.

Drug–Drug Interactions

Alfentanil

The interaction of ketamine with the respiratory depressant effect of alfentanil has been studied in eight healthy men, who received alfentanil as a continuous computer-controlled infusion aiming at a plasma concentration of 50 ng/ml and either an infusion of racemic ketamine increasing step-wise through 50, 100, and 200 ng/ml or placebo (47). Alfentanil caused hypoventilation by reducing respiratory rate, and this was antagonized by ketamine in a concentration-dependent manner. This combination may be effective in overcoming the adverse effects of either agent individually.

Eight healthy men participated in a 2-day study in which alfentanil was given to a constant plasma concentration of 50 ng/ml followed by the addition of ketamine at escalating plasma concentrations of 50, 100, and 200 ng/ml (48). The resting hypoventilation induced by alfentanil was antagonized by ketamine 200 ng/ml, but not 50 ng/ml.

Atracurium dibesilate

Ketamine has been shown to prolong the action of atracurium slightly (49).

Haloperidol

The interaction of the dopamine antagonist haloperidol 5 mg orally with subanesthetic doses of ketamine has been studied in a placebo-controlled study in 20 healthy volunteers over 4 days (50). Haloperidol pretreatment reduced impairment of executive cognitive functions produced by ketamine and reduced the anxiogenic effects of ketamine. However, it failed to block the ability of ketamine to produce psychosis, perceptual changes, negative symptoms, or euphoria, and it increased the sedative and prolactin responses to ketamine. These results imply that ketamine may impair executive cognitive functions via dopamine receptor activation in the frontal cortex, but that the psychoactive effects of ketamine are not mediated via dopamine receptors, but rather via NMDA receptor antagonism.

References

1. Epstein FB. Ketamine dissociative sedation in pediatric emergency medical practice. Am J Emerg Med 1993;11(2):180–2.
2. Weksler N, Ovadia L, Muati G, Stav A. Nasal ketamine for paediatric premedication. Can J Anaesth 1993;40(2):119–21.
3. Murray Wilson A. Multiple ketamine anaesthesia. Saudi Med J 1979;1:19.
4. Kohrs R, Durieux ME. Ketamine: teaching an old drug new tricks. Anesth Analg 1998;87(5):1186–93.
5. Adams HA. The use of (S)-ketamine in intensive care medicine. Acta Anaesthesiol Scand 1998;42:S212–3.
6. Kremer M. What's new with reactive airways and anesthesia? CRNA 1995;6(3):118–24.
7. Jahangir SM, Islam F, Aziz L. Ketamine infusion for postoperative analgesia in asthmatics: a comparison with intermittent meperidine. Anesth Analg 1993;76(1):45–9.
8. Kathirvel S, Sadhasivam S, Saxena A, Kannan TR, Ganjoo P. Effects of intrathecal ketamine added to bupivacaine for spinal anaesthesia. Anaesthesia 2000;55(9):899–904.
9. Jaksch W, Lang S, Reichhalter R, Raab G, Dann K, Fitzal S. Perioperative small-dose S(+)-ketamine has no incremental beneficial effects on postoperative pain when standard-practice opioid infusions are used. Anesth Analg 2002;94(4):981–6.
10. Adam F, Chauvin M, Du MB, Langlois M, Sessler DI, Fletcher D. Small-dose ketamine infusion improves postoperative analgesia and rehabilitation after total knee arthroplasty. Anesth Analg 2005;100:475–80.
11. Bell RF, Dahl JB, Moore RA, Kalso E. Peri-operative ketamine for acute post-operative pain: a quantitative and qualitative systematic review (Cochrane review). Acta Anaesthesiol Scand 2005;49:1405–28.
12. Bell RF, Dahl JB, Moore RA, Kalso E. Perioperative ketamine for acute postoperative pain. Cochrane Database Syst Rev 2006;CD004603.
13. Zsigmond EK, Kothary SP, Kumar SM, Kelsch RC. Counteraction of circulatory side effects of ketamine by pretreatment with diazepam. Clin Ther 1980;3(1):28–32.
14. Cabbabe EB, Behbahani PM. Cardiovascular reactions associated with the use of ketamine and epinephrine in plastic surgery. Ann Plast Surg 1985;15(1):50–6.
15. Waxman K, Shoemaker WC, Lippmann M. Cardiovascular effects of anesthetic induction with ketamine. Anesth Analg 1980;59(5):355–8.

16. Tarnow J, Hess W. Pulmonale Hypertonie und Lungenödem nach Ketamin. [Pulmonary hypertension and pulmonary edema caused by intravenous ketamine.] Anaesthesist 1978;27(10):486–7.

17. Taittonen MT, Kirvela OA, Aantaa R, Kanto JH. The effect of clonidine or midazolam premedication on perioperative responses during ketamine anesthesia. Anesth Analg 1998;87(1):161–7.

18. Ward J, Standage C. Angina pain precipitated by continuous subcutaneous infusion of ketamine. J Pain Symptom Manage 2003;25:6–7.

19. Handa F, Tanaka M, Nishikawa T, Toyooka H. Effects of oral clonidine premedication on side effects of intravenous ketamine anesthesia: a randomized, double-blind, placebo-controlled study. J Clin Anesth 2000;12(1):19–24.

20. Smith JA, Santer LJ. Respiratory arrest following intramuscular ketamine injection in a 4-year-old child. Ann Emerg Med 1993;22(3):613–5.

21. Gardner AE, Dannemiller FJ, Dean D. Intracranial cerebrospinal fluid pressure in man during ketamine anesthesia. Anesth Analg 1972;51(5):741–5.

22. Himmelseher S, Durieux ME. Revising a dogma: ketamine for patients with neurological injury? Anesth Analg 2005;101:524–34.

23. Fontana M, Mastrostefano R, Pietrangeli A, Madonna V. Acute intracranial hypertension syndrome due to ketamine in a patient with delayed radionecrosis simulating an expansive process. J Neurosurg Sci 1980;24(2):93–8.

24. Enarson MC, Hays H, Woodroffe MA. Clinical experience with oral ketamine. J Pain Symptom Manage 1999;17(5):384–6.

25. Haines DR, Gaines SP. N of 1 randomised controlled trials of oral ketamine in patients with chronic pain. Pain 1999;83(2):283–7.

26. Stotz M, Oehen HP, Gerber H. Histological findings after long-term infusion of intrathecal ketamine for chronic pain: a case report. J Pain Symptom Manage 1999;18(3):223–8.

27. Lahti AC, Warfel D, Michaelidis T, Weiler MA, Frey K, Tamminga CA. Long-term outcome of patients who receive ketamine during research. Biol Psychiatry 2001;49(10):869–75.

28. Pfenninger EG, Durieux ME, Himmelseher S. Cognitive impairment after small-dose ketamine isomers in comparison to equianalgesic racemic ketamine in human volunteers. Anesthesiology 2002;96(2):357–66.

29. Adler CM, Goldberg TE, Malhotra AK, Pickar D, Breier A. Effects of ketamine on thought disorder, working memory, and semantic memory in healthy volunteers. Biol Psychiatry 1998;43(11):811–6.

30. McCartney C, Sinha A, Katz J. A qualitative systematic review of N-methyl-D-aspartate receptor antagonists in preventive analgesia. Anesth Analg 2004;98:1385–400.

31. Honey GD, Honey RA, Sharar SR, Turner DC, Pomarol-Clotet E, Kumaran D, Simons JS, Hu X, Rugg MD, Bullmore ET, Fletcher PC. Impairment of specific episodic memory processes by sub-psychotic doses of ketamine: the effects of levels of processing at encoding and of the subsequent retrieval task. Psychopharmacology (Berl) 2005;181(3):445–57.

32. Klausen NO, Wiberg-Jorgensen F, Chraemmer-Jorgensen B. Psychomimetic reactions after low-dose ketamine infusion. Comparison with neuroleptanaesthesia. Br J Anaesth 1983;55(4):297–301.

33. Rabben T. Effects of the NMDA receptor antagonist ketamine in electrically induced A delta-fiber pain. Methods Find Exp Clin Pharmacol 2000;22(3):185–9.

34. Bowdle TA, Radant AD, Cowley DS, Kharasch ED, Strassman RJ, Roy-Byrne PP. Psychedelic effects of ketamine in healthy volunteers: relationship to steady-state plasma concentrations. Anesthesiology 1998; 88(1):82–8.

35. Krystal JH, Karper LP, Bennett A, D'Souza DC, Abi-Dargham A, Morrissey K, Abi-Saab D, Bremner JD, Bowers MB Jr, Suckow RF, Stetson P, Heninger GR, Charney DS. Interactive effects of subanesthetic ketamine and subhypnotic lorazepam in humans. Psychopharmacology (Berl) 1998;135(3):213–29.

36. Sherwin TS, Green SM, Khan A, Chapman DS, Dannenberg B. Does adjunctive midazolam reduce recovery agitation after ketamine sedation for pediatric procedures? A randomized, double-blind, placebo-controlled trial. Ann Emerg Med 2000;35(3):229–38.

37. Anand A, Charney DS, Oren DA, Berman RM, Hu XS, Cappiello A, Krystal JH. Attenuation of the neuropsychiatric effects of ketamine with lamotrigine: support for hyperglutamatergic effects of N-methyl-D-aspartate receptor antagonists. Arch Gen Psychiatry 2000;57(3):270–6.

38. Lauretti GR, Ramos MBP, De Mattos AL, De Oliveira AC. Emergence phenomena after ketamine anesthesia: influence of a selected recorded tape and midazolam. Rev Bras Anesthesiol 1996;46:329–34.

39. Grace RF. The effect of variable dose diazepam on dreaming and emergence phenomena in 400 cases of ketamine-fentanyl anaesthesia. Anaesthesia 2003;58:904–10.

40. Hergovich N, Singer E, Agneter E, Eichler HG, Graselli U, Simhandl C, Jilma B. Comparison of the effects of ketamine and memantine on prolactin and cortisol release in men. a randomized, double-blind, placebo-controlled trial. Neuropsychopharmacology 2001;24(5):590–3.

41. Darlong V, Shende D, Subramanyam MS, Sunder R, Naik A. Oral ketamine or midazolam or low dose combination for premedication children. Anaesth Intensive Care 2004;32:246–9.

42. Dundee JW, Fee JP, Moore J, McIlroy PD, Wilson DB. Changes in serum enzyme levels following ketamine infusions. Anaesthesia 1980;35(1):12–6.

43. Hall CH, Cassidy J. Young drug users adopt "bad trip" anesthetic. Independent 1992;2:1.

44. Ricaurte GA, McCann UD. Recognition and management of complications of new recreational drug use. Lancet 2005;365(9477):2137–45.

45. Narendran R, Frankle WG, Keefe R, Gil R, Martinez D, Slifstein M, Kegeles LS, Talbot PS, Huang Y, Hwang DR, Khenissi L, Cooper TB, Laruelle M, Abi-Dargham A. Altered prefrontal dopaminergic function in chronic recreational ketamine users. Am J Psychiatry 2005;162(12):2352–9.

46. Tao Y, Chen XP, Qin ZH. A fatal chronic ketamine poisoning. J Forensic Sci 2005;50(1):173–6.

47. Persson J, Scheinin H, Hellstrom G, Bjorkman S, Gotharson E, Gustafsson LL. Ketamine antagonises alfentanil-induced hypoventilation in healthy male volunteers. Acta Anaesthesiol Scand 1999;43(7):744–52.

48. Persson J, Scheinin H, Hellstrom G, Bjorkman S, Gotharson E, Gustafsson LL. Ketamine antagonises alfentanil-induced hypoventilation in healthy male volunteers. Acta Anaesthesiol Scand 1999;43(7):744–52.

49. Toft P, Helbo-Hansen S. Interaction of ketamine with atracurium. Br J Anaesth 1989;62(3):319–20.

50. Krystal JH, D'Souza DC, Karper LP, Bennett A, Abi-Dargham A, Abi-Saab D, Cassello K, Bowers MB Jr, Vegso S, Heninger GR, Charney DS. Interactive effects of subanesthetic ketamine and haloperidol in healthy humans. Psychopharmacology (Berl) 1999;145(2):193–204.

Midazolam

General Information

Midazolam is used mainly in parenteral form in anesthesia, as a sedative adjunct to medical and dental procedures, and in status epilepticus (1). Its pharmacology and therapeutics have been extensively reviewed (2). It produces greater amnesia than diazepam, useful in terms of its anesthetic use, but carries a risk of cardiorespiratory depression and death (SED-12, 99), particularly at the extremes of age and when combined with the opioid fentanyl (SEDA-22, 42), which can cause accumulation of midazolam (see Drug–Drug Interactions in this monograph). Vomiting has been reported in 10% of children having midazolam sedation before radiology (SEDA-22, 41). Behavioral disinhibition (SEDA-18, 44), acute withdrawal, and hiccups appear to be relatively common (SEDA-22, 41); hallucinations, flumazenil-reversible dystonia, and hypersensitivity have all been observed (SED-12, 99) (SEDA-17, 44).

Observational studies

The pharmacology and adverse effects of midazolam in infants and children have been reviewed (3).

Clinical electrophysiological procedures can be very complex and prolonged, requiring safe and effective conscious sedation. A study in 700 patients has shown that intermittent midazolam plus fentanyl in electrophysiological procedures is safe and efficacious (4). All the staff were ACLS-certified and had successfully completed conscious sedation training courses, but none was an anesthetist; one team member was dedicated to monitoring conscious sedation and providing rescue defibrillation if required.

Midazolam has been carefully evaluated for adverse effects when used in critically ill infants and children; several difficulties, including prolonged obtundation and paradoxical behavioral and withdrawal reactions, have been noted (SEDA-19, 35) (5). Midazolam by the buccal route has been evaluated in children with persistent seizures; it was both effective and well tolerated (6), offering obvious practical advantages to rectal or parenteral administration. The availability of flumazenil, a specific benzodiazepine antagonist, to correct any adverse or overdose effects from injected midazolam should not encourage laxity in its use. Recent reports have highlighted kinetic interactions between midazolam and a variety of other drugs, and its effects can be magnified or prolonged in patients with hepatic or renal insufficiency (SEDA-20, 32).

Midazolam was used in a wide range of doses (0.03–0.6 mg/kg) in 91 children undergoing diagnostic or minor operative procedures with intravenous midazolam sedation (7). Opioids were co-administered in 84% and oxygen desaturation occurred in 32%, most of whom had received high doses of opioids in addition to the midazolam. Other adverse events included airway obstruction ($n = 3$) and vomiting ($n = 1$). The presence of independent appropriate trained personnel not directly involved in performing the procedure, appropriate resuscitation equipment, and monitoring were recommended whenever midazolam and opioids are co-administered for intravenous sedation.

A cherry-flavored midazolam syrup was evaluated for premedication in 85 children requiring general anesthesia (8). The patients received a randomly assigned dose of 0.25, 0.5, or 1 mg/kg. All clinicians and observers were blinded to the treatment group. There was satisfactory dose-related sedation in 81%, and 83% had satisfactory non-dose-related anxiolysis at separation from parents and at anesthetic induction. One or more adverse events occurred in 36%, but only 31% of these were judged as possibly related to midazolam (hiccups 6%, hypoxemia 6%, vomiting 5%, hallucinations 4%, drooling 4%, agitation 2%, coughing 2%, diplopia 2%, dizziness 2%, and hypotension 2%). The authors suggested that although adverse effects were common, they were minor.

In a 1-year retrospective survey of the use of intramuscular midazolam in a 30-bed acute inpatient general adult unit in Sydney, Australia, 212 doses of intramuscular midazolam were given, predominantly 5 mg (48%) or 10 mg (50%) (9). An antipsychotic drug was co-administered in 2.4%. Adverse effects were documented in eight episodes (3.8%), seven cases of excess sedation and one of urinary incontinence. None of the adverse effects required medical intervention.

In 27 children with refractory generalized convulsive status epilepticus, midazolam 0.2 mg/kg as a bolus followed by 1–5 (mean 3.1) micrograms/kg/minute as a continuous infusion achieved complete control of seizures in 26 children within 65 minutes (10). There were no adverse effects, such as hypotension, bradycardia, or respiratory depression. In one patient with acute meningoencephalitis, status epilepticus could not be controlled. Five patients died of the primary disorders, one with progressive encephalopathy.

Comparative studies

Intranasal midazolam 0.2 mg/kg and intravenous diazepam 0.3 mg/kg have been compared in a prospective randomized study in 47 children (aged 6 months to 5 years) with febrile seizures that lasted over 10 minutes (11). Intranasal midazolam controlled seizures significantly earlier than intravenous diazepam. None of the children had respiratory distress, bradycardia, or other adverse effects. Electrocardiography, blood pressure, and pulse oximetry were normal in all children during seizure activity and after cessation of seizures.

In a Canadian multicenter, open, randomized trial in 156 patients to determine whether sedation with propofol would lead to shorter times to tracheal extubation and length of stay in ICU than sedation with midazolam, the patients who received propofol spent longer at the target sedation level than those who received midazolam (60 versus 44% respectively) (12). Propofol allowed clinically significantly earlier tracheal extubation than midazolam (6.7 versus 25 hours). However, this did not result in earlier discharge from the ICU.

Comparative studies

In a randomized trial of intramuscular midazolam 15 mg (n = 151) or intramuscular haloperidol 10 mg plus promethazine 50 mg (n = 150) in agitated patients in three psychiatric emergency rooms, both treatments were effective (13). Midazolam was more rapidly sedating than haloperidol + promethazine, reducing the time people were exposed to aggression. One important adverse event occurred in each group; a patient given midazolam had transient respiratory depression, and one given haloperidol + promethazine had a generalized tonic-clonic seizure.

In a comparison of intranasal midazolam 0.2 mg/kg and intravenous diazepam 0.2 mg/kg in the treatment of acute childhood seizures in 70 children aged 2 months to 15 years with acute seizures (febrile or afebrile), the two drugs were equally effective and there were no significant adverse effects in either group (14). Although intranasal midazolam was as safe and effective as diazepam, seizures were controlled more quickly with intravenous diazepam.

In a multicenter, randomized controlled comparison of buccal midazolam and rectal diazepam for emergency-room treatment of 219 separate episodes of active seizures in 177 children aged 6 months and older with and without intravenous access, the dose varied with age, from 2.5 to 10 mg (15). The primary end point was therapeutic success—cessation of seizures within 10 minutes and for at least 1 hour without respiratory depression requiring intervention. The therapeutic response was 56% (61 of 109) for buccal midazolam and 27% (30 of 110) for rectal diazepam. When center, age, known diagnosis of epilepsy, use of antiepileptic drugs, prior treatment, and length of seizure before treatment were taken into account by logistic regression, buccal midazolam was more effective than rectal diazepam. The rates of respiratory depression did not differ.

Randomizes studies

In a double-blind, randomized, placebo-controlled study during coronary angiography in 90 patients, midazolam with or without fentanyl and local anesthesia provided better hemodynamic stability than placebo (16).

In a randomized study in 301 agitated or aggressive patients, intramuscular midazolam was more rapidly sedating than a mixture of haloperidol + promethazine (17). There was only one important adverse event, transient respiratory depression, in one of the 151 patients who were given midazolam.

Sevoflurane often causes postoperative delirium and agitation in children, and this may be severe. The effect of intravenous clonidine 2 µg/kg on the incidence and severity of postoperative agitation has been assessed in a double-blind, randomized, placebo-controlled trial in 40 boys who had anesthetic induction with sevoflurane after oral midazolam premedication (18). There was agitation in 16 of those who received placebo and two of those who received clonidine; the agitation was severe in six of those given placebo and none of those given clonidine.

The effect of a single bolus dose of midazolam before the end of sevoflurane anesthesia has been investigated in a double-blind, randomized, placebo-controlled trial in 40 children aged 2–7 years (19). Midazolam significantly reduced the incidence of delirium after anesthesia. However, when it was used for severe agitation, midazolam only reduced the severity of agitation without abolishing it.

In the presence of acute neurological injuries, midazolam produces a high risk of raised intracranial pressure (20), and the risk of airway obstruction (21) is a further concern.

Recovery after propofol or midazolam has been compared in two studies (22,23). Memory was significantly impaired by midazolam, an effect that was reminiscent of the problems experienced with short-acting oral benzodiazepine hypnotics, such as triazolam.

In a double-blind, randomized, placebo-controlled trial 130 patients were randomized to either midazolam 7.5 mg of orally (n = 65) or a placebo (n = 65) as premedication before upper gastrointestinal endoscopy (24). The median anxiety score during the procedure was significantly reduced by midazolam. Significantly more of those who took midazolam graded overall tolerance as "excellent or good" and reported a partial to complete amnesia response. Those who took midazolam were more willing to repeat the procedure if necessary. Midazolam significantly prolonged the median recovery time. There were no significant effects on satisfaction score or hemodynamic changes.

Organs and Systems

Cardiovascular

Midazolam is often used for conscious sedation during transesophageal echocardiography. In a prospective study of the effects of midazolam or no sedation in addition to pharyngeal local anesthesia with lidocaine on the cardiorespiratory effects of transesophageal echocardiography in patients in sinus rhythm midazolam (median dose 3.3, range 1-5 mg) caused significantly higher heart rates and significantly lower blood pressures and oxygen saturations (25).

Nervous system

Forty anxious day-case patients undergoing extraction of third molar teeth under local anesthesia with sedation, were studied in a randomized, double-blind, controlled trial (26). A target-controlled infusion of propofol was compared with patient-controlled propofol for sedation, combined with a small dose of intravenous midazolam (0.03 mg/kg) to improve amnesia. Five patients became over-sedated in the target-controlled group compared with none in the patient-controlled group.

The potential of intrathecal midazolam to produce symptoms suggestive of neurological damage has been investigated in a comparison of patients (n = 1100) who received intrathecal anesthesia with or without intrathecal midazolam 2 mg (27). Eighteen risk factors were evaluated with respect to symptoms representing potential neurological complications. Intrathecal midazolam was not associated with an increased risk of neurological symptoms. In contrast, neurological symptoms were increased in patients aged over 70 years and in those with a blood-stained spinal tap.

Psychological

In a placebo-controlled study of the effects of midazolam 0.5 mg/kg as a premedicant in 40 children aged 4-6 years having myringotomy, midazolam caused significant *amnesia* on a cued recall task (28). In addition, free recall for post-drug events was also impaired by midazolam, suggesting that benzodiazepine-induced amnesia occurs even for highly salient information.

Sedation, cognition, and mood during midazolam infusion in 20 volunteers with red hair and 19 with non-red (blond or brown) hair were studied in a randomized, placebo-controlled, cross-over design, to test the hypothesis that patients with red hair may require more drug to attain desired degrees of sedation (29). The red-haired volunteers had significantly greater alertness and lower drowsiness scores than non-red-haired subjects during midazolam infusion. Visuospatial scores were significantly higher in the subjects with red hair than in those with non-red hair during both placebo and midazolam trials. Delayed memory scores were significantly higher during midazolam infusion in subjects with red hair than in those with non-red hair. Midazolam appears to cause significantly less sedation and cognitive impairment in red-haired subjects.

Body temperature

Hypothermia is common during anesthesia, and adversely affects outcome. It primarily results from internal redistribution of body heat from the core to the periphery. Premedication with sedative agents can affect perioperative heat loss by altering core-to-peripheral heat distribution. This has been analysed in a prospective randomized study in 45 patients undergoing arthroscopic knee ligament reconstruction surgery (30). Heavy premedication caused initial hypothermia. Moderate premedication reduced perioperative heat loss. No premedication was associated with significantly lower intraoperative core temperatures than in sedated patients.

Drug-Drug Interactions

Pharmacokinetic and pharmacodynamic interactions of midazolam with fluoxetine, fluvoxamine, nefazodone, and ketoconazole have been investigated in 40 healthy subjects (31). The mean AUC of midazolam was increased 772% by ketoconazole and 444% by nefazodone. However, fluoxetine and fluvoxamine had no significant effects. Nefazodone and ketoconazole caused significant increases in midazolam-related cognitive impairment, reflecting changed midazolam clearance.

Midazolam is metabolized by CYP3A4, as is atorvastatin. In a matched-pair study the effects of long-term atorvastatin on the pharmacokinetics of midazolam 0.15 mg/kg intravenously as a single dose were studied in 14 patients undergoing general anesthesia for elective surgery (32). Atorvastatin significantly reduced the clearance of midazolam by 33% and increased the AUC by 40%.

References

1. Parent JM, Lowenstein DH. Treatment of refractory generalized status epilepticus with continuous infusion of midazolam. Neurology 1994;44(10):1837–40.
2. Lauven PM. Pharmacology of drugs for conscious sedation. Scand J Gastroenterol Suppl 1990;179:1–6.
3. Blumer JL. Clinical pharmacology of midazolam in infants and children. Clin Pharmacokinet 1998;35(1):37–47.
4. Pachulski RT, Adkins DC, Mirza H. Conscious sedation with intermittent midazolam and fentanyl in electrophysiology procedures. J Interv Cardiol 2001;14(2):143–6.
5. Hughes J, Gill A, Leach HJ, Nunn AJ, Billingham I, Ratcliffe J, Thornington R, Choonara I. A prospective study of the adverse effects of midazolam on withdrawal in critically ill children. Acta Paediatr 1994;83(11):1194–9.
6. Scott RC, Besag FM, Neville BG. Buccal midazolam and rectal diazepam for treatment of prolonged seizures in childhood and adolescence: a randomised trial. Lancet 1999;353(9153):623–6.
7. Karl HW, Cote CJ, McCubbin MM, Kelley M, Liebelt E, Kaufman S, Burkhart K, Albers G, Wasserman G. Intravenous midazolam for sedation of children undergoing procedures: an analysis of age- and procedure-related factors. Pediatr Emerg Care 1999;15(3):167–72.
8. Marshall J, Rodarte A, Blumer J, Khoo KC, Akbari B, Kearns G. Pediatric pharmacodynamics of midazolam oral syrup. Pediatric Pharmacology Research Unit Network. J Clin Pharmacol 2000;40(6):578–89.
9. Bradley N, Malesu RR. The use of intramuscular midazolaman acute psychiatric unit. Aust NZ J Psychiatry 2003;37:111–2.
10. Ozdemir D, Gulez P, Uran N, Yendur G, Kavakli T, Aydin A. Efficacy of continuous midazolam infusion mortality-childhood refractory generalised convulsive status epilepticus. Seizure 2005;14:129–32.
11. Wassner E, Morris B, Fernando L, Rao M, Whitehouse WP. Intranasal midazolam for treating febrile seizures in children. Buccal midazolam for childhood seizures at home preferred to rectal diazepam. BMJ 2001;322(7278):108.
12. Hall RI, Sandham D, Cardinal P, Tweeddale M, Moher D, Wang X, Anis AH. Propofol vs midazolam for ICU sedation: a Canadian multicenter randomized trial. Chest 2001;119(4):1151–9.
13. Huf G, Coutinho ESF, Adams CE, Borges RVS, Ferreira MAV, Silva FJF, Pereira AJCR, Abreu FM, Lugao SM, Santos MPCP, Gewandsznajder M, Mercadante VRP, Lange W Jr. Dias CI. Rapid tranquillisation for agitated patientsemergency psychiatric rooms: a randomised trial of midazolam versus haloperidol plus promethazine. BMJ 2003;327:708–11.
14. Mahmoudian T, Zadeh MM. Comparison intranasal midazolam with intravenous diazepam for treating acute seizureschildren. Epilepsy Behav 2004;5(2):253–5.
15. McIntyre J, Robertson S, Norris E, Appleton R, Whitehouse WP, Phillips B, Martland T, Berry K, Collier J, Smith S, Choonara I. Safety efficacy of buccal midazolam versus rectal diazepam for emergency treatment of

seizureschildren: a randomised controlled trial. Lancet 2005;366:205–10.

16 Baris S, Karakaya D, Aykent R, Kirdar K, Sagkan O, Tur A. Comparison of midazolam with or without fentanyl for conscious sedation and hemodynamics in coronary angiography. Can J Cardiol 2001;17(3):277–81.

17 TREC Collaborative Group. Rapid tranquillisation for agitated patients in emergency psychiatric rooms: a randomised trial of midazolam versus haloperidol plus promethazine. BMJ 2003;327(7417):708–13.

18 Kulka PJ, Bressem M, Tryba M. Clonidine prevents sevoflurane-induced agitation in children. Anesth Analg 2001;93(2):335–8.

19 Kulka PJ, Bressem M, Wiebalck A, Tryba M. Prophylaxe des "Postsevoflurandelirs" un Midazolam. [Prevention of "post-sevoflurane delirium" with midazolam.] Anaesthesist 2001;50(6):401–5.

20 Eldridge PR, Punt JA. Risks associated with giving benzodiazepines to patients with acute neurological injuries. BMJ 1990;300(6733):1189–90.

21 Montravers PH, Dureuil B, Desmonts JM. Effects of midazolam on upper airway resistances. Anesthesiology 1988;69:A824.

22 Atanassoff PG, Alon E, Pasch T. Recovery after propofol, midazolam, and methohexitone as an adjunct to epidural anaesthesia for lower abdominal surgery. Eur J Anaesthesiol 1993;10(4):313–8.

23 Crawford M, Pollock J, Anderson K, Glavin RJ, MacIntyre D, Vernon D. Comparison of midazolam with propofol for sedation in outpatient bronchoscopy. Br J Anaesth 1993;70(4):419–22.

24. Mui L, Teoh AYB, Enders KWN, Lee Y, Au Yeung ACM, Chan Y, Lau, JYW, Chung SCS. Premedication with orally administered midazolam in adults undergoing diagnostic upper endoscopy: a double-blind, placebo-controlled randomised trial. Gastrointest Endosc 2005;61(2):195–200.

25. Blondheim DS, Levi D, Marmor AT. Mild sedation before transesophageal echo induces significant hemodynamic and respiratory depression. Echocardiography 2004;21(3):241–5.

26. Burns R, McCrae AF, Tiplady B. A comparison of target-controlled with patient-controlled administration of propofol combined with midazolam for sedation during dental surgery. Anaesthesia 2003;58:170–6.

27. Tucker AP, Lai C, Nadeson R, Goodchild CS. Intrathecal midazolam I: A cohort study investigating safety. Anesth Analg 2004;98:1512–20.

28. Buffett-Jerrott SE, Stewart SH, Finley GA, Loughlan HL. Effects of benzodiazepines on explicit memory in a paediatric surgery setting. Psychopharmacology 2003;168:377–86.

29. Chua MV, Tsueda K, Doufas AG. Midazolam causes less sedation in volunteers with red hair. Can J Anaesth 2004;51:25–30.

30. Toyota K, Sakura S, Saito Y, Ozasa H, Uchida H. The effect of pre-operative administration of midazolam on the development of intra-operative hypothermia. Anaesthesia 2004;59:116–21.

31. Lam YWF, Alfaro CL, Ereshefsky L, Miller M. Pharmacokinetic and pharmacodynamic interactions of oral midazolam with ketoconazole, fluoxetine, fluvoxamine, and nefazodone. J Clin Pharmacol 2003;43:1274–82.

32. McDonnell CG, Harte S, O'DriscollJ, O'Loughlin C, Van Pelt FD, Shorten GD. The effects of concurrent atorvastatin therapy on the pharmacokinetics of intravenous midazolam. Anaesthesia 2003;58:899–904.

Propanidid

General Information

Propanidid was used as an intravenous anesthetic for rapid induction and for maintenance of general anesthesia of short duration. However, it was withdrawn because of safety considerations regarding the solvent used, polyethoxylated castor oil (Cremophor EL) (SED-15, 1016) (1).

Reference

1. Dye D, Watkins J. Suspected anaphylactic reaction to Cremophor EL. BMJ 1980;280(6228):1353.

Propofol

General Information

Propofol is a short-acting intravenous induction agent, which is dissolved in a mixture of long-chain triglycerides and soya bean emulsion. It is now in general use in day-care anesthesia and is being increasingly used in infusions in intensive care units. Recovery from anesthetic doses compares favorably with that after enflurane and isoflurane (1).

It has been claimed that propofol produces good recovery after anesthesia. A review of the literature has shown that, for operations that last under 30 minutes, propofol seems to give the best recovery, but for longer operations isoflurane gave better quality recovery (2).

Observational studies

Gastrointestinal endoscopy is one of the most common invasive procedures (for example, about 500 000 procedures per year in Australasia). Propofol is a short-acting intravenous anesthetic with a rapid onset of action, a short half-life, and very favourable recovery characteristics, making it particularly suitable for day procedures. However, the use of propofol by non-anesthetists has been controversial because of the perceived risks of its smaller therapeutic ratio.

The incidence of adverse events related to the use of propofol has been examined in three prospective audits of nurse-administered endoscopy sedation regimens that primarily used propofol.

In the first study, adverse events were assessed in 300 patients over 3 months in a unit that already had experience with 8000 patients (3). The patients were carefully monitored with clinical observation, pulse oximetry, automated sphygmomanometry, and sidestream capnography via a nasal cannula sampling device. All received supplementary oxygen at 2 l/minute. There were no episodes of apnea, and assisted ventilation was not necessary. There were short periods of hypoxemia (defined as an oxygen saturation below 90%) in 11 patients. Three patients required an increase in supplementary oxygen to 4 l/minute. Hypotension (defined as a mean arterial pressure below 50mmHg) occurred briefly in 22 patients. Two patients required a 500 ml infusion of isotonic saline. The authors concluded that propofol may be safely administered by non-anesthetists who are familiar with its pharmacological properties and use.

In the second publication, nurses trained by an anesthesiologist gave propofol to 9152 patients in a private ambulatory setting (4). There were seven cases of airway or ventilation problems (three of prolonged apnea, three of laryngospasm, and one case of aspiration requiring hospitalization), all with upper endoscopy. Five patients required face-mask ventilation, but none required tracheal intubation. Monitoring did not include capnography.

The third study examined 1435 elderly patients aged 70-85 years and 351 aged over 85 years who received propofol sedation over 17 months (5). Four patients (0.3%) required airway manipulations and two required face-mask ventilation. There was bradycardia requiring atropine in four patients (0.3%), and a heart rate below 50/minute in 72 patients (5.7%). There was hypoxemia (SaO_2 below 90%) in 52 patients (4.7%) and hypotension (systolic pressure below 90mmHg) in 162 (11%). Capnography was not used routinely. The authors concluded that nurse-administered propofol in elderly patients is as safe as in younger ones.

The safety and efficacy of propofol sedation by an emergency physician (a non-anesthetist) for painful procedures (mostly fractures and joint dislocation reductions) in 393 children has been examined (6). The children also received morphine 0.1 mg/kg and/or fentanyl 1-2 micrograms/kg. There was hypoxemia in 19 (5%), 11 (3%) needed airway manipulation, and three (0.8%) required face-mask ventilation. Hypotension was very common (92%) but only required treatment with intravenous fluid boluses in two children (0.67%).

Comparative studies

Propofol versus midazolam

A combination of midazolam plus propofol has been compared with midazolam only for sedation in colonoscopy (7). Midazolam alone produced less profound amnesia, and patients took longer to recover. There were no differences in cardiovascular or respiratory parameters. Oxygen saturation was poor in both groups, with saturations less than 85% in 22% of patients given midazolam and in 19% of patients given propofol, although the patients did not initially receive supplementary oxygen. In a similar comparison of midazolam and propofol as sedative agents for diagnostic endoscopy in 80 patients, endoscopy was judged successful in 98% of patients given propofol (mean total dose 354 mg) and 80% of patients given midazolam (mean total dose 8 mg) (8). Patients in the propofol group recovered consciousness more quickly and had complete amnesia. One patient in the propofol

group suffered an apneic phase with impaired circulation, requiring manual ventilation and drug therapy.

In a Canadian multicenter, open, randomized trial in 156 patients to determine whether sedation with propofol would lead to shorter times to tracheal extubation and length of stay in ICU than sedation with midazolam, the patients who received propofol spent longer at the target sedation level than those who received midazolam (60 versus 44% respectively) (9). Propofol allowed clinically significantly earlier tracheal extubation than midazolam (6.7 versus 25 hours). However, this did not result in earlier discharge from the ICU.

Anesthetist-administered midazolam and patient-controlled propofol have been compared for sedation during vitreoretinal surgery (10). The patients received propofol 15–18 mg according to age, with a 1-minute lockout, or 0.25–0.5 mg of midazolam as judged necessary by the anesthetist. Few patients were amnesic for the procedure and both techniques produced satisfactory sedation and comfort. Non-anesthetists need to be extremely wary if using propofol for sedation, since propofol has a low therapeutic index and commonly causes unconsciousness, respiratory depression, and cardiovascular collapse, particularly when it is used in combination with either midazolam or alfentanil (11). Adequate staff, training, and facilities for resuscitation of patients must be available before considering propofol sedation. Propofol can cause deep sedation, and the episode reported in one of these studies is not surprising. Extreme caution must be exercised in recommending these techniques to non-anesthetists.

Acute withdrawal syndromes, including agitation and prolonged weaning, are common after long-term sedation with midazolam. It has been proposed that the sequential use of propofol following midazolam may have advantages over midazolam alone, reducing adverse effects while preserving the potential benefits ("co-sedation"). A midazolam-propofol sequence has been compared with midazolam alone for sedation for long-term mechanical ventilation in a prospective, randomized trial in 26 patients (12). The time from stopping sedation to tracheal extubation was significantly shorter in the midazolam-propofol group (1.3 hours) than in the midazolam group (4.0 hours). Agitation occurred in only 8% of the midazolam-propofol group, but in 54% of the midazolam group.

Organs and Systems

Cardiovascular

Propofol is a cardiodepressant and resets the baroreflex setpoint, with a tendency to bradycardia (which occurs in some 5% of cases), hypotension (16%), or both (1.3%) (13). The hypotension may be brought about by peripheral vasodilatation, reduced myocardial contractility, and inhibition of sympathetic nervous system outflow (14). Four deaths due to cardiovascular collapse during induction have been reported in patients aged 78–92 years given propofol 1.1–1.8 mg/kg (15). The patients were of ASA classes 3 or 4.

Total intravenous anesthesia with propofol resulted in a reduced heart rate and a higher frequency of oculocardiac reflex bradycardia than thiopental/isoflurane anesthesia, with a higher sensitivity of children younger than 6 years in all groups (16).

Hemodynamic effects
The cardiovascular effects of propofol have been examined in a randomized trial in 40 healthy subjects using transthoracic echocardiography (17). Propofol was given to the same total dose (2.5 mg/kg) at two different rates, 2 mg/second or 10 mg/second. In both groups, global and segmental ventricular function was unchanged, but propofol caused a markedly reduced end-systolic quotient, presumably related to reduced afterload. With the higher infusion rate, there was a significant reduction in fractional shortening, thought to be related principally to reduced preload.

There has been a prospective, double-blind, controlled comparison of propofol, midazolam, and propofol + midazolam for postoperative sedation in 75 patients who received low-dose opioid-based anesthesia for coronary bypass grafting (18). Mean induction doses of propofol and midazolam used alone were 2.5 times higher than when both were used together. The single agents caused significant reductions in blood pressure, left atrial filling pressure, and heart rate after induction. These hemodynamic changes returned to normal after 15 minutes with midazolam and after 30 minutes with propofol, except for the bradycardia, which remained for the duration of the sedation. The combination of propofol + midazolam had no significant hemodynamic effects, but was also associated with bradycardia lasting the duration of the sedation. There was a greater than 68% reduction in maintenance doses with the combination. Propofol and propofol + midazolam were associated with comparable times to awakening and extubation, while with midazolam alone recovery was slower. This study clearly showed a reduction in adverse effects from exploiting the sedative synergism between propofol and midazolam.

In a placebo-controlled study of induction of anesthesia with a combination of propofol + fentanyl in 90 patients aged over 60 years, prophylactic intravenous ephedrine 0.1 or 0.2 mg/kg given 1 minute before induction of anesthesia significantly attenuated the fall in blood pressure and heart rate that is usually observed (19). Prophylactic use of ephedrine may be useful in preventing the occasional instances of cardiovascular collapse recorded after induction of anesthesia using these agents in elderly people.

The hemodynamic effects of combining ephedrine with propofol in an effort to prevent hypotension and bradycardia have been investigated in 40 elderly patients of ASA grades III and IV, who received ephedrine 15, 20, or 25 mg added to propofol 200 mg (20). The hypotensive response to propofol was effectively prevented, but marked tachycardia in the majority of patients meant that the technique may not be beneficial, given the high incidence of ischemic heart disease in this age group.

In a double-blind, randomized, placebo-controlled study of the effects of ephedrine 70 micrograms/kg and ketamine 0.5 mg/kg in 75 patients, both drugs attenuated hypotension caused by propofol (21).

The effects of giving calcium chloride 10 mg/kg after induction of anesthesia with propofol, fentanyl, and pancuronium have been investigated in 58 patients undergoing elective coronary artery bypass grafting (22). Calcium chloride reduced the fall in arterial blood pressure and prevented the reductions in heart rate, stroke volume index, cardiac index, and cardiac output, compared with placebo. Propofol reduces the availability of calcium to the myocardial cells, and calcium chloride effectively minimizes the hemodynamic effects of propofol. However, given that intravenous calcium can be locally toxic when given via peripheral veins, the technique may have limited applicability.

Cardiac dysrhythmias
Propofol causes bradydysrhythmias by reducing sympathetic nervous system activity.

- A four-year-old patient developed a nodal bradycardia while receiving propofol 6 mg/kg/hour + remifentanil 0.25 microgram/kg/minute (23). The bradycardia responded to atropine 0.3 mg.
- Complete atrioventricular heart block occurred in a 9-year-old boy with Ondine's curse who received a single bolus injection of propofol (24).

The authors questioned the safe use of propofol in congenital central hypoventilation syndrome, which is a generalized disorder of autonomic function.

- Propofol caused marked prolongation of the QT_c interval in a 71-year-old woman with an acute myocardial infarction who required ventilatory support (25). Substituting midazolam for propofol was associated with normalization of the QT_c interval. Rechallenge with propofol was associated with further prolongation. There were no malignant ventricular dysrhythmias.

Pain on injection
Propofol can cause severe pain on injection, especially when injected into a small vein (26); the incidence is 25–74% (27). Administration of the lipid solvent in which propofol dissolved has confirmed that the solvent is responsible for this adverse effect (28).

- Severe pain on injection of propofol occurred in a 36-year-old man with severe Raynaud's phenomenon, including a history of skin ulceration when he was given a 2% propofol + lidocaine mixture into a vein on the back of his hand (29).

The author suggested that selecting a larger antecubital vein might be a wiser choice in these patients.

The effectiveness of lidocaine in preventing pain on injection has been confirmed, and a concentration of 0.1% was optimal (30). The kallikrein inhibitor nafamostat mesilate was as effective as lidocaine.

A controlled study in 100 women showed that pretreatment with intravenous ketamine 10 mg reduced the incidence of injection pain from 84 to 26% of patients (31).

Warming propofol to 37°C had no effect on the incidence of pain (32,33).

The effects of different doses of ketorolac, with or without venous occlusion, on the incidence and severity of pain after propofol injection have been studied in a randomized, double-blind study in 180 patients (34). Pretreatment with intravenous ketorolac 15 mg and 30 mg reduced the pain after propofol injection. A lower dose of ketorolac 10 mg with venous occlusion for 120 seconds achieved the same effect.

Ondansetron, tramadol, and metoclopramide were less effective than lidocaine in preventing pain on injection (35–37). Ondansetron and tramadol have been compared in patients being given propofol in a randomized, double-blind study in 100 patients (38). Tramadol 50 mg intravenously was as effective as ondansetron 4 mg intravenously with 15 seconds of venous occlusion at preventing propofol injection pain. However, there was significantly less nausea and vomiting in those given ondansetron.

Respiratory

Respiratory depression due to propofol is well recognized; apnea can result, especially with rapid injection (39).

Pulmonary fat embolism after the use of propofol has been attributed to the milky emulsion in which the propofol was dissolved (40).

Two cases of propofol-induced bronchoconstriction have been reported (41). Both patients had allergic rhinitis and had taken antihistamines during the hay fever season, but were otherwise healthy.

Propofol is often the induction agent of choice in people with asthma, as it causes bronchodilatation.

- A 45-year-old woman with sick building syndrome developed bronchospasm after induction of anesthesia with propofol (42). She had taken oral aminophylline and inhaled fluticasone for 6 years and had a raised eosinophil count (17%). She received methylprednisolone 80 mg and aminophylline 125 mg preoperatively, but still went on to develop bronchospasm that eventually responded to sevoflurane. Four weeks later, she underwent intradermal skin tests that were negative for propofol, vecuronium, and other anesthetic drugs. Drug lymphocyte stimulation tests were weakly positive for propofol.

Sick building syndrome associated bronchial hyper-reactivity is thought to be due to volatile organic compounds such as formaldehyde, toluene and xylene. In this case it seems to have been exacerbated by propofol.

Nervous system

Mutism has been attributed to propofol total intravenous anesthesia.

- A 56-year-old otherwise well woman underwent femoral fracture surgery, awoke, and was extubated after obeying commands and opening her eyes spontaneously, but was unable to speak (43). Clinical examination, blood tests, and a CT scan were otherwise unremarkable. There was no evidence of cerebral infarction on repeat imaging. She made a spontaneous recovery after 11 days.

Dystonias

Dystonic movements induced by propofol occurred in a patient undergoing elective cardioversion (44). Benzatropine 2 mg intravenously terminated the abnormal movements. The authors also reviewed all other reports of abnormal movements after propofol.

- Acute dystonia has been reported in a 14-year-old girl after the administration of propofol 150 mg + fentanyl 50 mg for dental anesthesia (45). The intraoperative course was uneventful, but she developed non-rhythmic and non-symmetrical shaking in her upper limbs, unresponsive to diazepam and paraldehyde. A CT scan of the brain was normal. Her symptoms were eventually relieved by procyclidine 2.5 mg.

This adverse effect has been reported many times with propofol in adults, but rarely in children.

Seizures

Myoclonus and opisthotonos, especially in children (46), and choreoathetosis (47) have been attributed to propofol. However, in experimental studies propofol has been shown to be effective against drug-induced seizures (48,49). It has been suggested that propofol inhibits efferent inhibitory neurons in the midbrain and reticular activating system, producing movements that originate subcortically and in the spinal cord (50).

- An otherwise healthy 63-year-old man was anesthetized with propofol 2 mg/kg + fentanyl 1 micrograms/kg followed by an infusion of propofol 6 mg/kg/hour (51). Three minutes after induction he developed myoclonus in his legs. This continued for 10 minutes and the anesthetic was abandoned. When he awoke 10 minutes later, the myoclonus stopped. A repeat anesthetic with propofol soon after caused the same response. When the procedure was performed 12 days later under regional block with propofol infusion for sedation, the myoclonus recurred, and lasted for 2 hours. The patient was alert after each anesthetic and did not appear to be post-ictal. An MRI scan of the spinal cord was normal.

Myoclonus after propofol does not appear to be associated with an adverse outcome.

Myoclonic movements during induction of propofol anesthesia have been described in a 1-year-old boy undergoing adenotonsillectomy (52). Anesthetic maintenance, emergence, and neurological outcome were uneventful. Similar symptoms have been reported during emergence of a 14-year-old boy after propofol anesthesia for suturing of an upper limb laceration (53). Although the pathophysiological mechanisms are not known, it has been proposed that the seizure activity that occurs is subcortical in origin, as it is not related to electroencephalographic changes (54). Seizure activity has also been reported in a

78-year-old man who was given propofol and had no subsequent evidence of epileptic activity (55).

Convulsions have been reported in two patients with no history of epilepsy after induction of anesthesia with propofol (56). However, in a crossover comparison in 20 epileptic patients undergoing cortical resection, in which the effects on the electrocorticogram of either propofol or thiopental during isoflurane + nitrous oxide anesthesia were studied, propofol caused no greater proconvulsive effect than thiopental, which is used to treat status epilepticus (57). In spite of occasional reports, a true epileptogenic effect of propofol remains to be proven.

A generalized tonic–clonic seizure has been attributed to propofol in a patient with tonic–clonic seizures after surgery for subarachnoid hemorrhage (58).

Pain due to propofol injection

The most common adverse effect of propofol is pain on injection. It is particularly the case when propofol is injected into the small veins on the back of the hand, compared with the forearm or antecubital fossa. The incidence is 25–74%; in one series of 18 patients, mean age 46 years, to whom propofol was given into a vein in the back of the hand over 30 seconds, pain was reported in 10 cases (59).

The mechanism of propofol-induced pain is not known, but it is probably related to the concentration of aqueous propofol at the site of injection (see drug formulations below). Other proposed mechanisms involve the generation of bradykinin, although there are conflicting results (60) (61), and pH, since the addition of lidocaine reduces the pH of propofol solution (62).

Many strategies to prevent propofol-induced pain have been tried. It may be reduced by rapid injection (63). In 100 patients anesthesia was induced with propofol injected in a sterile ground-glass syringe at a rate of 10 ml over 10–15 seconds; only 16% complained of pain; of the 24 patients aged under 50 years, 33% complained of pain (64).

Warming propofol to 37°C has no effect on the incidence of pain (65) (66).

Effect of formulation

The effect of altering the lipid emulsion carrier in propofol formulations on pain after injection has been evaluated in several studies. In particular, a modified lipid emulsion of propofol containing a mixture of medium-chain and long-chain triglycerides (MCT/LCT; Propofol-Lipuro) has been compared with the usual formulation (LCT; Diprivan), which contains long-chain triglycerides only.

The effects of altering the lipid emulsion carrier have been analysed in two prospective randomized studies in 222 and 80 patients respectively, in which a modified lipid emulsion of propofol containing a mixture of medium-chain and long-chain triglycerides (MCT/LCT) was compared with the usual formulation, which contains long-chain triglycerides (LCT) only (67,68). MCT/LCT propofol was equivalent to LCT propofol with lidocaine

pretreatment. Lidocaine before MCT/LCT propofol confers an additional advantage.

In 130 adults randomly assigned to a propofol emulsion containing medium-chain triglycerides or a lipid-free formulation, the latter caused more pain on injection (69).

In a comparison of MCT/LCT propofol and LCT propofol in 60 healthy subjects there was significantly less pain with MCT/LCT (70). However, when MCT/LCT was given first there was no significant difference. The authors concluded that MCT/LCT propofol is associated with less injection pain than LCT propofol and also seems to attenuate subsequent injection pain of LCT propofol when administered first. The mechanism is unknown, but they suggested that it might be related to a reduction in the concentration of propofol in the aqueous phase.

In 80 adults the maximal intensity of propofol-induced local pain was significantly lower after MCT/LCT propofol than after LCT propofol (71).

In a randomized, double-blind comparison of MCT/LCT propofol and LCT propofol in 194 patients, the former produced a significantly lower incidence of moderate injection pain (11% versus 26%) (72). Similar results were reported in 200 adults in whom the mechanism of the pain was also sought; bradykinin concentrations were the same after the two types of formulations and the authors concluded that the pain was probably due to propofol in the aqueous phase (Ohmizo).

In a randomized double-blind comparison of MCT/LCT propofol and LCT propofol + lidocaine in 83 children undergoing day case surgery, the former was associated with significantly less pain (73).

In 75 patients the addition of lidocaine to MCT/LCT propofol further reduced the incidence of pain (74).

A lipid formulation ("Ampofor") that contains 50% less soybean oil and egg lecithin (5% and 0.6% respectively) has been compared with the most commonly available propofol formulations in two randomized studies in 63 and 60 patients respectively (75) (76). Ampofor was associated with an increased incidence of pain on injection.

Lidocaine Lidocaine is the most extensively studied treatment for propofol-induced pain (77) (78) and is usually used as a comparator for other compounds. It should be given about half a minute before the propofol or mixed with the propofol immediately before administration.

In a double-blind, randomized study in 310 patients undergoing anesthesia three doses of lidocaine were compared, 0.1, 0.2, and 0.4 mg/kg; the lowest dose significantly reduced the incidence of pain and there was no improvement when the dose was increased (79).

In 183 patients aged 15–65 years who were given propofol into a vein on the back of the hand, lidocaine was added to the solution before injection in concentrations of 0.05, 0.10, 0.15, and 0.20% and compared with saline in the same concentrations (80). Severe pain in those given lidocaine occurred in 11–30% compared with 35–67% in those given saline, and overall the incidence of pain was reduced significantly by lidocaine. However, there was no benefit in using lidocaine in a concentration above 0.05%, although in another study a 0.1% strength was optimal (81).

Intravenous lidocaine + prilocaine in 70 patients aged 19–65 years, given either separately or together, reduced the amount of pain produced by propofol (82).

Topical anesthesia using 60% lidocaine tape also reduces the incidence of propofol-induced pain (83) (84), but in a double-blind, randomized, placebo-controlled study in 90 patients, topical 5% lidocaine + prilocaine cream (Emla) was not effective, whereas the addition of lidocaine to propofol was (85). However, Emla was applied for only 1 hour before the administration of propofol, and there is evidence that longer exposure is required; in 65 propofol anesthetics in 28 children during lumbar puncture and/or bone marrow aspiration, application of Emla 4 hours before propofol was effective (86).

Alfentanil In 22 patients the pain caused by propofol was modified by a bolus intravenous dose of alfentanil 1 mg (87).

Dexamethasone In a randomized, placebo-controlled, double-blind study in 70 patients, 18–60 years of age, intravenous dexamethasone 0.15 mg/kg up to a maximum of 8 mg reduced the incidence of propofol injection pain significantly when it was given 1 minute before propofol (88). However, it was associated with perineal itching and pain in some cases.

Dexmedetomidine In a randomized, placebo-controlled comparison of the α_2-adrenoceptor agonist dexmedetomidine 0.25 micrograms/kg and lidocaine 0.5 mg/kg in 90 patients, both drugs reduced pain from propofol (89).

Glyceryl trinitrate Glyceryl trinitrate ointment applied to the back of the hand reduced the incidence of propofol-induced pain in a placebo-controlled study in 60 women (90). There was no pain in 18 of 30 women who were pretreated with glyceryl trinitrate compared with 10 of 30 women who were pretreated with placebo. There was moderate or severe pain in 11 of those treated with placebo compared with only one of those who were treated with glyceryl trinitrate. The pain occurred 10 seconds or more after the start of injection in more than half the subjects, and in more than half the patients the site at which the pain was felt was above the injection site. No patient had a headache or postural hypotension.

5HT3 receptor antagonists In a double-blind, randomized, placebo-controlled study in 150 patients, intravenous granisetron 2 mg was as effective as intravenous lidocaine 40 mg with 120 seconds of venous occlusion at preventing propofol-induced pain and significantly better than placebo (91).

In a double-blind, randomized, placebo-controlled study in 80 patients, ondansetron reduced propofol-induced pain (92). Ondansetron and tramadol have been compared in 100 patients being given propofol in a randomized, double-blind study (93). Tramadol 50 mg intravenously was as effective as ondansetron 4 mg intravenously with 15 seconds of venous occlusion at preventing propofol injection pain. However, there was significantly less nausea and vomiting in those given ondansetron.

Ketamine In a placebo-controlled study in 100 women, pretreatment with intravenous ketamine 10 mg reduced the incidence of propofol-induced injection pain from 84% to 26% of patients (94).

Metoclopramide In a randomized, double-blind, placebo-controlled study in 90 patients, the addition of metoclopramide improved the analgesic effect of lidocaine in patients given intravenous propofol (95). However, in another study metoclopramide was less effective than lidocaine (96).

Nafamostat In a double-blind, randomized, placebo-controlled study in 213 patients, nafamostat mesilate 0.02 mg/kg significantly reduced propofol-induced pain (97). Nafamostat is an inhibitor of bradykinin generation from kallikrein, and in another study the same authors found increased bradykinin concentrations after injection of the lipid solvent of propofol, an effect that was attenuated by nafamostat (Nakane). They suggested that the effect of bradykinin on the injected vein increases contact between aqueous propofol and the free nerve endings of the vessel.

Nitrous oxide In a randomized, double-blind study in 90 patients, 50% nitrous oxide in oxygen + lidocaine 40 mg mixed in 1% propofol 20 ml was compared with 50% nitrous oxide in oxygen without lidocaine and 50% oxygen in air + lidocaine (98). The combination of 50% nitrous oxide + lidocaine was the most effective treatment. A similar result was found in a randomized, double-blind study in 102 adults (99).

NSAIDs In 250 patients intravenous flurbiprofen 50 mg immediately before propofol injection completely abolished injection pain and was more effective than lidocaine; when flurbiprofen was given 1 minute before propofol injection it was less effective (100).

In a randomized, double-blind study in 180 patients pretreatment with intravenous ketorolac 15 mg and 30 mg reduced propofol-induced pain (101). A lower dose of ketorolac 10 mg with venous occlusion for 120 seconds achieved the same effect. However, in another study in 22 patients, ketorolac 30 mg given before propofol had no effect (Eriksson).

Remifentanil In 225 patients aged 19–73 years, remifentanil 0.25 or 1 micrograms/kg immediately before propofol, remifentanil 0.25 micrograms/kg 1 minute before propofol, and pethidine (meperidine) 40 mg immediately before propofol were compared with saline; remifentanil 1 micrograms/kg provided the most effective pain relief (102).

The effects of remifentanil on the incidence and severity of pain after propofol injection have been compared with those of lidocaine in a double-blind, randomized, placebo-controlled study in 155 patients (103). Pretreatment with intravenous remifentanil infusion 0.25 micrograms/kg/minute significantly reduced the pain after propofol injection. Lidocaine 40 mg achieved the same effect.

Thiopental In 90 women aged 15–34 years who were given propofol into a vein in the back of the hand, coinduction with thiopental reduced the severity of the pain but not its frequency (104). However, lidocaine reduced both the severity (to a greater extent than thiopental) and the frequency.

Tramadol Tramadol was less effective than lidocaine in preventing propofol-induced pain (105), but equivalent to ondansetron (Memis).

Conclusions Propofol-induced pain has been reviewed (106). The authors reached the following conclusions:

- guaranteed pain-free propofol injection is not possible;
- single preventive interventions are not as effective as combinations of different measures;
- the application of a venous tourniquet improves the pain-reducing effect of drugs such as lidocaine;
- a propofol MCT/LCT emulsion should be used;
- for general anesthesia opioids or ketamine can be used and for sedation a subanesthetic dose of thiopental;
- for children Emla cream (lidocaine + prilocaine) is suitable, because it reduces the pain of both propofol injection and venous cannulation (it should be applied for several hours before the administration of propofol).

Psychological, psychiatric

The association of propofol with a range of excitatory events is well recognized. Behavioral disturbances with repeated propofol sedation have been reported in a 30-month-old child (107). Propofol was well tolerated initially, but the child then became increasing irritable, aggressive, and uncooperative during awakening from subsequent sedations, including screaming, kicking, hitting, and biting. The next two sedations were performed using methohexital and were not followed by any behavioral disturbances.

Prolonged delirium after emergence from propofol anesthesia has also been reported (108).

A psychotic reaction has been reported (109).

- A 37-year-old man who had abused metamfetamine, paint thinner, psychotomimetic drugs, and alcohol for 20 years was given chlorpromazine, haloperidol, and flunitrazepam just before surgery. After spinal anesthesia he was given propofol 5 mg/kg/hour intravenously. However, euphoria and excitement occurred 10 minutes after the start of the infusion and he had excitement, hallucinations, and delirium. His symptoms were suppressed by intravenous haloperidol 5 mg.

The authors speculated that propofol may produce psychotic symptoms when it is used in patients with a history of drug abuse.

Hallucinations have been attributed to propofol in a 70-year-old man (110).

Metabolism

Hyperlipidemia

Five cases of hyperlipidemia have been reported in 12 patients who received propofol infusions 3–8 mg/kg/hour for 10–187 hours for sedation in an intensive care unit (111). Propofol was their only source of lipids.

Propofol 2% has been compared with midazolam for sedation in 63 ventilated patients in intensive care (112). They were randomly assigned to either propofol 1.5–6.0 mg/kg/hour or midazolam 0.10–0.35 mg/kg/hour. Sedation was considered a failure if greater rates were required or if triglyceride concentrations were over 5.7 mmol/l (500 mg/dl) on one occasion or greater than 4.0 mmol/l (350 mg/dl) on two occasions. Hemodynamic, respiratory, and neurological variables were similar. Sedation failure occurred in 15 patients given propofol, three with increased triglyceride concentrations and 12 with poor sedation. In comparison, sedation failed in only one of the patients given midazolam. Average serum triglyceride concentrations were higher in the propofol group. In a separate retrospective comparison, triglyceride concentrations were lower than in similar patients treated with 1% propofol, and the sedation failure rate was lower using 2% propofol (9 versus 36%). The authors concluded that 2% propofol is safe but may be less efficient than midazolam. It should be noted that the dose ranges that they used may not have been comparable, leading to an artificially high rate of failure to provide adequate sedation in the propofol group.

Propofol infusion syndrome

A constellation of clinical symptoms including rhabdomyolysis, metabolic acidosis, cardiac dysrhythmias, cardiovascular collapse, and death associated with long-term administration of propofol has been termed the propofol infusion syndrome. Although it was initially recognized in children, the propofol infusion syndrome is now known to occur in both children (113) (114) and adults (115).

Five fatal cases of propofol infusion syndrome have been reported (116,117):

- A 27-year-old woman developed a metabolic acidosis, hypotension, and bradycardia.
- A 64-year-old man developed a metabolic acidosis, hypotension, and rhabdomyolysis.
- A 24-year-old woman developed hypotension, metabolic acidosis, and bradydysrhythmias.
- Two men, aged 7 and 17 years, presented with refractory status epilepticus. Both were treated with high-dose propofol infusions to achieve burst suppression on the electroencephalogram. During the second day of propofol infusion there was progressive severe lactic acidosis, hypoxia, pyrexia, and rhabdomyolysis, followed by hypotension, bradydysrhythmias, and renal dysfunction, leading to death. The total doses of propofol were 1275 mg/kg over 2.7 days and 482 mg/kg over 2 days.

Lactic acidosis and rhabdomyolysis have been reported in a child receiving an infusion of propofol for sedation in an intensive care unit (118).

- A previously healthy 10-month-old boy with an esophageal foreign body was given endotracheal intubation to protect his airway. Midazolam and morphine did not produce satisfactory sedation and he was given propofol by infusion, increased from 3.5 to 7 mg/kg/hour over 2 hours to a total dose of about 500 mg/kg over the next 2 days. Other drugs given included cefotaxime, flucloxacillin, and ranitidine. He developed green urine, triglyceridemia of 907 mg/dl (10 mmol/l), and lactic acidosis, with a peak lactate concentration of 18 mmol/l. He also developed hypotension, with first-degree atrioventricular block and right bundle branch block, unresponsive to atropine, external cardiac pacing, or isoprenaline. Continuous venovenous hemofiltration was instituted. He slowly improved over the next 2 days, but developed a raised creatine kinase activity (over 30 000 U/l) and myoglobinuria. A liver biopsy showed 10% necrosis of zone 3, with fatty infiltration characteristic of a toxic effect. A muscle biopsy showed large areas of muscle necrosis. Extensive investigations showed no underlying infectious or metabolic causes. He slowly recovered over 10 days and appeared to have completely recovered at 3 months.

Lactic acidosis without rhabdomyolysis has been reported in another case (119).

- A 61-year-old woman undergoing mitral valve surgery received fentanyl, midazolam, nitrous oxide, and propofol infusion 3 mg/kg/hour during a 5-hour anesthetic. She developed lactic acidosis soon after the completion of surgery and required reintubation and ventilation. The peak lactate concentration, which occurred 1 day later, was 14.3 mmol/l. There was also mild disturbance of liver function. She eventually recovered.

These cases are important because, unlike previous reports of metabolic acidosis after propofol infusion, the patients had no documented infections and, in at least one case, extensive investigation showed no other causes of the acidosis. The role of propofol in causing the metabolic problems appears to have been more likely in these than in previous reports. In the first three cases the doses of propofol used, both per hour and in all, were extremely high compared with normal therapeutic practice. The subject has also been reviewed, and it was pointed out that, although suggestive, the association of fatal metabolic acidosis with propofol infusion in sick patients is as yet unproven and to date hinges on 11 case reports of patients who had multiple problems (120).

Propofol infusion syndrome may present with one component only, such as lactic acidosis (115) or rhabdomyolysis (121). Initially, it was thought to result from cumulative toxicity, with reports after high-dose infusion as well as after prolonged administration of lower doses. However, later reports suggested that it can occur even after short-term use and low-dose administration (122). It has been suggested that patients who are susceptible to metabolic acidosis or rhabdomyolysis after propofol administration may have subclinical forms of mitochondrial diseases that affect either the respiratory chain complex or fatty acid oxidation (123). In order to minimize the development of propofol infusion syndrome as a potentially lethal complication, a maximum dose of 3 mg/kg/hour has been recommended for sedation in intensive care patients.

- Severe lactic acidosis occurred in a 7-year-old child with osteogenesis imperfecta during short-term (150 minutes) propofol infusion anesthesia (mean infusion rate 13.5 mg/kg/hour) (124). The peak arterial lactate

concentration occurred 160 minutes after withdrawal of propofol (lactate 9.2 mmol/l, bicarbonate 16 mmol/l, base deficit 8.3 mmol/l). The hyperlactatemia settled within 18 hours.

The authors suggested that the combination of a prolonged preoperative fast and a high dose of propofol had contributed to the lactic acidosis. Osteogenesis imperfecta is also associated with malignant hyperthermia, but the temperature was not raised in this case.

Short-term, low-dose infusions are usually thought to be safe. However, two cases of isolated severe lactic acidosis in adults during short-term (6–7 hours) propofol infusion sedation and anesthesia (infusion rates 1.5–7.5 mg/kg/hour) have been reported (125,126). Lactic acidosis resolved on withdrawal of propofol. These two reports were accompanied by an editorial, in which anesthesiologists were advised to check arterial blood gases and lactate concentrations in the event of unexpected tachycardia during propofol anesthesia (127). The authors concluded that in adults propofol can occasionally produce cytopathic hypoxia by impairing the electron transport chain or fatty acid oxidation.

It has been proposed that the mechanism of propofol toxicity might be attributed to impaired fatty acid oxidation, causing increased concentrations of malonyl-carnitine and C5-carnitine. Disturbed fatty acid oxidation might be caused by impaired entry of long-chain acylcarnitine ester into mitochondria. This, in turn, may be due to effects of propofol on mitochondrial electron transport, which has been shown in animals (particularly in cardiac myocytes). Support for this theory has been obtained in an investigation of the stored serum of a 5-month-old child who developed life-threatening propofol infusion syndrome after a mean infusion rate of 11.7 mg/kg/hour for 62hours (128). The baby recovered after withdrawal of propofol, charcoal hemoperfusion, and continuous venovenous hemofiltration. Serum samples taken while the baby was critically ill showed increased concentrations of acetyl and hydroxybutyryl species, with generalized increases in fatty acylcarnitine intermediates, especially medium-chain unsaturated and dicarboxylic species. A follow-up sample taken when the child had recovered was entirely normal.

Propofol infusion syndrome might be precipitated by a combination of prolonged propofol infusion and carbohydrate intake insufficient to suppress fat metabolism. Support for this hypothesis has come from a case report of a child with catastrophic epilepsy who developed fatal propofol infusion syndrome after a ketogenic diet was introduced in an attempt to control severe intractable epilepsy (129).

- A 10-year-old child had status epilepticus controlled with a combination of valproate, oxcarbazepine, and 48 hours of propofol infusion in a dose of 5.5 mg/kg/hour. After weaning from propofol, a classic ketogenic diet was instituted in an attempt to provide long-term control of the seizures. A day later status epilepticus recurred and propofol was restarted at a rate of 6–9 mg/kg/hour to suppress seizure activity (the diet, valproate, and oxcarbazepine were also continued). Shortly thereafter, he developed the classical constellation of malignant ventricular arrhythmias, hyperlipidemia, rhabdomyolysis, lactic acidosis, and biventricular cardiac failure. He did not survive.

The use of extracorporeal cardiac support in the successful management of the cardiac failure associated with propofol infusion syndrome has been described (130).

- A 13-year-old boy underwent a 17-hour craniotomy in an attempt to resect an arteriovenous malformation with propofol-based anesthesia. He developed frank propofol infusion syndrome after 74 hours of postoperative propofol sedation in the neurosurgical ICU (used to manage intracranial hypertension). Echocardiography showed severe biventricular dysfunction despite extraordinary pharmacological support. Extracorporeal circulation with membrane oxygenation (ECMO) was instituted at the bedside via cannulation of the left femoral vessels. Hemofiltration was added to the circuit. ECMO was discontinued 60 hours later, as there was normal ventricular function on echocardiography. He made a full recovery and returned to school.

Several case reports have ascribed survival to the early use of hemofiltration, but this case shows that very aggressive invasive cardiovascular support can also be useful.

Hypertriglyceridemia

The frequency and severity of hypertriglyceridemia and pancreatitis have been studied in 159 adults in intensive care who were given propofol for 24 hours or longer (131). There was hypertriglyceridemia in 29 (18%), of whom six had a serum triglyceride concentration of 11 mmol/l or more; the median maximum serum triglyceride concentration was 8.0 (range 4.6–20) mmol/l. At the time when hypertriglyceridemia was detected, the median infusion rate of propofol was 50 (range 5–110) micrograms/kg/minute. The median time from the start of propofol therapy to identification of hypertriglyceridemia was 54 (range 14–319) hours. Pancreatitis developed in three of the 29 patients with hypertriglyceridemia.

Porphyria

An acute attack of porphyria has been reported in association with propofol (132).

- A 23-year-old man, with a past history of Fallot's tetralogy repaired at age 2, had catheter ablation of an aberrant conduction pathway causing right ventricular tachycardia, a procedure that took 16 hours. He was sedated with propofol at an average rate of 100 micrograms/kg/minute, and required intubation for respiratory insufficiency half way through the procedure. He also received caffeine and isoprenaline during the procedure to induce ventricular tachycardia. After the procedure he could not be roused or extubated for a further 10 hours and remained drowsy for a further day. He had weakness of an arm and a leg and had lancinating abdominal and shoulder pains. Urinary concentrations of porphyrins, aminolevulinic acid, porphobilinogen, and coproporphyrin III were markedly raised. He made a good recovery after administration of dextrose.

Propofol is regarded as being safe in patients with different types of porphyria. This is the first reported case in which propofol had a possible role in causing raised porphyrin concentrations perioperatively. However, severe illness can also precipitate porphyria, so the association with propofol may have been incidental.

Hematologic

In 10 patients, propofol, but not intralipos, its solvent, inhibited platelet aggregation both in vivo and in vitro (134). This defect was not associated with a change in bleeding time, and it was assumed that the effect is not clinically significant. The cause was probably suppression of calcium influx and release from platelets.

Fat emulsions affect coagulation and fibrinolysis (135). In a study of 36 patients undergoing aortocoronary bypass operations with midazolam + fentanyl or propofol + alfentanil anesthesia, factor XIIa concentrations and kallikrein-like activity were about 30% higher in the propofol group. The authors suggested that there had been stronger activation of the contact phase at the start of recirculation and stronger fibrinolysis in the propofol group. They also found more hypotension in the propofol group, which they assumed to be due to release of kallikrein, resulting in release of bradykinin. Propofol has not been shown to cause increased perioperative bleeding.

Gastrointestinal

Propofol in subhypnotic doses is a potent antiemetic. In a double-blind, randomized study, a small dose of propofol (0.5 mg/kg) was compared with droperidol (20 micrograms/kg) or metoclopramide (0.2 mg/kg) given at the completion of surgery performed in 90 patients under standard anesthesia with thiopental, fentanyl, and sevoflurane (135). Follow-up was to 24 hours. The incidence of emesis at 24 hours was significantly lower in those who received propofol (10 versus 33% and 40% for droperidol and metoclopramide respectively).

Liver

Hepatocellular injury has been reported after the sole use of propofol for outpatient anesthesia (136).

- A young woman with multiple allergies underwent femoral hernia repair and the next day developed acute hepatitis, with severe nausea and vomiting and diffuse abdominal tenderness. She had very high transaminase activities and the prothrombin time was slightly raised. No viral cause could be demonstrated. Antinuclear antibody and smooth muscle antibody titers were not raised and the ceruloplasmin concentration was normal. Abdominal ultrasound did not show gallstones or any other abnormality. The urine was normal and did not contain porphyrins or porphobilinogen. She recovered spontaneously and refused liver biopsy.

Pancreas

There have been several reports of postoperative pancreatitis in association with propofol-induced anesthesia

(137–139). In view of the very widespread use of propofol for induction of anesthesia, the very rare reports, and the complexity of establishing the cause of acute pancreatitis, a causal relation between propofol and pancreatitis has not been clearly established.

- A healthy 35-year-old man developed acute pancreatitis a few hours after receiving a 15-minute propofol anesthetic for laser treatment of a urethral stricture (140). He spent 3 weeks in an intensive care unit, requiring both respiratory and renal support. There was no evidence of gallstones on abdominal imaging. There was no defect of lipid metabolism.
- A 51-year-old woman with a past medical history of a seizure disorder, schizophrenia, and asthma, who had been admitted with pneumonia, was sedated using a propofol infusion to assist mechanical ventilation (141). Over 7 days she received a total of 26.5 g of propofol at a maximum rate of 0.2 mg/kg/minute. When pancreatitis, which was associated with hypertriglyceridemia, was diagnosed, the propofol infusion was stopped. In addition to raised amylase activity, serum triglyceride concentrations peaked at 17 mmol/l and lipase activity at 564 U/l. She recovered over the next 7 days. On day 17 she underwent tracheostomy revision, during which she received propofol 200 mg. The subsequent postoperative period was complicated by another episode of pancreatitis, this time without associated hypertriglyceridemia. She recovered over the next several days. An ultrasound examination ruled out gallstone pancreatitis, despite the presence of cholelithiasis.
- A healthy 21-year-old woman developed acute pancreatitis a day after an anesthetic that lasted 138 minutes, with propofol for induction (142). She recovered after supportive therapy for 6 days. There was no evidence of gallstones on abdominal imaging and there was no defect in lipid metabolism.
- A 12-year-old girl developed acute pancreatitis within hours after exposure to a single dose of propofol (143). In the context of two cases of pancreatitis due to propofol in young patients with Cushing's syndrome, it has been suggested that such patients may be at increased risk (144). Propofol is often the agent of choice in sedation of critically ill patients, particularly in neurological illnesses, as it allows rapid assessment on withdrawal.
- A 27 year-old woman with pneumococcal meningitis developed pancreatitis after sedation with propofol (145). This resolved slowly after withdrawal of propofol.

The association between propofol and pancreatitis has been listed as "probable" in 25 reports of pancreatitis associated with propofol to the FDA registry. However, the features of this case, which included resolution of pancreatitis on drug withdrawal and recurrence on rechallenge, suggested that the association should be upgraded to "definitely causal."

Skin

A fixed drug eruption has been attributed to propofol (146).

Musculoskeletal

In an in vitro experiment using uterine muscle strips from 10 consenting parturients undergoing cesarean section, therapeutic concentrations of propofol had no effect on isometric tension developed during contraction of the muscle (147). However, higher than therapeutic concentrations did reduce the peak muscle tension that developed. These results confirm that propofol is free of this adverse effect, which is a known cause of postpartum bleeding after the use of volatile anesthetic drugs.

Rhabdomyolysis

Rhabdomyolysis has been reported in two patients receiving propofol for sedation while being ventilated for severe asthma (148).

- A 47-year-old woman had an infusion of propofol 200 micrograms/kg/minute for 4 days. On day 2 she developed hematuria, and laboratory investigations showed renal insufficiency with hyperkalemic metabolic acidosis. She died as a result of rhabdomyolysis with cardiac involvement.
- A 41-year-old man, who received propofol at rates of up to 222 micrograms/kg/minute for 2 days, developed oliguria, and the propofol was withdrawn. He was also receiving fentanyl and low molecular weight heparin for prophylaxis of deep vein thrombosis. He subsequently developed a very high creatine kinase activity (over 170 000 IU/l). Echocardiography showed globally depressed myocardial dysfunction. He subsequently recovered. The rates of propofol infusion were high and this was thought to be a contributing factor.

A similar death, possibly relating to propofol, has been reported.

- An 18-year-old man suffered multiple trauma (149). He was sedated for 98 hours with propofol 530–700 mg/hour. On day 5 he developed a metabolic acidosis with hyperkalemia and his serum was lipemic. An echocardiogram showed global hypokinesia. He deteriorated and died shortly afterwards.

Although in none of these cases was a definitive link between propofol and the pathology established, the authors pointed out that several other cases have been reported, especially in children. Clinicians should be more aware that propofol may cause rhabdomyolysis, which appears to occur particularly at high doses.

Rhabdomyolysis and the propofol infusion syndrome

The propofol-infusion syndrome consists of a metabolic acidosis, rhabdomyolysis, and cardiovascular collapse. It occurs after prolonged infusion of propofol (over 48 hours) and has generally been reported in children, but also occasionally in adults.

Propofol infusion syndrome mimics the mitochondrial myopathies, in which there are specific defects in the mitochondrial respiratory chain. The clinical features of mitochondrial myopathy result from a disturbance in lipid metabolism in cardiac and skeletal muscle. These patients generally remain well until stressed by infection or starvation, although subclinical biochemical abnormalities of mitochondrial transport can be demonstrated. It has been suggested that early management of critically ill children may not include adequate calorific intake to balance the increase in metabolic demands, and that in susceptible children the diversion of metabolism to fat substrates may cause the propofol infusion syndrome. It is unclear if the dose or duration of propofol infusion alters this effect. As adults have larger carbohydrate stores and require lower doses of propofol for sedation, this may account for the relative rarity of the syndrome in adults. The authors suggested that adequate early carbohydrate intake may prevent the propofol infusion syndrome (150).

• Five adults with head injuries inexplicably had fatal cardiac arrests in a neurosurgical intensive care unit after the introduction of a sedation formulation containing an increased concentration of propofol (151). There were striking similarities with the previously reported syndrome of myocardial failure, metabolic acidosis, and rhabdomyolysis in children who received high-dose propofol infusions for more than 48 hours.

In a subsequent retrospective cohort analysis the odds ratio for the propofol infusion syndrome was 1.93 (95% CI = 1.12, 3.32) for every 1 mg/kg/hour increase in mean propofol dose above 5 mg/kg/hour. The authors suggested that propofol infusion at rates over 5 mg/kg/hour should be discouraged for long-term sedation.

• A 13-year-old girl with a head injury, who received a high-dose infusion of propofol for 4 days, developed the propofol infusion syndrome (152).

In an accompanying editorial, aspects of the propofol infusion syndrome were reviewed, and the author suggested that prolonged high-dose propofol infusions (over 4.8–6.0 mg/kg/hour for over 48–72 hours) should be avoided and that if high-dose metabolic suppression is required for more than 3 days in head injury, the alternative of a barbiturate should be considered (153). However, these long-acting agents have well-known potent myocardial depressant effects of their own, which are difficult to manage.

• A 2-year-old boy with a gunshot head injury developed the propofol infusion syndrome after receiving propofol in an average dosage of 5.2 mg/kg/hour for 72 hours (150). On the fourth day he became oliguric, with raised potassium, urea, and creatinine concentrations, and then developed a nodal bradycardia (28 minute). Propofol was withdrawn and an isoprenaline infusion was started, but only emergency transvenous pacing restored his heart rate. Hemofiltration was begun, on the basis of another case report, and the acidosis cleared and cardiovascular function was restored. In a blood sample taken before hemofiltration malonylcarnitine, C5-acylcarnitine, creatine kinase, troponin T, and myoglobinemia were raised. The child made a complete recovery and 9 months later all markers of fatty-acid oxidation were normal.

These findings are consistent with impaired fatty-acid oxidation: reduced mitochondrial entry of long-chain acylcarnitine esters due to inhibition of the transport protein (carnitine palmityl transferase 1) and failure of the respiratory chain at complex II. Another previously reported abnormality of the respiratory chain in propofol-infusion syndrome is a reduction in cytochrome C oxidase activity, with reduced complex IV activity and a reduced cytochrome oxidase ratio of 0.004. Propofol can also impair the mitochondrial electron transport system in isolated heart preparations.

During administration of propofol 3 mg/kg/hour, a 40-year-old man developed a fever of 41°C, resistant to diclofenac and physical cooling (154). Propofol was replaced by midazolam. His urine darkened and his urinary output fell and eventually ceased completely. His serum creatine kinase activity was 708 nmol/1 and his serum myoglobin concentration 4625 nmol/1. His serum creatinine rose from 130 to 480 µmol/1 during the next 12 hours and he developed hyperkalemia (5.9 mmol/1) and a metabolic acidosis. Histological examination of skeletal muscle showed vacuole formation and cytochrome oxidase-negative fibers. Biochemical examination of the muscle fibers showed an increased free carnitine concentration and NADH-CoQ-oxidoreductase activity.

Sexual function

Sexual illusions and disinhibition were a problem in two women (aged 20 and 47 years) after sedation with propofol (155).

Immunologic

True anaphylaxis to propofol has been observed (156).

Infection risk

Soon after the introduction of propofol in 1989, clusters of infections related to its use were reported, and there have since been several reports (157,158). The complications include hypotension, tachycardia, septic shock, convulsions, and death. Ethylenediaminetetra-acetic acid (EDTA) was added to the formulation to retard microbial growth. However, there have been concerns over the effects of this additive on trace element homeostasis, particularly when it is used in intensive care units for long-term sedation. Five randomized controlled trials have been reviewed, and minimal or no effects have been found on zinc, magnesium, or calcium homeostasis. However, there is no evidence to suggest that cluster infection has been or will be reduced with this formulation and there is still a need for care with sterility when using this product.

Long-Term Effects

Drug withdrawal

Excitation, including generalized tonic–clonic seizures, has been observed on withdrawal of a propofol infusion in intensive care (159).

Genotoxicity

Propofol negatively affects very early development (first cell to blastocyst stage) in the mouse embryo. Cytogenetic assay systems based on the detection of sister chromatid exchanges in peripheral blood T lymphocytes have been widely advocated as a sensitive screening method for assessing genotoxic potential. The formation of sister chromatid exchanges in mitogen-stimulated T lymphocytes from 40 children undergoing propofol infusion anesthesia for minor operations has been investigated (160). There was no evidence to support propofol-induced genotoxicity.

Susceptibility Factors

Age

Propofol has previously been associated with death after prolonged infusion in seriously ill children. An in vitro study of the effects of propofol on GABA neurons in a cell culture showed evidence of toxicity after exposure for 8 hours (161). The authors proposed that this toxicity could be the cause of the problems observed in children.

In 21 critically ill children aged 1 week to 12 years, who were also receiving morphine by infusion, propofol kinetics were altered in very small babies and in children of all ages recovering from cardiac surgery (162). Increased volume of distribution and reduced metabolic clearance caused a prolonged half-life. The combination of morphine 20–40 micrograms/kg and 2% propofol 4–6 mg/kg/hour for up to 28 hours appears to be safe.

Drug Administration

Drug formulations

The problems of formulating propofol have been reviewed (163). It was originally formulated in Cremophor EL, which was later replaced by 10% soybean oil because of non-IgE-mediated anaphylactic reactions. However, such formulations can cause injection pain, sepsis, and hyperlipidemia and this has led to the development of propofol emulsions with altered propofol and lipid contents, the addition of different excipients to emulsions for antimicrobial activity, and non-emulsion formulations including cyclodextrin and polymeric micelle formulations. In addition, propofol prodrugs have been evaluated. The effects of different formulations of propofol on injection pain are discussed above.

A lipid-free solution of propofol avoids bacterial contamination but is associated with a high incidence of thrombophlebitis (164) 1% solution in Intralipid 10% has been associated with hyperlipidemia, especially raised triglycerides, when given by prolonged infusion to the critically ill, particularly children or patients with liver disease (165). A formulation of propofol 6% in lipofundin (medium-chain + long-chain triglycerides 10%) has been developed to reduce the risk of hyperlipidemia. In 24 patients who received an induction dose of propofol 2.5 mg/kg over 60 seconds of either the new formulation

in 6% or 1% solution and of the original 1% formulation, the pharmacokinetics, induction time, dosage requirements, and safety profile of the three agents were similar. Pain on injection was reported by 17% of the patients, and did not vary between formulations. The 6% solution may be safer for long-term infusion, when reducing the fat load is important.

Drug-Drug Interactions

It has been suggested that seizures in a 48-year-old man who was given intravenous propofol were potentiated by concurrent therapy with baclofen (166).

References

1. Millar JM, Jewkes CF. Recovery and morbidity after day-case anaesthesia. A comparison of propofol with thiopentone–enflurane with and without alfentanil. Anaesthesia 1988;43(9):738–43.
2. Carpentier JP, Riou O, Petrognani R, Seignot P, Aubert M. Étude comparée du reveil après entretien de l'anesthésie par propofol ou isoflurane. Essai de synthese des données actuelles. [A comparative study of recovery following maintenance of anesthesia with propofol or isoflurane. An attempt to synthesize current data.] Cah Anesthesiol 1993;41(4):327–30.
3. Külling D, Rothenbuhler R, Inauen W. Safety of nonanesthetist sedation with propofol for outpatient colonoscopy and esophagogastroduodenoscopy. Endoscopy 2003;35:679–82.
4. Walker JA, McIntyre RD, Schleinitz PF, Jacobson KN, Haulk AA, Adesman P, Tolleson S, Parent R, Donnelly R, Rex DK. Nurse-administered propofol sedation without anesthesia specialists in 9152 endoscopic cases in an ambulatory surgery center. Am J Gastroenterol 2003;98:1744–50.
5. Heuss LT, Schnieper P, Drewe J, Pfilmin E, Beglinger C. Conscious sedation with propofol in elderly patients: a prospective evaluation. Aliment Pharmacol Ther 2003;17:1493–501.
6. Bassett KE, Anderson JL, Pribble CG, Guenther EG. Propofol for procedural sedation in children in the emergency department. Ann Emerg Med 2003;42:773–82.
7. Reimann FM, Samson U, Derad I, Fuchs M, Schiefer B, Stange EF. Synergistic sedation with low-dose midazolam and propofol for colonoscopies. Endoscopy 2000;32(3):239–44.
8. Jung M, Hofmann C, Kiesslich R, Brackertz A. Improved sedation in diagnostic and therapeutic ERCP: propofol is an alternative to midazolam. Endoscopy 2000;32(3):233–8.
9. Hall RI, Sandham D, Cardinal P, Tweeddale M, Moher D, Wang X, Anis AH. Study Investigators. Propofol vs midazolam for ICU sedation: a Canadian multicenter randomized trial. Chest 2001;119(4):1151–9.
10. Morley HR, Karagiannis A, Schultz DJ, Walker JC, Newland HS. Sedation for vitreoretinal surgery: a comparison of anaesthetist-administered midazolam and patient-controlled sedation with propofol. Anaesth Intensive Care 2000;28(1):37–42.
11. Bell GD, Charlton JE. Colonoscopy—is sedation necessary and is there any role for intravenous propofol? Endoscopy 2000;32(3):264–7.

12. Saito M, Terao Y, Fukusaki M, Makita T, Shibata O, Sumikawa K. Sequential use of midazolam and propofol for long-term sedation in postoperative mechanically ventilated patients. Anesth Analg 2003;96:834–8.

13. Hug CC Jr, McLeskey CH, Nahrwold ML, Roizen MF, Stanley TH, Thisted RA, Walawander CA, White PF, Apfelbaum JL, Grasela TH, et al. Hemodynamic effects of propofol: data from over 25,000 patients. Anesth Analg 1993;77(Suppl 4):S21–9.

14. Searle NR, Sahab P. Propofol in patients with cardiac disease. Can J Anaesth 1993;40(8):730–47.

15. Warden JC, Pickford DR. Fatal cardiovascular collapse following propofol induction in high-risk patients and dilemmas in the selection of a short-acting induction agent. Anaesth Intensive Care 1995;23(4):485–7.

16. Wilhelm S, Standl T. Bietet Propofol Vorteile gegeniiber Isofluran für die sufentanil-supplementierte Auästhesie bei kindern in des strabismuschirurgie?. [Does propofol have advantages over isoflurane for sufentanil supplemented anesthesia in children for strabismus surgery?.] Anasthesiol Intensivmed Notfallmed Schmerzther 1996;31(7):414–9.

17. Bilotta F, Fiorani L, La Rosa I, Spinelli F, Rosa G. Cardiovascular effects of intravenous propofol administered at two infusion rates: a transthoracic echocardiographic study. Anaesthesia 2001;56(3):266–71.

18. Carrasco G, Cabre L, Sobrepere G, Costa J, Molina R, Cruspinera A, Lacasa C. Synergistic sedation with propofol and midazolam in intensive care patients after coronary artery bypass grafting. Crit Care Med 1998;26(5):844–51.

19. Michelsen I, Helbo-Hansen HS, Kohler F, Lorenzen AG, Rydlund E, Bentzon MW. Prophylactic ephedrine attenuates the hemodynamic response to propofol in elderly female patients. Anesth Analg 1998;86(3):477–81.

20. Gamlin F, Freeman J, Winslow L, Berridge J, Vucevic M. The haemodynamic effects of propofol in combination with ephedrine in elderly patients (ASA groups 3 and 4). Anaesth Intensive Care 1999;27(5):477–80.

21. Ozkoak I, Altunkaya H, Ozer Y, Ayoglu H, Demirel CB, Ciek E. Comparison of ephedrine and ketamine in prevention of injection pain and hypotension due to propofol induction. Eur J Anaesthesiol 2005;22(1):44–8.

22. Tritapepe L, Voci P, Marino P, Cogliati AA, Rossi A, Bottari B, Di Marco P, Menichetti A. Calcium chloride minimizes the hemodynamic effects of propofol in patients undergoing coronary artery bypass grafting. J Cardiothorac Vasc Anesth 1999;13(2):150–3.

23. Bagshaw O. TIVA with propofol and remifentanil. Anaesthesia 1999;54(5):501–2.

24. Sochala C, Deenen D, Ville A, Govaerts MJ. Heart block following propofol in a child. Paediatr. Anaesth 1999;9(4):349–51.

25. Sakabe M, Fujiki A, Inoue H. Propofol induced marked prolongation of QT interval in a patient with acute myocardial infarction. Anesthesiology 2002;97(1):265–6.

26. Tan CH, Onsiong MK. Pain on injection of propofol. Anaesthesia 1998;53(5):468–76.

27. Sear JW, Jewkes C, Wanigasekera V. Hemodynamic effects during induction, laryngoscopy, and intubation with eltanolone (5 beta-pregnanolone) or propofol. A study in ASA I and II patients. J Clin Anesth 1995;7(2):126–31.

28. Nakane M, Iwama H. A potential mechanism of propofol-induced pain on injection based on studies using nafamostat mesilate. Br J Anaesth 1999;83(3):397–404.

29. Gilston A. Raynaud's phenomenon and propofol. Anaesthesia 1999;54(3):307.

30. Ho CM, Tsou MY, Sun MS, Chu CC, Lee TY. The optimal effective concentration of lidocaine to reduce pain on injection of propofol. J Clin Anesth 1999;11(4):296–300.

31. Tan CH, Onsiong MK, Kua SW. The effect of ketamine pretreatment on propofol injection pain in 100 women. Anaesthesia 1998;53(3):302–5.

32. Uda R, Kadono N, Otsuka M, Shimizu S, Mori H. Strict temperature control has no effect on injection pain with propofol. Anesthesiology 1999;91(2):591–2.

33. Ozturk E, Izdes S, Babacan A, Kaya K. Temperature of propofol does not reduce the incidence of injection pain. Anesthesiology 1998;89(4):1041.

34. Huang YW, Buerkle H, Lee TH, Lu CY, Lin CR, Lin SH, Chou AK, Muhammad R, Yang LC. Effect of pretreatment with ketorolac on propofol injection pain. Acta Anaesthesiol Scand 2002;46(8):1021–4.

35. Ambesh SP, Dubey PK, Sinha PK. Ondansetron pretreatment to alleviate pain on propofol injection: a randomized, controlled, double-blinded study. Anesth Analg 1999;89(1):197–9.

36. Pang WW, Huang PY, Chang DP, Huang MH. The peripheral analgesic effect of tramadol in reducing propofol injection pain: a comparison with lidocaine. Reg Anesth Pain Med 1999;24(3):246–9.

37. Mok MS, Pang WW, Hwang MH. The analgesic effect of tramadol, metoclopramide, meperidine and lidocaine in ameliorating propofol injection pain: a comparative study. J Anaesthesiol Clin Pharmacol 1999;15:37–42.

38. Memis D, Turan A, Karamanlioglu B, Kaya G, Pamukcu Z. The prevention of propofol injection pain by tramadol or ondansetron. Eur J Anaesthesiol 2002;19(1):47–51.

39. Gillies GW, Lees NW. The effects of speed of injection on induction with propofol. A comparison with etomidate. Anaesthesia 1989;44(5):386–8.

40. el-Ebiary M, Torres A, Ramirez J, Xaubet A, Rodriguez-Roisin R. Lipid deposition during the long-term infusion of propofol. Crit Care Med 1995;23(11):1928–30.

41. Nishiyama T, Hanaoka K. Propofol-induced bronchoconstriction: two case reports. Anesth Analg 2001;93(3):645–6.

42. Hattori J, Fujimura N, Kanaya N, Okazaki K, Namiki A. Bronchospasm induced by propofol in a patient with sick house syndrome. Anesth Analg 2003;96:163–4.

43. Kati I, Demirel CB, Anlar O, Huseyinoglu UA, Silay E, Elcicek K. An unusual complication of total intravenous anesthesia: mutism. Anesth Analg 2003;96:168–70.

44. Schramm BM, Orser BA. Dystonic reaction to propofol attenuated by benztropine (Cogentin). Anesth Analg 2002;94(5):1237–40.

45. Bragonier R, Bartle D, Langton-Hewer S. Acute dystonia in a 14-yr-old following propofol and fentanyl anaesthesia. Br J Anaesth 2000;84(6):828–9.

46. Saunders PR, Harris MN. Opisthotonus and other unusual neurological sequelae after outpatient anaesthesia. Anaesthesia 1990;45(7):552–7.

47. McHugh P. Acute choreoathetoid reaction to propofol. Anaesthesia 1991;46(5):425.

48. Hasan MM, Hasan ZA, al-Hader AF, Takrouri MS. The anticonvulsant effects of propofol, diazepam, and thiopental, against picrotoxin-induced seizure in the rat. Middle East J Anesthesiol 1993;12(2):113–21.

49. Heavner JE, Arthur J, Zou J, McDaniel K, Tyman-Szram B, Rosenberg PH. Comparison of propofol with thiopentone for treatment of bupivacaine-induced seizures in rats. Br J Anaesth 1993;71(5):715–9.

50. Borgeat A, Dessibourg C, Popovic V, Meier D, Blanchard M, Schwander D. Propofol and spontaneous movements: an EEG study. Anesthesiology 1991;74(1):24–7.

51. Kiyama S, Yoshikawa T. Persistent intraoperative myoclonus during propofol–fentanyl anaesthesia. Can J Anaesth 1998;45(3):283–4.

52. Nimmaanrat S. Myoclonic movements following induction of anesthesia with propofol: a case report. J Med Assoc Thai 2005;88:1955–7.

53. Saravanakumar K, Venkatesh P, Bromley P. Delayed onset refractory dystonic movements following propofol anesthesia. Paediatr Anaesth 2005;15:597–601.

54. Borgeat A, Dessibourg C, Popovic V, Meier D, Blanchard M, Schwander D. Propofol and spontaneous movements: an EEG study. Anesthesiology 1991;74:24–7.

55. Hickey KS, Martin DF, Chuidian FX. Propofol-induced seizure-like phenomena. J Emerg Med 2005;29(4):447–9.

56. Yasukawa M, Yasukawa K. [Convulsion in two non-epileptic patients following induction of anesthesia with propofol.] Masui 1999;48(3):271–4.

57. Sneyd JR. Propofol and epilepsy. Br J Anaesth 1999; 82(2):168–9.

58. Iwasaki F, Mimura M, Yamazaki Y, Hazama K, Sato Y, Namiki A. [Generalized tonic-clonic seizure induced by propofol in a patient with epilepsy.]Masui 2001;50(2):168–70.

59. Sear JW, Jewkes C, Wanigasekera V. Hemodynamic effects during induction, laryngoscopy, and intubation with eltanolone (5Ã-pregnanolone) or propofol. A study in ASA I and II patients. J Clin Anesth 1995;7:126–31.

60. Nakane M, Iwama H. A potential mechanism of propofol-induced pain on injection based on studies using nafamostat mesilate. Br J Anaesth 1999;83:397–404.

61. Ohmizo H, Obara S, Iwama H. Mechanism of injection pain with long and long-medium chain triglyceride emulsive propofol. Can J Anaesth 2005;52(6):595–9.

62. Eriksson M, Englesson S, Niklasson F, Hartvig P. Effect of lignocaine and pH on propofol-induced pain. Br J Anaesth 1997;78(5):502–6.

63. Shimizu T, Inomata S, Kihara S, Toyooka H, Brimacombe JR. Rapid injection reduces pain on injection with propofol. Eur J Anaesthesiol 2005;22(5):394–6.

64. Lomax D. Propofol injection pain. Anaesth Intensive Care 1994;22:500–1.

65. Ozturk E, Izdes S, Babacan A, Kaya K. Temperature of propofol does not reduce the incidence of injection pain. Anesthesiology 1998;89:1041.

66. Uda R, Kadono N, Otsuka M, Shimizu S, Mori H, Ozturk E, Izdes S, Babacan A, Kaya K. Strict temperature control has no effect on injection pain with propofol. Anesthesiology 1999;91:591–2.

67. Adam S, von Bommel J, Pelka M, Dirckx M, Jonsson D, Klein J. Propofol-induced injection pain: comparison of a modified propofol emulsion to standard propofol with premixed lidocaine. Anesth Analg 2004;99:1076–9.

68. Kunitz O, Losing R, Schulz-Stubner S, Haaf-von-Below S, Rossaint R, Kuhlen R. Propofol-LCT versus propofol MCT/LCT with or without lidocaine - a comparison on pain on injection. Anaesthesiol Intensivmed Notfallmed Schmerzther 2004;39:10–4.

69. Dubey PK, Kumar A. Pain on injection of lipid-free propofol and propofol emulsion containing medium-chain triglyceride: a comparative study. Anesth Analg 2005;101(4):1060–2.

70. Sun NC, Wong AY, Irwin MG. A comparison of pain on intravenous injection between two preparations of propofol. Anesth Analg 2005;101(3):675–8.

71. Liljeroth E, Akeson J. Less local pain on intravenous infusion of a new propofol emulsion. Acta Anaesthesiol Scand 2005;49(2):248–51.

72. Nagao N, Uchida T, Nakazawa K, Makita K. Medium-/long-chain triglyceride emulsion reduced severity of pain during propofol injection. Can J Anaesth 2005;52(6):660–1.

73. Nyman Y, von Hofsten K, Georgiadi A, Eksborg S, Lnnqvist PA. Propofol injection pain in children: a prospective randomized double-blind trial of a new propofol formulation versus propofol with added lidocaine. Br J Anaesth 2005;95(2):222–5.

74. Yew WS, Chong SY, Tan KH, Goh MH. The effects of intravenous lidocaine on pain during injection of medium- and long-chain triglyceride propofol emulsions. Anesth Analg 2005;100(6):1693–5.

75. Song D, Hamza MA, White PF, Byerly SI, Jones SB, Macaluso AD. Comparison of a lower-lipid propofol emulsion with the standard emulsion for sedation during monitored anesthesia care. Anesthesiology 2004;100:1072–5.

76. Song D, Hamza MA, White PF, Klein K, Recart A, Khodaparasat O. The pharmacodynamic effects of a lower-lipid emulsion of propofol: a comparison with the standard propofol emulsion. Anesth Analg 2004;98:687–91.

77. Scott RP, Saunders DA, Norman J. Propofol: clinical strategies for preventing the pain of injection. Anaesthesia 1988 43(6):492–4.

78. King SY, Davis FM, Wells JE, Murchison DJ, Pryor PJ. Lidocaine for the prevention of pain due to injection of propofol. Anesth Analg 1992;74(2):246–9.

79. Gehan G, Karoubi P, Quinet F, Leroy A, Rathat C, Pourriat JL. Optimal dose of lignocaine for preventing pain on injection of propofol. Br J Anaesth 1991;66(3):324–6.

80. Tham CS, Khoo ST. Modulating effects of lignocaine on propofol. Anaesth Intensive Care 1995;23:154–7.

81. Ho C-M, Tsou M-Y, Sun M-S, Chu C-C, Lee T-Y. The optimal effective concentration of lidocaine to reduce pain on injection of propofol. J Clin Anesth 1999;11:296–300.

82. Eriksson M. Prilocaine reduces injection pain caused by propofol. Acta Anaesthesiol Scand 1995;39:210–13.

83. Uda R, Ohtsuka M, Doi Y, Inamori K, Kunimasa K, Ohnaka M, Minami T, Akatsuka M, Mori H. [Sixty percent lidocaine tape alleviates pain on injection of propofol after diminishing venipuncture pain.] Masui 47(7):843–7.

84. Yokota S, Komatsu T, Komura Y, Nishiwaki K, Kimura T, Hosoda R, Shimada Y. Pretreatment with topical 60% lidocaine tape reduces pain on injection of propofol. Anesth Analg 1997;85(3):672–4.

85. McCluskey A, Currer BA, Sayeed I. The efficacy of 5% lidocaine-prilocaine (EMLA) cream on pain during intravenous injection of propofol. Anesth Analg 2003;97(3):713–4.

86. Von Heijne M, Bredlv B, Sderhll S, Olsson GL. Propofol or propofol–alfentanil anesthesia for painful procedures in the pediatric oncology ward. Paediatr Anaesth 2004;14(8):670–5.

87. Fletcher JE, Seavell CR, Bowen DJ. Pretreatment with alfentanil reduces pain caused by propofol. Br J Anaesth 1994;72:342–4.

88. Singh M, Mohta M, Sethi AK, Tyagi A. Efficacy of dexamethasone pretreatment for alleviation of propofol injection pain. Eur J Anaesthesiol 2005;22(11):888–90.

89. Turan A, Memis D, Kaya G, Karamanlioglu B. The prevention of pain from injection of propofol by dexmedetomidine and comparison with lidocaine. Can J Anaesth 2005;52(5):548–9.

90. Wilkinson D, Anderson M, Gauntlett IS. Pain on injection of propofol. Modification by nitroglycerin. Anesth Analg 1993;77:1139–42.

91. Dubey PK, Prasad SSPain on injection with propofol: the effect of granisetron pre-treatment.. Clin J Pain 2003;19:121–4.

92. Ambesh SP, Dubey PK, Sinha PK. Ondansetron pretreatment to alleviate pain on propofol injection: a randomized, controlled, double-blinded study. Anesth Analg 1999;89:197–9.

93. Memis D, Turan A, Karamanlioglu B, Kaya G, Pamukcu Z. The prevention of propofol injection pain by tramadol or ondansetron. Eur J Anaesthesiol 2002;19:47–51.

94. Tan CH, Onsiong MK, Kua SW. The effect of ketamine pretreatment on propofol injection pain in 100 women. Anaesthesia 1998;53:296–307.

95. Fujii Y, Nakayama M. A lidocaine/metoclopramide combination decreases pain on injection of propofol. Can J Anaesth 2005;52(5):474–7.

96. Mok MS, Pang W-W, Hwang M-H. The analgesic effect of tramadol, metoclopramide, meperidine and lidocaine in ameliorating propofol injection pain: a comparative study. J Anaesthesiol Clin Pharmacol 1999;15:37–42.

97. Iwama H, Nakane M, Ohmori S, Kaneko T, Kato M, Watanabe K, Okuaki A. Nafamostat mesilate, a kallikrein inhibitor, prevents pain on injection with propofol. Br J Anaesth 1998;81(6):963-4:.

98. Sinha PK, Neema PK, Rathod RC. Effect of nitrous oxide in reducing pain of propofol injection in adult patients. Anaesth Intensive Care 2005;33(2):235–8.

99. Niazi A Galvin E, Elsaigh I, Wahid Z, Harmon D, Leonard I. A combination of lidocaine and nitrous oxide in oxygen is more effective in preventing pain on propofol injection than either treatment alone. Eur J Anaesthesiol 2005;22(4):299–302.

100. Nishiyama T. How to decrease pain at rapid injection of propofol: effectiveness of flurbiprofen. J Anesth 2005;19(4):273–6.

101. Huang YW, Buerkle H, Lee TH, Lu CY, Lin CR, Lin SH, Chou AK, Muhammad R, Yang LC. Effect of pre-treatment with ketorolac on propofol injection pain. Acta Anaesthesiol Scand 2002;46:1021–4.

102. Basaranoglu G, Erden V, Delatioglu H, Saitoglu L. Reduction of pain on injection of propofol using meperidine and remifentanil. Eur J Anaesthesiol 2005;22(11):890–2.

103. Roehm KD, Piper SN, Maleck WH, Boldt J. Prevention of propofol-induced injection pain by remifentanil: a placebo-controlled comparison with lidocaine. Anaesthesia 2003;58:165–70.

104. Haugen RD, Vaghadia H, Waters T, Merrick PM. Thiopentone pretreatment for propofol injection pain in ambulatory patients. Can J Anaesth 1995;42:1108–12.

105. Pang W-W, Huang P-Y, Chang D-P, Huang M-H. The peripheral analgesic effect of tramadol in reducing propofol injection pain: a comparison with lidocaine. Reg Anesth Pain Med 1999;24:246–9.

106. Auerswald K, Pfeiffer F, Behrends K, Burkhardt U, Olthoff D. Injektionsschmerzen nach Propofolgabe. Anasthesiol Intensivmed Notfallmed Schmerzther 2005;40(5):259–66.

107. Gozal D, Gozal Y. Behavior disturbances with repeated propofol sedation in a child. J Clin Anesth 1999;11(6):499.

108. Seppelt IM. Neurotoxicity from overuse of nitrous oxide. Med J Aust 1995;163(5):280.

109. Yamaguchi S, Mishio M, Okuda Y, Kitajima T. [A patient with drug abuse who developed multiple psychotic symptoms during sedation with propofol.]Masui 1998;47(5):589–92.

110. Venkatesh KH, Chandramouli BA. Postoperative hallucinations following propofol infusion in a neurosurgical patient: a diagnostic dilemma. J Neurosurg Anesthesiol 2005;17(3):176–7.

111. Mateu J, Barrachina F. Hypertriglyceridaemia associated with propofol sedation in critically ill patients. Intensive Care Med 1996;22(8):834–5.

112. Sandiumenge Camps A, Sanchez-Izquierdo Riera JA, Toral Vazquez D, Sa Borges M, Peinado Rodriguez J, Alted Lopez E. Midazolam and 2% propofol in long-term sedation of traumatized critically ill patients: efficacy and safety comparison. Crit Care Med 2000;28(11):3612–9.

113. Martin PH, Murthy BV, Petros AJ. Metabolic, biochemical and haemodynamic effects of infusion of propofol for long-term sedation of children undergoing intensive care. Br J Anaesth 1997;79:276–9.

114. Hansen TG. [Propofol infusion syndrome in children.] Ugeskr Laeger 167(39):3672–5.

115. Liolios A, Guerit JM, Scholtes JL, Raftopoulos C, Hantson P. Propofol infusion syndrome associated with short-term large-dose infusion during surgical anesthesia in an adult. Anesth Analg 2005;100:1804–6.

116. Hanna JP, Ramundo ML. Rhabdomyolysis and hypoxia associated with prolonged propofol infusion in children. Neurology 1998;50(1):301–3.

117. Kumar MA, Urrutia VC, Thomas CE, Abou-Khaled KJ, Schwartzman RJ. The syndrome of irreversible acidosis after prolonged propofol infusion. Neurocrit Care 2005;3(3):257–9.

118. Cray SH, Robinson BH, Cox PN. Lactic acidemia and bradyarrhythmia in a child sedated with propofol. Crit Care Med 1998;26(12):2087–92.

119. Watanabe Y. Lactic acidosis associated with propofol in an adult patient after cardiovascular surgery. J Cardiothorac Vasc Anesth 1998;12:611–2.

120. Susla GM. Propofol toxicity in critically ill pediatric patients: show us the proof. Crit Care Med 1998;26(12):1959–60.

121. Betrosian AP, Papanikoleou M, Frantzeskaki F, Diakalis C, Georgiadis G. Myoglobinemia and propofol infusion. Acta Anaesthesiol Scand 2005;49:720.

122. Haase R, Sauer H, Eichler G. Lactic acidosis following short-term propofol infusion may be an early warning of propofol infusion syndrome. J Neurosurg Anesthesiol 2005;17:122–3.

123. Farag E, Deboer G, Cohen BH, Niezgoda J. Metabolic acidosis due to propofol infusion. Anesthesiology 2005;102:697–8.

124. Kill C, Leonhardt A, Wulf H. Lactic acidosis after short-term infusion of propofol for anaesthesia in a child with osteogenesis imperfecta. Paediatr Anaesth 2003;13:823–6.

125. Burow BK, Johnson ME, Packer DL. Metabolic acidosis associated with propofol in the absence of other causative factors. Anesthesiology 2004;101:239–41.

126. Salengros J-C, Velghe-Lenelle C-E, Bollens R, Engelman E, Barvais L. Lactic acidosis during propofol-remifentanil anesthesia in an adult. Anesthesiology 2004;101:243–5.

127. Funston JS, Prough DS. Two reports of propofol anesthesia associated with metabolic acidosis in adults. Anesthesiology 2004;101:6–8.

128. Withington DE, Decell MK, Al Ayed T. A case of propofol toxicity. Pediatr Anesth 2004;14: further evidence for a causal mechanism.505–8.

129. Baumeister FAM, Oberhoffer R, Liebhaber GM, Kunkel J, Eberhardt J, Holthausen H, Peters J. Fatal propofol infusion syndrome in association with ketogenic diet. Neuropediatrics 2004;35:250–2.

130. Culp KE, Augoustides JG, Ochroch AE, Milas BL. Clinical management of cardiogenic shock associated with prolonged propofol infusion. Anesth Analg 2004;99:221–6.

131. Devlin JW, Lau AK, Tanios MA. Propofol-associated hypertriglyceridemia and pancreatitis in the intensive care unit: an analysis of frequency and risk factors. Pharmacotherapy 2005;25(10):1348–52.

132. Asirvatham SJ, Johnson TW, Oberoi MP, Jackman WM. Prolonged loss of consciousness and elevated porphyrins following propofol administrations. Anesthesiology 1998;89(4): 1029–31.

133. Aoki H, Mizobe T, Nozuchi S, Hiramatsu N. In vivo and in vitro studies of the inhibitory effect of propofol on human platelet aggregation. Anesthesiology 1998;88(2):362–70.

134. Schulze HJ, Wendel HP, Kleinhans M, Oehmichen S, Heller W, Elert O. Effects of the propofol combination anesthesia on the intrinsic blood-clotting system. Immunopharmacology 1999;43(2–3):141–4.

135. Fujii Y, Tanaka H, Kobayashi N. Prevention of postoperative nausea and vomiting with antiemetics in patients undergoing middle ear surgery: comparison of a small dose of propofol with droperidol or metoclopramide. Arch Otolaryngol Head Neck Surg 2001;127(1):25–8.

136. Anand K, Ramsay MA, Crippin JS. Hepatocellular injury following the administration of propofol. Anesthesiology 2001;95(6):1523–4.

137. Leisure GS, O'Flaherty J, Green L, Jones DR. Propofol and postoperative pancreatitis. Anesthesiology 1996;84(1):224–7.

138. Wingfield TW. Pancreatitis after propofol administration: is there a relationship? Anesthesiology 1996;84(1):236.

139. Goodale DB, Suljaga-Petchel K. Pancreatitis after propofol administration: is there a relationship? In reply. Anesthesiology 1996;84(1):236–7.

140. Betrosian AP, Balla M, Papanikolaou M, Kofinas G, Georgiadis G. Post-operative pancreatitis after propofol administration. Acta Anaesthesiol Scand 2001;45(8):1052.

141. Kumar AN, Schwartz DE, Lim KG. Propofol-induced pancreatitis: recurrence of pancreatitis after rechallenge. Chest 1999;115(4):1198–9.

142. Jawaid Q, Presti ME, Neuschwander-Tetri BA, Burton FR. Acute pancreatitis after single-dose exposure to propofol: a case report and review of literature. Dig Dis Sci 2002;47(3):614–8.

143. Gottschling S, Larsen R, Meyer S, Graf N, Reinhard H. Acute pancreatitis induced by short-term propofol administration. Paediatr Anaesth 2005;15(11):1006–8.

144. Priya G, Bhagat H, Pandia MP, Chaturvedi A, Seth A, Goswami R. Can propofol precipitate pancreatitis in patients with Cushing's syndrome? Acta Anaesthesiol Scand 2005;49(9):1381–3.

145. Manfredi R, Dentale N, Fortunato L, Pavoni M, Calza L, Chiodo F. Pancreatoxicity of propofol sedation during purulent meningitis. Clin Drug Invest 2004;24:181–3.

146. Jamieson V, Mackenzie J. Allergy to propofol? Anaesthesia 1988;43(1):70.

147. Shin YK, Kim YD, Collea JV. The effect of propofol on isolated human pregnant uterine muscle. Anesthesiology 1998;89(1):105–9.

148. Stelow EB, Johari VP, Smith SA, Crosson JT, Apple FS. Propofol-associated rhabdomyolysis with cardiac involvement in adults: chemical and anatomic findings. Clin Chem 2000;46(4):577–81.

149. Perrier ND, Baerga-Varela Y, Murray MJ. Death related to propofol use in an adult patient. Crit Care Med 2000;28(8):3071–4.

150. Wolf A, Weir P, Segar P, Stone J, Shield J. Impaired fatty acid oxidation in propofol infusion syndrome. Lancet 2001;357(9256):606–7.

152. Cannon ML, Glazier SS, Bauman LA. Metabolic acidosis, rhabdomyolysis, and cardiovascular collapse after prolonged propofol infusion. J Neurosurg 2001;95(6):1053–6.

153. Kelly DF. Propofol-infusion syndrome. J Neurosurg 2001;95(6):925–6.

154. Machata AM, Gonano C, Birsan T, Zimpfer M, Spiss CK. Rare but dangerous adverse effects of propofol and thiopental in intensive care. J Trauma 2005;58:643–5.

155. Kent EA, Bacon DR, Harrison P, Lema MJ. Sexual illusions and propofol sedation. Anesthesiology 1992;77(5):1037–8.

156. Laxenaire MC, Gueant JL, Bermejo E, Mouton C, Navez MT. Anaphylactic shock due to propofol. Lancet 1988;2(8613):739–40.

157. Cremer OL, Moons KG, Bouman EA, Kruijswijk JE, de Smet AM, Kalkman CJ. Long-term propofol infusion and cardiac failure in adult head-injured patients. Lancet 2001;357(9250):117–8.

157. Zaloga GP, Teres D. The safety and efficacy of propofol containing EDTA: a randomised clinical trial programme focusing on cation and trace metal homeostasis in critically ill patients. Intensive Care Med 2000;26(Suppl 4):S398–9.

158. Mehta U, Gunston GD, O'Connor N. Serious consequences to misuse of propofol anaesthetic. S Afr Med J 2000;90(3): 240.

159. Shearer ES. Convulsions and propofol. Anaesthesia 1990;45(3):255–6.

160. Krause TKW, Jansen L, Scholz J, Boettcher H, Wappler F, Burmeister M-A, Schulte am Esch J. Propofol anaesthesia in children does not induce the formation of sister chromatid exchanges in lymphocytes. Mutation Res 2003;542:59–64.

161. Matthieu JM, Honegger P. Le propofol est toxique pour les neurones GABAergiques immatures. [Propofol is toxic for immature GABAergic neurons.] Rev Med Suisse Romande 1996;116(12):971–3.

162. Rigby-Jones AE, Nolan JA, Priston MJ, Wright PM, Sneyd JR, Wolf AR. Pharmacokinetics of propofol infusions in critically ill neonates, infants, and children in an intensive care unit Anesthesiology 2002;97(6): 1393–400.

163. Baker MT, Naguib M. Propofol: the challenges of formulation. Anesthesiology 2005;103(4):860–76.

164. Paul M, Dueck M, Kampe S, Fruendt H, Kasper SM. Pharmacological characteristics and side effects of a new galenic formulation of propofol without soyabean oil. Anaesthesia 2003;58:1056–62.

165. Manikandan S, Sinha PK, Neema PK, Rathod RC. Severe seizures during propofol induction in a patient with syringomyelia receiving baclofen. Anesth Analg 2005;100(5):1468–9.

166. Knibbe CA, Voortman HJ, Aarts LP, Kuks PF, Lange R, Langemeijer HJ, Danhof M. Pharmacokinetics, induction of anaesthesia and safety characteristics of propofol 6% SAZN vs propofol 1% SAZN and Diprivan-10 after bolus injection. Br J Clin Pharmacol 1999;47(6):653–60.

LOCAL ANESTHETICS

General Information

Local anesthetics typically contain a hydrophilic tertiary amine group linked to a lipophilic ester or amide. The most commonly used local anesthetics are either amides or esters, as shown in Table 1. The aminoester anesthetics cause adverse reactions more commonly than local anesthetics in the amide group. The esters are typically metabolized by de-esterification by esterases, such as pseudocholinesterase in the plasma or esterases in the liver. Metabolism occurs rapidly, and so these agents have short durations of action after they reach the systemic circulation. The amides are mainly metabolized in the liver, by N-dealkylation followed by oxidation by CYP isozymes. Metabolism of these drugs occurs more slowly.

The potency of a local anesthetic depends on its lipophilicity (Table 2) (1); the more lipophilic, the more potent.

Table 1 Structural groups of some commonly used local anesthetics (durations of action in parentheses)

Amides
  Articaine
  Bupivacaine (2–8 hours)
  Cinchocaine (2–3 hours)
  Etidocaine (2–6 hours)
  Levobupivacaine
  Lidocaine (1–2 hours)
  Mepivacaine (1.5–3 hours)
  Prilocaine (1–2 hours)
  Ropivacaine (4–6 hours)

Esters of benzoic acid
  Cocaine

Esters of meta-aminobenzoic acid
  Proxymetacaine

Esters of para-aminobenzoic acid
  Benzocaine
  Chloroprocaine
  Oxybuprocaine
  Procaine (30–45 minutes)
  Propoxycaine
  Tetracaine

Table 2 Partition coefficients (n-octanol/water) of some local anesthetics

Local anesthetic	Partition coefficient
Benzocaine	1.44
Procaine	2.51
Mepivacaine	2.69
Prilocaine	2.73
Lidocaine	3.40
Bupivacaine	4.05
Etidocaine	4.19
Tetracaine	4.32
Oxybuprocaine	4.38

Local anesthetics can be classified as follows (2):

(a) low potency, short duration of action (for example procaine);
(b) intermediate potency, intermediate duration of action (for example lidocaine, prilocaine);
(c) high potency, long duration of action (for example ropivacaine).

Local anesthetics have a wide range of effects. They inhibit sodium, potassium, and calcium ion channels, alpha-adrenoceptors, and phosphatidylinositol signalling. They also cause dysrhythmias when injected directly into the brain. Local anesthetics are also mitochondrial poisons and impair oxidative phosphorylation.

The adverse effects of local anesthetics are well established (3,4). The safety advantages claimed for newer agents have to be treated with much reserve. With increasing experience, discovery of optimal doses, and understanding of potency differences, the tolerability of newer agents is often found to be similar to that of substances that have been used for much longer.

The adverse effects of local anesthetics fall broadly into four groups (5):

(a) Effects attributable to the technique itself rather than to the agent used, for example needle damage to a vessel or nerve.
(b) Local and regional effects of the drug, which may be related to its anesthetic activity or a consequence of irritation or allergy.
(c) Systemic effects, most usually seen if the agent is inadvertently injected into a blood vessel in sufficient quantities.
(d) Effects of additives, notably vasoconstrictors to prolong the local effect, hyaluronidase to promote penetration, and preservatives to prevent bacterial contamination or degradation (6).

The possibility must always be anticipated that when a local anesthetic is administered, some of it will reach organs or tissues for which it was not originally destined, either because it has been incorrectly administered or because some anatomical or other idiosyncrasy of the patient has resulted in unexpected diffusion or leakage of the agent beyond its intended location. The main problems that result relate either to effects on the nervous system or adverse effects resulting from unintended entry into the general circulation. Very occasionally, infections are transmitted (SEDA-16, 129).

Systemic toxicity is most likely to occur if a local anesthetic is accidentally injected into a vessel in sufficient quantity (7). Even with appropriate local administration, there is inevitably some diffusion of the local anesthetic into the body from the site at which it is applied, varying with local blood flow and the technique; intercostal block, for example, rapidly produces high plasma concentrations, while subcutaneous infiltration leads to much lower concentrations more slowly. The amount of local anesthetic used is another contributory factor.

Although the effects are usually mild, systemic toxicity related to local anesthesia can be fatal: in one study of 53 deaths after the use of local anesthetics there was no evidence of allergy (SED-11, 217) (8). In preventing systemic complications from local anesthesia, such measures as close monitoring of patients, the administration of intravenous fluids before major regional block, the immediate availability of drugs and equipment to treat systemic toxicity, preoxygenation, injection of a test dose, and incremental dosing are important measures.

Some distinction must be made between the main groups of local anesthetics as to the frequency of complications. Hypersensitivity reactions, for example, are relatively less common with the aminoamides, such as bupivacaine, cinchocaine, etidocaine, lidocaine, mepivacaine, prilocaine, and ropivacaine, than with the aminoesters. However, the systemic toxic effects of individual local anesthetics differ: bupivacaine, cinchocaine, and tetracaine are the most toxic. Furthermore, the individual characteristics of the patient (for example age, sex, body weight, and cardiac, renal, and hepatic function) are important (SEDA-17, 134).

The early recognition of complications can be very difficult if a local anesthetic is administered during general anesthesia, to prevent postoperative pain, since unconscious or sedated patients will not recognize the early signs of problems, such as traumatic paresthesia (9).

In a general review of the systemic toxicity of local anesthetics interesting trends were identified (10). The incidence of systemic toxicity has been falling during the last 20 years, most probably due to increased awareness of the potential cardiotoxicity of long-acting aminoamide local anesthetics. Steps to guard against unintentional intravascular injection have been increasingly used. These include aspiration, incremental injection, dose limitation, and the use of test doses. The most studied test dose is adrenaline 15 micrograms, which reliably produces a tachycardia in healthy subjects within 20 seconds of intravascular injection. Specifically, the incidence of cardiotoxicity has also fallen; several case series of systemic toxicity have been published in recent years, reporting only nervous system toxicity but no cases of cardiotoxicity. This contradicts previous estimates of the risk of cardiotoxicity, which suggested an incidence of 10% of all systemic toxicity reactions, reconfirming the impression of increased carefulness of healthcare professionals.

Organs and Systems

Cardiovascular

Cardiovascular complications are not uncommon in the course of local anesthesia; however, most changes are moderate, involving mild peripheral vasodilatation and reduced cardiac output with a change in heart rate.

Local anesthetics reduce myocardial contractility and rate of conduction (11). They also cause direct vasoconstriction or vasodilatation of vascular smooth muscle (12) and central stimulation of the autonomic nervous system (13).

Cardiac arrest and marked myocardial depression, in which hypoxia plays a critical role, have been reported.

Cardiovascular collapse can be severe and refractory to treatment; most fatal cases involve bupivacaine.

The cardiovascular system is more resistant to the toxic effects of local anesthetics than the nervous system. Mild circulatory depression can precede nervous system toxicity, but seizures are more likely to occur before circulatory collapse. The intravenous dose of lidocaine required to produce cardiovascular collapse is seven times that which causes seizures. The safety margin for racemic bupivacaine is much lower. The stereospecific levorotatory isomers levobupivacaine and ropivacaine are less cardiotoxic, and have a higher safety margin than bupivacaine, but not lidocaine; in the case of ropivacaine this may be at the expense of reduced anesthetic potency (14,15). Toxicity from anesthetic combinations is additive.

A comparison of the cardiotoxicity of the two stereoisomers of ropivacaine and bupivacaine on the isolated heart showed that both compounds had negative inotropic and negative chronotropic effects irrespective of the stereoisomer used, but bupivacaine had greater effects compared with ropivacaine at equal concentrations (16). Atrioventricular conduction time showed stereoselectivity for bupivacaine at clinical concentrations; the R(+) isomer had a greater effect in lengthening atrioventricular conduction time, but the less fat-soluble ropivacaine only showed stereoselectivity at concentrations far greater than those used clinically. Similar to the negative inotropic and chronotropic effects, bupivacaine produced greater effects on atrioventricular conduction time than ropivacaine at equal concentrations. This important study has confirmed speculations that not only the stereospecificity of ropivacaine but also its physicochemical properties contribute to its cardiac safety.

Current concepts of resuscitation after local anesthetic cardiotoxicity have been reviewed (17). Vasopressin may be a logical vasopressor in the setting of hypotension, rather than adrenaline, in view of the dysrhythmogenic potential of the latter. Amiodarone is probably of use in the treatment of dysrhythmias. Calcium channel blockers, phenytoin, and bretyllium should be avoided. In terms of new modes of therapy targeted at the specific action of local anesthetics, lipid infusions, propofol, and insulin/glucose/potassium infusions may all have a role, but further research is necessary.

Nervous system

Central nervous system effects of low concentrations of local anesthetics are mainly sedation and confusion; high concentrations are more likely to cause seizures (18).

The first sign of systemic toxicity can be mild sedation or diminished alertness. Dizziness, tinnitus, metallic tastes, muscle twitching, perioral numbness, visual disturbances, disorientation, and light-headedness are the most frequently reported adverse nervous system effects (19).

However, as the blood concentrations achieved are sometimes higher than one would anticipate, toxicity can occasionally prove much more severe than expected, for example frank convulsions, sometimes progressing to respiratory arrest and loss of consciousness. The management of local anesthetic-induced convulsions has been reviewed (20).

Local anesthetic-induced seizures have been reported more often with bupivacaine, particularly in combination with chloroprocaine (SEDA-20, 123). Ropivacaine-induced seizures have also been reported (21,22).

Severe seizures have been reported after topical use of TAC, a combination of tetracaine, adrenaline, and cocaine, in children (23,24).

Endocrine

Local anesthetics generally have only slight endocrine and metabolic adverse effects, without clinical repercussions.

Hematologic

Methemoglobinemia has been reported with benzocaine, Cetacaine (a mixture of benzocaine, butyl aminobenzoate, and tetracaine), cocaine, lidocaine, novocaine, and prilocaine. Acquired methemoglobinemia can result from exposure to chemicals that contain an aniline group, such as benzocaine and procaine, or to those that are transformed to metabolites that contain an aniline group, such as lidocaine and prilocaine. Toxic blood concentrations of local anesthetics, aberrant hemoglobin, and NADH-methemoglobin reductase deficiency are critical factors that favor the onset of methemoglobinemia. However, methemoglobinemia can occur even in the absence of such risk factors. Young children are most likely to experience clinical effects, but topical use (for example of Cetacaine) has very occasionally caused severe problems even in adults (25). Intravenous methylthioninium chloride (methylene blue) 1–2 mg/kg and oxygen are usually recommended when methemoglobinemia exceeds 30%.

There have again been several reports of methemoglobinemia following topical anesthesia (26,27). Most have been associated with topical benzocaine, and the patients recovered fully after the administration of methylthioninium chloride.

- A neonate born at 24 weeks had a rectal biopsy under general anesthesia and was intubated with an endotracheal tube that had been lubricated with lidocaine jelly 1 g and after the biopsy a rectal pack soaked in about 1 g of benzocaine lubricant; 30 minutes after surgery she developed cyanosis, with a methemoglobin concentration of 45% (28).

The authors postulated that either local anesthetic could have been responsible, but that the oxidant effects of the two agents may have been additive. They highlighted the need for awareness of seemingly minor uses of medications in neonates.

Liver

Reduced hepatic clearance, as well as relative overdosage, of local anesthetics can lead to systemic toxicity, as illustrated by three patients who underwent topicalization of the oropharynx for transesophageal echocardiography with lidocaine 10% spray or 2% viscous and subsequently became confused and drowsy (SEDA-21, 135).

Immunologic

Systemic hypersensitivity reactions are not a frequent problem in local anesthesia. Systemic toxicity or allergy to additives (hyaluronidase, bisulfate, parabens) has sometimes been mistakenly classified as hypersensitivity to local anesthetics (SEDA-17, 135) (29). Well-documented case reports are very few, relating particularly to the older aminoesters; this appears to be because these agents have the highly antigenic para-aminobenzoic acid as a metabolite (SEDA-13, 98). The incidence of true allergy is actually very low, probably less than 1% of all the adverse effects attributable to these substances (SEDA-20, 123).

Allergic reactions to aminoamide local anesthetics are unusual, but type I hypersensitivity reactions are described, and life-threatening anaphylaxis can rarely occur (SEDA-21, 136) (SEDA-22, 134). Cross-reaction between amides also occurs, for example articaine, bupivacaine, lidocaine, and prilocaine (SEDA-22, 134).

The extreme rarity of allergic reactions to local anesthetics has been confirmed in a study of 236 patients with suspected hypersensitivity to local anesthetics referred to an allergy clinic for intradermal testing and subcutaneous challenge; none tested positive (30). This paper was accompanied by a useful editorial outlining the role of the allergologist in assessing reactions to local anesthetics (31).

- A 54-year-old woman developed a type IV hypersensitivity reaction to lidocaine 2% and mepivacaine 2% on two separate occasions (32). Skin patch tests showed positive reactions at 48 and 96 hours to both agents and cross-reactivity to bupivacaine and prilocaine.
- A 35-year-old pregnant woman with a history of multiple allergies to local anesthetics underwent provocative challenge testing with preservative-free bupivacaine at 38 weeks gestation (33). The procedure was performed with full monitoring in the labor suite. There was no evidence of a reaction. She subsequently went on to have a cesarean section with preservative-free bupivacaine and fentanyl, with excellent analgesia throughout labor, delivery, and repair of her first-degree tear.

Nevertheless, reservations regarding skin testing during pregnancy were expressed in correspondence following this publication, on the grounds that fetal well-being may be greatly endangered during such procedures (34). In response, the authors of the initial case report pointed out that according to the American Academy of Allergy, Asthma, and Immunology, "patients who are pregnant·····should be tested only if the results are contemplated to have substantial and immediate therapeutic implications". They suggested that the provision of regional anesthesia using local anesthetics for labor has substantial and immediate therapeutic implications for the parturient sufficient to justify their approach (35).

Type IV delayed hypersensitivity reactions are uncommon, but allergic contact dermatitis and localized erythema and blistering have been reported (SEDA-21, 136).

- A 58-year-old man with a urological stoma used a catheter lubricated with Braum Monodose ointment (36). After almost 2 years, he developed severe pruritus and squamous erythematous plaques in the peristomal skin. Patch tests were positive with the lubricant ointment and one of its constituents, tetracaine.

Both anaphylactoid reactions and bronchospasm have occasionally been reported, although the latter may have been due to sympathetic nervous blockade leading to unopposed parasympathetic effects (SEDA-18, 143) (37).

Contact hypersensitivity also occurs. Benzocaine is a potent skin sensitizer, and several cases of contact dermatitis to lidocaine have been reported. In many cases there is no cross-reactivity between different local anesthetics.

- A 79-year-old man developed a weeping dermatitis of the perianal skin, buttocks, and proximal thighs (38). In the previous 3 weeks, he had used Proctosedyl cream which contains cinchocaine (dibucaine). Patch tests were positive with Proctosedyl cream and 5% cinchocaine in petrolatum, while benzocaine, lidocaine, and clioquinol were negative.
- A 62-year-old woman had a systemic contact dermatitis several days after topical administration of DoloPosterine ointment for hemorrhoids (39). She had erythematous vesicular lesions on her perianal area and an edematous erythematous rash on her upper thighs, elbow flexures, axillae, and face. Patch tests with the ointment and its constituents were positive with DoloPosterine and dibucaine 5% in petrolatum; patch tests with benzocaine and other local anesthetics were negative.
- A 71-year-old Japanese man developed an itchy erythematous papular eruption after using an over-the-counter medicament for skin wounds (Makiron) for 1 month (40). Patch tests with the constituents showed positive reactions to dl-chlorphenamine maleate and cinchocaine hydrochloride (both 1% in petrolatum). Patch tests with lidocaine hydrochloride and mepivacaine hydrochloride showed no cross-sensitization.

However, some sensitized patients do cross-react with various related local anesthetic agents or chemically similar compounds, including some muscle relaxants (SEDA-15, 117). On the other hand, cross-reactivity between aminoesters and aminoamides seems unlikely and does not appear to be on record. Although cross-reactivity between amide local anesthetics is uncommon, it has been reported.

- A 26-year-old woman, 6 months pregnant, developed local redness and itching after exposure to topical agents containing lidocaine, and a further similar reaction to bupivacaine, also with swelling, 8 hours after injection (41). She had a history of anaphylaxis to an unidentified agent, and a patch test was performed using mepivacaine, lidocaine, and ropivacaine; all resulted in strong reactions after 48 hours, while patch testing was negative with chloroprocaine. She subsequently had a cesarean section under spinal anesthesia with chloroprocaine with no adverse reaction.
- A 39-year-old man was investigated for three episodes of facial swelling following dental procedures over 2 years. The swelling always occurred on the same side

as the dental procedure and about 12 hours after it, took a couple of days to resolve, did not respond to antihistamines, and was not associated with a rash, laryngeal edema, or bronchospasm. He was admitted twice and treated with intravenous antibiotics for cellulitis. He also reported a history of a rash after penicillin but no previous reactions to local anesthetics. All blood tests, including full blood count, C3 and C4 concentrations, and C1 esterase inhibitor activity and function were normal; an antinuclear antibody test was negative, IgE concentrations were not raised, and latex-specific IgE was not detected. Skin prick, intradermal, and subcutaneous tests were carried out with isotonic saline, lidocaine, prilocaine, and procaine; these did not show immediate reactions, but 2 days later a wheal appeared at the lidocaine site. There was a less intense reaction with prilocaine and none with saline or procaine.

The authors concluded that sensitization to lidocaine must have taken place during previous procedures and that cross-reactivity with another amide type local anesthetic, prilocaine, had also occurred.

Contact dermatitis was reported in three hemodialysis patients who used Emla cream repeatedly as analgesia for AV fistula cannulation (SEDA-21, 136).

Twenty patients with a prior history of generalized and/or local skin reactions after local anesthetics were examined with intradermal testing and patch testing; in 10 of them a lymphocyte transformation test was performed to investigate whether they had T cell sensitization to local anesthetics, which might have been responsible for their symptoms (42). Only two had a positive intradermal test, whereas six had a positive patch test and six had a positive lymphocyte transformation test, suggesting that allergic skin symptoms could be mediated by T cells in some patients who do not have evidence of an IgE-mediated reaction.

- A 20-year-old woman, who had had eight previous uneventful exposures to local anesthetics for dental procedures, received an injection of 1% lidocaine for treatment of an in-growing toenail; 12 hours later she developed widespread urticaria lasting a week accompanied by bronchospasm and abdominal discomfort (43). A skin prick test gave a slight positive reaction, and later a positive intradermal injection provided evidence of a true type I hypersensitivity reaction. Following negative skin and intradermal tests with prilocaine, subsequent dental treatment 12 months later was performed using prilocaine with no untoward effects.
- A 70-year-old woman received a peribulbar block using 10 ml of 2% lidocaine, 0.75% bupivacaine (50/50), and hyaluronidase 500 units for cataract extraction; 12 hours later she awoke with a painful, swollen eye (44). There was marked swelling, erythema, tenderness of the eyelids, and a tense orbit, with reduced visual acuity, marked restriction of eye movements, and conjunctival chemosis. There was no hematoma or evidence of infection, but allergy could not be ruled out. Four days later, she received tetracaine eye drops and local infiltration with lidocaine for further suturing and again developed similar symptoms and signs in that eye, with swelling

extending to the cheek; follow-up showed persistent ocular dysfunction.

The second patient had had previous exposure to prilocaine, lidocaine, and bupivacaine without problems. The author proposed a diagnosis of lidocaine allergy, although hyaluronidase as the antigen could not be excluded.

- A 23-year-old woman developed an allergic contact dermatitis after applying an over-the-counter proprietary antipruritic jelly containing 0.1% cinchocaine chloride, and a "caine" mixture (5% benzocaine, 1% cinchocaine hydrochloride, 1% procaine hydrochloride) (45). She had positive patch testing to both components.

Allergic reactions attributed to local anesthetics can be due to excipients in the formulation (46).

- A 69-year-old woman developed hypesthesia of all four limbs lasting several hours after three gastroscopies using lidocaine jelly; although the symptom was not typical of an allergic reaction, intradermal tests and nasal provocation tests were performed. The intradermal tests were negative, but the nasal provocation tests were positive for carboxymethylcellulose, a suspending agent used in lidocaine jelly; this caused ipsilateral nasal congestion and dysesthesia of the tongue and the ipsilateral temporal region within 30 minutes. A drug-induced lymphocyte stimulation test was also positive for carboxymethylcellulose.

Hypersensitivity to carboxymethylcellulose may have contributed to this patient's unusual symptoms.

The use of skin testing to identify a causative drug allergen has been repeatedly advocated by several groups, but their advice has not always been followed. Intradermal testing can be helpful in distinguishing between safe and unsafe agents in patients with a history of allergy to local anesthesia.

Various types of immunodepressant effects of local anesthetics can be detected by laboratory testing, although they may have no clinical significance. Lidocaine dose-dependently inhibits EA rosetting by human lymphocytes. In vitro depression of human leukocyte random motility and phagocytosis has also been reported (SED-11, 220) (47).

When injected into the skin, local anesthetics often cause pseudo-allergic reactions, with similar symptoms to immediate type allergy (48). However, true immediate hypersensitivity to local anesthetics is extremely rare.

- A 50-year-old man had local infiltrations a few days after an injection of lidocaine and dexamethasone (49). Prick and intradermal tests were negative after 20 minutes. However, lidocaine produced a positive patch test after 2 days, with erythema and papules.

Second-Generation Effects

Fertility

The use of in vitro fertilization has raised the question of whether the use of local anesthetics during oocyte removal is innocuous or not. Pharmacological concentrations of anesthetic agents are found in follicular fluid (50). No clinical effects have been noted, but knowledge of the

behavioral effects of lidocaine on offspring in rats must cause some concern (SEDA-15, 117).

Pregnancy

It seems most unlikely that local anesthetics have any adverse effect on the fetus when used during pregnancy (51). However, the risks of local anesthetic toxicity may be greater in pregnancy because an increase in the unbound fraction of local anesthetic and physiological changes increase the transfer of local anesthetic into the central nervous system. The authors of a report of systemic symptoms in a pregnant patient suggested the precautionary use of a lower dose of local anesthetic than usual and a longer tourniquet time, to increase the safety of this technique during pregnancy (52).

Susceptibility Factors

Age

Children
Neonates and infants absorb local anesthetics more rapidly after topical application to the airways, and peak plasma concentrations can be reached within 1 minute of application. In the first few months of life they have a larger volume of distribution, reduced hepatic clearance, and lower concentrations of albumin and alpha$_1$-acid glycoprotein (53).

Drug Administration

Drug administration route

Local anesthetics can be given by many different routes, each of which has its own particular adverse effects. In this section the following routes of administration are covered:

- Airway anesthesia
- Brachial plexus anesthesia
- Buccal anesthesia
- Caudal anesthesia
- Cervical plexus anesthesia
- Dental anesthesia
- Digital anesthesia
- Epidural anesthesia
- Femoval anesthesia
- Infiltration anesthesia
- Intercostal nerve anesthesia
- Interpleural anesthesia
- Intra-articular anesthesia
- Intradermal anesthesia
- Intrathecal (spinal) anesthesia
- Intravenous regional anesthesia
- Laryngeal anesthesia
- Leg anesthesia
- Lumbar plexus anesthesia
- Nasal anesthesia
- Neck anesthesia
- Obstetric anesthesia
- Ocular anesthesia

- Oropharyngeal anesthesia
- Otic anesthesia
- Paravertebral anesthesia
- Perianal anesthesia
- Peritonsillar anesthesia
- Respiratory anesthesia
- Sciatic nerve anesthesia
- Skin anesthesia
- Stellate ganglion anesthesia
- Subcutaneous anesthesia
- Submucosal anesthesia
- Urinary tract anesthesia

When injecting local anesthetics to achieve regional blockade, a test dose is recommended in order to exclude intravascular placement of the needle or catheter. However, newer local anesthetics, such as ropivacaine and levobupivacaine, are supposed to have less systemic toxicity than bupivacaine. A study was therefore undertaken in 120 patients to determine whether test doses of these agents cause sufficient nervous system symptoms to identify accidental intravenous injection (54). The patients were randomized to one of four different intravenous treatments: saline, 2% lidocaine (100 mg), 0.5% ropivacaine (25 mg), or 0.5% levobupivacaine (25 mg). Compared with ropivacaine and levobupivacaine, lidocaine caused more reliably recognizable nervous system symptoms. The authors therefore could not recommend plain ropivacaine or levobupivacaine for test dose purposes.

Airway anesthesia
Respiratory
Laryngospasm is a serious event that results in partial or complete upper airway obstruction. It can occur after airway anesthesia by local anesthetic spray.

A 54-year-old patient scheduled for flexible fiberoptic bronchoscopy, following a lung transplantation 18 months before, had intravenous induction with propofol (55). The vocal cords and vocal folds adducted immediately after a rapid injection of 2 ml of 2% lidocaine via a bronchoscope injection port. Ventilation ceased and the end-tidal carbon dioxide concentration fell to zero. There was spontaneous recovery after 40 seconds and ventilation resumed.

The authors postulated that direct application of a drug on the vocal cords has the potential to induce laryngospasm, although this has never been described before in clinical practice.

There has been a report of total airway obstruction after topical anesthesia of the larynx before fiberoptic intubation (56).

A 69-year-old man with a neck cancer had inspiratory and expiratory stridor, and it was decided to perform an awake fiberoptic intubation. Four minutes after topicalization of the larynx using 7.5 ml of lidocaine 2% he had total airway obstruction. An attempt at cricothyroidotomy failed, but oral fiberoptic intubation finally succeeded. The vocal cords were abducted and not swollen.

The authors speculated that either laryngospasm or depression of laryngeal muscle tone due to the use of lidocaine could have caused sudden obstruction.

Nervous system
Seizures can occur after airway anesthesia.

- A 70-year-old man was given lidocaine 1200 mg to anesthetize the airway before bronchoscopy and 5 minutes later had a tonic–clonic seizure lasting 2 minutes before self termination (57). There were no long-term harm sequelae. The lidocaine concentration 30 minutes later was 33 µmol/l and may have been as high as 40 µmol/l during the procedure.

Lidocaine is potentially toxic at concentrations over 30 µmol/l. The authors stressed that local anesthetics should be used sparingly in airway anesthesia.

Transient cerebellar ataxia a few minutes after the topical use of lidocaine on mucosal surfaces has been described in two patients, a 58-year-old man who had lidocaine 10% spray for bronchoscopy and a 66-year-old woman who received lidocaine 2% orally for transesophageal echocardiography (58). In neither case was another cause of cerebellar ataxia identified. The second patient had previously had a similar reaction to lidocaine.

Sensory systems
Permanent anosmia after topical nasal anesthesia with lidocaine 4% has been described.

- A 62-year-old man had fiberoptic endoscopy with lidocaine 4% spray and 10 minutes later complained of anosmia (59). Computed tomography ruled out tumor, infection, and obstruction.

The authors postulated, in the absence of other obvious causes, that lidocaine had caused mitochondrial dysfunction, with activation of apoptotic pathways. They concluded that endoscopic topical local anesthesia should be done with the subject sitting and the head upwards to reduce contact of the anesthetic with the olfactory cleft.

Brachial plexus anesthesia
The systemic complications of brachial plexus anesthesia are similar to those seen with others if sufficient drug enters the circulation. Injections outside the axillary sheath result in higher plasma concentrations of local anesthetic than intrasheath injection (SEDA-22, 135). However, several other complications are specific to this route. Local complications include hematoma and infection. Horner's syndrome, temporary phrenic nerve blockade, and peripheral neuropathies have been reported (SEDA-18, 142).

The adverse effects of ropivacaine and bupivacaine have been compared in 104 patients who received 30 ml of either 0.75% ropivacaine or 0.5% bupivacaine for subclavian perivascular brachial plexus block (60). There were similar incidences of nausea (33 and 28%), vomiting (8 and 14%), and Horner's syndrome (8 and 6%), and one patient who received bupivacaine developed a tonic-clonic generalized seizure 8 minutes after injection, suggestive of systemic toxicity.

Patient-controlled interscalene analgesia (PCIA) with ropivacaine 0.2% has been compared with patient-controlled intravenous analgesia (PCIVA) with an opioid in 35 patients after elective major shoulder surgery (61). Although hemidiaphragmatic excursion on the non-operated side was increased in the PCIA group 24 and 48 hours after the initial block, pulmonary function was similar in both groups. Pain was significantly better controlled in the PCIA group at 12 and 24 and the PCIA group had a lower incidence of nausea and vomiting (5.5 versus 60%).

Cardiovascular

Cardiovascular complications can arise from unintended stellate ganglion block (SEDA-21, 131).

- A 67-year-old man had an axillary plexus block for a right palmar fasciectomy with mepivacaine 850 mg and adrenaline 225 micrograms. Twenty minutes later he became agitated and confused and an electrocardiogram showed fast atrial fibrillation. Rapid systemic absorption of the combination of high-dose mepivacaine and adrenaline in a patient who was also taking amiodarone, sotalol, captopril, and amiloride for pre-existing cardiac disease was felt to be responsible (62).

Pulmonary embolism has been attributed to brachial plexus block.

- A 43-year-old man with end-stage renal disease became acutely hypoxic after an interscalene brachial plexus block with 35 ml of 1.5% mepivacaine for primary placement of an arteriovenous fistula in the left arm (63). He had been undergoing hemodialysis for 1 month using subclavian and internal jugular vascular catheters for temporary access. Immediately after an apparently straightforward block, his oxygen saturation fell from 99 to 85%, he complained of chest pain and shortness of breath, and he developed hemoptysis. A CT scan suggested acute pulmonary embolism.

The authors proposed that manipulations and vasodilatation related to the interscalene block may have facilitated the dislodgement of a pre-existing thrombus in the arm.

- A 34-year-old man undergoing acromioplasty of the right shoulder had a sudden cardiac arrest after an interscalene brachial plexus block with a mixture of ropivacaine 150 mg and lidocaine 360 mg (64). After successful resuscitation, severe hypotension persisted, necessitating the use of an adrenaline infusion. The patient developed pulmonary edema and was mechanically ventilated for 22 hours. He eventually made a good recovery.

A similar report with the use of a combination of lidocaine and levobupivacaine has been published (65). Tachycardia was the only cardiovascular symptom, while seizures were easily treatable. Both reports are in line with the improved cardiovascular safety reported with enantiomer-specific local anesthetics as discussed below.

Transient vascular insufficiency has been reported after axillary brachial plexus block (66).

In a 3-year-old child, an axillary plexus block using 7 ml of bupivacaine 0.5% and 3 ml of lidocaine 2% with adrenaline 1:200 000 was established to allow re-implantation of an amputated thumb. After the injection, the hand became pale and no pulses were palpable; 15 minutes later the color and pulses returned.

The author noted that this is a rare event, with only one previous published report, and proposed that several mechanisms may have been causative: intra-arterial injection of adrenaline or local anesthetic, mechanical obstruction from subintimal injection into the arterial wall, severe vasospasm, and a pressure effect on the axillary sheath.

Respiratory

Large volumes (30–40 ml) of local anesthetics for interscalene block cause hemidiaphragmatic paresis in nearly all patients. An interscalene brachial plexus block in 11 volunteers using 10 ml of either 0.25% bupivacaine or 0.5% bupivacaine, both with adrenaline 1:200 000, resulted in significant impairment of lung function (forced vital capacity fell by 75% and FEV_1 by 78%) and in hemidiaphragmatic excursion in those given 0.5% bupivacaine, but not 0.25% bupivacaine (67). The authors suggested that 10 ml of 0.25% bupivacaine provides adequate anesthesia, with only occasional interference with respiratory function.

However, reducing the volume of local anesthetic (1.5% mepivacaine) from 40 to 20 ml, and applying proximal digital pressure, did not reduce the incidence or intensity of diaphragmatic paralysis during interscalene block in 20 patients, in whom arterial oxygen saturation fell significantly (68).

- A 55-year-old man with newly diagnosed non-small-cell lung cancer developed difficulty in breathing, cyanosis, agitation, and confusion, 10 minutes after interscalene supplementation of an axillary nerve block with only 3 ml of 2% mepivacaine with adrenaline (69). He was anesthetized, intubated, and ventilated. Surgery proceeded and postoperative radiographic examination of the lungs showed ipsilateral elevation of the diaphragm with reduced respiratory excursion. Phrenic nerve block after the interscalene injection was the postulated cause of the deterioration in respiratory function. He was successfully extubated at the end of the procedure.

Pneumothorax has occasionally been observed (70). The axillary technique is recommended to prevent this complication (71).

Phrenic nerve palsy, resulting in paralysis of the ipsilateral hemidiaphragm, can rarely cause severe respiratory compromise, depending on pre-existing lung dysfunction. In unpremedicated patients who underwent supraclavicular brachial plexus block for upper limb surgery, blocks were performed using a peripheral nerve stimulator and 0.5 ml/kg of bupivacaine 0.375% (72). Spirometric and ultrasonographic assessments of diaphragmatic function were made at intervals. Of 30 patients, 15 had complete paralysis of the hemidiaphragm, 5 had reduced diaphragmatic movement, and 10 had no change. Those with complete paralysis all had significant reductions in pulmonary function and those with reduced or normal movement had minimal changes. Only one of the patients had respiratory symptoms and the oxygen saturation remained unchanged. This may not be the case, however, in patients with significant pre-existing respiratory disease or in obese people; the authors therefore suggested caution in choosing this approach as a safer alternative to general anesthesia in such individuals.

Two cases of respiratory compromise after infraclavicular brachial plexus blockade have been described (73).

- An 84-year-old woman weighing 74 kg had a past history of hypertension, emphysema, and ischemic heart disease. She had an infraclavicular brachial plexus block with 40 ml (400 mg) of prilocaine 1% and 10 ml (75 mg) of ropivacaine 0.75%, and 20 minutes later developed difficulty in breathing and became desaturated. She had received midazolam 2 mg before the block.
- A 47-year-old woman with a history of hypertension, gastric reflux, and obesity was premedicated with oxazepam 10 mg and had an infraclavicular brachial plexus block with the same doses of ropivacaine and prilocaine as in the first case; 10 minutes later she developed dyspnea and became desaturated.

Each patient's symptoms settled with supplementary oxygen, and surgery proceeded uneventfully. In both instances a chest X-ray showed a raised hemidiaphragm on the side of the block, but pneumothorax was excluded. The respiratory compromise was probably caused by paresis of the ipsilateral diaphragm due to blockade of the phrenic nerve, which is likely to occur after an infraclavicular plexus block but is well tolerated in most patients. Dyspnea in these two patients may have resulted from several factors. Both had been lightly sedated with benzodiazepines (although both were alert and cooperative, so this probably had a minimal contribution). The first had emphysema, which may have been an important factor; in such patients diaphragmatic function is important for sufficient gas exchange and a 50% loss of function can result in significant impairment. The second woman was obese, and obesity is associated with a reduction in functional residual capacity and respiratory function, so she may have had reduced respiratory reserve. The authors suggested that in patients with reduced pulmonary reserve, infraclavicular brachial plexus blockade should be avoided and an axillary approach considered. In addition they speculated that a smaller volume of local anesthetic may reduce the risk of phrenic nerve blockade.

Ear, nose, throat

Vocal cord paralysis can occur when local anesthesia is used after previous damage.

- A 71-year-old patient with unrecognized pre-existing left vocal cord paralysis developed severe stridor and airway compromise after right-sided subclavian plexus block (74). The paralysis was the consequence of partial

glossectomy and neck dissection 18 months earlier for squamous cell carcinoma of the tongue.

The authors recommended evaluation of vocal cord function before brachial plexus block in patients with previous surgery or radiotherapy to the neck.

Nervous system

Neurological injury after peripheral blockade has an incidence of less than 1%. However, it has been suggested that for axillary nerve blocks, neurological damage is more likely if paresthesia is the endpoint for location of the nerve sheath, in contrast to the transarterial method. This is probably due to the increased likelihood of direct damage from a needle, intraneural injection of local anesthetic, or toxicity of the local anesthetic to the nerve (75). However, published results on this issue remain contradictory (76).

Ropivacaine is less toxic than bupivacaine. However, there have been reports of brachial plexus blockade after ropivacaine, associated with unusual symptoms of nervous system toxicity; none of the patients recalled the events and there were no subsequent sequelae (77).

- A 46-year-old man received an axillary nerve block using 40 ml of 0.5% ropivacaine with 1:200 000 adrenaline and 45 seconds later developed a sinus tachycardia and started screaming, appearing terrified. He struck out violently with all limbs and sat upright, attempting to leave the bed. The pulse oximeter reading (SpO_2) fell to 90% and his symptoms were interpreted as a seizure and treated successfully with 100% oxygen, sodium thiopental, and intubation.
- A 60-year-old woman received an interscalene block using 30 ml of 0.5% ropivacaine with 1:200 000 adrenaline. Immediately after the injection, she sat up and began screaming in a loud high-pitched voice, appearing terrified and enraged. She then attempted to get off the stretcher in an uncoordinated manner and became unresponsive to verbal commands. She had a sinus tachycardia and hypotension. Treatment with 100% oxygen and propofol was effective.
- A 76-year-old woman received an interscalene block using 20 ml of 0.75% ropivacaine with 1:400 000 adrenaline. At the end of the injection, she sat up and appeared extremely terrified; she screamed twice, fell back on the stretcher, and began moving the unblocked arm and both legs in clonic movements, remaining unresponsive to verbal command. She had a sinus tachycardia and hypertension (205/70 mmHg). The seizure abated with thiopental.

The authors suggested that these signs of anxiety, vocalization, and agitation may have been due to the administration of ropivacaine formulated exclusively as the $S(-)$ enantiomer, which has a spectrum of nervous system and cardiovascular toxicity different from the racemic mixture.

Reverse arterial flow can cause nervous system toxicity, even during peripheral regional blocks with only small volumes of local anesthetic (78).

- A 47-year-old woman received an axillary brachial plexus block with 3 ml of 1% lidocaine after negative aspiration. She became dysphoric 30 seconds later, with muscle twitching in the face and distal arms, became unresponsive, and required ventilation.

During a study of 104 adults to compare the efficacy and safety of 40 ml of 0.75% ropivacaine (300 mg) and 40 ml of 0.5% bupivacaine (200 mg) for axillary plexus block, significantly more patients reported postoperative dizziness in the ropivacaine group (5 versus 0) (79). However, this occurred 4–5 hours after the injection in two patients and the day after in the other three, and was therefore unlikely to have been due to high serum concentrations. One patient developed dizziness, dysarthria, and unconsciousness, with convulsions shortly after an injection of ropivacaine, indicating an intravenous injection.

In some cases adjuvants should be considered as well as the local anesthetic after a toxic reaction (80).

- A 52-year-old woman received an axillary plexus block with 20 ml of 1% ropivacaine, clonidine 70 micrograms, and 15 ml of 1% mepivacaine with 1:400 000 adrenaline. Generalized tonic-clonic seizure activity developed, even though careful incremental aspiration was performed. She was still comatose 90 minutes later, but this was reversed by intravenous naloxone.

The authors suggested that clonidine could have been responsible for the maintenance of her unconscious state.

Axillary blockade using high-dose mepivacaine with adrenaline was performed in 50 patients, each of whom received 850 mg of mepivacaine; two patients had symptoms of toxicity associated with this combination (euphoria, dizziness, and tinnitus) 13 and 15 minutes after the procedure with doses of 14.1 and 16.4 mg/kg of mepivacaine respectively (81). One patient who received 10.9 mg/kg developed hypertension and atrial fibrillation, became agitated, and lost consciousness 12 minutes after the block was performed, and required beta-blockade and midazolam before waking up 15 minutes later. Another received 6.5 mg/kg, became light-headed, agitated, and hypertensive, and reported whole body numbness 18 minutes later, with resolution of symptoms after 10 minutes with beta-blockade. The author thought that adrenaline had probably been responsible for the reaction in the first patient. As high-dose mepivacaine did not greatly improve the quality of the block and can obviously produce serious systemic reactions, it would be prudent to limit the dose to under 10 mg/kg.

Horner's syndrome is a well-recognized complication of interscalene brachial plexus block, stellate ganglion block, and occasionally epidural blockade. It occurs when the local anesthetic reaches the cervical sympathetic trunk and is usually transient. However, persistent Horner's syndrome is a rare complication, and may represent traumatic interruption of the cervical sympathetic chain. Cases of prolonged Horner's syndrome related to prevertebral hematoma formation at the site of continuous interscalene blockade have been described (82).

- A 48-year-old obese woman had a 22G interscalene catheter inserted under local anesthesia via a short-bevel stimulating needle. Anesthesia was achieved using 0.6% ropivacaine 40 ml followed by an infusion of ropivacaine 0.2% for effective analgesia. On day 3, she reported blurred vision and a painful neck swelling. She had developed a hematoma around the catheter insertion site (confirmed by ultrasound) and had an ipsilateral Horner's syndrome including myosis, ptosis, enophthalmos, ipsilateral anhidrosis, and conjunctival hyperemia.
- An interscalene catheter was inserted in an awake 20-year-old woman for analgesia after shoulder surgery. Analgesia was achieved with ropivacaine 0.2% as a 30 ml bolus followed by an infusion of the same solution. One day later she had visual disturbance and neck swelling due to a hematoma between the prevertebral and scalene muscles.

Neither patient was taking NSAIDs, aspirin, or anticoagulants. Catheters were removed immediately on diagnosis of hematoma formation. There was no neurological or sympathetic fiber damage to the upper limb in either patient, as tested by electroneuromyography and sympathetic skin response. Remission in both cases occurred within 1 year. There has been one previous report of prolonged Horner's syndrome in the absence of any obvious technical complication (83). Further studies into the use of interscalene catheters are needed to assess their propensity to cause this rare complication.

In 60 patients receiving patient-controlled interscalene analgesia with either ropivacaine 0.2% or bupivacaine 0.15%, there was a significant reduction in hand motor function and an increased incidence of paresthesia in the bupivacaine group, with no difference in pain scores (84). This finding contrasts with that in a comparison of epidural bupivacaine or ropivacaine, in which there was no difference in motor function between the two groups (85).

Inadvertent injection into the subarachnoid space, occasionally causing cerebral or neurological problems, is a life-threatening complication of brachial plexus anesthesia. It can also cause postdural puncture headache (SEDA-21, 131).

Interscalene block can cause paralysis of the arm.

- A 33-year-old woman received combined regional and general anesthesia for a shoulder repair (86). Preoperatively an interscalene catheter was placed uneventfully. The next day, she had almost complete paralysis of the arm with hypesthesia of dermatomes C5–7. The symptoms persisted and 4.5 months later, during surgical exploration of the brachial plexus, electrical stimulation of the three trunks was possible and there were electrophysiological signs of recovery. Despite extensive neurophysiological tests a clear cause could not be established and there was no improvement at 2 years.

Sensory systems

- An intolerable metallic taste appeared and disappeared in a 48-year-old woman within hours of infusion of bupivacaine via an axillary catheter, and its severity changed with the rate of infusion (87). The mechanism was postulated to be through sodium channels or taste bud disturbances.

Psychological, psychiatric

- A 59-year-old woman, grade ASA I, had psychiatric effects associated with local anesthetic toxicity after receiving bupivacaine 50 mg and mepivacaine 75 mg for an axillary plexus block. She complained of dizziness and a "near death experience" (88).

Hematologic

Methemoglobinemia has been reported in a woman who received a combination of local anesthetics (89).

- A 60-year-old woman with medical problems including severe coronary vascular disease and anemia, taking multiple medications, including isosorbide dinitrate, received axillary plexus blockade with bupivacaine 150 mg + 10 ml of 1% lidocaine injected into the operative field; 90 minutes later her SpO_2 fell to 85–89% on oxygen 10 l/minute. She became drowsy, disoriented, and tachypneic, and an arterial blood gas showed a metabolic acidosis and a methemoglobin concentration of 6.4%. Her mental status improved 10 minutes after methylthioninium chloride and sodium bicarbonate; her $SpO2$ rose to 96% on air, her methemoglobin concentration fell to 1.6%, and her acidosis partly resolved.

The authors assumed that displacement of lidocaine from protein binding by bupivacaine, in combination with metabolic acidosis and treatment with nitrates, had caused methemoglobinemia.

Susceptibility factors

Mepivacaine toxicity has been studied in 10 patients with end-stage chronic renal insufficiency undergoing vascular access surgery (90). These patients represent a high-risk group for general anesthesia, as they often have concomitant coronary artery disease, hypertension, and diabetes. Brachial plexus block is often used: as well as avoiding systemic effects, it enhances regional blood flow. However, high doses of local anesthetic are required, and this block carries one of the highest rates of seizures. In this study, following axillary block with mepivacaine 650 mg, plasma concentrations were greater than the threshold of 6 micrograms/ml, above which signs of nervous system toxicity reportedly occur. The authors suggested that the absence of nervous system signs may have been due to slow systemic absorption of the local anesthetic. Peak concentrations occurred after 60–90 minutes, but were still high at 150 minutes, raising the question of more prolonged monitoring after these blocks.

Buccal anesthesia

Persistent hiccup, paralysis of cranial nerves, and systemic toxicity are the main complications of local anesthesia in the mouth (91–93). Trismus has been seldom reported (94–96).

Caudal anesthesia

Caudal anesthesia is commonly used for children undergoing operations below the diaphragm. Bupivacaine has for a long time been the most common local anesthetic in use. However, the long-acting aminoamide ropivacaine is reported to have a better safety profile than bupivacaine; being a single enantiomer it carries less risk of nervous system and cardiovascular toxicity. The authors of a review article concluded that, based on current evidence, ropivacaine 0.2% is the optimal concentration for pediatric caudal block (97).

The levorotatory enantiomer of bupivacaine, levobupivacaine, is being more widely used. Like ropivacaine it has a wider margin of safety for cardiovascular and central nervous system effects. In an open study the efficacy and safety of caudal levobupivacaine 0.25% (2 mg/kg) was studied in 49 children under 2 years of age undergoing subumbilical surgery (98). In 90% there was adequate analgesia. One patient had an adverse event, a mild rash, which was possibly related to levobupivacaine.

In a study in 60 anesthetized children undergoing minor subumbilical surgery caudal blocks, 0.2% ropivacaine, 0.25% racemic bupivacaine, and 0.25% levobupivacaine (all 1 ml/kg) were compared (99). All the blocks were successful in terms of intraoperative and early postoperative analgesia. Ropivacaine, but not levobupivacaine, was associated with less motor block during the first postoperative hour compared with racemic bupivacaine. However, the lower concentration of ropivacaine will have biased this result.

Caudal block with bupivacaine in children provides adequate analgesia in the early postoperative period, but additional analgesia is often required as the block wears off. Two studies have looked at adjuvants to prolong the analgesic effect.

The first was a randomized, controlled trial in 60 boys undergoing unilateral herniorrhaphy (100). They received 0.25% bupivacaine 1 ml/kg or the same dose of bupivacaine plus 1.5 mg/kg tramadol, or tramadol 1.5 mg/kg alone made up to the same volume. Caudal administration of bupivacaine plus tramadol resulted in more effective analgesia, with a longer period without demand for additional analgesia postoperatively without increases in any adverse effects. The second was a study of the addition of midazolam to caudal bupivacaine in 30 children undergoing genitourinary surgery (101). They randomly received 0.25% bupivacaine 0.5 ml/kg or the same dose of bupivacaine plus midazolam 50 micrograms/kg. There were no untoward events in either group. Fewer required additional analgesia in the first 6 hours postoperatively in the bupivacaine plus midazolam group than with bupivacaine alone: 27% compared with 60%. Midazolam prolonged analgesia with no increase in adverse effects.

In 165 children receiving caudal anesthesia with fentanyl 1 mg/kg and bupivacaine 4 mg/kg, there were adverse effects in only six, two of whom required postoperative ventilation. This was felt to be due to their pathology and not the anesthetic. However, there was no comment on the presence or absence of specific local anesthetic adverse effects, and an unusually high dose of bupivacaine was used, 4 mg/kg, twice that recommended by the manufacturers and greater than that used by most pediatric anesthetists (2.5–3 mg/kg) (SEDA-20, 124).

Caudal bupivacaine has been successfully combined with clonidine, ketamine, diamorphine, and buprenorphine, with increased duration of anesthesia and a low incidence of adverse effects (SEDA-20, 124) (SEDA-21, 131).

Awake regional anesthesia for inguinal hernia repair in former preterm infants has been suggested, in order to avoid life-threatening respiratory complications that can occur after general anesthesia. Caudal anesthesia is becoming a more popular technique for this purpose. To prolong the duration of anesthesia and to reduce the postoperative need for analgesics in these infants, caudal clonidine has been considered useful.

- A former preterm infant had two awake caudal anesthetics for herniotomy within 3 weeks (102). The first was uneventful with bupivacaine 0.25% at 35 weeks of age. At 38 weeks, the baby had intraoperative and postoperative bouts of apnea after inadvertent administration of bupivacaine 0.125% plus clonidine.

Cardiovascular

There has been a report of T wave changes on the electrocardiogram during caudal administration of local anesthetics (103).

- A 4.2 kg 2-month-old baby was given a caudal injection under general anesthesia for an inguinal hernia repair. A mixture of 1% lidocaine 2 ml and 0.25% bupivacaine 2 ml was injected. Every 1 ml was preceded by an aspiration test and followed by observation for electrocardiographic changes for 20 seconds. On administration of the third 1 ml dose, there was a significant increase in T wave amplitude. The aspiration test was repeated and was positive for blood. The caudal injection was stopped and the electrocardiogram returned to normal after 35 seconds. The baby remained cardiovascularly stable with no postoperative sequelae.

Previous reports have suggested that an increase in T wave amplitude could result from inadvertent intravascular administration of adrenaline-containing local anesthetics. This is the first case report of local anesthetics alone causing significant T wave changes.

Nervous system

Inadvertent dural puncture is a recognized complication in up to 1% of caudal anesthetics. It can be due to excessive needle insertion or sacral abnormalities. Potentially serious consequences, such as total spinal anesthesia, can result (SEDA-21, 131).

Neuromuscular

In a controlled, randomized study in 60 children undergoing subumbilical surgery three different concentrations of levobupivacaine were used for caudal anesthesia (104). The caudal block was performed with levobupivacaine 0.125%, 0.2%, or 0.25% (total volume 1 ml/kg). The 0.125% solution was associated with significantly less early motor blockade but also a significantly shorter duration of postoperative analgesia.

Hematolog

In eight episodes of toxic methemoglobinemia in seven premature infants after the combination of caudal anesthesia (prilocaine 5.4–6.7 mg/kg) and Emla cream (prilocaine 12.5 mg) for herniotomy, the highest methemoglobin concentration 5.5 hours after anesthesia was 31% (105). All the infants were symptomatic, with mottled skin, pallor, cyanosis, and poor peripheral perfusion. The most severe symptoms occurred at 3–8 hours and disappeared within 10–20 hours. The authors stressed the importance of recognizing the poor tolerance of premature infants to methemoglobinemia and that whereas topical prilocaine is relatively safe, caudal administration is not.

Susceptibility factors

Children

Caudal anesthesia is a common regional technique in children. Both ropivacaine and bupivacaine are widely used in regional anesthesia. Unlike in adults, there are conflicting pharmacokinetic data in children.

In a randomized study of the unbound plasma concentrations of bupivacaine and ropivacaine for caudal block, 38 children were randomized to 0.5ml/kg of bupivacaine or ropivacaine 0.25% (106). After bupivacaine the unbound concentrations were 47 and 24 ng/ml at 1 and 2 hours respectively. After ropivacaine group the corresponding unbound concentrations were 61 and 50 ng/ml. The differences between the groups were statistically significant. These concentrations are far below the toxic concentrations quoted in the literature for bupivacaine (unbound plasma concentrations >250 ng/ml) and ropivacaine (>150–600 ng/ml).

Cervical plexus anesthesia
Nervous system

Deep cervical plexus block can cause ipsilateral phrenic nerve palsy. A patient with pre-existing respiratory disease and a contralateral raised hemidiaphragm developed hypoxia and respiratory distress when given 20 ml of plain bupivacaine 0.375% by this route for carotid endarterectomy (107). Local anesthetic spread resulted in presumed stellate ganglion block, which caused nasal congestion and aggravated the respiratory distress. The symptoms resolved without intubation, but the authors advised against deep cervical plexus block in patients with diaphragmatic motion abnormalities or chronic respiratory disease.

Nerve palsies can occur during deep cervical plexus anesthesia.

- A woman complained of being unable to clear secretions effectively from her throat, had a paroxysm of coughing, and developed a large neck hematoma requiring surgical re-exploration (108).

- A 71-year-old man complained of difficulty in breathing and was desaturated on pulse oximetry for 5 minutes after cervical plexus blockade (109). He required tracheal intubation, was ventilated for 110 minutes, and was then successfully extubated. It was thought that the most likely diagnosis was cardiorespiratory failure exacerbated by phrenic nerve blockade.
- A 67-year-old man developed transient hemiparesis and facial nerve palsy before becoming unconscious and apneic 10 minutes after a right cervical plexus block (109). His trachea was intubated without the need for anesthetic drugs and he was ventilated. Hypotension was treated with intravenous ephedrine. He woke up, started breathing, and was extubated 75 minutes later. The authors postulated brainstem anesthesia following accidental injection of local anesthetic into a dural cuff as a cause of loss of consciousness.

Hemidiaphragmatic paralysis can occur with cervical plexus anesthesia and can be particularly risky in cases of pre-existing airways obstruction (110).

Infiltration of even small doses of a local anesthetic in the region of the carotid artery is likely to cause nervous system toxicity if injected intra-arterially (111).

- A 76-year-old man had already received a deep and superficial cervical plexus block for an awake carotid endarterectomy. One hour later, during manipulation of the carotid artery discomfort was treated with infiltration of 1 ml of 0.5% lidocaine in that region. Immediately he became unresponsive, with generalized tonic-clonic seizure activity of the face and arms. He was given 100% oxygen and within 30 seconds the seizure terminated spontaneously with no sequelae.

This demonstrates the requirement for constant vigilance in a patient undergoing awake carotid endarterectomy.

Dental anesthesia

Dental anesthesia is generally safe and effective. However, it can cause adverse effects, ranging from mild to severe, perhaps a reflection of the number of dental anesthesias performed.

Systemic effects, such as dizziness, tachycardia, agitation, nausea, tremor, syncope, seizures, and bronchospasm, are a definite risk with local anesthesia in a vascular area. A wide range of patients present for dental surgery, and it is important that an adequate medical history be taken and accurate doses calculated on an individual basis. Low concentrations of adrenaline should be used.

Complication rates increase with premedication at home, and pre-existing disease or risk factors, such as pregnancy, cardiovascular disease, and allergies. Articaine and lidocaine with epinephrine 1:200 000 were associated with a low incidence of complications (3.1 and 0%), whilst mepivacaine and articaine with adrenaline 1:100 000 caused the most frequent complications (7.2 and 6.1%) (SEDA-22, 135).

Cardiovascular

Acute hypertension leading to myocardial infarction and pulmonary edema has been described after the use of mepivacaine with levonordefrin (112).

Nervous system

An unexplained case of permanent neurological deficit, consisting of left facial palsy, right sensorineural hearing loss, gait ataxia, and hemisensory loss in the body and face, has been described after inferior alveolar nerve block (113).

Facial paralysis is occasionally reported and is not necessarily due to poor technique; in one case vascular spasm seemed to provide an explanation (SED-12, 252).

- An 8-year-old girl received prilocaine for a dental procedure performed under 70% oxygen/30% nitrous oxide (114). The dose of 288 mg was 2.7 times higher than the recommended safe dose of 6 mg/kg. Toward the end of the procedure, she became unconscious and had a convulsion.

Two reviews have highlighted the fact that the degree and incidence of neurological damage after dental anesthesia is probably underestimated. Some drugs, such as articaine and prilocaine, seem to cause a higher incidence of paresthesia than others (SEDA-20, 124).

In seven subjects articaine with adrenaline caused distortion of lingual nerve function with effects on vowel pronunciation and therefore the potential to impair speech (115).

- A 49-year-old man developed uvular deviation as a result of palatal muscle paralysis following intraoral mandibular block of the inferior alveolar nerve with 1.8 ml of 2% lidocaine with adrenaline 1 in 100 000 (116). A few minutes after injection he had swallowing difficulties and a foreign body sensation in his throat. There was paralysis of the velum palatinum, with deviation of the uvula towards the non-paralysed side opposite the point of anesthetic infiltration. This resolved after the anesthetic had worn off.

The authors suggest that a high inferior alveolar nerve block can easily affect the mandibular nerve if the anesthetic solution diffuses to the internal trunk of the third trigeminal branch and the supply to the tensor veli palatini.

Paresthesia associated with the use of local anesthetics as part of dental care is infrequent, although its incidence has increased over the last 30 years.

Prolonged dysesthesia has been reported in seven cases of inferior alveolar nerve block injection, all associated with articaine (117). The author recommended a widespread survey of the relation between prolonged dysesthesia and particular local anesthetic choices to clarify this apparent adverse effect.

In fact, such a review was published in 2003 (118). The use of articaine, and to a lesser extent prilocaine, for lingual and inferior alveolar nerve blocks is associated with a higher incidence of paresthesia in these nerves compared with lidocaine, bupivacaine, or mepivacaine.

This raises doubts about the suitability of articaine and prilocaine for local anesthesia in dentistry. The incidence of paresthesia associated with the use of these agents should be considered when selecting a local anesthetic for anesthesia of the mandible and associated structures.

Sensory systems

Adverse ocular effects, such as ptosis, are on record (SEDA-15, 118). Transient dizziness, diplopia, and partial blindness have been reported after the entry of lidocaine with adrenaline into the ophthalmic artery following mandibular block (119). A similar case after posterior alveolar block resulted in dizziness and diplopia for 3 hours when the patient stood up, possibly due to the entry of local anesthetic into the ophthalmic artery (SEDA-22, 135).

Ophthalmological complications after intraoral anesthesia occurred in 14 cases over 15 years (120). The most common symptom was diplopia. Three patients developed Horner's syndrome, with ptosis, enophthalmos, and miosis on the same side as the anesthesia. Three patients developed mydriasis and ptosis. There was complete resolution in all patients. The authors postulated that direct diffusion of anesthetic solution from the pterygomaxillary fossa through the sphenomaxillary cavity to the orbit had caused the ophthalmological effects.

- A 45-year-old man developed temporary monocular blindness, ophthalmoplegia, ptosis, and mydriasis immediately after a mandibular block injection (121). Unidentified intra-arterial injection into the maxillary artery, with backflow of the local anesthetic solution to the middle meningeal artery was the postulated cause.
- A 73-year-old man with a history of infective endocarditis was admitted for multiple dental extractions and received prilocaine 144 mg after aspiration (122). Within 2 minutes he reported that he could not see in his left eye. Fundoscopy showed diffusely obstructed retinal vessels, with multiple segmented clear fluid emboli and an incomplete cherry-red spot. There was no evidence of choroidal abscess or central nervous system signs of recent thromboembolism. Anterior chamber ocular paracentesis with ocular massage was attempted without improvement. Five days later his visual acuity remained at light perception only. Two months later his vision was unchanged.

The authors noted that this is a rare event and proposed causative mechanisms: intra-arterial injection causing retrograde flow in an abnormal anatomy or injection through vascular abnormalities from previous trauma or inflammation. It was difficult to implicate endocarditis, in the absence of calcific or platelet fibrin emboli. They concluded that delivery of local anesthetic must be done with aspiration before and care during injection. This will possibly prevent intravascular injection.

Immunologic

True allergic reactions to amide local anesthetics are extremely rare. Anaphylaxis after local lidocaine administration has been reported (123).

- A 4-year-old child, previously healthy, received an intrapulpal injection of 0.5 ml of lidocaine 2% with 1:100 000 adrenaline for a dental procedure; 15 minutes later he became severely cyanotic and short of breath, and had a respiratory arrest and sinus bradycardia. Cardiopulmonary resuscitation was started immediately, followed by rapid blood volume expansion and adrenaline administration. After 24 hours his vital; signs stabilized and he recovered completely.

Allergic reactions to lidocaine in dental cartridges and reusable vials can occur because of preservatives such as parabens. However, in this case the preservative was sodium sulfite, which has not been reported to cause anaphylactic reactions. The cause of the anaphylaxis was not determined in this case, as the parents refused tests.

Additives

Additives in local anesthetic solutions can cause allergic reactions (124).

- A 34-year-old man developed swelling and redness of the face after receiving lidocaine as Lignospan® for dental treatment. Patch testing showed allergic contact dermatitis due to the preservative disodium ethylene-diamine tetra-acetic acid (EDTA).

Digital anesthesia

Digital anesthesia with 1% lidocaine plus adrenaline was performed on 23 patients for surgery to finger injuries; 11 patients received adrenaline 1:200 000, and 12 received 1:100 000 (125). A digital tourniquet was also used, but no patient developed ischemic symptoms. The authors discussed the usefulness of adrenaline as an additive to local anesthetic solutions in prolonging regional block, reducing the dose of local anesthetic required. They stated that an extensive search of the literature had revealed no sound clinical evidence to support the widely held opinion that adrenaline contributes to the risk of gangrene when it is used in digital blocks.

Epidural anesthesia

The accidental transformation of epidural to subarachnoid block can be dramatic, and tracheal intubation and ventilatory support may be necessary (126). Severe hypotension can result after inadvertent intrathecal local anesthesia (SEDA-21, 131). In women in labor, fetal bradycardia can occur. Postdural puncture headache can also be a sign of catheter migration.

Long-term epidural catheters can be highly effective in the management of chronic pain of malignant and non-malignant origin, but they can also cause complications. Infection and extravasation of fluid to the paraspinal tissue resulting in inadequate analgesia have been described in a patient with non-Hodgkin's lymphoma (127). Another patient with non-Hodgkin's lymphoma had a tunnelled thoracic epidural for analgesia and presented with spinal cord compression. Laminectomy showed a mass consisting of white chalk-like drug-related precipitate around the catheter tip. As the solvent for bupivacaine contains sodium hydroxide and sodium chloride, the authors assumed that the mass was a precipitate of sodium hydroxide (128).

- A 1-year-old boy inadvertently received ropivacaine 6 mg intravenously over 2 hours when his epidural infusion was incorrectly connected to his intravenous cannula (46). He had already received ropivacaine 28 mg via his epidural catheter. He suffered no overt adverse effects.

In a dose-finding study for the combination of 0.2% ropivacaine with fentanyl for thoracic epidural analgesia in 224 patients undergoing major abdominal surgery, each received fentanyl in concentrations of 0, 1, 2, or 4 micrograms/ml; effective pain relief was provided by all the combinations and the degree of motor block was low overall and did not differ significantly among the groups (129). Hypotension was most common during the first postoperative 24 hours and was most frequent in those given fentanyl 4 micrograms/ml. Although the combination with fentanyl 4 micrograms/ml improved the quality of analgesia, there was a higher incidence of adverse effects, such as hypotension, nausea, and pruritus.

Patient-controlled epidural analgesia is increasingly being used, as it reduces the need for adjustment of epidural infusion rates by anesthetic personnel. In a retrospective survey of 1057 patients who received postoperative patient-controlled epidural analgesia using bupivacaine 0.1% plus fentanyl 5 micrograms/ml, on the first postoperative day 93% of the patients had adequate analgesia and 96% reported no nausea; two patients had an episode of respiratory depression and one patient was unrousable (130). Hypotension occurred in 4.3%, but there were no cases of epidural hematoma or abscess. Despite these adverse events, the authors concluded that patient-controlled epidural analgesia was effective and safe on surgical wards. The large amount of fentanyl in the solution they used is most probably the reason for the rare, potentially life-threatening adverse effects.

The amount of bupivacaine with fentanyl used in patient-controlled epidural analgesia was significantly less than with a continuous infusion of the same mixture in a group of 54 patients (mean age 71 years) after total knee arthroplasty (131). However, 10% of the patients were too confused to use the PCEA device. Despite the advantages of analgesic dosage reductions, a constant infusion may prove more appropriate in this age group.

Patient-controlled epidural analgesia (0.05% bupivacaine and fentanyl 4 micrograms/ml) has been studied prospectively in 1030 patients requiring postoperative analgesia (132). Pruritus was the most common adverse effect, with an incidence of 17%, with two susceptibility factors: age (under 58 years) and increased consumption of analgesia (over 9 ml/hour). The incidence of nausea was 15% and of sedation 13%; female sex was a slight risk factor for both. Hypotension had an incidence of 6.8% and motor block of 2%; lumbar placement of the epidural catheter was the strongest risk factor. Respiratory depression occurred in 0.3%.

The effects of single-dose epidural analgesia with lidocaine and morphine have been studied in 60 women undergoing elective cesarean section (133). The patients received morphine sulfate 4 mg and 2% lidocaine 18–20 ml. Four patients proceeded to general anesthesia owing to failure of the epidural block to reach T6, 48% of patients complained of discomfort during surgery, and 23% needed supplementary analgesia. Perioperative adverse effects were hypotension 29%, bradycardia 3.6%, and shivering 5.4%. Postoperative adverse effects were pruritus 45% and nausea and vomiting 35%. Apgar scores at 1 and 5 minutes were 8 or over. At 2 hours and 24 hours, two babies had transient tachypnea and one had mild respiratory distress. Maternal and neonatal venous concentrations of morphine, measured at delivery, were low. The authors recommended this technique for elective cesarean section in uncomplicated obstetric patients. This study had no control group and reported a high incidence of unwanted effects and a high perioperative failure rate. Mean analgesic duration of morphine was reported as 24 hours. However, 75% of patients required additional analgesia after 12 hours. There was no record of the incidence of postoperative maternal respiratory depression.

Comparative studies

After thoracotomy, 106 patients received a thoracic epidural infusion of either 0.1% or 0.2% bupivacaine, both with fentanyl 10 micrograms/ml, compared with epidural fentanyl alone; there was no difference in the number of episodes of postoperative hypotension (systolic pressure below 90 mmHg) or in the number of interventions for postoperative hypotension, but intraoperative vasopressors were used significantly more in the bupivacaine groups (134). In addition, two patients given 0.2% bupivacaine reported slight weakness of both hands and another asided Horner's syndrome and weakness of the right hand. There was a similar incidence of nausea and pruritus in all the groups; however, the incidence of respiratory depression with fentanyl was high (4.2%).

Random allocation of 150 women in labor to either an intermittent epidural bolus, a continuous epidural infusion, or patient-controlled epidural analgesia with 0.125% bupivacaine and sufentanil 0.5 micrograms/ml resulted in significantly more frequent motor blockade with continuous infusion compared with intermittent boluses (22 versus 4%), with similar frequencies of pruritus, hypotension, and high sensory level in each group (135).

In 52 patients who received either epidural bupivacaine (0.10–0.28 mg/kg/hour) or lidocaine (0.44–0.98 mg/kg/hour), both with epidural morphine, there were no significant differences in the times to mobilize, motor function (as measured by the Bromage grade), and the incidence of hypotension (136). Most of the patients had no motor blockade, and the Bromage grade did not help predict which of them could be mobilized.

In 90 parturients who received epidural analgesia during labor with bolus administration of either 10 ml of 0.125% bupivacaine or 0.125% ropivacaine, each with sufentanil 7.5 micrograms, there were comparable onset times and duration of analgesia in the two groups, but patients given ropivacaine had significantly less motor blockade after the third and subsequent epidural injections compared with those given bupivacaine: 93% of those given ropivacaine had no motor impairment compared with 66% of those given bupivacaine (137). There were no differences in hemodynamic effects and pruritus.

An epidural infusion of 0.2% ropivacaine plus sufentanil has been compared with 0.175% bupivacaine plus sufentanil in 86 patients postoperatively after major gastrointestinal surgery; there was no statistically significant difference in the incidence of adverse effects (respiratory depression, sedation, nausea, vomiting, pruritus, and motor blockade), but those given ropivacaine mobilized more quickly (138).

In 60 women who underwent elective cesarean section under epidural anesthesia, 0.5% levobupivacaine or 0.5% bupivacaine (30 ml) were equally efficacious in terms of anesthesia (139). The incidence and severity of motor blockade, hypotension, changes in QT interval, nausea, and vomiting were not significantly different, and neither were the neonatal Apgar scores.

Drug combinations are often used in epidural anesthesia to enhance the analgesic effect and minimize adverse effects. Continuous epidural analgesia (0.125% bupivacaine 12.5 mg/hour and morphine 0.25 mg/hour) has been compared with patient-controlled analgesia (morphine) in 60 patients after major abdominal surgery. Analgesia was superior in the epidural group, satisfaction and sedation scores were similar in both groups, whilst episodes of moderate nocturnal postoperative hypoxemia (SaO_2 85–90%) were more frequent in the epidural group (140).

The addition of opioids to local anesthetic to improve the efficacy of epidural analgesia for cesarean section has been advocated (133,141). A test dose of lidocaine 60 mg was given to 24 patients undergoing elective cesarean section, followed by either bupivacaine 45 mg or bupivacaine 45 mg plus fentanyl 50 micrograms (141). Sensory blockade to T6 was achieved in both groups, but pain scores were significantly lower in the fentanyl group. Rescue fentanyl on uterine exteriorization was required in 40% of the control group, but in none in the fentanyl group. There were no significant differences in adverse effects, specifically pruritus, hypotension, nausea and vomiting, maternal respiratory depression, and Apgar scores.

Analgesia after major surgery has been evaluated in a prospective study in 2696 patients, who received either epidural or intravenous analgesia for postoperative pain relief (142). Epidural analgesia consisted of bupivacaine 0.25% with morphine 0.05 mg/ml and was used in 1670 patients. Intravenous analgesia with morphine 1 mg/ml was used in 1026 patients. The patients with epidural analgesia had better pain relief both at rest and during mobilization compared with intravenous analgesia. However, orthostatic dysregulation in 6%, pruritus in 4.4%, and technical problems in 6.2% were more frequent with epidural analgesia. In comparison, intravenous morphine analgesia had a higher frequency of opioid related adverse effects, such as sedation/hallucinations/nightmares/confusion in 2.5% and respiratory depression in 1.2%. This study used background infusion plus patient-controlled analgesia in both groups, which might have affected the adverse effects in the intravenous group; perhaps another choice of epidural solution would have caused less hypotension.

Cardiovascular

Hypotension is a frequent adverse effect of epidural anesthesia. In a comparison of the effects of bupivacaine and ropivacaine in 60 women undergoing cesarean section, 90% had a fall in blood pressure to below 90 mmHg, or by more than 30% of baseline (143).

Abrupt onset of arterial hypotension is also a complication of cervical epidural anesthesia, particularly in elderly patients (144). However, supplementation with adrenaline in this high-risk group is no longer defensible; it is better to be cautious with dosage and to monitor the patient closely.

- Severe hypotension during a lumbar epidural anesthetic in a 61-year-old woman taking amitriptyline was refractory to high doses of ephedrine and other indirect alpha-adrenergic agents (145). It eventually responded to one dose of noradrenaline 200 micrograms, illustrating the importance of the choice of vasopressor for treating hypotension in the presence of chronic tricyclic antidepressant use.
- A 27-year-old woman developed significant myocardial depression and pulmonary edema after administration of 5 ml of bupivacaine 0.5% via an epidural catheter (146). The bupivacaine followed a test dose of 3 ml lidocaine 2%.

Although initial aspiration on the epidural catheter was negative, the most likely explanation must be inadvertent intravascular administration of lidocaine and bupivacaine.

Hypotension during epidural anesthesia can be due to functional hypovolemia. It is usually treated with intravenous fluids and/or vasopressors. In order to validate the changes in intravascular volumes after thoracic epidural anesthesia over a longer time, a study was undertaken in 12 healthy volunteers, who were randomized to receive either colloidal fluid (hydroxyethyl starch 7 ml/kg) or a vasopressor (ephedrine 0.2 mg/kg) 90 minutes after the administration of 10 ml of bupivacaine 0.5% through a thoracic epidural inserted at T7–10 (147). Thoracic epidural anesthesia in itself did not lead to any changes in blood volume, despite a fall in blood pressure. The authors concluded that fluid administration leads to dilution and recommended that hydroxyethyl starch may be preferred to ephedrine in patients with cardiopulmonary disease, in order to avoid perioperative fluid overload.

In a randomized double-blind study of the cardiovascular effects and neonatal outcome of epidural blockade in healthy parturients scheduled for elective cesarean section, the patients were allocated to either epidural ropivacaine 0.75% or bupivacaine 0.5% (148). The two agents produced equally satisfactory blockade, but ropivacaine 0.75% produced a more pronounced reduction in maternal heart rate. However, this had no effect on neonatal outcome. The authors concluded that both bupivacaine 0.5% and ropivacaine 0.75% could be recommended for epidural anesthesia in elective cesarean section.

Unusually, a mother and her child died after repeated administration of a local anesthetic for cesarean section;

pulmonary edema was believed to have been the cause (149).

Intracardiac conduction disturbances should not be considered as absolute contraindications to epidural anesthesia: there were only nine cases of sinus bradycardia, easily reversed with atropine sulfate, in 66 patients (150). However, rare cases of complete heart block and complete left bundle branch block have occurred (SEDA-21, 132) (151).

Unexpected cardiopulmonary arrest can result from accidental dural puncture during epidural blockade (SEDA-22, 136).

- Asystolic cardiac arrest has been described in a 55-year-old man who underwent partial hepatectomy under combined general and epidural anesthesia (152). During postoperative recovery he developed asystole followed by ventricular fibrillation. Resuscitation was unsuccessful.

The authors concluded that in the absence of any other abnormality the arrest had been the result of an autonomic imbalance due to spreading sympathetic block, although other postoperative causes of death should not be discarded.

Prolongation of the QT interval can predispose to dysrhythmias with local anesthetics.

- Intraoperative cardiac arrest occurred in a 9-year-old child with Pfeiffer syndrome (craniosynostosis, mild syndactyly of hands and feet, and dysmorphic facial features) undergoing reversal of a colostomy (153). All previous anesthetics had been uneventful. The child received an epidural catheter at the L3/4 interspace. A test dose of 2 ml of lidocaine 1% with adrenaline 1: 200 000 was administered and aspiration for spinal fluid was negative. One minute after the first dose of bupivacaine 0.25% 3 ml with adrenaline 1: 200 000 he developed cardiac dysrhythmias and 3 minutes later, and before surgical incision, ventricular fibrillation. After chest compression, 100% oxygen, adrenaline, and sodium bicarbonate, sinus rhythm returned. Blood was aspirated from the epidural catheter. Postoperative investigation showed a long QT syndrome.

Prolongation of the QT interval predisposes to ventricular dysrhythmias and can be triggered by adrenaline. In this case the authors concluded that accidental intravascular injection of bupivacaine and adrenaline may have triggered the dysrhythmia.

Brugada syndrome (right bundle branch block and raised ST segments), can cause sudden cardiac death, potentially hastened by class I antidysrhythmic drugs. Intravenous sodium channel blockers such as local anesthetics can unmask Brugada syndrome.

- A 77-year old man with no previous symptoms of ischemic heart disease underwent elective gastrectomy for carcinoma of the stomach (154). Preoperative electrocardiography showed partial right bundle branch block. An epidural catheter was inserted at interspace T9/10 before induction. Aspiration of the catheter was negative for blood and cerebrospinal fluid. Bupivacaine

0.25% 10 ml was given in 2 ml increments, and an infusion of 0.125% bupivacaine and fentanyl 2.5 µg/ml was begun at 8 ml/hour. The operation was uneventful. Three epidural bolus doses were given postoperatively over 11 hours, consisting of 0.125% bupivacaine with fentanyl 2.5 µg/ml, 8 ml, 5 ml, and 5 ml. After the last dose, his systolic blood pressure fell to 80 mmHg. An electrocardiogram showed right bundle branch block with new convex-curved ST segment elevation in V1-V3. Acute myocardial infarction was ruled out and a diagnosis of Brugada syndrome was made. Bupivacaine was withdrawn after a total infusion time of 17 hours (total dose of bupivacaine 443 mg). The patient made a complete and uneventful recovery.

This is the first reported case of Brugada syndrome unmasked by bupivacaine. Cocaine was the only local anesthetic to show this before. As Class Ib drugs such as lidocaine do not induce the characteristic electrocardiographic changes, the authors suggested that bupivacaine causes greater inhibition of the rapid phase of depolarization in Purkinje fibers and ventricular muscle, and remains bound to sodium channels for longer than lidocaine.

Respiratory

Respiratory depression was noted in 0.24% of patients in a Chinese series of 10 978 epidural blocks (SED-12, 254) (155). Direct paralysis of respiration probably plays an important role. Respiratory depression with adverse cardiovascular effects after miscalculated dose requirements or a misplaced catheter has also been described (SEDA-22, 136).

In 15 patients receiving lidocaine 300 mg plus adrenaline by cervical epidural injection, the upper cervical nerve roots C3, 4, and 5 were anesthetized. None of the patients had pre-existing pulmonary disease. Only one had symptoms of impaired pulmonary function at 20 minutes after epidural, and complained of dyspnea, with a reduction in maximum inspiratory pressure, FEV_1, FVC, and SpO_2. Four patients had a bradycardia requiring atropine, eight complained of nausea, and one developed hypotension requiring ephedrine. At 20 minutes after the epidural, all the patients had a maximum reduction in FEV_1 and FVC, ranging from 12 to 16% of preanesthetic measurements. The authors felt that as the maximum inspiratory pressure was virtually unchanged, this suggested that the motor function of the phrenic nerve was mostly intact, despite analgesia of the C3, 4, and 5 dermatomes (156).

Hiccups that last longer than 48 hours are referred to as persistent hiccups, and those lasting more than 2 months are considered intractable. Persistent or intractable hiccups can lead to fatigue, sleep disturbances, dehydration, and even wound dehiscence in the perioperative period.

- A 65-year-old man received a series of three epidural injections, each with 11 ml of a mixture of 0.08% bupivacaine and triamcinolone 80 mg, in an anesthesia pain clinic for evaluation and treatment of lumbar spinal stenosis (157). After the first two injections he developed leg weakness, which resolved after about 4 hours. After the third injection he developed mild urinary retention, which resolved without consequence 6 hours later. All three injections were associated with hiccups after about 1 hour and persisting for 5–7 days. He received two further epidural injections of a glucocorticoid in isotonic saline and did not develop hiccups. All the procedures were 8 weeks apart. A year later, after an epidural injection for a total knee replacement he developed hiccups, which resolved 9 days later.

There are many causes of hiccups. They are most commonly gastrointestinal in origin, such as gastric distention or gastro-esophageal reflux disease. Metabolic derangements and drugs are also frequently implicated. Two cases of hiccups after thoracic epidural injections of glucocorticoids have previously been reported, but in this case a glucocorticoid injection without bupivacaine did not lead to hiccups.

During pregnancy and labor there are important respiratory changes. In a prospective study to clarify whether minor motor blockade brought on by lumbar epidural anesthesia in laboring women further compromises respiratory function, 60 parturients received lumbar epidural anesthesia at L2–4 (158). After a test dose of 3 ml of lidocaine 2% and then a total dose of 10–15 ml of bupivacaine 0.125%, followed by a bolus of fentanyl 50 micrograms, a continuous infusion of 10 ml/hour of bupivacaine 0.125% with fentanyl 0.0001% was started, when sensory blockade at T10 was reached. Most of the patients (87%) had significant improvements in respiratory function, suggesting benefits of epidural analgesia in parturients.

Nervous system

Three case reports have illustrated the neurological consequences of epidural anesthesia in predisposed patients.

- A 51-year-old man, ASA grade II, with non-insulin-dependent diabetes, underwent radical prostatectomy and enterocystoplasty under general anesthesia, before which a lumbar epidural catheter was inserted at L3–4 but was not used during surgery (159). In the recovery room, a test dose of 3 ml of lidocaine 1% with adrenaline 1:200 000 was administered, followed by a bolus dose of 10 ml of ropivacaine 0.75%, which resulted in a block that reached T10. One hour later an infusion of ropivacaine 0.2% was started at 5 ml/hour. Ten hours later he complained of pain, and the pump rate was increased to 10 ml/hour. The treatment was continued for 72 hours without any more dosage adjustments. Eight hours after the end of the epidural treatment he described a burning sensation and pain in the back, spreading to the legs and feet. These symptoms increased with movement, but there were no motor abnormalities. The symptoms persisted, and electromyography showed a sensory polyneuropathy in all four limbs. Eight weeks after the operation he described diminished pain and paresthesia.

The author suggested that local anesthesia in patients with pre-existing diabetic polyneuropathy may result in additional ischemic insult and intraneural edema. Patients with diabetes may therefore be at higher risk of local anesthetic toxicity.

- A 64-year-old man, with a history of multiple spinal operations, chronic low-back pain, and a transient cauda equina syndrome after the most recent operation, was given a left L2 transforaminal epidural injection, unsuccessfully (160). A further attempt at L1 was successful, and 5 ml of bupivacaine 0.125% and 40 mg of triamcinolone was injected. Two minutes later his legs became paralysed. An MRI scan showed signal changes consistent with acute spinal infarction. Four years later he showed no improvement.

Direct injury to the vascular supply of the spinal cord may have been one explanation for this adverse outcome; other reasons included vasospasm caused by either bupivacaine or the glucocorticoid, end-capillary occlusion by glucocorticoid particles, or needle-related factors.

- A 27-year-old primipara was admitted to hospital at week 36 because of a 10-day history of progressive weakness and numbness in all limbs (161). Guillain–Barré syndrome was diagnosed and she was given large doses of intravenous immunoglobulin. Her neurological symptoms improved after 5 days. Five weeks later she spontaneously delivered under epidural analgesia (L2–3), after a test dose of 3 ml of lidocaine 2% with 1:200 000 adrenaline and then 25 mg of ropivacaine 0.2% with 16 micrograms of sufentanil over 3 hours. At this stage she had increased sensory and motor block. Twelve hours postpartum she was unable to walk and had augmented symptoms from the arms, together with facial weakness. She was given large doses of intravenous immunoglobulin. Four months later her status had improved but she still depended on a walker.

The authors speculated that the worsening of the patient's symptoms could have been due to local anesthetic toxicity, since local anesthetics can cause morphological changes in neurons in vitro, impairing their growth.

Peripheral paresthesia, in 1.13% of patients in a Chinese series (SED-12, 254) (155) and 0.16% of patients in a Japanese study of 15 884 epidurals (162), is the most frequent neurological deficit attributed to spinal and epidural analgesia.

High spinal block has previously been reported as a rare complication of epidural anesthesia.

- A 31-year-old woman in labor had an epidural catheter sited at L3/4 (163). A test dose of 0.25% bupivacaine 10 ml was followed 90 minutes later by another 10 ml. After a further 90 minutes she required cesarean section, had a block to T7, and was topped up with 0.75% ropivacaine 10 ml. Within minutes she developed arm weakness, and over the next 15 minutes developed further ascending block requiring intubation. Three hours later the block had regressed to T8 and she had no further complications.

The cause was thought to be subdural injection, although other mechanisms could not be excluded; for example the catheter could have been partly intrathecal and the ultimate distribution of the dose could have been related to the speed of injection or catheter migration before the final dose was given.

Lumbar extradural analgesia with bupivacaine increases intracranial pressure in some patients, apparently those who already have some reduced intracranial compliance, and who may be at risk (164). A sudden increase in intracranial pressure, due to an increased volume in the caudal space, can precipitate respiratory arrest because of direct midbrain stimulation.

- A watershed cerebral infarct with subsequent full recovery occurred in a 70-year-old man 8 hours after a hypotensive event following an incremental bolus of 1% lidocaine 10 ml via an established epidural catheter (165).

A cause-and-effect relation cannot be established in such cases.

Epidural anesthesia can mask a neurological deficit, such as nerve compression of the femoral nerve and lateral femoral cutaneous nerve of the thigh from the lithotomy position (SEDA-22, 137).

- Neurological effects after accidental intravenous injection of a large dose of levobupivacaine (142 mg) have been described during epidural anesthesia (166).
- A 77-year-old woman had epidural anesthesia, following negative aspiration, with a 3 ml test dose of 0.75% levobupivacaine with 1:200 000 adrenaline and then incremental doses up to a total of 17 ml of 0.75% levobupivacaine. During the final 5 ml of injection, she became disoriented and drowsy, with slurred speech, immediately followed by excitation with shouting and writhing about. She was given thiopental for seizure prophylaxis with high-flow oxygen, and the excitatory signs abated. The catheter was withdrawn 1 cm and blood was freely aspirated. The serum levobupivacaine concentration 14 minutes later was 2.7 micrograms/ml.

Transient radicular irritation

Transient radicular irritation has been reported (SEDA-21, 130) (SEDA-22, 137).

- A 38-year-old woman underwent cystoscopy and urethral dilatation in the lithotomy position under continuous epidural anesthesia at the L3–4 interspace with 3 ml of 1.5% lidocaine with adrenaline 1:200 000 as a test dose, followed by a total of 15 ml of 2% lidocaine with adrenaline 1:200 000 in incremental doses (167). The operation was uneventful, but 4 hours later she developed severe bilateral buttock and posterior leg pain, described as "deep, aching, and excruciating," worse when immobile, and better when standing; there were no other symptoms and ibuprofen gave immediate relief.

The authors stressed that transient radicular irritation can occur after epidural administration, despite the lower concentrations of lidocaine in the cerebrospinal fluid.

- Transient neurological symptoms have been reported in two parturients who received lidocaine 45 mg with adrenaline 5 micrograms/ml as a test dose followed by bupivacaine (168). One patient received a single dose of bupivacaine 12.5 mg and the other received a total of 62 mg bupivacaine administered as two 5 ml and one 3 ml bolus of 0.25% bupivacaine followed by an infusion of 0.125% bupivacaine at 5 ml/hour for 4 hours 40 minutes. Both patients later developed reversible burning lower back, buttock pain, and leg pain; there was nothing to suggest intrathecal administration of local anesthetic in either case. Both patients gave birth in the lithotomy position, which may have been contributory.
- Severe burning pain in the buttocks, thighs, and calves has been described in a 5-year-old boy who was given 0.25% bupivacaine and morphine epidurally for perioperative and postoperative analgesia (169).

Two unexplained cases of back and leg pain have been separately described (SEDA-20, 125).

Motor block

Prolonged profound motor block occurred in two patients using patient-controlled epidural analgesia with 0.1% ropivacaine subsequent to spinal bupivacaine for cesarean section (170). One of them developed pressure sores on both heels. The authors hypothesized that epidural ropivacaine may interact with intrathecal bupivacaine to prolong its effects and advised caution when this combination is used, as unexpected motor block can ensue.

The optimal concentration of lumbar epidural ropivacaine in terms of adverse effects and quality of analgesia has been studied in 30 patients using patient-controlled epidural analgesia after lower abdominal surgery (171). Each solution provided comparable analgesia, but motor block was significantly more common and more intense with 0.2% ropivacaine + 4 micrograms/ml fentanyl than with 0.1% ropivacaine + 2 micrograms/ml fentanyl or 0.05% ropivacaine + 1 microgram/ml fentanyl. The amount of ropivacaine used by the 0.1% ropivacaine group was significantly higher than in the other two groups, implying that the concentration rather than the amount of ropivacaine is a primary determinant of motor block with patient-controlled epidural analgesia. The authors recommended the use of ropivacaine in concentrations under 0.2% to reduce motor blockade while still providing effective analgesia.

Epidural solutions containing 0.125% levobupivacaine with and without fentanyl 4 micrograms/ml produced a greater degree of motor blockade only in the first 6 hours of patient-controlled epidural analgesia compared with fentanyl alone in groups of 22 patients after total hip or knee arthroplasty (172).

- An 85-year-old woman undergoing elective right total knee replacement had prolonged motor blockade of her left leg when her epidural ropivacaine (0.2% at 8–10 ml/hour) infusion was discontinued on the third postoperative day; normal motor function had returned by the sixth postoperative day (173).

Paraplegia can result, and can be prevented by early recognition, appropriate investigation, and immediate surgical intervention.

- Delayed onset, prolonged coma, and flaccid quadriplegia occurred in a 22-year-old woman 2 hours after an injection of fentanyl 100 micrograms and 10 ml bupivacaine 0.25%, given in divided doses (4, 3, and 3 ml) via an epidural catheter (174). At the time of the initial attempt at insertion she had complained of severe cervico-occipital pain with loss of resistance to air injection. Despite negative aspiration of CSF, the physician suspected intrathecal injection of air and abandoned the attempt at epidural catheter placement at that level. An epidural catheter was successfully inserted one level higher. Within 1 hour of the original epidural injection, she developed hypotension requiring ephedrine, and a surprisingly high sensory block to T6 with profound lower limb motor blockade. This progressed 2 hours later to upper limb weakness, with respiratory failure requiring intubation and ventilation. She remained unconscious for 9 hours after the initial intubating dose of thiopental. She was able to move all of her limbs 26 hours later and was successfully extubated 43 hours later.

In this case the authors felt that although the initial picture looked like the effects of subdural injection of bupivacaine and fentanyl, the prolonged coma with high motor blockade was more reminiscent of total spinal injection. They postulated that delayed total spinal anesthesia had occurred in this patient as a result of the epidural administration of a large quantity of bupivacaine and fentanyl via a hole made in the dura during the first attempt at epidural insertion.

Accidental subdural block can also lead to rapidly developing high block, patchy block, and symptoms such as myoclonus and anxiety (SEDA-20, 125) (SEDA-22, 136).

Total spinal anesthesia

Permanent or temporary deficits of spinal cord function are caused either by cord ischemia after arterial hypotension, or by cord compression due to an epidural or subdural hematoma or infection, or injury to the spinal cord and nerve roots as a consequence of needle puncture, introduction of a catheter, or chemical irritation.

Total spinal anesthesia is a potentially life-threatening complication of epidural anesthesia.

- A 68-year-old man developed total spinal anesthesia after the administration of 20 ml of ropivacaine 1% without a prior test dose via an epidural catheter, which was inadvertently placed intrathecally (101). Initial aspiration of both the Touhy needle and the catheter failed to identify the intrathecal position of the catheter. The patient noted weakness in his right leg immediately after the end of the injection. This was followed by weakness in his right arm, asystole, apnea, and loss of consciousness. Ventricular escape beats

were noted and sinus rhythm returned after mask ventilation with 100% oxygen and the administration of atropine 1 mg and ephedrine 50 mg. He was able to open his eyes, but remained apneic and was therefore intubated and ventilated. Cardiovascular stability was maintained with incremental boluses of ephedrine to a total of 60 mg. He regained consciousness and was successfully extubated 145 minutes later. All sensory and motor deficits had resolved within 8 hours and no neurological deficit or transient neurological symptoms were detected 5 days later.

This complication emphasizes the fact that aspiration is not sufficient to identify an intrathecal catheter position and that a large dose of a local anesthetic should never be administered without a prior test dose.

- Total spinal anesthesia was suspected in a 46-year-old man who was found unconscious and apneic with no palpable cardiac output 20 minutes after a high thoracic (T2/3) epidural injection of 3 ml lidocaine 1% and 3 ml bupivacaine 0.125% (175). Following initial cardiopulmonary resuscitation he was admitted to the intensive care unit, where treatment included mechanical lung ventilation, thiamylal infusion, and cooling to a core temperature of 33–34°C. The thiamylal was withdrawn after 17 days and he was warmed and successfully extubated the next day. He was discharged after a further 4 months of rehabilitation with no relevant neurological consequences.

Horner's syndrome

Horner's syndrome (miosis, ptosis, anhidrosis, and vasodilatation, with increased temperature of the affected side) can result from epidural anesthesia. A report of Horner's syndrome due to a thoracic epidural catheter has highlighted the fact that small doses of local anesthetic can block the sympathetic fibers to the face, particularly when the catheter tip is close to T2 (176). The same symptoms have been reported after obstetric epidural anesthesia (177).

Horner's syndrome has been reported after lumbar epidural block in two other patients who were having lumbar epidural anesthesia for chronic pain treatment (178). The authors suggested that this complication had probably occurred through anatomical changes in the epidural space, leading to a high degree of sympathetic blockade.

A left-sided Horner's syndrome has been reported following a lumbar epidural with ropivacaine for cesarean section (179). The symptoms resolved after 5 hours. The most likely cause was high sympathetic block, possibly facilitated by left lateral positioning, leading to cephalad spread of the local anesthetic. The authors also wondered whether the physicochemical properties of ropivacaine favor its effect on sympathetic fibers over bupivacaine.

Even a dilute solution, such as 0.04% bupivacaine, can cause Horner's syndrome through high cephalad spread (180).

- A 32-year-old woman in labor had an epidural catheter inserted at L3/4. A test dose of total 5 ml lidocaine 1.5% with adrenaline 1: 200 000 was followed by

15 ml of 0.04% bupivacaine with fentanyl (1.66 micrograms/ml) with the patient in the left lateral position. An infusion of the same mixture at 15 ml/hour was started. After 1 hour she developed miosis, conjunctival injection, and ptosis of the left eye. The upper sensory level was T3/T2. The epidural infusion was stopped for 1 hour and restarted at 12 ml/hour. The signs of Horner's syndrome resolved completely after 2 hours.

Sensory systems

Hearing loss after epidural block has been reported (181).

- A 30-year–old woman with a body mass index of 54 received an epidural catheter at the L3/4 interspace during labor. The procedure was uneventful. A test dose of 3 ml lidocaine 2% was administered. The first top-up dose consisted of 10 ml plain bupivacaine 0.25%. The sensory level was T10 bilaterally after 15 minutes. With the first top-up and every subsequent top-up dose (bupivacaine 0.1% with fentanyl 2 micrograms/ml) she complained of bilateral hearing loss, disappearing spontaneously after 30-60 seconds. After 10 hours a cesarean section was performed. Anesthesia was achieved with two injections of 10 ml of bupivacaine 0.5%. Transient deafness occurred with each top-up dose. The postoperative period was uneventful.

Transient hearing loss after epidural block occurs because the perilymph in the inner ear is in continuity with the cerebrospinal fluid and any pressure wave in the epidural space is conducted to affect the inner ear (182).

Metabolism

A small reduction in glucose concentrations, rarely leading to hypoglycemic coma, can occur (SEDA-16, 130). This effect is in keeping with the finding that the catabolic stress response to surgery may be suppressed by epidural analgesia (SED-12, 254) (183). However, in one study, thoracic epidural administration produced a degree of hyperglycemia (SED-12, 252) (184).

- Symptomatic hypoglycemia occurred in a healthy 30-year-old primigravida after a second 5 ml bolus of 0.25% bupivacaine administered epidurally during labor (185). She developed an altered mental state, which responded rapidly to 50 ml of 50% dextrose administered intravenously.

Urinary tract

Epidural anesthesia increases the risk of urinary retention (186).

Skin

Delayed-type hypersensitivity to epidural ropivacaine has been described.

- A 74-year-old man with postherpetic neuralgia and no history of drug allergies developed a purpuric rash and widespread blotchy erythema on his legs, trunks, and arms following continuous epidural blockade with ropivacaine 0.2% without preservatives (up to 96 ml/day) (187). He had normal white cell and platelet counts and

a slight eosinophilia (640×10^6/l). The epidural infusion and other drugs (amitriptyline, alprazolam, and laxoprofen) were withheld and the eruptions completely resolved within 7 days. Intradermal ropivacaine 0.2% produced erythema (maximum size 23 mm×13 mm) at 8–72 hours. Histology showed perivascular infiltrates of lymphocytes and eosinophils in the dermis. Patch testing with amitriptyline, alprazolam, and loxoprofen induced no eruptions, and neither did restarting the drugs.

This report led to a correspondence questioning the duration of the infusion and also possible cumulative toxicity of ropivacaine (188).

Musculoskeletal

Occasionally orthopedic patients have developed compartment syndrome postoperatively during epidural infusions of bupivacaine/fentanyl mixtures. However, although "aggressive analgesia" was blamed for the resulting disasters, there seems to have been a remarkable lack of adequate pressure area care, correct positioning, and regular review of both patients and splints (SEDA-22, 136).

Infection risk

Contamination of catheters, with subsequent clinical infection, is a potential hazard of epidural analgesia. But not every suspected infection is what it seems; aseptic meningitis has been described after an intradural injection of bupivacaine with methylprednisolone acetate (189).

Death

Inadvertent intravenous administration, due to the accidental placement of an epidural catheter in a vein, is a high-risk complication; deaths have been reported (190).

Pregnancy

Patient-controlled epidural analgesia using either 0.125% ropivacaine with fentanyl 2 micrograms/ml or 0.125% bupivacaine with fentanyl 2 micrograms/ml was studied in 50 patients during labor. Significantly more patients receiving bupivacaine developed motor blockade; 68% of patients in the bupivacaine group developed minimal motor block (Bromage score = 1), while the majority (68%) of patients in the ropivacaine group had no motor blockade. The incidences of adverse effects were similar in both groups. Hypotension occurred in 24% of the ropivacaine group and 16% of the bupivacaine group. Pruritus occurred in 56% of the ropivacaine group and 52% of the bupivacaine group (191).

In 122 women who received 20 ml of either ropivacaine 7.5 mg/ml or bupivacaine 5 mg/ml for epidural anesthesia during elective cesarean section, there were no significant differences in adverse effects, such as the incidence of hypotensive episodes, bradycardia, or nausea and vomiting; however, there was a greater median fall in systolic blood pressure in those given ropivacaine (24 versus 16%) (192). Efficacy and neonatal tolerability were similar in the two groups. This, together with its lesser cardiotoxicity, favors ropivacaine as an alternative to bupivacaine in this setting.

The possibility of increased maternal mortality is a topic of debate. In 1979 there were 150 maternal deaths (0.27 per 1000 births) in Germany, of which 15–25% were apparently related to regional anesthesia, with such complications as hypotension, systemic toxicity, total spinal block, hematoma, catheter rupture, and uterine injury (SED-12, 253) (193). However, obstetric regional anesthesia is regarded as being safer than general anesthesia, whatever the choice of drug, if competently and carefully performed.

Fetotoxicity

Maternal hypotension and excessive placental transfer of local anesthetics and other drugs, for example narcotics or sedatives, given to the mother before or during delivery are the main causes of neonatal death related to the use of these agents in obstetrics. However, deaths are very infrequent (194).

In about 10% of cases, obstetric use of epidural anesthesia will cause some bradycardia in the fetus, but this is not always a clinical problem (SEDA-15, 119). However, accidental intravenous injection of bupivacaine can lead to both maternal convulsions and severe fetal bradycardia (195).

The question of possible neurobehavioral effects in the child as a consequence of obstetric analgesia is still debated; although impairment of visual and neurological performance, reduced alertness, and alterations in walking and muscle tone have all been reported, most authors have found normal Apgar scores and psychomotor development after obstetric anesthesia (SED-12, 253) (196,197), and any functional defects noted at birth are likely to be transient (198).

The effects of low concentrations of epidural bupivacaine on the developing neonatal brain has been studied in infant rhesus monkeys, to decide if there was a detrimental relation between perinatal analgesia with epidural bupivacaine and later infant development (199). The monkeys, whose mothers had been given epidurals at term (but not during labor) were subjected to a battery of neurobehavioral tests for 1 year. The authors concluded that epidural bupivacaine did not cause neonatal abnormalities or specific cognitive defects, but that it may delay the normal course of behavioral development. It is difficult to extrapolate the results of this small study to human obstetrics.

Susceptibility factors

Epidural infusions of bupivacaine are often used in children. However, there are concerns about the increased incidence of adverse effects in infants, owing to reduced hepatic clearance and serum protein binding. In 22 infants aged 1–7 months who received a continuous infusion of bupivacaine 0.375 mg/kg/hour for 2 days during and after surgery, the unbound and total serum concentrations of bupivacaine were measured, along with presurgical and postsurgical concentrations of alpha$_1$ acid glycoprotein (200). The concentrations of alpha$_1$ acid glycoprotein increased markedly after surgery. However, because of reduced clearance unbound concentrations of bupivacaine increased to over 0.2 micrograms/ml in two infants younger than 2 months. The authors proposed a maximum dosage rate of 0.25 mg/kg/hour in infants younger than 4 months and 0.3 mg/kg/hour in older infants.

Femoral block
Infection risk

- Psoas abscess complicating femoral nerve block has been reported (201).
- A 35-year-old woman was admitted for arthroscopic arthrolysis of the knee. A femoral catheter was placed before induction of general anesthesia under strict aseptic conditions. The catheter was connected via a 0.2 μm bacterial filter to an infusion device containing ropivacaine. The catheter remained in place for 4 days with no sign of infection at the site of insertion. On the fifth day she complained of lower quadrant abdominal pain and developed a fever and a raised leukocyte count. A pelvic scan showed a psoas abscess, which was drained under CT guidance. The aspirate contained *Staphylococcus aureus*. After antibiotic therapy the abscess resolved completely.

The authors conclude that the abscess had probably esulted from catheter colonization at a superficial site that had spread to the psoas space.

Infiltration anesthesia

Forty adverse events during direct local anesthetic infusion into surgical wounds have been reported to the US FDA (202). These reports included 17 cases of necrosis, 13 of cellulitis, 15 surgical wound infections, and 10 unspecified infections. Of four patients who received bupivacaine and adrenaline as continuous wound infiltration after total knee procedures, two developed full thickness sloughs and two developed partial thickness sloughs; all required plastic surgery. In their discussion, the FDA pointed out that these reports had not been verified for accuracy and completeness. The authors concluded that there was not an established causal link between surgery, the use of an infusion device or the infusion of bupivacaine (with or without adrenaline), and the adverse events. Nevertheless, the reports were considered to constitute an important signal.

Cardiovascular

Hemodynamic changes due to additives in local anesthetics have been described. Local anesthetics containing adrenaline are routinely used in functional endoscopic sinus surgery (FESS) for achieving hemostasis. In a prospective double-blind study of the hemodynamic effects of infiltration with lidocaine + 1:200,000 adrenaline 76 patients were randomly allocated to three groups (203). Group I received 2% lidocaine 2 ml with adrenaline, group II received saline 2 ml with adrenaline, and group III received saline 2 ml without adrenaline. Adrenaline, with and without lidocaine, caused significant hemodynamic changes compared with saline. The changes lasted no more than 4 minutes. The authors concluded that the changes were due to the effects of adrenaline on β_2 adrenoceptors.

Nervous system

Spinal cord infarction is an extremely rare but catastrophic complication of paravertebral injection.

- A 66–year-old man with a painful cervical spine received a paravertebral cervical infiltration of lidocaine + cortisone at C5-6 (204). He developed respiratory failure 2.5 hours later and was successfully resuscitated. However, he developed a tetraplegia with full consciousness and was ventilation for the next 2 months, when he died. An MRI scan confirmed an ischemic lesion of the upper anterior cervical myelin. Neuropathology confirmed anterior infarction of the cervical myelin at C2/C3, with obstruction of the anterior spinal artery by an epithelialized fibrocartilaginous embolus.

It was not possible to conclude with absolute certainty, for legal purposes, that the cervical infiltration had caused the fibrocartilaginous embolism. However, the authors suggested that without any other relevant evidence anatomically or at post-mortem, there was a strong suggestion that puncture of an intervertebral fibrous disc and subsequent transportation of the material into an arterial lumen by the cannula caused the ultimately fatal outcome.

Facial paralysis can be the consequence of local anesthetic administration in the laryngeal area.

- A 4-year-old boy was given a peritonsillar infiltration of bupivacaine hydrochloride 0.5%, in a volume of 2–3 ml per tonsil, and both tonsils were removed uneventfully (205). A few minutes later, he developed right-sided peripheral facial paralysis, which worsened over the next hour. There was neither laceration nor bleeding. The facial paralysis improved slowly and completely resolved after 8 hours.

The authors assumed that the paralysis had been caused by a direct effect of the local anesthetic agent on the facial nerve.

Sensory systems

Tumescent anesthesia is a form of protracted infiltration anesthesia using large volumes of diluted local anesthetics. It is used for liposuction, which has become the most frequently performed cosmetic procedure in the world. In eight consecutive patients of ASA grade I, plasma concentrations and objective/subjective symptoms over 20 hours after tumescent anesthesia with lidocaine 35 mg/kg (3 liters of a buffered solution of 0.08% lidocaine with adrenaline) at an average rate of 116 ml/minute were noted (206). Peak plasma concentration of 2.3 µg/ml of lidocaine occurred after 5–17 hours. There was no correlation between peak concentrations and dose per kg or total amount of lidocaine infiltrated. One patient had tinnitus after 14 hours at a plasma concentration of

3.3 µg/ml. The authors suggested that even though no fluid overload or toxic symptoms occurred in this small group of patients, there is still a risk of toxicity in association with peak concentrations of lidocaine that may occur after discharge.

Intercostal nerve anesthesia
Nervous system
High spinal anesthesia after inadvertent injection is a possible complication of intercostal nerve block (SED-12, 252). Pneumothorax is another reported complication (70).

Respiratory
Unilateral bronchospasm after interpleural block with bupivacaine has been described.

- A 55-year-old man received an interpleural block with 20 ml of bupivacaine 0.5% + adrenaline 100 µg (1:200000) after a test dose and 45 minutes later there was a fall in SpO_2 from 98 to 93% accompanied by a rise in respiratory rate to 30/minute and mild respiratory distress (207). On auscultation there were expiratory wheezes on the right side and normal breath sounds on the left. The unilateral bronchospasm resolved spontaneously, coinciding with a three-segment regression of analgesia to T4.

Anesthetic techniques that can cause bronchospasm in non-asthmatic patients include: interscalene brachial plexus block, interpleural block, spinal and general anesthesia, and intercostal nerve block. Bronchospasm can be initiated by any technique that interrupts sympathetic innervation in the lungs but spares the parasympathetic.

Interpleural anesthesia
Interpleural administration of local anesthetics has been followed by Horner's syndrome and increased skin temperature, apparently pointing to an effect on the sympathetic nervous system (208). Pneumothorax or infection can also result. Interpleural administration of local anesthetics can produce high serum drug concentrations and a risk of systemic toxicity (SEDA-21, 13), possibly increased by the addition of adrenaline (SEDA-20, 126).

Intra-articular anesthesia
Intra-articular anesthesia has been used successfully in many patients, with few adverse effects (SEDA-20, 126). However, it is not always safe; at least one death has occurred from bupivacaine used in this way (209). Intra-articular anesthesia in the knee joint was followed in one case by necrosis of the knee ligament and the skin, apparently due to localized drug-induced embolism (210).

Intradermal anesthesia
Intradermal local anesthetic solutions can cause considerable pain on injection. Additives, such as hyaluronidase, which are used to enhance the analgesic effect of local anesthetics, can often exacerbate this (211). Infiltration

from the inside of a wound can be less painful than through intact skin (212).

The order of injection can affect the pain of local anesthetic infiltration with buffered lidocaine; in a sequence of two injections the second injection was consistently reported to be more painful than the first. This finding has important consequences with regard to trial design in this area of research (213). Buffered lidocaine warmed to 37°C was less painful than warmed plain lidocaine, plain lidocaine, and buffered lidocaine in a randomized controlled trial in 26 volunteers (214).

Intrathecal (spinal) anesthesia

Intrathecal anesthesia has been compared with general anesthesia in 33 patients with pre-eclamptic toxemia undergoing cesarean section (215). The complications after general anesthesia were more serious, with a 4.3% mortality, whereas complications after spinal anesthesia were less serious and easily manageable, notably intraoperative hypotension (47%), difficulty in locating the subarachnoid space (29%), and intraoperative vomiting (6%).

Hyperbaric ropivacaine 0.25% has been compared with hyperbaric bupivacaine 0.25% in a crossover study in 18 volunteers who received an intrathecal anesthetic; the doses were 4, 8, or 12 mg (216). More patients had lumbosacral back pain after intrathecal ropivacaine compared with bupivacaine (5 versus 1), although this difference was not significant; the back pain lasted 3–5 days and was mild to moderate in intensity.

Intrathecal isobaric ropivacaine (15 mg) has been compared with intrathecal isobaric bupivacaine (10 mg) in 100 patients having transurethral resection of the bladder or prostate (217). Median cephalad spread of blocks was two segments higher for both pinprick and cold with bupivacaine compared with ropivacaine. Onset time to anesthesia was the same in both groups. Significantly more patients in the ropivacaine group complained of painful sensations at the surgical site (16 versus 0%). There was no difference in anesthetic duration, the incidence, intensity, onset, and duration of motor blockade, or the incidence of hypotension in the two groups. There were no cases of transient neurological symptoms. The authors concluded that ropivacaine 15 mg is less potent than bupivacaine 10 mg for intrathecal analgesia.

Continuous intrathecal anesthesia with 10 ml of 0.25% bupivacaine over 24 hours has been compared with continuous epidural anesthesia with 48 ml of 0.25% bupivacaine over 24 hours during the first 2 days after hip replacement in 102 patients (218). Continuous spinal anesthesia provided better analgesia and more patient satisfaction, but significantly more patients had motor blockade during the day of surgery and the first postoperative day. There was a significantly higher incidence of nausea and vomiting with continuous epidural anesthesia (39 versus 21).

When a pneumatic tourniquet was used in intrathecal anesthesia, pain was twice as frequent with tetracaine (60%) as with bupivacaine (25%) (219). However, using bupivacaine and tetracaine together seems to produce a more prolonged analgesic effect without inducing more hypotension than either agent alone (SEDA-18, 143).

In 80 patients undergoing lower extremity or lower abdominal surgery randomized to receive hyperbaric bupivacaine 10 mg alone or in combination with fentanyl 12.5 micrograms intrathecally, those given fentanyl had significantly longer duration of analgesia with no reported sedation or respiratory depression (220). Pruritus occurred in 20% of patients given fentanyl and shivering occurred significantly more often in those given bupivacaine only (30 versus 12.5%).

The addition of low doses of clonidine and neostigmine to intrathecal bupivacaine + fentanyl in 30 patients in labor significantly increased the duration of analgesia but was associated with significantly more emesis (221).

In a comparison of intrathecal bupivacaine 10 mg and bupivacaine 7.5 mg combined with ketamine 25 mg, in 30 healthy women there was no extension of postoperative analgesia or reduction in postoperative analgesic requirements in those given ketamine (222). Those given ketamine had a shorter duration of motor blockade, but had an increased incidence of adverse effects, and the study was abandoned after 30 patients.

Intrathecal blockade with 0.5% isobaric bupivacaine 10 mg has been compared with 0.5% isobaric bupivacaine 5 mg combined with fentanyl 25 micrograms (diluted to 2 ml with isotonic saline) in 32 patients undergoing elective cesarean section (223). The bupivacaine + fentanyl combination was associated with significantly less hypotension than bupivacaine alone (31 versus 94%) and a near 10-fold reduction in the mean ephedrine requirement (2.8 versus 23.8 mg). There were also significant differences in the incidence of nausea (31 versus 69%) and the median time to peak block (8 versus 10 minutes) with bupivacaine plus fentanyl. The authors advised further large-scale studies to quantify the minimum dose of bupivacaine plus fentanyl for single-dose spinal anesthesia.

An isobaric solution of sameridine given intrathecally in doses of 15, 20, and 23 mg has been compared with hyperbaric lidocaine 100 mg in 100 volunteers (224). Sameridine has both local anesthetic and opioid analgesic properties. There was one incident of transient paresthesia with sameridine 20 mg and two cases of bradycardia with lidocaine; the incidence of hypotension was more frequent with lidocaine, but pruritus was more common with sameridine.

A technique for the reversal of an unintentional total spinal anesthetic has been described (225). The epidural catheter, positioned in the intrathecal space, was used to wash out the overdose of local anesthetic by "cerebrospinal lavage", leading to rapid recovery.

Comparative studies

Hyperbaric ropivacaine 0.5% and hyperbaric bupivacaine 0.5% for spinal anesthesia, 3 ml of either, have been compared in 40 randomized patients undergoing lower-abdominal, perineal, or lower-limb surgery (226). The onset time with bupivacaine was significantly faster than with ropivacaine. The mean duration of sensory block was significantly longer with bupivacaine. The patients given ropivacaine mobilized and passed urine significantly faster than those who received bupivacaine. There was also more hypotension with bupivacaine. The authors concluded that ropivacaine 15 mg in glucose 50 mg/ml provides reliable spinal anesthesia with less hypotension than bupivacaine.

Cardiovascular

Hypotension is the most frequent adverse effect of spinal anesthesia; in one very large series it occurred in 22% of the subarachnoid group (227), but the actual figures differ with the anesthetic, its concentration, and the definition of hypotension used. For example single-dose spinal anesthesia causes significantly more hypotension and bradycardia than continuous spinal anesthesia (228). Hypotension may be more of a problem with tetracaine or lidocaine than with bupivacaine in equivalent doses (SEDA-12, 35), and the incidence is less when the patient is in the lateral rather than the sitting position. However, using bupivacaine and tetracaine together seems to produce a more prolonged analgesic effect without inducing more hypotension than either agent alone (SEDA-18, 143). Hypotension is also reported with intrathecal opioids and opioid/local anesthetic combinations; sufentanil appears to predominate in these reports (SEDA-21, 132) (SEDA-22, 137).

The adverse effects of spinal anesthesia have been evaluated in a large prospective study in 1132 children aged 6 months to 14 years undergoing lower body surgery (229). Spinal blocks were performed with 0.5% bupivacaine at doses of 0.2 mg/kg at interspace L3–4 or L5–S1. Only 27 patients required some form of anesthetic supplementation. There was hypotension in 17 patients. The incidences of headache (n = 5) and low back pain (n = 9) were low. There were no other neurological complications.

Intra-operative hypotension is common and potentially dangerous in elderly patients undergoing spinal anesthesia for repair of hip fractures. Combining an intrathecal opioid with a local anesthetic allows a reduction in the dose of local anesthetic and causes less sympathetic block and hypotension, while still maintaining adequate anesthesia.

In a double-blind, randomized comparison in 40 patients of glucose-free bupivacaine 9.0 mg with added fentanyl 20 micrograms with glucose-free bupivacaine 11.0 mg alone, the incidence and frequency of hypotension was reduced by the addition of fentanyl (230). Similarly, falls in systolic, diastolic, and mean blood pressures were all less. However, there were four failed blocks in those given fentanyl compared with one in those given bupivacaine alone.

Cerebral blood flow has been evaluated prospectively in former preterm infants who underwent inguinal hernia repair with spinal anesthesia (231). There was a significant reduction in diastolic cerebral blood flow velocities, explained by reduced arterial blood pressure secondary to spinal anesthesia and impaired cerebral autoregulation.

However, the clinical relevance of these findings was unclear.

Hypotension can be prevented or treated with vasopressors and/or fluids (SED-12, 254) (SEDA-18, 143) (232–234). A comparison of these approaches showed that ephedrine alone is less effective than ephedrine and colloid (235), and metaraminol, with or without colloid, is better than colloid alone (236).

The effect of baricity on the hemodynamic effects of intrathecal 0.5% bupivacaine has been measured by recording invasive systolic blood pressure and central venous pressure in 36 men given plain bupivacaine 0.5%, heavy bupivacaine 0.5% (in dextrose 8%), or a mixture of the two (in dextrose 4%) (237). Heavy bupivacaine caused more rapid falls in central venous pressure and systolic blood pressure than plain bupivacaine. However, it was subsequently remarked that both 4 and 8% dextrose are significantly hyperbaric relative to adult cerebrospinal fluid, implying that the 4% solution should have behaved more like the 8% solution (238).

In 191 women who had had cesarean sections under spinal anesthesia using hyperbaric bupivacaine 12–15 mg and morphine 0.25 mg, who were transferred to the recovery room on a stretcher with the upper body either flexed 30° or supine during transport 10% of each group had a greater than 20% fall in systolic blood pressure unaffected by position (239). The authors recommended routine monitoring of the blood pressure and pulse after transfer to the stretcher, and suggested that raising the head for the comfort of the mother during transport does not increase the risk of hypotension.

Isobaric bupivacaine 4 mg combined with fentanyl 20 micrograms has been compared with isobaric bupivacaine 10 mg alone in 20 patients over the age of 70 undergoing surgery for fractured neck of femur (138). Hypotension was defined as a systolic blood pressure less than 90 mmHg or a fall in mean arterial pressure of more than 25%. Significantly more patients given bupivacaine only had hypotension (90 versus 10%). The mean dosage requirement of ephedrine was higher with bupivacaine only (32 versus 0.5 mg) and two patients in this group required phenylephrine, while no patient given bupivacaine plus fentanyl did. No patient in either group complained of perioperative pain or required supplementary analgesia intraoperatively.

In young infants similar problems with blood pressure occur, and some changes in heart rate may be found, but tend to be transient (SEDA-12, 154) (240).

Intrathecal blockade for cesarean section using 0.5% hyperbaric bupivacaine at three different doses of 7.5 mg, 8.75 mg, and 10 mg has been studied in a double-blind comparison in 60 patients (241). There was no significant difference in maximum block height, but more of the patients who were given the two lower doses had moderate visceral pain requiring rescue ketamine. Bupivacaine 10 mg was associated with significantly more bradycardia, and 7.5 and 8.75 mg with significantly more hypotension. Motor block lasted significantly longer with 10 mg. The outcome was good in all the infants, although one baby whose mother had received bupivacaine 10 mg had an

Apgar score below 10 at 5 minutes. The authors concluded that the use of bupivacaine 7.5 mg avoids hypotension, bradycardia, and prolonged block.

Bradycardia occurs in some 3% of spinal anesthetics in adults. Bradycardia can lead to cardiac arrest, either by direct block of the sympathetic innervation of the heart (in unintended high block) or as a consequence of insufficient venous return. In 900 cases of major anesthetic mishaps giving rise to compensation claims, there were 14 cases of cardiac arrest under spinal anesthesia, of which six were fatal (242). Myocardial infarction and cardiac arrest preceded by atrioventricular block have also been described.

- A 68-year-old man was given 0.5% bupivacaine 4 ml or spinal anesthesia, and 5 minutes later complained of nausea and developed hypotension, loss of consciousness, and a tonic-clonic seizure. He had first-degree heart block 4 minutes after subarachnoid injection, followed 1 minute later by third-degree heart block, and then asystole. He was successfully resuscitated. Proposed theories included a reflex bradycardia resulting from reduced venous return and/or unopposed vagal tone due to thoracic sympathectomy induced by spinal anesthesia (243).

Bradycardia has been reported to follow spinal anesthesia in association with urinary retention (244).

- A receding spinal block to level L1–2 gave rise to acute bradycardia (34–40/minute) and transient loss of consciousness in a 31-year-old man 5 hours after spinal anesthesia; on waking he complained of severe low back pain, and although he had no symptoms of urinary retention, urinary catheterization yielded 900 ml of urine with immediate relief of symptoms.

Slow injection of hyperbaric bupivacaine 8 mg has been compared with hyperbaric bupivacaine 15 mg used to achieve bilateral block in 30 patients of ASA grades I–II (245). There was significantly greater cardiovascular stability in the patients who had a unilateral spinal block.

Respiratory

Respiratory arrest is one of the most serious potential adverse effects of spinal anesthesia, either due to brainstem depression in high block or rostral spread of opioids after the use of combined techniques (SEDA-21, 132) (SEDA-22, 137).

Immediate respiratory arrest has been reported after the administration of intrathecal bupivacaine and fentanyl (246).

- A 26-year-old woman in labor was given an epidural for analgesia. After 2 hours and total doses of bupivacaine 77.5 mg and fentanyl 190 micrograms, the epidural was removed owing to failure. A subsequent intrathecal injection of bupivacaine 2.5 mg plus fentanyl 10 micrograms was followed 4 minutes later by apnea and loss of consciousness. She was rapidly intubated and regained consciousness after 15 minutes, at which time her

sensory level was T8 to pinprick. She was extubated after 30 minutes.

The authors concluded that the respiratory depression had been due to excessive cephalad spread of fentanyl, possibly facilitated by the volume of bupivacaine that had previously been injected epidurally.

Bronchospasm has been reported in two obstetric patients, possibly due to thoracic sympathetic blockade in one and hypersensitivity in the other (SEDA-21, 132).

There is a potential risk that spinal anesthesia will cause apnea in premature infants. However, spinal anesthesia with a sound technique has been used safely in high-risk infants. Tetracaine was used in 142 such cases; only two infants had serious adverse effects, one with unexplained but treatable apnea and one in whom too high a block resulted in respiratory arrest (247).

Two former preterm infants (postconceptual age 38 weeks) both received spinal anesthetics for inguinal herniorrhaphy (block level T4–6) (248). No other medications were given. Both infants had frequent episodes of perioperative apnea and associated bradycardia. One had a 20-second bout of apnea, with an oxygen saturation of 70% and a heart rate of 80/minute, the other a 30-second bout of apnea, with a saturation of 70% and a heart rate of 60/minute. These episodes persisted for 8 hours into the postoperative period in one of the infants.

The frequency of transient neurological symptoms and neurological complications after spinal anesthesia with lidocaine compared with other local anesthetics has been reviewed (249). Lidocaine causes transient neurological symptoms in one in seven patients receiving spinal anesthesia and the relative risk is about seven times higher for lidocaine than for bupivacaine, prilocaine, and procaine. While the latter anesthetics are associated with a lower risk of transient neurological symptoms, their longer duration or lower quality of anesthesia may limit their suitability for ambulatory surgery.

- A patient who was receiving modified-release morphine for malignant pain had a respiratory arrest after intrathecal bupivacaine 12.5 mg. She recovered after treatment with naloxone. Another patient who was taking modified-release morphine was given intrathecal morphine 10 mg and bupivacaine 7.5 mg. He had respiratory distress and became comatose. Morphine-induced respiratory depression was not diagnosed and the patient subsequently died. In both cases, respiratory distress and sedation was probably due to opioid action in the absence of the stimulating effect of pain on respiration, due to the intrathecal bupivacaine (250).
- A 20-year-old woman who received a combined spinal epidural for labor had a respiratory arrest 23 minutes after the administration of sufentanil 10 micrograms and bupivacaine 2.5 mg (251).

Nervous system

The incidence of transient neurological symptoms with lidocaine compared with other local anesthetics has been the subject of a systematic review of 14 randomized, controlled trials in 1347 patients, 117 of whom developed transient neurological symptoms (252). Of the 117, 94 developed the symptoms after the use of lidocaine (out of 674 patients treated with lidocaine). The clinical picture was typically bilateral pain in the buttocks, thighs, and legs, which started within 24 hours after the initiation of spinal anesthesia and after complete recovery from spinal anesthesia. The pain varied in intensity from mild to severe (visual analogue scale score 2–9.5), and most patients complained of mild to moderate pain. A nonsteroidal anti-inflammatory drugs was the treatment of choice and a few patients were given opioids as well. In most cases the pain disappeared by the second day and the maximum duration was 5 days; only one patient had symptoms for 10 days. None had any neurological symptoms. The relative risk of transient neurological symptoms after spinal anesthesia with lidocaine was 4.35 (95% CI = 1.98, 9.54) and therefore significantly higher than with other local anesthetics (bupivacaine, prilocaine, procaine, and mepivacaine). This increased risk must be weighed against the benefit of rapid, short-acting anesthesia when considering whether to use lidocaine for ambulatory anesthesia.

As early ambulation after spinal anesthesia has been described as a risk factor for transient neurological symptoms, the effects of ambulation after subarachnoid lidocaine have been subjected to a randomized, double-blind study in 60 patients, comparing early ambulation with 6 hours recumbent position postoperatively (253). There was no significant difference between the groups in the incidence of transient neurological symptoms (23% versus 27%). In all patients the symptoms resolved spontaneously. The authors proposed that there is no correlation between the time of ambulation and the incidence of transient neurological symptoms.

While lidocaine is primarily regarded as the agent causing transient neurological symptoms, mepivacaine has also infrequently been implicated (254). In a prospective single-center study of 1273 patients who received spinal or combined spinal–epidural anesthesia with plain mepivacaine 1.5% for ambulatory surgery, transient neurological symptoms occurred in 78 patients (6.4%) (255). None of the 372 combined spinal–epidural anesthetics was inadequate for surgery, but 14 of 838 spinal anesthetics (1.7%) were inadequate. The mean age of patients who developed transient neurological symptoms was 48 years, older than that of patients without symptoms, 41 years. Transient neurological symptoms were not influenced by sex or intraoperative position. None of the patients had permanent neurological sequelae. The authors concluded that spinal anesthesia with mepivacaine is associated with a high success rate and infrequent transient neurological symptoms, making it likely to be a safe and effective technique for ambulatory patients.

Unusually prolonged spinal anesthesia has also been reported.

• A 67-year-old man with significant peripheral arterial disease scheduled for femoropopliteal bypass surgery had an uneventful spinal injection with hyperbaric bupivacaine 15 mg (256). A sensory level was recorded bilaterally at T10. Nine hours later there was complete motor blockade and no sensory level regression. A CT scan with contrast was negative. About 24 hours later there was sensory regression to L1-L2 and complete spontaneous recovery from sensory and motor blockade occurred at 29 hours. There was no permanent neurological deficit or pain.

Negative radiology and complete resolution of symptoms ruled out spinal hematoma in this case. The authors assumed caudal maldistribution of hyperbaric solution hypothetically related to a low volume of CSF, reduced elimination from the subarachnoid space secondary to atherosclerosis, or an unknown cause, although transient spinal artery syndrome could not be ruled out.

Neurological defects and arachnoiditis after neuroaxial anesthesia has been reviewed (257). Arachnoiditis in the context of epidural anesthesia can be caused by epidural abscess, traumatic puncture, local anesthetics, detergents, and other substances unintentionally injected into the spinal canal. Severe burning pain in the lower back and legs and dysesthesia and numbness in a non-dermatomal distribution suggest direct injury to the spinal cord. Patients with these symptoms should be thoroughly examined by a neurologist, followed by an MRI scan of the affected area. The author suggested that immediate administration of glucocorticoids and NSAIDs should be considered, to prevent inflammation, which might develop into arachnoiditis.

Combined spinal-epidural analgesia for labor has a well-established safety record. However, there have been reports of unusual complications including, in one case, aphonia and aphagia (258).

• A 21-year-old otherwise healthy woman at 37 weeks gestation, with no drug allergies and no previous anesthesia, received combined spinal-epidural analgesia in the sitting position at vertebral interspace L2/3. There were no technical problems and there was free flow of cerebrospinal fluid. She was given fentanyl 10 micrograms combined with 1 ml of bupivacaine 2.5 mg/ml, and an epidural catheter was inserted to 5 cm. No blood or spinal fluid was aspirated. She reported pain relief after 2 minutes. About 4 minutes after the subarachnoid injection her voice became weak and she then lost the ability to talk and swallow. She was alert and conscious and had normal vital signs; no treatment was given and she became able talk and swallow again after 20 minutes. Uneventful epidural analgesia was later used for labor and delivery.

The authors speculated that there had been extensive cephalad spread of fentanyl in the subarachnoid space, since there has been one previous report of dysphagia after the administration of fentanyl combined with bupivacaine using combined spinal-epidural analgesia in conjunction with labor analgesia.

Seven patients with chronic pain receiving intrathecal analgesics and/or local anesthetics were screened for catheter associated masses (259). Three of the seven had intraspinal masses; two were asymptomatic. Patients with intraspinal masses were significantly younger and were receiving significantly higher doses of morphine than the patients without masses; it is unclear whether local anesthetics contribute to this complication. The authors concluded that patients receiving long-term intrathecal analgesia should undergo periodic radiographic surveillance to look for catheter-associated masses and to allow intervention before neurological deficits occur.

Spinal myoclonus can develop as a result of stimulation of the spinal cord, which can be caused by spinal cord compression, tumors, vascular myelopathy, infections, demyelinating diseases, trauma, and paraneoplastic syndromes, but also by medications such as contrast media, local anesthetics, and analgesics. Segmental spinal myoclonus after spinal bupivacaine has been described (260).

- A 56-year-old woman underwent surgery for bilateral leg varices; she received 3 ml of 0.5% hyperbaric bupivacaine at the L4/5 interspace. Two hours postoperatively she started to have bilateral rhythmic myoclonic movements of the legs. The frequency gradually increased and reached a maximum after 30 minutes then disappeared after another 30 minutes without any neurological sequelae.

A toxic spinal cord lesion has been described after long-term treatment of chronic pain via an intrathecal catheter (261).

A 45-year-old man with severe right sciatic trunk compression neuropathy had a programmable pump system implanted, connected to a catheter in the intrathecal space advanced to the level of T12. The pump delivered bupivacaine in a concentration of 20 then 40 mg/ml, at daily doses of 24–27 mg for 459 days. After 13 months reduced efficacy made it necessary to add clonidine 200 micrograms/day. This combination continued for the next 600 days. After nearly 3 years he developed lower back pain and neurological symptoms, including gait ataxia and loss of proprioception. An MRI scan showed a small round cavity within the spinal cord associated with widespread cord edema. Three months later a scan showed complete resolution of the medullary edema, accompanied by marked improvement of neurological function. However, a centromedullary lesion at T9 and a hyperdense posterolateral lesion at T10–11 persisted.

The authors were unable to suggest a precise cause of this complication, but they discussed potential neurotoxic effects of bupivacaine, possibly related to high local concentrations. This caser reinforces recommendations that drug concentrations be kept low in these cases and that patients with intrathecal drug systems should have brief neurological evaluations at every pump refill.

- A 40-year-old woman developed acute aphasia and a change in mental status 15 minutes after the intrathecal administration of sufentanil 10 micrograms and isobaric bupivacaine 2.5 mg as part of a combined spinal epidural anesthetic for analgesia during labor (262). She appeared to be in a dissociated state, had apparent difficulty swallowing, and was aphasic, but able to follow simple commands. She had sensory block to T6 on the right and T8 on the left, with no motor block. The neurological picture resolved about 100 minutes after the anesthetic; an exact etiology could not be established.

- A similar case has been reported 20 minutes after the intrathecal administration of 0.5% hyperbaric bupivacaine 2 ml for cesarean section (263). She became unresponsive then apneic for a short time. There were no changes in heart rate or blood pressure and no loss of airway protection. She slowly regained consciousness over the next hour without any consequences.

The authors were unclear about the cause and suggested subdural injection, as the slow onset, stable hemodynamics, and rapid recovery were suggestive of this complication. However, other causes, including a psychogenic response, are possibilities.

- New onset, severe lightning pain after repeated subarachnoid blockade occurred in a 48-year-old man with pre-existing neuropathic pain after incomplete spinal cord injury, similar to previous reports in patients with phantom limb pain (264).

Postural headache is a common complication of spinal anesthesia (so-called postdural puncture headache). It is caused by CSF leakage through the puncture site. The incidence has been greatly reduced by the use of smaller-gauge and pencil-point spinal needles. However, headache (or psychosis) can be the presenting sign of subdural hematoma, which has twice been observed in women given spinal anesthesia for childbirth (SEDA-18, 143).

- A 30-year-old patient developed aseptic meningitis 24 hours after spinal anesthesia with bupivacaine plus fentanyl; it resolved without sequelae within 48 hours (265).

Conus medullaris syndrome has been reported after consecutive intrathecal injections of hyperbaric 1% tetracaine, followed by hyperbaric 5% lidocaine with adrenaline, in a patient with diabetic neuropathy (SEDA-21, 130).

Less frequent neurological complications are bladder dysfunction or sphincter paresis (266), intracranial hypertension, and convulsions, the latter reflecting systemic toxicity.

- A 36-year-old man had two generalized tonic-clonic convulsions after receiving intrathecal tetracaine 8 mg to supplement inadequate block established by intrathecal administration of tetracaine 10 mg (267). His seizures were controlled with intravenous thiamylal sodium. He regained consciousness, but complained of dizziness and blurred vision. He had a sensory block to T4–5.

The authors excluded total spinal anesthesia as a cause of the seizures, on the basis of the sensory level and the lack of hypotension.

Cauda equina syndrome
Cauda equina syndrome is the triad of bilateral paraparesis or paraplegia of the muscles of the legs and buttocks, saddle anesthesia plus sensory deficits below the groin, and incompetence of bladder and rectal sphincters, causing incontinence of urine and feces.

Cauda equina syndrome has been reported after the use of microcatheters for continuous intrathecal anesthesia. The concern was sufficient reason for the FDA to withdraw microcatheters from the US market after 11 cases of cauda equina in 1992 (SEDA-21, 129) (268). It has now become obvious that a confounding factor was the use of hyperbaric solutions pooling around lumbosacral nerve roots, aggravated by the poor mechanics of microcatheters and the use of inappropriate amounts; the authors of one study argued that the problem was not evident with the use of low concentrations of isobaric local anesthetics administered via microcatheters (269).

Six cases of the syndrome have also been reported after "single-shot" spinal anesthesia at the L3–4 interspace with 5% hyperbaric lidocaine (270).

- A 55-year-old man was given 5% hyperbaric lidocaine 100 mg intrathecally in the sitting position for transurethral resection of the prostate in the lithotomy position, with no complications. However, the next day he complained of persistent numbness of the perianal, scrotal, penile, and sacral regions, and both legs. He also had difficulty in defecation and weakness of both quadriceps muscles. Despite normal MRI scanning, electromyography, and electroneurography, he had no neurological improvement, even 1.5 years after the operation.
- A 59-year-old woman received 5% hyperbaric lidocaine 60 mg for an operation on a toe. That evening she complained of urinary and bowel incontinence; 5 months later she had urinary stress incontinence and bowel incontinence, with absent anal reflexes. There was also reduced sensation over the medial side of the foot.
- A 48-year-old woman had spinal anesthesia for hallux valgus surgery and had pain radiating to the left buttock during insertion of the needle. Hyperbaric 5% lidocaine 100 mg was injected, with no associated paresthesia. One month later, she complained of persistent numbness of the perianal and sacral regions and had sensory loss in these regions, which failed to improve over 6 months.
- A 31-year-old man had spinal anesthesia with 5% hyperbaric lidocaine 100 mg for fasciotomy. His systolic blood pressure briefly fell to 90 mmHg and he was given ephedrine. He later complained of persistent numbness of the entire right leg, right scrotum, right side of the penis, and right buttock, and had difficulty in micturition; there was no improvement one month later, and he had reduced pain and temperature sensation in the right leg, intact touch sensation, and weakness of right hip extension. His neurological state did not improve over a year.
- A 37-year-old woman had varicose vein surgery under spinal anesthesia with 5% hyperbaric lidocaine 120 mg in two injections followed by a general anesthesia, because the spinal block was inadequate. Postoperatively she complained of persistent numbness in the right buttock, difficulty in micturition, and bowel incontinence. She had reduced sensation in the perianal region and both labia majora, with a large residual urine volume. An MRI scan was normal, but electromyography, electroneurography,

and cystometry 4 months later showed denervation of the pelvic muscles, partial denervation of the detrusor muscle, and signs of re-innervation. After 5 months her condition remained much the same.
- A 59-year-old man had spinal anesthesia for hallux valgus surgery with 5% hyperbaric lidocaine 75 mg. The next day he had persistent perianal numbness, difficulty in micturition, and a large residual urine volume. An MRI scan was normal and he had reduced perianal and scrotal sensation, difficulty in defecation, and erectile impotence. He was no better 5 months later.

The authors stated that at least some of the cases had probably resulted from neurotoxicity of hyperbaric lidocaine, most often in the absence of obvious maldistribution. They recommended that hyperbaric lidocaine should be used in concentrations not exceeding 2% and in a total dose no greater than 60 mg.

- A 75-year-old woman with a history of lumbar laminectomy, but no neurological deficit, received an intrathecal injection of 4 ml of 0.5% bupivacaine with preservatives at the L4–5 level using a 22-gauge spinal needle for a total knee replacement (271). Intraoperatively she complained of severe low back pain, which improved 8 hours later. In parallel, she developed persistent sensory loss to L1 and flaccid paralysis of both legs. An MRI scan was normal, but myelography showed inflammation of the cauda equina; 2 months later she developed hydrocephalus and had adhesive arachnoiditis of the thoracolumbar region. Her neurological condition did not improve over 2 years.
- A 72-year-old man of ASA status 1 had spinal anesthesia with hyperbaric bupivacaine 0.5% for an inguinal hernia repair, and anesthesia and surgery were uneventful (272). However, the next morning he had difficulty in defecating and complained of impaired ambulation and urinary retention, which required bladder catheterization. He had impaired sensation to pinprick in both L5 dermatomes, in the perineal region, and over the left calf, with reduced reflexes, gait changes, and sleep disturbances. Cauda equina syndrome was diagnosed.

The authors concluded that bupivacaine neurotoxicity had occurred, in view of the absence of any other identifiable cause for the neurological deficit. One previous case of persistent cauda equina syndrome after a single intrathecal dose of hyperbaric bupivacaine has been reported (273). This was attributed to maldistribution of local anesthetic due to spinal stenosis by adhesions secondary to meningitis. Local anesthetic neurotoxicity is believed to occur mainly in the cauda equina, because the sacral root sheaths are substantially longer (and larger for S1) than neighboring lumbar roots, are devoid of protective sheaths, and given their dorsal position in the thecal sac (in particular L5, S1, and S2), are more exposed to pooling of a hyperbaric anesthetic.

A retrospective review of 603 continuous spinal anesthetics (127 had microcatheters) showed three patients with postoperative paresthesia, one of whom was from the microcatheter group (274). One patient, who had received anesthesia via a macrocatheter with 5% lidocaine, developed sensory cauda equina syndrome.

- A 57-year-old man with pre-existing severe vascular disease was given bupivacaine 12.5 mg with 1:1000 adrenaline 0.2 ml for incision and drainage of a thigh abscess (275). After 2–3 minutes he complained of "severely painful warmth" on the anterior of both thighs. The pain resolved with onset of the block, but the next morning he had symptoms of cauda equina syndrome. Some perineal sensation returned over the next few days.

The authors suggested that the neurological deficit had been due to anterior spinal artery insufficiency secondary to intrathecal bupivacaine and adrenaline. They questioned the use of adrenaline in patients with multi-organ vascular disease.

- A man with severe vascular disease was given general and epidural anesthesia with 2% isobaric lidocaine plus adrenaline for a popliteal distal vein bypass graft (276). The epidural inadvertently became a total spinal, which was discovered at the end of the operation. He developed cauda equina syndrome, confirmed by electromyography. He was unable to turn or sit up by himself for a month and at 12 months was walking with a cane and needed self-catheterization and medication for neuropathic pain.

The cauda has a tenuous blood supply, and in this patient with pre-existing vascular disease, perioperative hypotension and the use of intrathecal adrenaline may have precipitated ischemia in an area with very poor reserve. To follow this with an accidental large dose of lidocaine, which is neurotoxic in animals when directly applied and theorized to cause interruption of nerve blood supply, would add insult to injury. The authors questioned the wisdom of performing continuous epidural anesthesia in such patients, when frequent neurological assessments cannot be performed.

Bupivacaine has recently been implicated in two cases of cauda equina syndrome (277). One patient was given 3.6 ml of a hyperbaric 0.5% solution, and the other, 3.5 ml of plain bupivacaine. Spinal stenosis was felt to have contributed to the first case, while the cause of the second was unclear.

- Cauda equina syndrome occurred in a 55-year-old woman who underwent spinal anesthesia with a 22 G needle in the L4–5 interspace (278). On needle insertion, she felt radiating pain in her right leg. The needle was immediately withdrawn and repositioned. Pain-free intrathecal injection of 2.0 ml of hyperbaric cinchocaine 0.24% with adrenaline 66 micrograms resulted in block to L1. Surgery was carried out in the supine position. Three days postoperatively, she had enuresis and reduced perineal sensation, without bowel dysfunction or lower limb symptoms. There was sensory loss at S2–5. The symptoms persisted, required self-catheterization and systemic steroids, and disappeared on the 19th postoperative day.

The cause of this transient neurological deficit was unclear, but the authors suggested that the following factors may have contributed:

- direct nerve damage;
- local anesthetic toxicity;
- adrenaline effects.

Transient radicular irritation

Neurological sequelae of intrathecal anesthesia are rare and usually minor. However, transient radicular irritation can occur with the use of both isobaric and hyperbaric solutions of local anesthetics. Hyperbaric 5% lidocaine is such a persistent offender that there is little to recommend its use in neuraxial blockade (SEDA-20, 125) (SEDA-21, 129) (SEDA-22, 138). However, others have suggested that lidocaine can be used for intrathecal anesthesia if a short-acting anesthetic is desired (279). There have also been reports with most other local anesthetics, including tetracaine and mepivacaine. High concentrations of hyperbaric 4% mepivacaine are likely to cause transient radicular irritation of the same order of magnitude as 5% lidocaine (280). A randomized study with isobaric mepivacaine 2% administered intrathecally to patients undergoing surgery in the supine position showed an incidence of 7.5% compared with 2.5% with isobaric lidocaine 2% (281). There is a low incidence of transient radicular irritation after intrathecal bupivacaine, but a few cases have been reported (SEDA-20, 125). Bupivacaine and tetracaine have toxic effects on chick neuron cultures in vitro (282).

Since the cause of transient radicular irritation after lidocaine intrathecal anesthesia has not been elucidated, and although non-neurotoxic mechanisms must be considered, it has been recommended that the lowest effective doses and concentrations for intrathecal injection should be used (283).

Presentation

Transient radicular irritation causes transient pain in the back, buttocks, and lower extremities, without formal neurological signs or symptoms. It can follow single-dose intrathecal anesthesia. Lidocaine has been reported as the predominant culprit. However, transient radicular irritation has also been reported with bupivacaine, mepivacaine, tetracaine, and prilocaine. Osmolarity, the addition of dextrose, and speed of injection do not contribute, and even reducing the concentration of lidocaine does not alter the incidence (284,285).

Cases involving lidocaine (286–288) and mepivacaine (289,290) have been reported.

- A 50-year-old woman had a right knee arthroscopy under spinal anesthesia with 1% lidocaine 4 ml. The anesthetic and procedure were uncomplicated. At 4 hours she complained of a mild cramp in her buttocks and went home at 6 hours. By the next morning the buttock pain was severe, cramp-like in nature, and radiated down the fronts of both thighs. Walking alleviated it, simple analgesics were ineffective, and lying down made the pain worse. Neurological examination was unremarkable and the pain was gone after 36 hours.
- A 74-year-old man who had a cystoscopy performed in the lithotomy position, reported dull pain in the hips,

buttocks, and legs, radiating to the toes after a spinal anesthetic with 5% hyperbaric lidocaine 75 mg. The pain occurred 30 hours after the dural puncture and disappeared after 18 hours. Three months before he had had a similar anesthetic for a transurethral resection of the prostate and complained of similar but more severe symptoms of transient radicular irritation.

- A 66-year-old woman with unrecognized spinal stenosis had six spinal anesthetics over 3 years. The first five were with lidocaine 2%. After 24–48 hours, she developed pain in the back, hips, buttocks, and thighs, which lasted for 2–3 days. On the sixth occasion she had a spinal anesthetic with 1.5% mepivacaine 4 ml and the next day again had severe back pain radiating bilaterally to the hips and thighs.
- Three patients undergoing minor surgical procedures in the lithotomy position were given a spinal anesthetic with 2% mepivacaine 3 ml. From 6 to 10 hours postoperatively they complained of burning pain in both buttocks radiating to both thighs and calves. Neurological examination in all cases was normal and all symptoms had resolved by 3–5 days postoperatively.
- A 30-year-old man had a left spermatic vein ligature performed in the supine position. He had uncomplicated unilateral spinal anesthesia with 1% hyperbaric bupivacaine 8 mg. Three days later he reported an area of hypesthesia in the L3–4 dermatomes of the left leg. Sensation returned to normal after 2 weeks.

Incidence

The incidence of transient radicular irritation varies depending on the local anesthetic used, its baricity, and its concentration. It has been reported to be as high as 37% in patients who receive 5% lidocaine. In a prospective study of 303 parturients undergoing intrathecal anesthesia using 0.75% hyperbaric bupivacaine or 5% lidocaine there were no cases of transient radicular irritation after lidocaine (291). This is remarkable, as significantly more procedures were performed in the lithotomy position in the lidocaine group; the authors wondered if such a low incidence of transient radicular irritation could have been explained by their use of a 1:1 dilution of lidocaine with cerebrospinal fluid.

Transient neurological symptoms have been studied in patients given intrathecal lidocaine 2% or intrathecal prilocaine 2%. In one study of 70 patients transient neurological symptoms occurred in 20% of patients given lidocaine, with no cases in those given prilocaine (292). In another study in 70 patients given intrathecal procaine or lidocaine in a 2:1 dose ratio there were significantly more transient neurological symptoms with lidocaine than with procaine (31 versus 6%) (293). However, in a similar study of 100 patients there was no significant difference in the incidence of transient neurological symptoms, although the trend suggested a lower incidence with prilocaine (4 versus 14.3%) (294).

In 110 patients presenting for knee arthroscopy who were randomized to receive either 1% hypobaric lidocaine 50 mg or 1% hypobaric lidocaine 20 mg + fentanyl 25 micrograms complaints of transient neurological symptoms were nearly ten times more frequent in those given lidocaine 50 mg (33 versus 3.6%) (295). Patients given lidocaine 50 mg also had a greater fall in systolic blood pressure and a greater need for ephedrine.

In a prospective study of 1045 patients receiving spinal anesthesia with 3% hyperbaric lidocaine for anorectal surgery in the prone position, 4 (0.4%) complained of aching, hypesthesia, numbness, and dull pain in both buttocks and legs on the third postoperative day. In three cases the symptoms resolved by day 5 and in one by day 7 (296).

In a retrospective audit of 363 patients receiving spinal anesthesia, of whom 322 received hyperbaric 5% lidocaine 75–100 mg and 41 hyperbaric 0.5% bupivacaine 12.5–15 mg, six patients given lidocaine reported back pain at 24 hours; five of them had undergone arthroscopy. One patient given bupivacaine, who underwent arthroscopy, complained of backache (297).

Over 14 months, 1863 patients received spinal anesthesia, of whom 40% were given bupivacaine, 47% lidocaine, and 13% tetracaine (298). Patients given lidocaine had a significantly higher risk of transient radicular irritation (relative risks 5.1 compared with bupivacaine and 3.2 compared with tetracaine). They were more likely to be men, have outpatient surgery, and have surgery in the lithotomy position. For those who were given lidocaine, the relative risk of transient radicular irritation was 2.6, for those in the lithotomy position 3.6, and for ambulatory surgery 1.6. Most of the patients had resolution of symptoms by 72 hours and all by 6 months.

The incidence of transient radicular irritation with two different local anesthetics used for single-dose spinal anesthesia has been studied in 60 ambulatory patients given spinal anesthesia for knee arthroscopy (299). None of those who were given 1.5% mepivacaine 45 mg developed transient radicular irritation. Six of those given 2% lidocaine 60 mg developed transient radicular irritation, but all symptoms resolved by 1–5 days. The difference between the two groups was significant.

Of 90 patients who received intrathecal hyperbaric lidocaine 5%, mepivacaine 4%, or bupivacaine 0.5%, none in the bupivacaine group developed transient radicular irritation, but 20% in the lidocaine group and 37% in the mepivacaine group complained of a mixture of back and leg pain, classified as transient radicular irritation (280).

When 90 patients received spinal anesthesia for gynecological procedures with 2% lidocaine, 2% prilocaine, or 0.5% bupivacaine (all 2.5 ml in 7.5% glucose), nine of the 30 patients who received lidocaine had transient radicular irritation, defined as pain or dysesthesia in the legs or buttocks, compared with none of the 30 patients who received bupivacaine (300). The symptoms resolved within 48 hours. One of the 30 patients who received prilocaine had transient radicular irritation that lasted for 4 days.

In 200 patients given hyperbaric 5% lidocaine or hyperbaric 5% prilocaine, four developed transient radicular irritation after lidocaine (the patients were supine or prone) compared with one after prilocaine (this patient had a knee arthroscopy) (301). There were no significant differences between the two groups.

When procaine 5% or procaine 5% with fentanyl 20 micrograms was given to 106 patients for spinal anesthesia, the incidence of transient radicular irritation was 0.9% (302). There was nausea and vomiting in 17% of men and 32% of women.

Procaine has been suggested as an alternative to lidocaine for intrathecal use in ambulatory surgery, as it also has a short duration of action. In a randomized, double-blind comparison of procaine 10% or lidocaine 5% in glucose 7.5% for spinal anesthesia, transient radicular irritation occurred in 27% of the lidocaine group compared with none of the patients in the procaine group (303). However, the failure rate in the procaine group was 14%. This was perhaps a reflection of the fact that the procaine was glucose-free.

Intrathecal hyperbaric lidocaine 1.5% has been compared with hyperbaric bupivacaine 0.75% for outpatient transvaginal oocyte retrieval (304). The time to voiding of urine and the time to discharge were significantly longer in the bupivacaine group, despite the fact that there were no differences in the time to recovery of sensory and motor function. The incidence of transient radicular irritation in the lidocaine group was 5%, compared with none of the women in the bupivacaine group. The authors concluded that bupivacaine was a useful alternative to lidocaine in outpatient spinal anesthesia.

There have been two studies of transient radicular irritation in the obstetric population. One was a randomized, double-blind comparison of intrathecal hyperbaric lidocaine 5% or bupivacaine 0.75% for postpartum tubal ligation (305). All the patients were supine for surgery. The incidence of transient radicular irritation was 3% with lidocaine and 7% with bupivacaine. The other was a prospective follow-up study of patients who had cesarean sections under spinal anesthesia using hyperbaric 0.5% bupivacaine; the incidence of transient radicular irritation was 8.8% (306).

In a careful meta-analysis, 29 randomized, controlled studies of the incidence of transient radicular irritation were identified (307). Lidocaine and mepivacaine were identified as the two local anesthetics that most commonly cause transient radicular irritation, while prilocaine, bupivacaine, and ropivacaine had the lowest incidences. Owing to insufficient data, definitive statements could not be made about the effects of the baricity of the local anesthetic, the concentration, and the effect of vasoconstrictors, although all these factors seemed not to be relevant. With regard to intrathecal ropivacaine, the incidence in the formal studies was zero. However, there has been one previous report after intrathecal administration, and one report of transient radicular irritation following epidural anesthesia with ropivacaine; the symptoms resolved within 24 hours (308).

Mechanism

The cause of transient radicular irritation is unclear but probably multifactorial. Several factors have been implicated (SEDA-21, 130) (284,309):

(a) high concentrations of local anesthetic producing neurological injury;
(b) possibly the high osmolarity and density of some solutions;
(c) the addition of vasopressors that compromise neural blood flow;

(d) pooling of anesthetic around nerve roots;
(e) the patient's position, with a significantly higher incidence in patients positioned for knee arthroscopy and the lithotomy position (stretching lumbosacral nerve roots);
(f) co-existing disease subarachnoid lidocaine;
(g) ambulatory surgery;
(h) stretching of nerve roots.

With the introduction of 25 gauge and 27 gauge spinal needles, it was suggested that slow injection may be an additional factor predisposing to transient radicular irritation, since layering of the hyperbaric fluid in the dependent portion may lead to areas of highly concentrated local anesthetic (310).

The high baricity of the local anesthetic solutions was thought to be chiefly responsible for transient radicular irritation. However, isobaric local anesthetics have also been implicated; commonly the concentrations are 2% or greater. From comparisons of 2 and 5% hyperbaric and isobaric lidocaine and hyperbaric 0.5% bupivacaine, it seems more likely that high concentrations of local anesthetic solutions are responsible for transient radicular irritation rather than the osmolarity of the solutions (311–313). That the concentration of lidocaine is not a contributory factor to transient radicular irritation has been shown in 109 patients who received hyperbaric spinal lidocaine 50 mg, as a 2, 1, or 0.5% solution (314). The incidence of transient radicular irritation did not differ (16, 22, and 17% respectively).

The importance of the patient's position has been illustrated by a study in which transient neurological symptoms occurred in five of 12 volunteers who were given 5% lidocaine 50 mg intrathecally and then placed in the low lithotomy position (315). No consistent abnormalities were detected by prespinal and postspinal electromyography, nerve conduction studies, or somatosensory evoked potentials. This is in line with the current opinion that transient neurological symptoms constitute neither a true neurological syndrome nor an expression of the neurotoxicity of local anesthetics.

In 70 patients undergoing surgery in the supine position, there were transient neurological symptoms in 26% of patients after intrathecal lidocaine, compared with 3% after intrathecal bupivacaine (316). The incidence of transient neurological symptoms after intrathecal lidocaine 5% in patients undergoing surgery in the supine position is therefore similar to the previously reported incidence in the lithotomy position.

Animal studies have highlighted the potential toxic effects of adding adrenaline to local anesthetics for intrathecal injection. In one study the effects of adding 0.01% adrenaline to intrathecal tetracaine 1% and 2% was investigated in rabbits (317). Although adrenaline had no neurotoxic effects when given alone, there was worsening of neurotoxicity when it was given in combination with tetracaine. The same group had previously shown an increase in glutamate concentrations in the CSF and dose-dependent neurotoxicity with tetracaine injected intrathecally in rabbits (318). In another study they looked at the effects of intrathecal lidocaine 5% with and without adrenaline 0.02% on the spinal cord and nerve roots of rats (318). They showed that lidocaine 5% caused persistent sensory impairment and histological damage that was significantly exacerbated by the addition of adrenaline.

Several explanations for the increased neurotoxicity of vasoconstrictors, such as adrenaline and phenylephrine, in combination with local anesthetics have been offered:

(a) vasoconstrictors may reduce the absorption of local anesthetics and thereby increase anesthetic exposure intrathecally;
(b) a reduction in blood flow caused by vasoconstrictors may cause ischemia in the spinal cord;
(c) bisulfite, used as a preservative in adrenaline formulations, which may have a role, although that would not explain the lack of toxicity seen with adrenaline alone.

A randomized study in 64 patients undergoing urological, gynecological, or lower limb surgery showed no significant difference in the incidence of transient neurological symptoms between hyperbaric tetracaine 0.5% with and without phenylephrine 0.025% (319). In fact, the neurological symptoms that were described (in 6.7% of the patients) occurred in the group without phenylephrine and could possibly have been explained by the patient's position or by the effects of plaster-cast compression postoperatively.

Early ambulation has previously been implicated in transient radicular irritation. However, in a randomized trial there was no difference between early and late mobilization in patients who received intrathecal lidocaine 2% for inguinal hernia repair; the incidence was 23% in both groups (320).

In a prospective audit of 100 patients having intrathecal anesthesia with 5% hyperbaric lidocaine in a mean dose of 73 mg, there was an unusually low incidence of 4% (321). All the patients recovered completely, which led the authors to conclude that 5% hyperbaric lidocaine is acceptable for intrathecal anesthesia in patients in whom rapid recovery from the block is desired. The low incidence in this study might have been due to the fact that the patients were placed in the supine or lateral position, as patient position has previously been reported to be a risk factor for the development of transient radicular irritation, the lithotomy position and knee arthroscopy having a higher incidence, possibly owing to excessive stretching of the nerve roots, leading to ischemic damage.

This impression has been confirmed by three recent reports of patients who developed transient radicular irritation after intrathecal anesthesia, as all these patients had surgery in positions that could have caused excessive stretching of nerve roots.

- A 44-year-old man developed transient pain in the buttocks and thighs 4 hours after 4% hyperbaric mepivacaine had been used to provide anesthesia for knee arthroscopy (322). The symptoms resolved after 2 days.
- A 46-year-old woman had an epidural placed at L4/5 (323). As there was insufficient block 20 minutes after injection of 300 mg mepivacaine, the epidural catheter

was removed and an intrathecal injection of 0.5% tetracaine 2 ml dissolved in 5% glucose was performed. She was then placed in the lithotomy position for 30 minutes. One day postoperatively she developed pain and numbness in her left leg, and the numbness spread to the lower back, buttocks, and thighs. The symptoms disappeared after 4 days.

- A 50-year-old man had an intrathecal injection of 2% lidocaine 40 mg diluted to 1% with sterile water, while in the prone jack-knife position for excision of a pilonidal cyst (324). About 7 hours after the start of the block he developed acute sharp lower back pain radiating to the right buttock. There were no accompanying neurological signs. The pain settled with ketorolac and was gone after 5 days.

The last case is the first report of transient radicular irritation after the use of hypobaric lidocaine, but it again suggests the importance of sciatic stretching.

A high concentration of tetracaine given intrathecally in rabbits caused neuronal injury and glutamate release in the CSF (318). The authors postulated that this might give some insight into the mechanisms of neurotoxicity of intrathecal local anesthetics.

An animal study of the histological and physiological effects of intrathecal lidocaine at varying concentrations from 3 to 20% showed the presence of lesions in the posterior roots and columns characterized by axonal degeneration (325). The lesions were severe at higher concentrations, but even at the lower concentration of 7.5% there were mild lesions that did not correlate with the presence of neurofunctional deficit.

In a study of the effect of clinically relevant concentrations of lidocaine, bupivacaine, mepivacaine, and ropivacaine on cultured neurons, the local anesthetics caused destruction of the growth cones, implying that they have a toxic effect on the growth and regeneration of neuronal tissue (326). Lidocaine had the most marked effect and mepivacaine the least. While this might not be of direct relevance to the etiology of transient radicular irritation, the authors pointed out the potential risks of using local anesthetics in very young children, taking into consideration the difficulties of extrapolating from in vitro studies to in vivo use.

Sensory systems

Hearing
In some series, transient hearing loss after anesthesia with bupivacaine was found with intrathecal but not epidural administration (SEDA-13, 99) (SEDA-16, 129)(327). It has been suggested that the cause could be a reduction in CSF pressure transmitted through the cochlear aqueduct (328), a hypothesis that has been both supported and criticized (SEDA-16, 129). Sensorineural hearing loss after spinal anesthesia with bupivacaine has been thought to be due to the entry of bupivacaine into the inner ear, resulting in a direct effect on its functional apparatus (329).

When 44 patients undergoing inguinal hernia repair were given intrathecal anesthesia with 2% prilocaine

6 ml or 0.5% bupivacaine 3 ml, those given prilocaine had an average hearing loss of about 10 dB and 1–3 days postoperatively and those given bupivacaine had an average hearing loss of about 15 dB (330). However, 10 of 22 in those given prilocaine developed hearing loss, compared with four of the 22 given bupivacaine.

Gastrointestinal

Dysphagia has been reported from the cephalad spread of a spinal anesthetic (331).

- A 26-year-old woman underwent cesarean section with an intrathecal injection of 12 mg of 0.75% hyperbaric bupivacaine, fentanyl 25 micrograms, and morphine 0.2 mg. After 4 minutes she developed hypotension, which was treated with ephedrine. Another 4 minutes later she became agitated and complained of difficulty in swallowing. At this stage she had a block to T4 with no dyspnea, her facial sensation was normal, and phonation was intact; the dysphagia resolved within 30 minutes.

Urinary tract

Urinary retention as a true transient neurological symptom developed after accidental total spinal anesthesia with mepivacaine, which is often considered to be the best agent for intrathecal anesthesia, owing to its low incidence of transient radicular irritation (332).

- A 71-year-old man received an intrathecal anesthetic with 2 ml of 0.3% hyperbaric mepivacaine using a 25-gauge Quincke needle at the L3–4 interspace, before which he had slight hypesthesia in the L5–S1 dermatomes in the right leg, reportedly having originated from the use of local anesthetic in the lumbar spine 16 years before to treat severe lumbago (333). When he was turned supine he started to complain of severe lightning pain in the region of his hypesthetic segments, which completely resolved 4 hours later.

Musculoskeletal

Profound musculoligamental relaxation by high doses of local anesthetics may contribute to the development of postoperative musculoskeletal pain. Of 60 patients who received either spinal anesthesia with hyperbaric 5% lidocaine (85–100 mg) or balanced general anesthesia with neuromuscular blockade, there was transient radicular irritation in eight patients who received spinal anesthesia and in one who received general anesthesia, a significant difference (334). However, there was non-radiating back pain in ten of the patients who received spinal anesthesia and in six of those who received general anesthesia.

Sexual function

For reasons that are not understood, intraoperative penile erection is sometimes observed with neuraxial blockade; it can be followed by prolonged priapism (SEDA-14, 110).

A long-standing belief that intrathecal anesthesia in young men reduces sexual potency was not confirmed in a retrospective study (SEDA-17, 139).

Fetotoxicity

Severe prolonged fetal bradycardia has been observed after intrathecal injection as a component of combined spinal epidural anesthesia in labor (335).

- A healthy 21-year-old gravida 1, para 0 at 39 weeks, with an uncomplicated pregnancy, received spinal epidural anesthesia at the level of L2–3 with a combined dose of bupivacaine 2.5 mg (1 ml of 2.5 mg/ml) and fentanyl 5 micrograms; 5 minutes later there was severe fetal bradycardia. An emergency cesarean section was performed under general anesthesia. Maternal and neonatal postoperative courses were uneventful.

In this case the maternal vital signs were stable and there was no circulatory hypotension or uterine hypotonia. The exact mechanism of this severe fetal bradycardia was unclear. The author stated that fetal bradycardia should be recognized as a complication after subarachnoid administration of lipid-soluble opioids and local anesthetics.

Intravenous regional anesthesia

Systemic toxic reactions are the most common complications of intravenous regional anesthesia, and they occur soon after the tourniquet is released. In cases of early accidental tourniquet release or rupture, deaths have resulted; prilocaine seems to be the safest agent for this technique (336).

- A 74-year-old woman was given prilocaine 400 mg for carpal tunnel surgery. Within 3 minutes, she developed signs of central nervous system toxicity, sweating, and tachycardia. Twenty minutes later, her symptoms had resolved and the cause was found to be a leak in the tourniquet.

The authors used this case to stress the importance of adequately functioning equipment and the relative safety of prilocaine (337).

Methods of reducing the dose of lidocaine used in intravenous regional anesthesia by adding fentanyl 0.05 mg, pancuronium bromide 0.5 mg, or both, have been evaluated in 60 patients undergoing elective forearm, wrist, and hand surgery; the dose of lidocaine used was 100 mg (338). None of the patients had signs of drug toxicity on release of the tourniquet; those who were given all three agents had better anesthesia and muscle relaxation. A separate group of volunteers, in whom the tourniquet was released immediately after injection of the lidocaine/fentanyl/pancuronium mixture, complained of minor adverse effects including mild dizziness and transient visual disturbances and one case of vomiting and moderate hypotension.

A study of lidocaine toxicity in intravenous regional anesthesia showed that two of 24 patients who were given 0.5% lidocaine 40 ml for carpal tunnel decompression had serum lidocaine concentrations above the target range 2 minutes before and 2, 5, and 10 minutes after distal tourniquet deflation (339). However, no patients had signs of central nervous system or cardiovascular toxicity.

Cardiovascular
Chloroprocaine, because of its rapid onset and ester hydrolysis, should be the ideal agent for intravenous regional anesthesia. However, there are reports that it can cause endothelial damage and dysrhythmias after tourniquet deflation (340).

- Phlebitis seems to have been triggered by intravenous regional anesthesia in a 32-year-old smoker who was also taking oral contraceptives (341).

Nervous system
In 15 volunteers, ropivacaine 1.2 and 1.8 mg/kg produced intravenous regional anesthesia as quickly as a conventional dose of lidocaine (3 mg/kg), but with more prolonged anesthesia (55 minutes before loss of pinprick analgesia) and motor block (120 minutes before return of hand grip strength) at the higher dose, suggesting that ropivacaine can provide a greater degree of residual analgesia (342). All the volunteers given lidocaine and only one patient receiving high-dose ropivacaine developed light-headedness and a hearing disturbance when the tourniquet was released after 30 minutes, but with individual peak arterial plasma ropivacaine concentrations lower than the mean values for the group. The authors pointed out the limitations of this study in terms of a small sample size and their inability to determine the safety of ropivacaine for intravenous regional anesthesia.

- A 56-year-old man developed unexplained acute aphasia when the tourniquet was released 20 minutes after the infusion of 0.75% lidocaine 20 ml for wrist surgery (343). He also had light-headedness, but no circumoral numbness or visual or auditory disturbances. He made a spontaneous recovery 20 hours later with no sequelae.

The correlation of nervous system adverse effects with plasma concentrations after the intravenous administration of 40 ml of lidocaine 0.5% plus ropivacaine 0.2% for regional anesthesia has been examined in 10 volunteers (344). The double-cuffed tourniquet was inflated for as long as it could be tolerated. The incidence, duration, and intensity of nervous system adverse effects were recorded at 3, 10, and 30 minutes after tourniquet release and correlated with venous samples. There was a lower incidence and shorter duration of nervous system adverse effects with ropivacaine than with lidocaine; however, the dose of ropivacaine was much lower than that of lidocaine and therefore no clear conclusions can be drawn. In view of the availability of safer and effective alternatives for intravenous regional anesthesia, such as prilocaine and lidocaine, the reasons for using ropivacaine are hard to comprehend.

Nervous system
A mixture of lidocaine and clonidine resulted in seizures when used for a Bier block (345).

- A 47-year-old man received lidocaine 150 mg with clonidine 30 micrograms for intravenous regional anesthesia to treat a complex regional pain syndrome of the arm. The tourniquet was deflated 60 minutes after the injection. Ten minutes later he felt unwell and had

rhythmic clonic movements accompanied by altered consciousness and vocal automatism. During the next 2 hours he had five similar episodes, which were interpreted as complex partial seizures.

Seizures are a well-known complication of intravenous injection of local anesthetics. By blocking voltage-gated sodium channels, lidocaine reduces neuronal excitability. Clonidine may reduce the threshold for seizures further, by reducing the availability of noradrenaline centrally. However, the mechanism of this interaction is not fully understood.

Patients should be given clear instructions to protect themselves from injury after local anesthesia, as emphasized in a recent case report (346).

- A 38-year-old woman had liposuction of the inner and outer thighs using tumescent local anesthesia and intravenous sedation. The treated areas were infiltrated with isotonic saline containing lidocaine 0.1%, 1: 1000 adrenaline, and 10 ml of sodium bicarbonate 8.4%. The procedure took 2.5 hours and the patient was discharged 2 hours later. At home she fell asleep with a lighted cigarette in her hand. The cigarette burned through her clothes to cause a full thickness burn on her upper thigh. She did not discover the burn until the following day. The burn was painless and was treated conservatively.

Sensory systems
Ears
It has been suggested that ropivacaine is a good choice for intravenous regional anesthesia because of its longer duration of action and lower risk of toxicity. In 20 patients scheduled for upper limb surgery who received 40 ml of either ropivacaine 0.2% or lidocaine 0.5% for intravenous regional anesthesia, both agents provided same onset and quality of surgical anesthesia, but ropivacaine gave longer-lasting analgesia in the immediate postoperative period (344). Additionally, one patient in the lidocaine group had tinnitus on release of the tourniquet, while there were no adverse effects in the ropivacaine group.

Taste
When 20 patients each received 40 ml of 0.5% chloroprocaine or 0.5% lidocaine for intravenous regional anesthesia, chloroprocaine caused a significantly higher incidence of a metallic taste (22 versus 0%) than lidocaine; when the study was repeated using alkalinized instead of plain chloroprocaine, there was no significant difference between the groups (347).

Skin
When 20 patients each received 40 ml of 0.5% chloroprocaine or 0.5% lidocaine for intravenous regional anesthesia, chloroprocaine caused a significantly higher incidence of urticaria (28 versus 0%) than lidocaine; when the study was repeated using alkalinized instead of plain chloroprocaine, there was no significant difference between the groups (347).

- A 41-year-old man was given 40 ml of lidocaine 0.5% for intravenous regional anesthesia for release of a trigger finger (348). He developed a uniform, circumferential, reddish brown and in places purple discoloration of the forearm below the tourniquet. Ultrasound and Doppler sonography ruled out a hematoma, a collection, or circulatory predicament. After 8 days the rash disappeared completely.

The authors observed that although this did not need any particular treatment, it caused undue psychological trauma and inconvenience to the patient.

Laryngeal anesthesia

Local anesthesia to the larynx, for example with 4% lidocaine, is generally safe. Laryngeal edema has been reported in a few cases, perhaps due to the propellant rather than to lidocaine itself (349). An unusual complication is mydriasis if part of the spray is accidentally directed to the eye (SEDA-18, 144).

- A 22-year-old man had a generalized tonic-clonic convulsion and loss of consciousness after an attempted superior laryngeal nerve block using 2% lidocaine 2 ml (350). The seizure was not terminated by intravenous diazepam 10 mg and he was intubated after intravenous thiopental and suxamethonium. He required two boluses of ephedrine 10 mg to maintain his blood pressure. Surgery proceeded uneventfully and he recovered without any sequelae.

The authors postulated vertebral artery injection of local anesthetic as the cause of the seizure and loss of consciousness.

Local anesthesia administered directly into a fracture hematoma can cause systemic absorption and toxicity (SED-12, 252) (351).

Leg anesthesia
Musculoskeletal

Avulsion of the Achilles tendon followed diagnostic tibial nerve block for spastic equinovarus (352).

- A 67-year-old woman with a 3-year history of left hemiplegia secondary to a hemorrhagic stroke underwent diagnostic tibial nerve block to confirm Achilles tendon shortening due to spasticity. A posterior popliteal fossa approach using nerve stimulation was used, resulting in successful block. However, avulsion of the Achilles tendon with an avulsion fracture of the osteoporotic calcaneum occurred after first contact of the foot with the ground. She was treated conservatively and was asymptomatic 4 months later.

The authors suggested that the tibial nerve block had suppressed the spasticity and weakened the triceps surae muscle, resulting in passive tension of the Achilles tendon. This increase in tension exceeded the mechanical strength of the tendon, resulting in the avulsion injury.

Lumbar plexus anesthesia

The combination of lumbar plexus and posterior sciatic nerve block represents an alternative to a neuraxial technique.

- An 80-year-old 41 kg woman was given a combination of a posterior lumbar plexus block and a posterior sciatic nerve block for dynamic hip screw repair of a fractured right neck of femur (353). The lumbar plexus block was technically difficult, requiring three attempts, and 25 ml of ropivacaine 0.75% (187.5 mg), adrenaline (1 in 400 000), and clonidine 50 micrograms was slowly injected, aspirating after every 3 ml. The sciatic nerve block was straightforward, and 20 ml of a solution containing mepivacaine 1.5% (300 mg), adrenaline 1 in 400 000, and clonidine 50 micrograms was injected slowly. She had seizures and dysrhythmias 20 minutes after completion of the block. Cardiopulmonary resuscitation was successful, surgery proceeded under general anesthesia, and she made a full recovery. Blood samples taken 5 minutes after the seizures contained ropivacaine 1.9 micrograms/ml and mepivacaine 3.7 micrograms/ml.

The authors suggested that the timing of events (the neurological signs preceded cardiac toxicity) suggested a toxic reaction to one of the local anesthetics or an overdose from their combination.

Nervous system

Phantom limb pain immediately after lumbar plexus block has been described (354).

- A 72-year-old woman with a left below-knee amputation and intermittent phantom limb pain, had a lumbar plexus block via a posterior lumbar approach before anesthesia and 30 ml of levobupivacaine 0.5% was injected after successful identification of the lumbar plexus with a nerve stimulator needle. Within 5 minutes, she had phantom limb pain in the distribution of the sciatic nerve similar to previous episodes but more severe. A sciatic nerve block was performed with 15 ml of levobupivacaine 0.5% with complete resolution of the pain within 5 minutes.

This report demonstrates unmasking of phantom limb pain in a sciatic distribution after lumbar plexus block not dissimilar from previous reports with spinal anesthesia. The authors concluded that neighboring peripheral nerves may play an inhibitory role in phantom limb pain.

Nasal anesthesia

Intranasal 4% lidocaine has been used for migraine and cluster headaches with success and few serious adverse effects: a bitter taste was common and some patients complained of nasal burning and oropharyngeal numbness

Unilateral mydriasis (anisocoria), suggesting serious neurological injury, has been attributed to topical cocaine (355).

- A 51-year-old man developed mydriasis in one eye, with loss of the accommodation reflex, immediately after endoscopic sinus surgery, before which 4% cocaine had been applied to the nasal mucosa on cotton pledglets. There were no surgical or anatomical complications.

The authors suggested a diagnosis of local anesthetic blockade of the nasociliary nerve.

Acute angle closure glaucoma has been attributed to local cocaine (356).

- A 46-year-old woman developed acute angle closure glaucoma 24 hours after the application of topical intranasal 25% cocaine (about 200 mg) for an elective antral washout under general anesthesia. She developed a severe headache around the right eye, with halos and blurring of vision on the same side and associated nausea and vomiting. The next day, when she awoke, she had completely lost the vision in that eye.

Neck anesthesia

With regional anesthesia in the neck there is a risk of inadvertent intra-arterial injection; this could explain one report of convulsions in an elderly woman (357). There is also a risk of subarachnoid injection and pneumothorax.

Obstetric anesthesia

When a local anesthetic is used for episiotomy, there is a risk that the needle will enter the child's scalp; in two cases involving prilocaine, this resulted in cyanosis, methemoglobinemia, and hemolytic anemia (358).

Retroperitoneal hematoma has been reported as a complication of pudendal block, probably due to pudendal artery perforation (SEDA-21, 134).

Prilocaine 3% + felypressin 0.03 IU/ml has been compared with lidocaine 2% + adrenaline 12.5 micrograms/ml in 300 women having large-loop excision of the cervical transformation zone (359). Those who received lidocaine had significantly less blood loss, but were more likely to have adverse effects, including shaking and feeling faint.

Fetotoxicity

Two cases of neonatal intoxication resulting from the administration of a local anesthetic to the mother for episiotomy during labor, initially diagnosed as perinatal asphyxia, have been reported (360).

- Within minutes of vaginal birth, two full-term neonates developed signs of central nervous and cardiovascular system toxicity, including hypertonia, convulsions, apnea, bradycardia, and hypotension. In neither case was there evidence of fetal distress, and fetal monitoring was normal. The first mother had received lidocaine (2.5%) + prilocaine (2.5%) cream and the second 10 ml of mepivacaine solution 2%. Blood samples from both babies at 2 hours showed high concentrations

of the respective local anesthetics. In both cases neurodevelopment at 12 months was normal.

The authors suggested that "unexplained perinatal asphyxia" could be ruled out by finding high concentrations of local anesthetic in the blood, urine, and cerebrospinal fluid. Therefore, if neonatal intoxication is suspected, an early urine specimen for toxicology screening is the cheapest and easiest way to secure the diagnosis.

Ocular anesthesia

Respiratory

Reports of apnea and seizures with retrobulbar anesthesia continue to appear (361).

Nervous system

A cluster of 25 cases of transient or permanent diplopia occurred after 13 retrobulbar blocks, 10 peribulbar blocks, and two unknown techniques, possibly related to the non-availability of hyaluronidase, highlighting the likely importance of hyaluronidase in preventing anesthetic-related myopathy in the extraocular muscles (362). Other reports of 21 cases of persistent postoperative diplopia following the peribulbar technique (363) and 4 cases following the retrobulbar technique during the period of non-availability of hyaluronidase support this theory (364). Bupivacaine and lidocaine may be contraindicated for peribulbar or retrobulbar injections without hyaluronidase.

Severe sneezing after ocular local anesthetic injection during intravenous sedation has been linked to photic sneezing. However, in 557 patients there was no relation between the two (365). Severe involuntary sneezing occurred after ocular blockade under thiopental sedation overall in 5.2% and only in 7.6% of those with a history of photic sneezing; peribulbar block had a significantly higher incidence of involuntary sneezing compared with retrobulbar block (24 versus 4.5%). Sneezing can occur with many hypnotics and after injections inside the muscle cone and outside the orbit, without pupillary dilatation or lid elevation (366). Awareness of this phenomenon can facilitate recognition and prompt needle withdrawal to avoid serious problems from sudden head movements during injection.

Sensory systems

A conjunctival cyst and orbital cellulitis have been described after sub-Tenon's block.

A 68-year-old man received a sub-Tenon's block for cataract surgery (367). During a routine follow up for glaucoma, a conjunctival cyst was noticed adjacent to the carbuncle of the right eye at the site of the sub-Tenon's injection. The cyst had apparently developed over the previous 4–6 months and was about 8 mm in diameter, transparent, and multiloculated. Although conspicuous, the cyst did not cause discomfort.

Sub-Tenon's block has become a popular anesthetic technique for cataract surgery because of its safety, faster onset of anesthetic effect, and patient preference. Inclusion cyst formation as a complication is a late event and has not previously been reported. While without consequences in this case, raised lesions of the eyeball, such as cysts, if close to the limbus, can prevent uniform coating of the cornea by tears, resulting in focal dryness and eventually thinning of the cornea. The authors proposed that simple and meticulous technique, including perpendicular positioning of the scissors, smaller snips, gentle holding of the conjunctival edges, and teasing the edges of inversion if present, will help to avoid this potential complication.

Two cases of orbital swelling after sub-Tenon's anesthesia have been reported (368).

- Two patients presented with proptosis and chemosis after the third post-operative day. Computed tomography showed non-specific inflammation of the orbital soft tissues. They were treated with oral glucocorticoids and antibiotics, and the inflammation subsided within 4 weeks. Both patients had otherwise uneventful cataract surgery, were apyrexial, and were generally well.

Possible explanations for these episodes were infection, reactions to povidone-iodine or local anesthetic, or trauma due to the sub-Tenon's cannula.

Sub-Tenon anesthesia is regarded as being safer than retrobulbar anesthesia in regard to the risk of optic nerve injury. However, optic neuropathy secondary to sub-Tenon anesthesia has been reported (369).

Drug abuse

A toxic keratopathy has been attributed to abuse of oxybuprocaine (370).

A 47-year-old woman with systemic lupus erythematosus and a corneal ulcer was given oxybuprocaine 0.05% qds, but instead used it every 5–10 minutes. Two weeks later she developed a toxic keratopathy, with persisting lesions for 6 months.

The authors concluded that local anesthetics should not be prescribed for patients with dry eyes, especially when the integrity of the ocular surface is altered.

Death

Misplacement or migration of a catheter can lead to unwanted effects, as illustrated by a recent case (371).

A 38-year-old woman was given 3 ml of bupivacaine 0.5% by her sister through an orbital catheter for analgesia at home around 7 hours after ambulatory surgery. She stopped breathing and could not be resuscitated. Autopsy showed that the catheter had migrated into the subarachnoid space through the superior orbital fissure, probably facilitated by deficiency of collagen II in this patient, who had Stickler syndrome.

The authors recommended that orbital indwelling catheters should be used for analgesia only in hospital.

Ocular explosion occurred in seven cases after periocular anesthetic injections (372). To minimize the incidence of ocular explosion, the authors recommended the following:

(a) use a blunt needle and a 12 ml syringe;
(b) aspirate the plunger and wiggle the syringe before injection;
(c) discontinue the injection if corneal edema or resistance to injection is noted;
(d) inspect the globe for evidence of intraocular injection before ocular massage or placement of a Honan balloon.

Contralateral amaurosis and third nerve palsy has been described after retrobulbar anesthesia (373).

- An 84-year-old woman received a retrobulbar block in the right eye with 3.5 ml of lidocaine 2% for cataract surgery; 15 minutes later she stated that she could not see from the other eye. On examination after surgery, the left eye had very limited motility and a dilated pupil unreactive to light. Over the next 2 hours her visual acuity improved to baseline without treatment.

The authors proposed that injection of local anesthetic into the subdural space of the optic nerve sheath was the underlying mechanism. They suggested that the local anesthetic had tracked along the ipsilateral optic nerve sheath posteriorly within the subdural space to the area of the chiasma, where it had compromised function of the contralateral optic nerve and the third cranial nerve.

Musculoskeletal

A series of 26 patients with persistent diplopia after retrobulbar anesthesia was carefully examined (374). The authors suggested that direct muscle trauma caused by the injection needle or myotoxicity of the local anesthetics (either lidocaine 2%, a mixture of lidocaine 2% and 4%, or a mixture of lidocaine 2% and bupivacaine 0.75%) could have caused the muscular imbalance in half of the cases. However, they also mentioned other causes, including surgical trauma or adhesions caused by gentamicin sulfate-derived inflammation.

A similar report of diplopia due to motility disturbance of the inferior oblique muscle after retrobulbar anesthesia has been reported (375). The authors suggested either damage caused by the needle tip or myotoxicity of the local anesthetic (a 4 ml mixture of lidocaine 2%, bupivacaine 0.5%, and 5 units of hyaluronidase) as the most likely explanations.

In contrast, in another study there were no myotoxic effects in 13 patients after retrobulbar block using lidocaine 2% compared with a control group who had topical anesthesia, despite the use of a sensitive tool (saccadic velocity) (376).

Retrobulbar anesthesia

Retrobulbar anesthesia, competently administered, is a safe procedure. In 13 000 patients in whom a curved needle technique was used, the only serious complication was a single case of postoperative ischemic neuropathy (377). However, other centers have experienced recurrent problems with chemosis (up to 30%), sub-conjunctival hemorrhage, and lid hemorrhage before perfecting their technique (SEDA-18, 144).

Inadvertent injection into the subarachnoid space surrounding the optic nerve has on various occasions led to bilateral impairment of vision and ophthalmoplegia, with varying degrees of nervous system and respiratory effects, ranging from pulmonary edema (378) to respiratory arrest (SED-12, 254) (SEDA-21, 133) (379). Similar adverse effects result from diffusion of the local anesthetic toward the cerebrospinal fluid (SEDA-14, 110). Several groups have shown that such complications can occur, especially with higher concentrations, independently of any fault in technique (SED-12, 254) (380). Patients must therefore be closely monitored during ocular anesthesia and surgery. Particular care should be taken in patients with orbital roof defects, as there is potential for local anesthetics to move rapidly into the nervous system, with severe toxic effects (SEDA-20, 126).

On the other hand, headache after bupivacaine-induced block has been traced to the use of a vasoconstrictor additive, and is more likely to occur with noradrenaline than adrenaline (381). Unwanted effects on the eye muscles, occurring in some 1% of retrobulbar blocks, extend to ptosis, horizontal rectus muscle palsy, and lagophthalmos; all recover spontaneously within a matter of weeks (382). It has been postulated that local anesthetics can be myotoxic, causing contracture and subsequent diplopia (383). Tissue pressure, causing ischemia, can also lead to muscle damage and subsequent contracture and strabismus (SEDA-22, 139).

Two cases of vitreous hemorrhage have been observed after retrobulbar block in patients with severe diabetic retinopathy (384).

- A retrobulbar injection in a 45-year-old woman with high myopia was complicated by globe perforation with vitreous and submacular hemorrhage (385).
- In another case, retrobulbar hemorrhage and raised intraocular pressure developed after subtenon block with lidocaine (386).

Retinal vascular occlusion is rare, but it can occur in patients with severe vascular disease, without retrobulbar or optic nerve sheath hemorrhage; the mechanism is unclear (SED-12, 254) (387).

There is a risk of traumatic optic nerve injury with retrobulbar block (SEDA-21, 134).

Complications from retrobulbar block can arise from accidental scleral perforation and intraocular injection of local anesthetic.

- An 86-year-old man scheduled for cataract surgery sustained an inadvertent occult single perforating needle injury with an intraocular injection of 0.5% plain bupivacaine during a retrobulbar block using a long (38 mm) needle (388). He had pain on injection and a raised intraocular pressure, with corneal edema, poor iris detail, and a reduced red reflex. Paracentesis

lowered the intraocular pressure and surgery proceeded uneventfully. At 6 weeks, he had a reduction in visual acuity, and a scan identified a vitreous hemorrhage and retinal detachment. Prompt vitreoretinal surgery was performed with reasonable success.

The authors added that retinal toxicity of the local anesthetic agent did not affect the visual outcome in this patient. Scleral perforation is a well-known complication of eye blocks for ophthalmic surgery. The incidence with retrobulbar techniques is 0.075% and with peribulbar blocks 0.0002%. When recognized, ocular perforation usually requires a vitreoretinal procedure and is associated with a poor visual outcome. Risk factors include an anxious or oversedated patient, long sharp needles, superior injection, incorrect angle of needle insertion, and myopic eyes. If the intraocular pressure is increased, paracentesis may acutely reduce it, preventing retinal and optic nerve ischemia and possible permanent visual loss.

Retrobulbar anesthesia can lead to serious systemic toxicity. However, in animal studies accidental intravitreous spread of lidocaine, bupivacaine, or a mixture of the two did not cause long-term retinal damage (389).

Possible techniques to reduce complications include avoiding Atkinson's position, the classical position for retrobulbar block (390), during injection, limiting the volume of solution injected, and the use of shorter needles (391,392).

Retrobulbar anesthesia can be complicated by brainstem anesthesia (393).

- A 79-year-old man received retrobulbar anesthesia using a 1:1 mixture of 2% lidocaine and 0.5% bupivacaine plus hyaluronidase, which was complicated by brainstem anesthesia presenting as dysarthria. Initially there was some resistance to injection and the syringe was withdrawn slightly before injection of 4 ml of solution; 5 minutes later he complained of a strange sensation in his throat, which progressed to difficulty in swallowing and not being able to speak above a whisper. His blood pressure rose to 210/118 and his pulse to 120/minute; he also had signs of involvement of cranial nerves III, VI, and XII. He received glyceryl trinitrate for the hypertension and by 24 hours all the cranial nerve symptoms and signs had resolved.

Two cases of cardiopulmonary arrest after retrobulbar block for corrective squint surgery have been described (394). Both the patients were fit, healthy young men and they received a retrobulbar block with 2% lidocaine 2 ml via a 23G 1.5″ needle after negative aspiration. Three minutes later both complained of breathlessness and rapidly became apneic and unresponsive, with unrecordable pulse and blood pressure. Both were resuscitated and became fully alert within 40 minutes. Possible reasons suggested were an allergic reaction, a direct toxic effect, a vasovagal attack, intra-arterial injection, or injection directly into the optic nerve sheath with spread of the local anesthetic into the CSF. The latter seemed to be the most likely in these cases. Since then the authors have altered their technique, including changing the position of gaze and using a short blunt needle. These cases illustrate the need for careful monitoring, knowledge of potential complications, and the ready availability of resuscitation facilities (including appropriately trained personnel familiar with the equipment), even when performing what many regard as minor local anesthetic blocks.

Contralateral amaurosis and third nerve palsy has been described after retrobulbar anesthesia (373).

An 84-year-old woman received a retrobulbar block in the right eye with 3.5 ml of lidocaine 2% for cataract surgery; 15 minutes later she stated that she could not see from the other eye. On examination after surgery, the left eye had very limited motility and a dilated pupil unreactive to light. Over the next 2 hours her visual acuity improved to baseline without treatment.

The authors proposed that injection of local anesthetic into the subdural space of the optic nerve sheath was the underlying mechanism. They suggested that the local anesthetic had tracked along the ipsilateral optic nerve sheath posteriorly within the subdural space to the area of the chiasma, where it had compromised function of the contralateral optic nerve and the third cranial nerve.

Musculoskeletal

A series of 26 patients with persistent diplopia after retrobulbar anesthesia was carefully examined (374). The authors suggested that direct muscle trauma caused by the injection needle or myotoxicity of the local anesthetics (either lidocaine 2%, a mixture of lidocaine 2% and 4%, or a mixture of lidocaine 2% and bupivacaine 0.75%) could have caused the muscular imbalance in half of the cases. However, they also mentioned other causes, including surgical trauma or adhesions caused by gentamicin sulfate-derived inflammation.

A similar report of diplopia due to motility disturbance of the inferior oblique muscle after retrobulbar anesthesia has been reported (375). The authors suggested either damage caused by the needle tip or myotoxicity of the local anesthetic (a 4 ml mixture of lidocaine 2%, bupivacaine 0.5%, and 5 units of hyaluronidase) as the most likely explanations.

In contrast, in another study there were no myotoxic effects in 13 patients after retrobulbar block using lidocaine 2% compared with a control group who had topical anesthesia, despite the use of a sensitive tool (saccadic velocity) (376).

Peribulbar anesthesia

Peribulbar anesthesia is generally considered safer than retrobulbar anesthesia, with a lower incidence of adverse effects. It avoids deep penetration of the orbit and therefore inadvertent subarachnoid injection. It also seems to be safer with regard to the risk of bulb perforation (396).

Cardiovascular

In addition to complications arising from the local anesthetic used during ocular anesthesia, complications can arise as a direct result of the injection. An arteriovenous fistula has been reported (397).

- An arteriovenous fistula of the supraorbital vessels developed in a 75-year-old man after peribulbar anesthesia with a supplementary supranasal injection. He elected to have conservative management and the lesion remained asymptomatic and static in size over 10 months follow-up.

Respiratory

Pulmonary edema has been attributed to lidocaine (398).

- A 74-year-old woman had peribulbar blockade with 4 ml of 2% lidocaine at the inferotemporal approach and then 3 ml at the medial approach. She had a history of mitral stenosis, occasional angina, and possibly myocardial infarction, but denied breathlessness on exertion, nocturnal dyspnea, or orthopnea. She had breathlessness and sweating 10 minutes after the medial injection. She then developed hypoxia and a few minutes later began to cough up pink frothy secretions, required intubation, and developed a sinus tachycardia without acute electrocardiographic or cardiac enzyme changes.

The authors assumed that she had developed neurogenic pulmonary edema, probably worsened by the co-existing myocardial disease.

Sensory systems

Nine patients developed prolonged symptomatic diplopia (predominantly vertical) after peribulbar anesthesia with ropivacaine 1% plus hyalase 750 units (399). The mean time to resolution of the diplopia was 24 hours. The authors stressed the importance of warning patients undergoing peribulbar blockade with ropivacaine of the possibility of prolonged diplopia and queried its future use in routine cataract surgery.

Six cases of global perforation have occurred during routine cataract surgery (SEDA-21, 134). It has incidentally led to contralateral mydriasis, hemiplegic coma, and damage to the infra-orbital nerve (SEDA-18, 144). The contralateral eye may exhibit oculomotor weakness (SEDA-16, 130). Three other reports have highlighted problems.

- A 76-year-old man undergoing trabeculectomy developed bilateral amaurosis after a peribulbar block with 6 ml of a mixture of 2% lidocaine, 0.5% bupivacaine, and hyaluronidase (400). The authors thought it unlikely that the optic nerve sheath had been penetrated and suggested that local spread to the optic nerves via the subarachnoid or subdural space had been responsible.
- A 49-year-old woman had a tonic-clonic seizure about 15 minutes after a peribulbar block for left trabeculectomy (401). She recovered and surgery continued uneventfully. However, she had severe permanent visual loss in that eye, and an MRI scan at 4 weeks showed swelling of the left optic nerve. The authors suggested that some prilocaine had been injected into the nerve sheath, causing the convulsions, local optic nerve swelling, and subsequent optic nerve atrophy.

In 60 patients, peribulbar blockade was performed with either 8 ml of 0.75% ropivacaine or a 1:1 mixture of 2%

lidocaine and 0.5% bupivacaine (402). Surgical block was achieved after a similar period of time in each group, but ropivacaine provided a better quality of postoperative analgesia, with no pain reported at 24 hours in 26 (87%) compared with 18 (60%) in the lidocaine + bupivacaine group. One patient given ropivacaine reported unbearable pain due to a high intraocular pressure, and the incidence of postoperative nausea and vomiting was under 7% in both groups.

In 54 patients who received peribulbar anesthesia with either 1% ropivacaine or a mixture of 0.75% bupivacaine + 2% lidocaine there was no significant difference in akinesia scores or adverse effects reported the following day, notably headache, dizziness, nausea, scalp anesthesia, and diplopia, the latter occurring in 26% and 30% respectively (403).

Peribulbar anesthesia with 1% etidocaine, 0.5% bupivacaine, and hyaluronidase has been evaluated in 300 patients (404). The mean volume administered was 17 ml. There was adequate analgesia in 85% of cases, and the other 15% required supplementation with a sub-tenon block. Akinesia occurred in 82% of cases. Two patients developed generalized seizures, and four developed severe hypotension.

- A rare case of hyphema after peribulbar block with 1% lidocaine 8 ml occurred in a 38-year-old woman with a history of Fuchs' heterochromic iridocyclitis (405).

Postoperative strabismus and diplopia occurred in two of 200 patients undergoing cataract extraction under peribulbar anesthesia; the symptoms resolved spontaneously by 6 months (406).

Hematologic

- A 27-year-old woman with diabetes mellitus, complicated by diabetic retinopathy and chronic renal insufficiency with anemia, developed methemoglobinemia (11%) after peribulbar blockade with prilocaine 80 mg, bupivacaine 30 mg, hyaluronidase, and naphazoline (407). She recovered uneventfully after methylthioninium chloride 1.5 mg/kg.

The authors concluded that she may have been at increased risk of methemoglobinemia as a result of the metabolic acidosis associated with renal insufficiency, since impaired protein binding of prilocaine could have increased the concentrations of ionized prilocaine. Furthermore, the patient was also taking isosorbide dinitrate, which may have predisposed her to methemoglobinemia.

Topical anesthesia in the eye
Topical anesthesia in the eye is relatively safe in controlled circumstances, when administered correctly (SEDA-20, 127). There does not seem to be any benefit in warming topical local anesthetic solutions before use (408).

Topical anesthetic abuse, mostly unintentional, remains a persistent cause of keratitis and epithelial defects, leading to continuing ocular pain, visual impairment, and at worst enucleation (SEDA-21, 134) (SEDA-22, 140) (409).

Mechanisms include direct toxicity of the local anesthetic or preservative and immunological causes.

In 14 patients, 0.5% proxymetacaine had similar efficacy to 0.4% oxybuprocaine and 0.5% tetracaine but was significantly better tolerated (410).

There have been reports of topical ocular anesthetic abuse.

- A 49-year-old woman developed repeated episodes of severe keratitis after radial keratotomy for myopia (411). After 18 months of repeated hospital admissions, several operations, and considerably reduced visual acuity, it eventually transpired that she had been self-medicating with 1% proparacaine mixed with artificial tears to control pain after her surgery.

Abuse of these medications often results in irreversible corneal damage and visual loss (412). Two patients continued to instil their topical 0.5% tetracaine eye-drops, despite medical advice. The result was bilateral corneal perforation in the first case and a large unilateral descemetocele in the second. Surgery was required to correct the perforations, but the long-term anatomical and functional results were poor. A third patient had obtained 0.5% tetracaine hydrochloride drops over the counter to relieve discomfort in his eye after colleagues at work had attempted to remove a foreign body from his eye. He had developed chronic toxic keratitis and was persuaded to discontinue the eye-drops. With appropriate treatment the cornea returned to normal.

Lidocaine gel 2% has been compared with 0.5% tetracaine drops for topical anesthesia in cataract surgery in 25 patients (413). There were no corneal epithelial or ocular surface complications, demonstrating the safety of the gel, which may provide a more practical and efficient method of anesthesia, because it needs to be applied only once as opposed to three applications of the drops.

Differences in the manufacture of unpreserved lidocaine formulations have been postulated as a cause of transient corneal clouding in patients who were given intraocular unpreserved lidocaine 1% as an adjunct to topical anesthesia (414). Independent analysis of the lidocaine solution associated with corneal clouding found it to be hypotonic and not buffered with bicarbonate compared with the solution that did not cause corneal clouding.

Intracameral anesthesia
Non-preserved intracameral lidocaine 1% is a useful adjunct to topical anesthesia for cataract surgery. In 631 patients, topical anesthesia alone was compared with combined topical and intracameral anesthesia (415) The combination had greater efficacy—only 1% of those given combined anesthesia needing to be converted to general anesthesia compared with 40% of those given topical anesthesia alone. The authors suggest that the key difference between the two methods is reduced sensitivity to the microscope light. Another prospective study in 93 patients showed that intracameral non-preserved lidocaine was both safe and efficacious; four patients

reported discomfort and none had measurable endothelial cellular changes (416).

The endothelial toxicity of local anesthetics has been assessed in pigs, as this might be relevant to the safety of agents given by intracameral injection (417). Lidocaine, mepivacaine, and prilocaine were safe, while bupivacaine in clinically effective concentrations resulted in significant cell reduction.

Sub-tenon anesthesia

Sub-tenon infiltration of local anesthesia has recently become increasingly popular for cataract and vitreoretinal surgery; presumed advantages are its safety, speed of onset, and patient compliance. Three cases of persistent diplopia following sub-tenon local anesthesia have been reported (418). Two of the patients were given injections of 4 ml of a mixture of lidocaine 1% or 2% with adrenaline 1 in 100 000 and hyaluronidase 1500 units, and the third was given 4 ml of 0.75% bupivacaine with lidocaine. All had vertical diplopia, consistent with restriction of the inferior rectus muscle, which persisted for 2–9 months. The authors suggested possible mechanisms, including direct trauma to the muscle, inflammation and adhesions, infection, and myotoxicity of local anesthetics. They have since modified their technique, reducing the rate and force of infiltration.

An infectious complication of sub-tenon anesthesia has been reported (419).

- A 63-year-old woman underwent phacoemulsification and lens implantation under sub-tenon block. After the local anesthetic was injected, the eye was prepared with an aqueous solution of povidone iodine and the surgery proceeded uneventfully. At the end, gentamicin and betamethasone were injected subconjunctivally. Over the next few days she developed orbital cellulitis, requiring intravenous antibiotics.

The authors concluded that bacterial contamination of the episcleral space from the ocular surface or skin flora had occurred during or after the sub-tenon injection. They recommended applying topical povidone iodine before the episcleral space is opened, in order to reduce this risk.

Eyelid and conjunctival anesthesia

Local infiltration with prilocaine 2% was significantly more comfortable than lidocaine 2% in a prospective randomized study in 125 patients undergoing minor eyelid procedures (420).

Two cases of transient blindness after subconjunctival injection of 2% mepivacaine 2 ml were reported in patients with advanced refractory glaucoma undergoing diode laser cyclophotocoagulation (421). The authors hypothesized that in patients with advanced optic neuropathy, even subconjunctival anesthesia can result in optic nerve block.

Oropharyngeal anesthesia

Reduced hepatic clearance, as well as relative overdosage, of local anesthetics can lead to systemic toxicity, as illustrated by three patients who underwent topical anesthesia of the oropharynx for transesophageal echocardiography and subsequently became confused and drowsy (SEDA-21, 135).

- Acute bilateral parotid swelling occurred after upper gastrointestinal endoscopy in a 53-year-old woman who had gargled 2% lidocaine solution beforehand; the swelling was associated with difficulty in swallowing and resolved after treatment with intravenous glucocorticoids for 4 days (422).
- A 21-year-old developed seizures, respiratory distress requiring tracheal intubation, severe hypotension, and then bradycardia culminating in asystole and death while gargling with 4% lidocaine 20 ml (800 mg) (423).

The authors strongly advised against exceeding the maximum recommended dose of lidocaine (200 mg), even when using it topically.

Otic anesthesia

Transient vestibular irritation without hearing loss after infiltration of the auditory canal has been incidentally attributed to diffusion of the local anesthetic from the site of injection (424).

Paravertebral anesthesia

Postural headache after thoracic paravertebral nerve anesthesia, and probably reflecting dural entry, has been reported (425). Nerve root damage is another possible complication. Hematuria due to injury to the kidney or ureter is an unusual complication of lumbar paravertebral sympathetic block (426).

An epidural abscess and paraplegia occurred after paravertebral lidocaine infiltration for back pain (SEDA-21, 133).

Among 44 women who received a single paravertebral block with 0.3 ml/kg of 0.5% bupivacaine at the level of T4 for breast surgery, there was one incident of epidural spread of the block with paraparesis for 280 minutes accompanied by unilateral Horner's syndrome for 170 minutes (427).

Post-thoracotomy pain can be treated with thoracic epidural or thoracic paravertebral blockade. In 100 adult patients allocated to receive one of these treatments with preoperative bolus doses of bupivacaine followed by a continuous infusion there was less postoperative respiratory morbidity and significantly better arterial oxygenation in the paravertebral group; nausea (10 versus 2), vomiting (7 versus 2), and hypotension (7 versus 0) were more problematic in the epidural group (428).

An interesting case is described where a catheter was inadvertently placed in the subdural space during intended cannulation of the paravertebral space (395).

- After induction of anesthesia a 49-year-old woman, scheduled for thoracotomy, was placed in the left lateral position in order to perform a right paravertebral block. After loss of resistance to air with a 16-gauge Tuohy needle, an epidural catheter was threaded 3 cm into what was thought to be the paravertebral space. Aspiration was negative and 3 ml of bupivacaine 0.5% with adrenaline 1: 200 000 was injected as a test dose.

After 10 minutes without hemodynamic compromise a further 12 ml of 0.5% bupivacaine was injected down the catheter. However, 15 minutes later the patient developed bradycardia (48/minute) and hypotension (70/40 mmHg) and required intravenous fluid 500 ml, ephedrine 30 mg, and noradrenaline to maintain arterial pressure. The noradrenaline infusion was tapered over the next 60 minutes. When she was extubated at the end of surgery over 3 hours later there was no motor or sensory block. Contrast medium injected down the catheter and subsequent X-rays and CT scans showed that the catheter was in the subdural space.

While total dural puncture and total spinal anesthesia have been reported after attempted paravertebral block, this is the first reported case of subdural catheter placement. The authors acknowledged that the diagnosis of a misplaced catheter was masked by the general anesthesia.

Perianal anesthesia
Local anesthetic ointments are widely used to relieve the symptoms of hemorrhoids and anal fissures. Absorption through the mucosa can be considerable; a case of convulsions as a suspected consequence of such treatment has been cited (SED-12, 253) (429).

Peritonsillar anesthesia
A stroke occurred after infiltration of the tonsillar bed with bupivacaine subsequent to tonsillectomy (430).

- A 16-year-old girl undergoing adenotonsillectomy had cardiac asystole for 10 seconds after injection of her adenoid bed with 0.5% bupivacaine 1 ml with adrenaline 5 micrograms/ml. She had already been given an unstated quantity of bupivacaine with adrenaline 5 micrograms/ml injected into her tonsillar fossae. Her cardiac output returned spontaneously, but she had a central medullopontine infarction, confirmed on MRI and CT brain scans. Magnetic resonance angiography showed an abnormal circle of Willis, with absence of both posterior communicating vessels. The authors were unclear as to the exact cause of the cardiac event and stroke, which resulted in a persistent neurological deficit.

Two cases of medullary injury after injections of local anesthetics intraoperatively have been reported (431).

- A 4-year-old child received injections of lidocaine plus adrenaline into the anterior tonsillar pillars and nasopharynx during adenotonsillectomy. After the procedure, he became agitated and dysarthric, vomited, and had abnormal eye movements. He was unable to stand and walk, owing to ataxia. An MRI scan showed a cavity in the right paramedian medulla.
- A 7-year-old boy underwent tonsillectomy, with an injection of lidocaine plus adrenaline into the operative field. After surgery he was lethargic, and during the next 24 hours he developed respiratory distress requiring mechanical ventilation. He was pyrexial (41.8°C) and had cardiomegaly and a left hemiparesis. A cranial

MRI scan showed a hemorrhagic lesion in the right paramedian medulla.

Both patients had lesions in the medial medulla supplied by branches of the anterior spinal and vertebral arteries, and although such cases are rare it seems wise, in the light of these reports, to avoid the routine use of adrenaline as an adjunct to local anesthesia for adenotonsillectomy.

Excessive volumes of local anesthetic in a confined space can lead to life-threatening upper airway obstruction. When glossopharyngeal nerve blocks are used for tonsillectomy, children under 15 kg should be given 1 ml or less of 0.25% bupivacaine per tonsil (432).

Respiratory anesthesia
Topical anesthesia of the airways is commonly used to facilitate endoscopy and sometimes manipulation of the airways. This can result in an increase in airway flow resistance, possibly due to laryngeal dysfunction (433). Lidocaine spray 10%, used for upper airways anesthesia for fiber optic intubation in a grossly obese patient, caused acute airway obstruction. The patient went on to have a percutaneous tracheotomy, and it was postulated that the local anesthetic had abolished laryngeal receptors responsible for airway maintenance, or that laryngospasm and reduced muscle tone due to the lidocaine might have been the cause (SEDA-22, 140).

- Unilateral bronchospasm has been described in a 19-year-old woman after the administration of lidocaine 4% 5 ml into the larynx via a Laryngojet injector (434).

Lidocaine gel is not recommended for lubrication of laryngeal masks. It confers no benefits and increases the incidence of adverse effects such as intraoperative hiccups, postoperative hoarseness, nausea, vomiting, and tongue paresthesia (435).

- A patient due to have a bronchoscopy was given an overdose of lidocaine to anesthetize the airway by an inexperienced health worker. He was then left unobserved and subsequently developed convulsions and cardiopulmonary arrest (436). He survived with severe cerebral damage. His lidocaine concentration was 24 micrograms/ml about 1 hour after initial administration (a blood concentration over 6 micrograms/ml is considered to be toxic).
- A 19-year-old healthy volunteer undergoing bronchoscopy was given about 1200 mg of lidocaine to anesthetize the airway and was sent home after the procedure, despite complaining of chest pain. Shortly afterwards she had a tonic-clonic seizure and cardiopulmonary arrest and died 2 days later. The research protocol had failed to specify an upper dose limit for lidocaine (437).

Sciatic nerve anesthesia
Sciatic nerve anesthesia can cause cardiovascular depression (438).

- A 74-year-old man was to receive a combined sciatic nerve and psoas compartment block for a total hip arthroplasty; the classic Labat's approach was used and 30 ml of 0.75% ropivacaine was injected over 1.5 minutes, after which he suddenly became unresponsive and developed tonic–clonic movements. Propofol was administered and the seizure resolved, but he developed sinus bradycardia with progressive lengthening of the QRS interval, which converted to nodal bradycardia. A ventricular escape rhythm at 20/minute with T wave inversion was treated with ephedrine 10 mg and adrenaline 0.1 mg, resulting in supraventricular tachycardia with transient atrial fibrillation.

The authors pointed out that an equipotent dose of bupivacaine would have resulted in worse cardiovascular depression with less chance of successful resuscitation.

Skin anesthesia

Topical local anesthetics play an important role in anogenital contact allergy (439–443). Cinchocaine is commonly used in topical antihemorrhoidal formulations and is a well-known sensitizer (444). Although benzocaine is not as widely used in topical anesthetic formulations in Germany, patients with anogenital dermatitis were at higher risk of sensitization. Amide-type local anesthetics, like lidocaine HCl and tetracaine, are less potent sensitizers (445). Contact allergy to local anesthetics is more often observed among patients with perianal complaints than patients with perianal and vulval or only vulval dermatitis (441).

Different types of topical reactions have been reported after the use of emla cream (a eutectic mixture of prilocaine 2.5% and lidocaine 2.5%).

- A 9-year-old boy with beta thalassemia major, who required subcutaneous infusions of deferoxamine 5 times a week, had been having emla cream applied to the injection sites and later developed an eczematous rash at these sites (446). Initial patch testing 4 months later elicited a positive response to emla cream. Subsequent testing confirmed a positive test to prilocaine. Lidocaine and related anesthetics gave negative results. He continued further treatment with tetracaine 4% cream with no problems, and an allergic contact dermatitis was diagnosed.
- A 2-year-old Caucasian boy developed purpuric reactions at the sites of application of emla cream, used for curettage of molluscum contagiosum (447). He had no other symptoms, but had a family history of atopy and had had mild atopic dermatitis since the age of 6 months. He was not treated and the purpura healed without sequelae in about 2 weeks.
- A 5-year-old girl with acute lymphoblastic leukemia developed a purpuric rash at sites where EMLA cream had been used to obtain local anesthesia before lumbar puncture (27). Her routine hematological tests showed thrombocytopenia with a platelet count of 38×10^9/l. The lesion was asymptomatic and completely resolved without treatment in about 2 weeks.

Patch tests were not performed in the second and third cases, but allergic contact dermatitis does not present with purpuric lesions. The mechanisms of action of local anesthetics, including a direct action on voltage-gated sodium channels, a direct effect on the membrane lipid matrix with subsequent structural alterations, and a direct effect on lipid-protein interfaces, all support a potential hypothesis of a direct toxic effect of EMLA cream on the blood vessels. The authors reported other factors that may be involved in the pathogenesis of such a condition, including atopic dermatitis, predisposition in children, prematurity, trauma, and thrombocytopenia.

Localized angioedema has been described subsequent to the use of emla.

- A 46-year-old man with idiopathic genital pain syndrome was given emla cream (448). After using it for 2 weeks, he complained of swelling of the glans penis associated with mild itching and edema. A patch test with emla cream, half diluted with white soft paraffin, lidocaine 2%, and cream base, gave a positive reaction to lidocaine+ prilocaine and not to lidocaine alone. The symptoms resolved with topical glucocorticoids.

The diagnosis was contact angioedema secondary to contact allergy to prilocaine.

Hematologic

Methemoglobinemia with systemic toxicity has been reported af6ter the use of emla cream (lidocaine + prilocaine) (449).

- A 30-year-old woman who came for laser epilation of the legs had successfully undergone the same procedure 1 week before. One hour before the procedure, a total of 150 g of emla (5 tubes, 30 g per tube) was applied to both legs under occlusive dressing. About 2 hours later she developed symptoms of systemic toxicity, including light-headedness, numbness of the tongue, muscle twitching, and dyspnea. She had a methemoglobin concentration of 20% and was given methylthioninium chloride (methylene blue) 50 mg intravenously.

The authors suggested that increased absorption of emla and subsequent toxicity could have been due to several mechanisms. Thermal injury from the first and current procedures and the occlusive dressing could have increased absorption; displacement of bound drug caused by contraceptive medication and inhibition of cytochrome P450 by sertraline could have produced increased plasma concentrations of lidocaine and prilocaine. In conclusion, excessive application of emla to damaged skin should be avoided.

A 3-year-old child had a seizure and methemoglobinemia (18%) after the use of emla (5 g spread on an area of about 1140 cm^2 on the back) before allergy testing (450).

This case differed from previous ones in that a reasonable amount of emla was used on normal skin.

Skin

In two patients the use of emla cream before skin biopsy resulted in the misdiagnosis of a lysosomal storage disease, because of ultrastructural features in the biopsy

(451). When repeated without emla the skin biopsies looked normal.

Death

A fatal reaction to topical use of a mixed local anesthetic gel has been described (452).

- A 22-year-old college student died after applying a topical gel containing lidocaine 10%, tetracaine 10%, and phenylephrine. She had seizures in her car and although the conclusion was death due to high dose of lidocaine, questions were raised about the relevance of tetracaine, which is better absorbed.

The author highlighted the variable doses of local anesthetics in compounded products, their easy availability as non-prescription items, and the unnecessary use of higher doses when alternatives with appropriate doses are available (453).

Drug formulations

A topical formulation of 4% or 5% lidocaine cream (ELA-max) has been reviewed and compared with emla for pediatric use (454). The author concluded that ELA-max has similar efficacy to emla and two main advantages: faster onset of action and a reduced risk of methemoglobinemia. Only minor adverse effects, such as erythema, have been reported.

Stellate ganglion anesthesia

Inadvertent spinal anesthesia and subsequent nervous system toxicity, for example with transient paralysis or apnea, are the main complications of stellate ganglion block (SEDA-22, 140). It has been suggested that ultrasound guidance when performing the block might improve safety (455). The use of very small test doses and an anterior approach to the stellate ganglion are recommended preventive measures.

Brachial plexus paresis has been reported (456). Accidental block of the recurrent laryngeal nerve can cause hoarseness and occasionally aspiration of saliva (457).

In two women with Raynaud's syndrome, the symptoms were aggravated contralaterally after stellate ganglion block (SEDA-18, 145).

Severe hypertension has been reported after a left-sided block, possibly due to vagal nerve block and unopposed sympathetic output (SEDA-21, 134).

Convulsions are a recognized complication of inadvertent intra-arterial injection during stellate ganglion block; two such cases have been described (458).

- A 28-year-old 75 kg woman underwent stellate ganglion block for symptomatic treatment of Raynaud's syndrome. An anterolateral approach was used, guarding the carotid artery and jugular vein. After an aspiration test was negative in two planes, 5 ml of 1% lidocaine was injected over 2–3 seconds using a 20 G needle. However, a second aspiration test was positive for blood, the needle was pulled back, and on reinjection the patient immediately had a severe generalized tonic-clonic seizure. The patient made a rapid recovery with no further treatment and was fully conscious after 2 minutes.

- A 31-year-old 72 kg man with diabetes, who had had a below-knee amputation in the past, developed Buerger's disease affecting his hands, particularly on the He underwent his third stellate ganglion block for symptomatic treatment. An anterior paratracheal approach was used with a 20 G 3.5 cm needle; after an aspiration test was negative in two planes, 1 ml of 1% lidocaine was injected every 2–3 seconds. After one injection, he had an abrupt seizure which was treated with diazepam 10 mg. He made a full recovery and later completed his course of stellate ganglion blocks uneventfully.

It was thought that inadvertent vertebral arterial injection had occurred, with subsequent rapid elimination due to high cerebral blood flow. The authors suggested several precautions to minimize this risk, including using a large-diameter needle and using less than the calculated minimum arterial toxic dose of lidocaine (16.8 mg) as the initial test dose; for subsequent doses they suggested 5 mg.

Subcutaneous anesthesia

When infiltrating local anesthetics into the skin there is always a risk of intravascular injection (SEDA-17, 140), but it can be avoided by back-aspiration of the syringe or continuous advancement of the needle during injection.

Skin infiltration with local anesthetics can cause pain. The pain experienced during skin infiltration of lidocaine, chloroprocaine, and buffered solutions of both has been studied in 22 volunteers in a double-blind, randomized study (459). The pH of the solutions was unrelated to the pain score, but both formulations of chloroprocaine were significantly less painful than lidocaine.

A weak solution of lidocaine has sometimes been injected into excess fat before liposuction, so that the procedure can be carried out without general anesthesia. The technique is generally regarded as safe (460). However, deaths are reported, associated with local anesthetic toxicity or drug interactions (461).

Of 30 volunteers who had subcutaneous slow infusion tumescent anesthesia at 250 ml/hour with three solutions containing lidocaine 2 mg/ml, ropivacaine 0.5 mg/ml mixed with lidocaine 1 mg/ml, and ropivacaine 1 mg/ml alone, all containing adrenaline 1:1 000 000, one had a tingling sensation in the tongue after lidocaine and another went into vasovagal shock (462). In the same paper, 5020 surgical procedures were reported in 3270 patients using different strengths of ropivacaine alone (0.05–0.2%) with a maximum dose of 300 mg, or with a mixture of ropivacaine and prilocaine (0.08–0.3%) with a maximum ropivacaine dose of 160 mg and a maximum prilocaine dose of 300 mg. There was no methemoglobinemia and there were no minor or major adverse effects related to the local anesthetic. The maximum plasma concentrations were low, suggesting that higher maximum doses may be possible, provided adrenaline is added.

- Ventricular tachycardia, severe hypertension, and pulmonary edema developed in a 53-year-old woman soon after she had a skin flap infiltrated with 4 ml of 0.5% lidocaine and 0.0005% adrenaline (20 micrograms) (463).

This has been previously described during general anesthesia but not with a local anesthetic alone, and the author emphasized the risk of severe cardiovascular compromise, even with a small dose of adrenaline.

Five patients with complex regional pain syndrome received a subcutaneous infusion of 10% lidocaine, with successful alleviation of many of their symptoms; initially 200 mg/kg was infused but symptoms of vertigo and slurred speech each occurred in four of them and stuttering in three, so the rate was adjusted to 100–190 mg/hour and serum lidocaine concentrations of 0.1–8.1 micrograms/ml (average 3.7 micrograms/ml); other symptoms, such as aphasia, nausea, fatigue, metallic taste, light-headedness, and perioral numbness, each occurred in over half of the patients (464).

An iatrogenic tension pneumothorax was the result of breast infiltration with lidocaine and adrenaline before an augmentation procedure (SEDA-20, 127).

Infiltration anesthesia has reportedly caused transient paralysis.

- Transient paraplegia occurred after wound site infiltration with bupivacaine in a 35-year-old woman during removal of a lumboperitoneal shunt that had been inserted 2 years previously for benign intracranial hypertension (465). Under general anesthesia with the patient in the left lateral position, a small incision was made over the right flank and the drain was easily removed. The site was infiltrated with 7.5 ml of 0.5% bupivacaine with adrenaline 1 in 200 000. During recovery, she was anxious and moderately hypotensive and had a flaccid paralysis from T4 down. An MRI scan was normal. She gradually recovered motor function, sensation, and pain at the wound site.

The authors concluded that the local anesthetic may have passed down a fistulous track into the subarachnoid space, producing spinal block.

Tumescent anesthesia is an infiltration technique now widely used in cosmetic surgery. It involves the infiltration of a relatively large volume of a solution containing lidocaine, adrenaline, sodium bicarbonate, and isotonic saline into the subdermal fat plane. There have been previous descriptions of severe and even fatal complications.

Plasma lidocaine concentrations and symptoms of local anesthetic toxicity have been reported in five oriental patients after tumescent local anesthesia (466). The patients received lidocaine in total doses of 20–35 mg/kg. The plasma lidocaine concentration 3 hours later did not exceed the toxic concentration of 5 µg/ml and was significantly lower at 8 hours.

Submucosal anesthesia

Complications noted at various times with submucosal use include allergic reactions to the parabens present in lidocaine, systemic effects due to general diffusion (which readily occurs), or necrosis (when adrenaline is included in the formulation) (SEDA-16, 131).

Urinary tract anesthesia

Urethral instillation of anesthetics is most likely to be needed in the elderly, in whom there may be marked absorption from the mucosa, especially if it is diseased or damaged. Seizures after instillation of lidocaine jelly (for example 20 ml of a 2% formulation) have been reported as a consequence of this (467).

Nervous system

Seizures after the application of local anesthetic gel for urological catheterization have been reported (468).

- A 40-year-old man received a spinal anesthetic with 3 ml of hyperbaric bupivacaine 0.5%. A gel containing lidocaine 2% (40 ml) was used for cystoscopy to aid bladder catheterization. He developed circumoral tingling followed by a generalized tonic–clonic seizure and was given a barbiturate and diazepam. The serum lidocaine concentration was 20 µg/ml (in the high toxic range) and fell to 12 µg/ml after 12 hours.

Absorption across the urethral mucosa would be expected to be rapid, because of the rich vascular supply, and that peak plasma concentrations would be higher by this route because of the absence of hepatic first-pass removal. In this case, the dose of lidocaine was high. The authors suggested that a gel without a local anesthetic should be used when the patient is given some form of regional anesthesia for catheterization.

Local anesthetic gels and creams used liberally on traumatized epithelium can be rapidly absorbed, resulting in systemic effects, such as convulsions, particularly if excessive quantities are used.

- A 40-year-old woman developed seizures after lidocaine gel 40 ml was injected into the ureter during an attempt to remove a stone (469).

Drug formulations

Plain aqueous gel and 2% lidocaine hydrochloride gel (Instagel ™) have been compared in 100 men attending for flexible cystoscopy in a double-blind study (470). They were randomized to receive either 11 ml of plain aqueous gel or 11 ml of 2% lidocaine gel intraurethrally and scored discomfort with a visual analogue scale. There was significantly less urethral discomfort in the patients who received the plain gel. The authors believed that the increased discomfort associated with lidocaine gel may have been due to excipients. They concluded that there is little rationale in using lidocaine gel for cystoscopy using fine-caliber flexible instruments. Competence with the cystoscope and good lubrication are essential for patient comfort during simple urethral instrumentation.

Drug–Drug Interactions

Neuromuscular blockers

The effects of non-depolarizing neuromuscular blocking drugs can be potentiated and their actions prolonged by large doses of local anesthetics, because of depression of nerve conduction, inhibition of acetylcholine formation, mobilization, and release, reduced postsynaptic receptor channel opening times, and reduced muscle contraction (471).

Opioids

Opioids potentiate the analgesic effect of neuraxial local anesthetics, with minimal adverse effects (SEDA-18, 141) (SEDA-20, 121) (SEDA-22, 135), as shown in several studies with clonidine, fentanyl, morphine, or pethidine as the systemic or neuraxial analgesic, and bupivacaine, lidocaine, and ropivacaine as the local anesthetic. The benefits have been shown in relief of long-term pain and postoperative pain, in adults and children (SEDA-18, 141) (SEDA-18, 146).

Sulfones/sulfonamides

Local anesthetics, sulfones, and sulfonamides are all aniline derivatives, exposure to which, particularly to two or three concurrently, can predispose patients to methemoglobinemia (5,472,473).

Suxamethonium

Procaine and cocaine are esters that are hydrolysed by plasma cholinesterase and can therefore competitively enhance the action of suxamethonium (474). Chloroprocaine may have a similar action. Lidocaine also interacts, although the mechanism is not clear unless very high doses are used (475).

Tubocurarine

Local anesthetics have diverse effects on the neuromuscular junction. In very large doses they produce paralysis on their own. When the recommended doses are used for local anesthesia, systemic absorption is small and interaction with relaxants is not to be expected. However, large doses injected intravascularly (accidentally, or therapeutically for dysrhythmias) can potentiate relaxants of both types (476,477).

Compounds added to local anesthetics

Adrenaline

Adrenaline has been largely abandoned as an adjuvant to local anesthetics, although in a 1:80 000 concentration it is still sometimes used in dental and in epidural anesthesia.

Ventricular dysrhythmias have been reported in a case of adrenaline overdose (478).

- A 5-year-old boy was given subcutaneous adrenaline 1:1000 after a severe allergic reaction to a bee sting. Inadvertently, 10 times the correct dose was given. He

developed extra beats and two brief runs of ventricular tachycardia, but recovered fully after about 20 minutes. Creatine kinase activity, both total and the MB fraction, was slightly raised in this patient (total 603 IU/l, MB fraction 161 IU/l; upper limits of the local reference range 243 and 15 IU/l), suggesting cardiac damage.

Life-threatening torsade de pointes has been observed when an epidural anesthetic was given using 20 ml of bupivacaine containing only 1:200 000 adrenaline (479).

When adrenaline 0.4 ml of a 1 mg/ml solution was inadvertently injected into the penile skin of a 12-hour-old neonate the skin blanched and the error was immediately understood (480). After repeated doses of phentolamine (total 0.65 mg) the skin regained its normal color. There were no sequelae.

Adrenaline is occasionally used as a hemostatic agent, with rare complications. However, they do occur, as noted in a report from Lyon (481).

- A 64-year-old man with diabetes and hypertension bled from a site in the lower rectum. A local injection of adrenaline 0.2 mg successfully stopped the hemorrhage, but very soon after he became hypotensive, with rapid atrial fibrillation (ventricular rate not given), the first time he had experienced this. He reverted spontaneously to sinus rhythm within 24 hours.

The authors suggested that if this type of procedure is contemplated in elderly patients with cardiovascular disease an anesthetist should be present to monitor cardiovascular status; it may in any case be wiser to avoid adrenaline altogether in favor of other means of hemostasis.

A more unusual site of adrenaline injection has been described in a Canadian report (482).

- A 79-year-old woman developed pituitary apoplexy in an adenomatous gland and was being prepared for *trans*-sphenoidal hypophysectomy. Topical adrenaline (1:1000) was applied to both nostrils and then 1.5 ml of 1% lidocaine containing 1:100 000 adrenaline was injected into the nasal mucosa. The blood pressure immediately rose from 100/50 to 230/148 mmHg and the pulse rate from 48 to 140/minute. Although she was treated immediately with esmolol and intravenous glyceryl trinitrate, resulting in normalization of her blood pressure, subsequent investigations showed that she had had a painless myocardial infarction. She made a full recovery after pituitary surgery.

The authors suggested that if adrenaline is to be used in such cases, even lower concentrations might be advisable. This is reasonable, although one also wonders in this case whether her blood pressure may have been lowered too rapidly.

Clonidine

Clonidine is used epidurally, in combination with opioids, neostigmine, and anesthetic and analgesic agents, to produce segmental analgesia, particularly for postoperative relief of pain after obstetrical and surgical procedures.

The use of clonidine in pediatric anesthesia has been reviewed (483).

Edetic acid and its salts

Disodium edetate can cause contact dermatitis, for instance when used in local anesthetics (484).

Ephedrine

Tricyclic antidepressants inhibit the uptake of catecholamines, such as ephedrine, into sympathetic neurons and can enhance their cardiovascular effects (485).

- A 61-year-old woman taking amitriptyline 25 mg/day underwent oophorectomy for ovarian cancer under combined general and epidural lumbar anesthesia. After the administration of the local anesthetic she developed hypotension refractory to high doses of ephedrine and dopaminergic drugs. Control was achieved with noradrenaline 200 µg.

The authors suggested that even the small amounts of ephedrine present as additives in some local anesthetics can have a marked effect on the cardiovascular system.

Fentanyl

The analgesic effect of fentanyl 1.5 µg/kg has been compared with that of tramadol 1.5 mg/kg in 61 patients receiving standardized anesthetics for day-case arthroscopic knee surgery (486). Opioid adverse effects and analgesia were similar in the two groups.

The analgesic effects and adverse effects profiles of subcutaneous fentanyl and subcutaneous morphine have been compared in a double-blind, crossover, 6-day study in 23 patients with cancer pain (487). There were no significant differences in pain scores between the two drugs and no changes in the level of acute confusion (using the Saskatoon Delirium Checklist) or cognitive impairment (in tests of semantic fluency and trail-making tests). Fentanyl caused significantly less constipation. The patients in this study were highly stable and compliant, and the results cannot be generalized.

The addition of fentanyl 1 µg/ml to ropivacaine 7.5 mg/ml did not improve nerve blockade by axillary brachial plexus anesthesia in a double-blind, randomized study in 30 patients undergoing orthopedic procedures (488). In another double-blind, randomized study, 60 patients receiving axillary brachial plexus blockade were given 0.25% bupivacaine 40 mg, 0.25% bupivacaine 40 mg plus fentanyl 2.5 µg/ml, or 0.125% bupivacaine 40 mg plus fentanyl 2.5 µg/ml (489). The addition of fentanyl 2.5 µg/ml prolonged sensory and motor blockade without any improvement in the onset of anesthesia and no significant increase in adverse effects. These two studies have reaffirmed the current position of conflicting results in studies of the benefits of adding fentanyl to local anesthetics for peripheral nerve blockade.

The ideal combination strength of ropivacaine with fentanyl for postoperative epidural analgesia has been investigated in two studies. In a double-blind, randomized study, 30 patients undergoing lower abdominal surgery received one of three solutions for PCA after a standardized combined epidural and general anesthetic: ropivacaine 0.2% plus fentanyl 4 µg, ropivacaine 0.1% plus

fentanyl 2 µg, or ropivacaine 0.05% plus fentanyl 1 µg (490). All three solutions produced equivalent analgesia. Motor block secondary to the ropivacaine was significantly more frequent and intense with ropivacaine 0.2% plus fentanyl 4 µg. Pruritus, nausea, sedation, and hypotension occurred equally often in the three groups and were mild. It was therefore inferred that ropivacaine 0.2% plus fentanyl 4 µg is preferable for analgesia after lower abdominal surgery.

The addition of clonidine or fentanyl to local anesthetics for single shot caudal blocks has been studied in 64 children undergoing bilateral correction of vesicoureteral reflux randomized into four groups (491). The control group received a mixture of 0.25% bupivacaine with adrenaline plus 1% lidocaine; other groups received the same combination plus 1.5 µg/kg of clonidine, or the control combination plus 1 µg/kg of fentanyl, or the control combination plus 0.5 µg/kg of fentanyl plus 0.75 µg/kg of clonidine. The addition of either clonidine or fentanyl significantly prolonged anesthesia, and during recovery the groups receiving local anesthetics alone or with the addition of fentanyl alone had significantly increased heart rates. Two of the children who received extradural fentanyl had a transient reduction in oxygen of saturation to 92% in the first hour of recovery. One of these was from those who received fentanyl alone, while one had received fentanyl plus clonidine. Vomiting occurred only in children exposed to fentanyl (nine of 29 subjects). This is the first report of respiratory depression in children after the caudal administration of fentanyl or clonidine, this adverse effect having been previously described with extradural opioids and clonidine in adults.

The relations between fentanyl and local anesthetics and their adverse effects profiles in epidural analgesia (492) further demonstrate the need for well-controlled, double-blind studies (493,494).

The use of a continuous epidural infusion of lidocaine 0.4% plus fentanyl 1 µg/ml in combination with intravenous metamizol 40 mg/kg provided significantly better analgesia than epidural morphine 20 µg/kg plus intravenous metamizol 40 mg/kg during the first 3 postoperative days in 30 children undergoing orthopedic surgery, without increasing the incidence of adverse effects; however, the difference in beneficial effect was small (495).

Prophylactic nalbuphine 4 mg and droperidol 0.625 mg with minidose lidocaine + fentanyl spinal anesthesia in a randomized, double-blinded, controlled study in 62 patients having outpatient knee arthroscopy provided significantly better analgesia and reduced nausea and pruritus than in another 62 patients who received only nalbuphine 4 mg with minidose lidocaine + fentanyl spinal anesthesia (496).

Noradrenaline

Like adrenaline, noradrenaline is also sometimes added to local anesthetics (for example in a 1:250 000 concentration) to prolong their effect; it should not be injected into extremities (finger, penis) for this purpose, since dangerous ischemia can result (497).

When infusing noradrenaline the infusion should always be ended very gradually, since otherwise a catastrophic fall in blood pressure can occur.

References

1. Grouls RJ, Ackerman EW, Korsten HH, Hellebrekers LJ, Breimer DD. Partition coefficients (n-octanol/water) of N-butyl-p-aminobenzoate and other local anesthetics measured by reversed-phase high-performance liquid chromatography. J Chromatogr B Biomed Sci Appl 1997;694(2):421–5.

2. Covino BG. Pharmacology of local anesthetic agents. Ration Drug Ther 1987;21(8):1–9.

3. McCaughey W. Adverse effects of local anaesthetics. Drug Saf 1992;7(3):178–89.

4. Young ER, MacKenzie TA. The pharmacology of local anesthetics—a review of the literature. J Can Dent Assoc 1992;58(1):34–42.

5. Reynolds F. Adverse effects of local anaesthetics. Br J Anaesth 1987;59(1):78–95.

6. Muller U, Bircher A, Bischof M. Allergisches Angioödem nach zahnärztlicher Applikation eines Lokalanästhetikum und Hyaluronidase enthaltenden Vorspritzmittels. [Allergic angioedema after local dental anesthesia and a hyaluronidase-containing preanesthetic injection solution.] Schweiz Med Wochenschr 1986;116(51):1810–3.

7. Covino BG. Toxicity of local anesthetic agents. Acta Anaesthesiol Belg 1988;39(3 Suppl 2):159–64.

8. Lalli AF, Amaranath L. A critique on mortality associated with local anaesthetics. Anesthesiol Rev 1982;9:29.

9. Ecoffey C, Samii K. Complication neurologique après anesthésie peridurale chez un garçon de 15 ans. [Neurologic complication after epidural anesthesia in a 15-year-old boy.] Ann Fr Anesth Réanim 1990;9(4):398.

10. Mulroy MF. Systemic toxicity and cardiotoxicity from local anesthetics: incidence and preventive measures. Reg Anesth Pain Med 2002;27(6):556–61.

11. Lynch C 3rd. Depression of myocardial contractility in vitro by bupivacaine, etidocaine, and lidocaine. Anesth Analg 1986;65(6):551–9.

12. Ashley EM, Quick DG, El-Behesey B, Bromley LM. A comparison of the vasodilatation produced by two topical anaesthetics. Anaesthesia 1999;54(5):466–9.

13. Zaugg M, Schulz C, Wacker J, Schaub MC. Sympatho-modulatory therapies in perioperative medicine. Br J Anaesth 2004;93(1):53–62.

14. Polley LS, Columb MO, Naughton NN, Wagner DS, van de Ven CJ. Relative analgesic potencies of ropivacaine and bupivacaine for epidural analgesia in labor: implications for therapeutic indexes. Anesthesiology 1999;90(4): 944–50.

15. Capogna G, Celleno D, Fusco P, Lyons G, Columb M. Relative potencies of bupivacaine and ropivacaine for analgesia in labour. Br J Anaesth 1999;82(3):371–3.

16. Graf BM, Abraham I, Eberbach N, Kunst G, Stowe DF, Martin E. Differences in cardiotoxicity of bupivacaine and ropivacaine are the result of physicochemical and stereo-selective properties. Anesthesiology 2002;96(6):1427–34.

17. Weinberg GL. Current concepts in resuscitation of patients with local anesthetic cardiac toxicity. Reg Anesth Pain Med 2002;27(6):568–75.

18. Brown DL, Ransom DM, Hall JA, Leicht CH, Schroeder DR, Offord KP. Regional anesthesia and local anesthetic-induced systemic toxicity: seizure frequency and accompanying cardiovascular changes. Anesth Analg 1995;81(2):321–8.

19. Mather LE, Cousins MJ. Local anaesthetics and their current clinical use. Drugs 1979;18(3):185–205.

20. d'Athis F. Comment traiter un accident toxique?. [How should a toxic accident be treated?.] Ann Fr Anesth Reanim 1988;7(3):227–32.

21. Korman B, Riley RH. Convulsions induced by ropivacaine during interscalene brachial plexus block. Anesth Analg 1997;85(5):1128–9.

22. Abouleish EI, Elias M, Nelson C. Ropivacaine-induced seizure after extradural anaesthesia. Br J Anaesth 1998;80(6):843–4.

23. Mofenson HC, Caraccio TR. Tack up a warning on TAC. Am J Dis Child 1989;143(5):519–20.

24. Daya MR, Burton BT, Schleiss MR, DiLiberti JH. Recurrent seizures following mucosal application of TAC. Ann Emerg Med 1988;17(6):646–8.

25. Ferraro L, Zeichner S, Greenblott G, Groeger JS. Cetacaine-induced acute methemoglobinemia. Anesthesiology 1988; 69(4):614–5.

26. Abdallah HY, Shah SA. Methemoglobinemia induced by topical benzocaine: a warning for the endoscopist. Endoscopy 2002;34(9):730–4.

27. Margulies DR, Manookian CM. Methemoglobinemia as a cause of respiratory failure. J Trauma 2002;52(4):796–7.

28. Voelker CA, Brown L, Hinson RM. Perioperatively acquired methaemoglobinaemia in a preterm infant. Paediatr Anaesth 2002;12(3):284–6.

29. Fisher MM, Bowey CJ. Alleged allergy to local anaesthetics. Anaesth Intensive Care 1997;25(6):611–4.

30. Berkun Y, Ben-Zvi A, Levy Y, Galili D, Shalit M. Evaluation of adverse reactions to local anesthetics: experience with 236 patients. Ann Allergy Asthma Immunol 2003;91:342-5.

31. Macy E. Local anesthetic adverse reaction evaluations: the role of the allergist. Ann Allergy Asthma Immunol 2003;91:319-20.

32. Duque S, Fernndez L. Delayed-type hypersensitivity to amide local anesthetics. Allergol Immunopathol (Madr) 2004;32(4):233-4.

33. Balestrieri PJ, Ferguson JE 2nd. Management of a parturient with a history of local anesthetic allergy. Anesth Analg 2003;96:1489-90.

34. Hepner DL, Castells MC, Tsen LC. Should local anesthetic allergy testing be routinely performed during pregnancy? Anesth Analg 2003;97:1853-4.

35. Balestrieri PJ, Ferguson JE 2nd. Author response. Anesth Analg 2003;97:1854.

36. Fernandez-Redondo V, Leon A, Santiago T, Toribio J. Allergic contact dermatitis from local anaesthetic on peri-stomal skin. Contact Dermatitis 2001;45(6):358.

37. McGough EK, Cohen JA. Unexpected bronchospasm during spinal anesthesia. J Clin Anesth 1990;2(1):35–6.

38. Kearney CR, Fewings J. Allergic contact dermatitis to cinchocaine. Australas J Dermatol 2001;42(2):118–9.

39. Erdmann SM, Sachs B, Merk HF. Systemic contact dermatitis from cinchocaine. Contact Dermatitis 2001;44(4):260–1.

40. Hayashi K, Kawachi S, Saida T. Allergic contact dermatitis due to both chlorpheniramine maleate and dibucaine hydrochloride in an over-the-counter medicament. Contact Dermatitis 2001;44(1):38–9.

41. Redfern DC. Contact sensitivity to multiple local anesthetics. J Allergy Clin Immunol 1999;104(4 Pt 1):890–1.

42. Orasch CE, Helbling A, Zanni MP, Yawalkar N, Hari Y, Pichler WJ. T-cell reaction to local anaesthetics:

relationship to angioedema and urticaria after subcutaneous application—patch testing and LTT in patients with adverse reaction to local anaesthetics. Clin Exp Allergy 1999;29(11):1549–54.

43. Ball IA. Allergic reactions to lignocaine. Br Dent J 1999;186(5):224–6.

44. Walters G, Georgiou T, Hayward JM. Sight-threatening acute orbital swelling from peribulbar local anesthesia. J Cataract Refract Surg 1999;25(3):444–6.

45. Nakada T, Iijima M. Allergic contact dermatitis from dibucaine hydrochloride. Contact Dermatitis 2000;42(5):283.

46. Kakuyama M, Toda H, Osawa M, Fukuda K. An adverse effect of carboxymethylcellulose in lidocaine jelly. Anesthesiology 1999;91(6):1969.

47. Hammer R, Dahlgren C, Stendahl O. Inhibition of human leukocyte metabolism and random mobility by local anaesthesia. Acta Anaesthesiol Scand 1985;29(5):520–3.

48. Gall H, Kaufmann R, Kalveram CM. Adverse reactions to local anesthetics: analysis of 197 cases. J Allergy Clin Immunol 1996;97(4):933–7.

49. Breit S, Rueff F, Przybilla B. "Deep impact" contact allergy after subcutaneous injection of local anesthetics. Contact Dermatitis 2001;45(5):296–7.

50. Bailey-Pridham DD, Reshef E, Drury K, Cook CL, Hurst HE, Yussman MA. Follicular fluid lidocaine levels during transvaginal oocyte retrieval. Fertil Steril 1990;53(1):171–3.

51. Friedman JM. Teratogen update: anesthetic agents. Teratology 1988;37(1):69–77.

52. Coleman M, Kelly DJ. Local anaesthetic toxicity in a pregnant patient undergoing lignocaine-induced intravenous regional anaesthesia. Acta Anaesthesiol Scand 1998;42(2):267–9.

53. Dalens BJ, Mazoit JX. Adverse effects of regional anaesthesia in children. Drug Saf 1998;19(4):251–68.

54. Owen MD, Gautier P, Hood DD. Can ropivacaine and levobupivacaine be used as test doses during regional anesthesia? Anesthesiology 2004;100(4):922–5.

55. Riley RH, Musk MT. Laryngospasm induced by topical application of lignocaine. Anaesth Intensive Care 2005;33(2):278.

56. Ho AM, Chung DC, To EW, Karmakar MK. Total airway obstruction during local anesthesia in a non-sedated patient with a compromised airway. Can J Anaesth 2004;51(8):838-41.

57. Rodins K, Hlavac M, Beckert L. Lignocaine neurotoxicity following fibre-optic bronchoscopy. NZ Med J 2003;116:U500.

58. Perney P, Blanc F, Mourad G, Blayac JP, Hillaire-Buys D. Transitory ataxia related to topically administered lidocaine. Ann Pharmacother 2004;38(5):828-30.

59. Salvinelli F, Casale M, Hardy JF, D'Ascanio L, Agro F. Permanent anosmia after topical nasal anaesthesia with lidocaine 4%. Br J Anaesth 2005;95(6):838-9.

60. Vaghadia H, Chan V, Ganapathy S, Lui A, McKenna J, Zimmer K. A multicentre trial of ropivacaine 7.5 mg × ml^{-1} vs bupivacaine 5 mg × ml^{-1} for supra clavicular brachial plexus anesthesia Can J Anaesth 1999;46(10): 946–51.

61. Borgeat A, Perschak H, Bird P, Hodler J, Gerber C. Patient-controlled interscalene analgesia with ropivacaine 0.2% versus patient-controlled intravenous analgesia after major shoulder surgery: effects on diaphragmatic and respiratory function Anesthesiology 2000;92(1):102–8.

62. Koscielniak-Nielsen ZJ. An unusual toxic reaction to axillary block by mepivacaine with adrenaline. Acta Anaesthesiol Scand 1998;42(7):868–71.

63. Rose M, Ness TJ. Hypoxia following interscalene block. Reg Anesth Pain Med 2002;27(1):94–6.

64. Reinikainen M, Hedman A, Pelkonen O, Ruokonen E. Cardiac arrest after interscalene brachial plexus block with ropivacaine and lidocaine. Acta Anaesthesiol Scand 2003;47:904-6.

65. Khan H, Atanassoff PG. Accidental intravascular injection of levobupivacaine and lidocaine during the transarterial approach to the axillary brachial plexus. Can J Anaesth 2003;50:95.

66. Bhat R. Transient vascular insufficiency after axillary brachial plexus block in a child. Anesth Analg 2004;98(5):1284-5.

67. al-Kaisy AA, Chan VW, Perlas A. Respiratory effects of low-dose bupivacaine interscalene block. Br J Anaesth 1999;82(2):217–20.

68. Sala-Blanch X, Lazaro JR, Correa J, Gomez-Fernandez M. Phrenic nerve block caused by interscalene brachial plexus block: effects of digital pressure and a low volume of local anesthetic. Reg Anesth Pain Med 1999;24(3):231–5.

69. Koscielniak-Nielsen ZJ. Hemidiaphragmatic paresis after interscalene supplementation of insufficient axillary block with 3 ml of 2% mepivacaine. Acta Anaesthesiol Scand 2000;44(9):1160–2.

70. Pichlmayr I, Galaske W. Auswertung von 821 supraklavikulären und subaxillären Plexus-Anästhesien in Bezug auf Effektivität. Nebenerscheinungen und Komplikationen, unter Berücksichtigung der Ausbildungs-Verpflichtungen einer medizinischer Hochschule. [Supraclavicular and subaxillar plexusanaesthesias in 821 patients. Efficiency, side-effects and complications under the aspect of the educational—engagement on a medical school.] Prakt Anaesth 1978;13(6):469–73.

71. Matthes H, Denhardt B. Erfahrungen bei Blockaden des Plexus brachialis. [Experiences with brachial plexus blocks.] Langenbecks Arch Chir 1977;345:505–10.

72. Mak PH, Irwin MG, Ooi CG, Chow BF. Incidence of diaphragmatic paralysis following supraclavicular brachial plexus block and its effect on pulmonary function. Anaesthesia 2001;56(4):352–6.

73. Heid FM, Kern T, Brambrink AM. Transient respiratory compromise after infraclavicular vertical brachial plexus blockade. Eur J Anaesthesiol 2002;19(9):693–4.

74. Rollins M, McKay WR, McKay RE. Airway difficulty after a brachial plexus subclavian perivascular block. Anesth Analg 2003;96:1191-2.

75. Herman N. Neurologic complications of regional anesthesia. Semin Anesth 1998;17:64–72.

76. Gibbons JJ, Lennon RL, Rose SH, Wedel DJ, Gibson BE. Axillary block of the brachial plexus: "you can't get there from here ···". Anesthesiology 1988;68(2):314–5.

77. Klein SM, Benveniste H. Anxiety, vocalization, and agitation following peripheral nerve block with ropivacaine. Reg Anesth Pain Med 1999;24(2):175–8.

78. Dominguez E, Garbaccio MC. Reverse arterial blood flow mediated local anesthetic central nervous system toxicity during axillary brachial plexus block. Anesthesiology 1999;91(3):901–2.

79. Raeder JC, Drosdahl S, Klaastad O, Kvalsvik O, Isaksen B, Stromskag KE, Mowinckel P, Bergheim R, Selander D. Axillary brachial plexus block with ropivacaine 7.5 mg/ml. A comparative study with bupivacaine 5 mg/ml Acta Anaesthesiol Scand 1999;43(8):794–8.

80. Botero M, Enneking FK. Reversal of prolonged unconsciousness by naloxone after an intravascular injection of

a local anesthetic and clonidine. Anesth Analg 1999;88(5): 1185–6.

81. Koscielniak-Nielsen ZJ, Nielsen PR, Nielsen SL, Gardi T, Hermann C. Comparison of transarterial and multiple nerve stimulation techniques for axillary block using a high dose of mepivacaine with adrenaline. Acta Anaesthesiol Scand 1999;43(4):398–404.

82. Ekatodramis G, Macaire P, Borgeat A. Prolonged Horner syndrome due to neck hematoma after continuous inter-scalene block. Anesthesiology 2001;95(3):801–3.

83. Sukhani R, Barclay J, Aasen M. Prolonged Horner's syn-drome after interscalene block: a management dilemma. Anesth Analg 1994;79(3):601–3.

84. Borgeat A, Kalberer F, Jacob H, Ruetsch YA, Gerber C. Patient-controlled interscalene analgesia with ropivacaine 0.2% versus bupivacaine 0.15% after major open shoulder surgery: the effects on hand motor function Anesth Analg 2001;92(1):218–23.

85. Sanchez-Conde P, Nicolas J, Rodriguez J, Garcia-Castano M, del Barrio E, Muriel C. Estudio comparativo entre ropivacaina y bupivacaina en analgesia epidural del parto. [Comparison of ropivacaine and bupivacaine for epidural analgesia during labor.] Rev Esp Anestesiol Reanim 2001;48(5):199–203.

86. Dullenkopf A, Zingg P, Curt A, Borgeat A. Funktionsverlust der oberen Extremität nach Bankart—Schulteroperation unter Interscalenus—blockade und Allgemeinanästhesie. [Persistent neurological deficit of the upper extremity after a shoulder operation under gen-eral anesthesia combined with a preoperatively placed interscalene catheter.] Anaesthesist 2002;51(7):547–51.

87. Lo AB. Bupivacaine-induced metallic taste. J Pharm Technol 1999;15:54–5.

88. Marsch SC, Schaefer HG, Castelli I. Unusual psychological manifestation of systemic local anesthetic toxicity. Anesthesiology 1998;88(2):531–3.

89. Schroeder TH, Dieterich HJ, Muhlbauer B. Methemoglobinemia after axillary block with bupivacaine and additional injection of lidocaine in the operative field. Acta Anaesthesiol Scand 1999;43(4):480–2.

90. Rodriguez J, Quintela O, Lopez-Rivadulla M, Barcena M, Diz C, Alvarez J. High doses of mepivacaine for brachial plexus block in patients with end-stage chronic renal fail-ure. A pilot study. Eur J Anaesthesiol 2001;18(3):171–6.

91. Gmyrek G, Hartmann H, Ludewig K, Modersohn D, Schottke C. Zur Vermeidung von Zwischenfällen bei der stomatologischen Lokalanästhesie. [The prevention of accidents in dental local anesthesia.] Stomatol DDR 1977;27(11):772–9.

92. Hyams SW. Oculomotor palsy following dental anesthesia. Arch Ophthalmol 1976;94(8):1281–2.

93. Dosseh MB, Dupiot M, Gueye MS. A propos d'un incident gravissime d'anesthésie locale à la xylocaine. [Apropos of a severe complication of local anesthesia using xylocaine.] Bull Soc Med Afr Noire Lang Fr 1977;22(3):318–20.

94. McDonogh T. An unusual case of trismus and dysphagia. Br Dent J 1996;180(12):465–6.

95. Stacy GC, Hajjar G. Barbed needle and inexplicable par-esthesias and trismus after dental regional anesthesia. Oral Surg Oral Med Oral Pathol 1994;77(6):585–8.

96. Stone J, Kaban LB. Trismus after injection of local anes-thetic. Oral Surg Oral Med Oral Pathol 1979;48(1):29–32.

97. de Beer DA, Thomas ML. Caudal additives in children-solutions or problems? Br J Anaesth 2003;90:487-98.

98. Taylor R, Eyres R, Chalkiadis GA, Austin S. Efficacy and safety of caudal injection of levobupivacaine, 0.25%, in children under 2 years of age undergoing inguinal hernia repair, circumcision or orchidopexy. Paediatr Anaesth 2003;13:114-21.

99. Ivani G, DeNegri P, Conio A, Grossetti R, Vitale P, Vercellino C, Gagliardi F, Eksborg S, Lonnqvist PA. Comparison of racemic bupivacaine, ropivacaine, and levo-bupivacaine for pediatric caudal anesthesia: effects on postoperative analgesia and motor block. Reg Anesth Pain Med 2002;27(2):157–61.

100. Senel AC, Akyol A, Dohman D, Solak M. Caudal bupiva-caine-tramadol combination for postoperative analgesia in pediatric herniorrhaphy. Acta Anaesthesiol Scand 2001;45(6):786–9.

101. Esteban JL, Gomez A, Gonzalez-Miranda F. Unintended total spinal anaesthesia with ropivacaine. Br J Anaesth 2000;84(5):697–8.

102. Fellmann C, Gerber AC, Weiss M. Apnoea in a former preterm infant after caudal bupivacaine with clonidine for inguinal herniorrhaphy. Paediatr Anaesth 2002;12(7): 637–40.

103. Tanaka M, Nitta R, Nishikawa T. Increased T-wave ampli-tude after accidental intravascular injection of lidocaine plus bupivacaine without epinephrine in sevoflurane-anesthetized child. Anesth Analg 2001;92(4):915–7.

104. Ivani G, De Negri P, Lonnqvist PA, Eksborg S, Mossetti V, Grossetti R, Italiano S, Rosso F, Tonetti F, Codipietro L. A comparison of three different concentrations of levo-bupivacaine for caudal block in children. Anesth Analg 2003;97:368-71.

105. Frey B, Kehrer B. Toxic methaemoglobin concentrations in premature infants after application of a prilocaine-con-taining cream and peridural prilocaine. Eur J Pediatr 1999;158(10):785–8.

106. Bozkurt P, Arslan I, Bakan M, Cansever MS. Free plasma levels of bupivacaine and ropivacaine when used for caudal block in children. Eur J Anaesthesiol 2005;22(8):640-1.

107. Stoneham MD, Wakefield TW. Acute respiratory distress after deep cervical plexus block. J Cardiothorac Vasc Anesth 1998;12(2):197–8.

108. Harris RJ, Benveniste G. Recurrent laryngeal nerve block-ade in patients undergoing carotid endarterectomy under cervical plexus block. Anaesth Intensive Care 2000;28(4):431–3.

109. Carling A, Simmonds M. Complications from regional anaesthesia for carotid endarterectomy. Br J Anaesth 2000;84(6):797–800.

110. Castresana MR, Masters RD, Castresana EJ, Stefansson S, Shaker IJ, Newman WH. Incidence and clinical signifi-cance of hemidiaphragmatic paresis in patients undergoing carotid endarterectomy during cervical plexus block anesthesia. J Neurosurg Anesthesiol 1994;6(1):21–3.

111. Stoneham MD, Bree SE. Epileptic seizure during awake carotid endarterectomy. Anesth Analg 1999;89(4):885–6.

112. Pearson AC, Labovitz AJ, Kern MJ. Accelerated hyper-tension complicated by myocardial infarction after use of a local anesthetic/vasoconstrictor preparation. Am Heart J 1987;114(3):662–3.

113. Shenkman Z, Findler M, Lossos A, Barak S, Katz J. Permanent neurologic deficit after inferior alveolar nerve block: a case report. Int J Oral Maxillofac Surg 1996;25(5): 381–2.

114. Virts BE. Local anesthesia toxicity review. Pediatr Dent 1999;21(6):375.

115. Niemi M, Laaksonen JP, Vahatalo K, Tuomainen J, Aaltonen O, Happonen RP. Effects of transitory lingual

nerve impairment on speech: an acoustic study of vowel sounds. J Oral Maxillofac Surg 2002;60(6):647–52.

116. Sanchis JM, Penarrocha M. Uvular paralysis after dental anesthesia. J Oral Maxillofac Surg 2002;60(11):1369–71.

117. Pedlar J. Prolonged paraesthesia following inferior alveolar nerve block using articaine. Br J Oral Maxillofac Surg 2003;41:202.

118. Dower JS, Jr. A review of paresthesia in association with administration of local anesthesia. Dent Today 2003;22:64-9.

119. Goldenberg AS. Transient diplopia as a result of block injections. Mandibular and posterior superior alveolar. NY State Dent J 1997;63(5):29–31.

120. Penarrocha–Diago M, Sanchis-Bielsa JM. Ophthalmologic complications after intraoral local anesthesia with articaine. Oral Surg Oral Med Oral Pathol Oral Radiol Endod 2000;90(1):21–4.

121. Wilkie GJ. Temporary uniocular blindness and ophthalmoplegia associated with a mandibular block injection. A case report. Aust Dent J 2000;45(2):131–3.

122. Rishiraj B, Epstein JB, Fine D, Nabi S, Wade NK. Permanent vision loss in one eye following administration of local anesthesia for a dental extraction. Int J Oral Maxillofac Surg 2005;34(2):220-3.

123. Chiu CY, Lin TY, Hsia SH, Lai SH, Wong KS. Systemic anaphylaxis following local lidocaine administration during a dental procedure. Pediatr Emerg Care 2004;20(3):178-80.

124. Bhushan M, Beck MH. Allergic contact dermatitis from disodium ethylenediamine tetra-acetic acid (EDTA) in a local anaesthetic. Contact Dermatitis 1998;38(3):183.

125. Wilhelmi BJ, Blackwell SJ, Miller J, Mancoll JS, Phillips LG. Epinephrine in digital blocks: revisited. Ann Plast Surg 1998;41(4):410–4.

126. Beck GN, Griffiths AG. Failed extradural anaesthesia for caesarean section. Complication of subsequent spinal block. Anaesthesia 1992;47(8):690–2.

127. Rauck RL, Colon J, Lesser GJ, Naveira FA, Speight KL. Paraspinal fluid extravasation from long-term epidural catheter delivery system. Anesthesiology 1998;88(6):1672–5.

128. Johnston MK, Harland SP. Spinal cord compression from precipitation of drug solute around an epidural catheter. Br J Neurosurg 1998;12(5):445–7.

129. Scott DA, Blake D, Buckland M, Etches R, Halliwell R, Marsland C, Merridew G, Murphy D, Paech M, Schug SA, Turner G, Walker S, Huizar K, Gustafsson U. A comparison of epidural ropivacaine infusion alone and in combination with 1, 2, and 4 micrograms/ml fentanyl for seventy-two hours of postoperative analgesia after major abdominal surgery Anesth Analg 1999;88(4):857–64.

130. Wigfull J, Welchew E. Survey of 1057 patients receiving postoperative patient-controlled epidural analgesia. Anaesthesia 2001;56(1):70–5.

131. Silvasti M, Pitkanen M. Patient-controlled epidural analgesia versus continuous epidural analgesia after total knee arthroplasty. Acta Anaesthesiol Scand 2001;45(4):471–6.

132. Liu SS, Allen HW, Olsson GL. Patient-controlled epidural analgesia with bupivacaine and fentanyl on hospital wards: prospective experience with 1,030 surgical patients. Anesthesiology 1998;88(3):688–95.

133. Niruthisard S, Somboonviboon W, Thaithumyanon P, Mahutchawaroj N, Chaiyakul A. Maternal and neonatal effects of single-dose epidural anesthesia with lidocaine and morphine for cesarean delivery. J Med Assoc Thai 1998;81(2):103–9.

134. Mahon SV, Berry PD, Jackson M, Russell GN, Pennefather SH. Thoracic epidural infusions for post-thoracotomy pain: a comparison of fentanyl–bupivacaine mixtures vs. fentanyl alone. Anaesthesia 1999;54(7):641–6.

135. Boutros A, Blary S, Bronchard R, Bonnet F. Comparison of intermittent epidural bolus, continuous epidural infusion and patient controlled-epidural analgesia during labor. Int J Obstet Anesth 1999;8(4):236–41.

136. Rygnestad T, Zahlsen K, Bergslien O, Dale O. Focus on mobilisation after lower abdominal surgery. A double-blind randomised comparison of epidural bupivacaine with morphine vs. lidocaine with morphine for postoperative analgesia. Acta Anaesthesiol Scand 1999;43(4):380–7.

137. Gautier P, De Kock M, Van Steenberge A, Miclot D, Fanard L, Hody JL. A double-blind comparison of 0.125% ropivacaine with sufentanil and 0.125% bupivacaine with sufentanil for epidural labor analgesia Anesthesiology 1999;90(3):772–8.

138. Brodner G, Mertes N, Van Aken H, Pogatzki E, Buerkle H, Marcus MA, Mollhoff T. Epidural analgesia with local anesthetics after abdominal surgery: earlier motor recovery with 0.2% ropivacaine than 0.175% bupivacaine Anesth Analg 1999;88(1):128–33.

139. Bader AM, Tsen LC, Camann WR, Nephew E, Datta S. Clinical effects and maternal and fetal plasma concentrations of 0.5% epidural levobupivacaine versus bupivacaine for cesarean delivery Anesthesiology 1999;90(6):1596–601.

140. Motamed C, Spencer A, Farhat F, Bourgain JL, Lasser P, Jayr C. Postoperative hypoxaemia: continuous extradural infusion of bupivacaine and morphine vs patient-controlled analgesia with intravenous morphine. Br J Anaesth 1998;80(6):742–7.

141. Shapiro A, Fredman B, Olsfanger D, Jedeikin R. Anaesthesia for caesarean delivery: low-dose epidural bupivacaine plus fentanyl. Int J Obstet Anesth 1998;7(1):23–6.

142. Flisberg P, Rudin A, Linner R, Lundberg CJ. Pain relief and safety after major surgery. A prospective study of epidural and intravenous analgesia in 2696 patients. Acta Anaesthesiol Scand 2003;47:457-65.

143. Datta S, Camann W, Bader A, VanderBurgh L. Clinical effects and maternal and fetal plasma concentrations of epidural ropivacaine versus bupivacaine for cesarean section. Anesthesiology 1995;82(6):1346–52.

144. Bonnet F, Derosier JP, Pluskwa F, Abhay K, Gaillard A. Cervical epidural anaesthesia for carotid artery surgery. Can J Anaesth 1990;37(3):353–8.

145. Boada S, Solsona B, Papaceit J, Saludes J, Rull M. Hipotension por bloqueo simpatico refractarie a efedrina en una paciente en tratamiento cronico con antidepresivos tricíclicos. [Hypotension refractory to ephedrine after sympathetic blockade in a patient on long-term therapy with tricyclic antidepressants.] Rev Esp Anestesiol Reanim 1999;46(8):364–6.

146. Cotileas P, Myrianthefs P, Haralambakis A, Cotsopoulos P, Stamatopoulou C, Ladakis C, Baltopoulos G. Bupivacaine-induced myocardial depression and pulmonary edema: a case report. J Electrocardiol 2000;33(3):291–6.

147. Holte K, Foss NB, Svens n C, Lund C, Madsen JL, Kehlet H. Epidural anesthesia, hypotension, and changes in intravascular volume. Anesthesiology 2004;100(2):281-6.

148. Kampe S, Tausch B, Paul M, Kasper SM, Bauer K, Diefenbach C, Kiencke P. Epidural block with ropivacaine and bupivacaine for elective caesarean section: maternal cardiovascular parameters, comfort and neonatal well-being. Curr Med Res Opin 2004;20(1):7-12.

149. Van Zundert AA, Scott DB. A fatal accident after epidural anesthesia for cesarean section. Acta Anaesthesiol Belg 1989;40(3):195–9.

150. Tarot JP, Coriat P, Samii K, Viars P. Peridural anesthesia and intracardiac conduction disturbance. Anesth Analg Reanim 1980;37:9–12.

151. Ng KP. Complete heart block during laparotomy under combined thoracic epidural and general anaesthesia. Anaesth Intensive Care 1996;24(2):257–60.

152. Lopez Galera S, Fernandez Galinski D, Echevarria Martin J, Aguilar Sanchez JL. Asistolia despues de anestesia combinada. [Asystole after combination anesthesia.] Rev Esp Anestesiol Reanim 2002;49(6):334–6.

153. Cucchiaro G, Rhodes LA. Unusual presentation of long QT syndrome. Br J Anaesth 2003;90:804-7.

154. Phillips N, Priestley M, Denniss AR, Uther JB. Brugada-type electrocardiographic pattern induced by epidural bupivacaine. Anesth Analg 2003;97:264-7.

155. Anonymous. Major complications in continuous dural anesthesia. Clin Med J 1980;93:194.

156. Stevens RA, Frey K, Sheikh T, Kao TC, Mikat-Stevens M, Morales M. Time course of the effects of cervical epidural anesthesia on pulmonary function. Reg Anesth Pain Med 1998;23(1):20–4.

157. McAllister RK, McDavid AJ, Meyer TA, Bittenbinder TM. Recurrent persistent hiccups after epidural steroid injection and analgesia with bupivacaine. Anesth Analg 2005;100(6):1834-6.

158. von Ungern-Sternberg BS, Regli A, Bucher E, Reber A, Schneider MC. The effect of epidural analgesia in labour on maternal respiratory function. Anaesthesia 2004;59(4):350-3.

159. Al-Nasser B. Toxic effects of epidural analgesia with ropivacaine 0.2% in a diabetic patient. J Clin Anesth 2004;16(3):220-3.

160. Huntoon MA, Martin DP. Paralysis after transforaminal epidural injection and previous spinal surgery. Reg Anesth Pain Med 2004;29(5):494-5.

161. Wiertlewski S, Magot A, Drapier S, Malinovsky JM, P r on Y. Worsening of neurologic symptoms after epidural anesthesia for labor in a Guillain-Barr patient. Anesth Analg 2004;98(3):825-7.

162. Tanaka K, Watanabe R, Harada T, Dan K. Extensive application of epidural anesthesia and analgesia in a university hospital: incidence of complications related to technique. Reg Anesth 1993;18(1):34–8.

163. Britts R, Wadsworth R. Unexpectedly high block during total lunar eclipse. Int J Obstet Anesth 2002;11:71–2.

164. Hilt H, Gramm HJ, Link J. Changes in intracranial pressure associated with extradural anaesthesia. Br J Anaesth 1986;58(6):676–80.

165. Wu CL, Francisco DR, Benesch CG. Perioperative stroke associated with postoperative epidural analgesia. J Clin Anesth 2000;12(1):61–3.

166. Kopacz DJ, Allen HW. Accidental intravenous levobupivacaine. Anesth Analg 1999;89(4):1027–9.

167. Freedman JM, Rudow MP. Bilateral buttock and leg pain after lidocaine epidural anesthesia. Anesth Analg 1999;88(5):1188.

168. Markey JR, Naseer OB, Bird DJ, Rabito SF, Winnie AP. Transient neurologic symptoms after epidural analgesia. Anesth Analg 2000;90(2):437–9.

169. Bourlon-Figuet S, Dubousset AM, Benhamou D, Mazoit JX. Transient neurologic symptoms after epidural analgesia in a five-year-old child. Anesth Analg 2000;91(4):856–7.

170. Buggy DJ, Allsager CM, Coley S. Profound motor blockade with epidural ropivacaine following spinal bupivacaine. Anaesthesia 1999;54(9):895–8.

171. Liu SS, Moore JM, Luo AM, Trautman WJ, Carpenter RL. Comparison of three solutions of ropivacaine/fentanyl for postoperative patient-controlled epidural analgesia. Anesthesiology 1999;90(3):727–33.

172. Kopacz DJ, Sharrock NE, Allen HW. A comparison of levobupivacaine 0.125%, fentanyl 4 microgram/ml, or their combination for patient-controlled epidural analgesia after major orthopedic surgery Anesth Analg 1999;89(6):1497–503.

173. Baldwin ES, Turner MA. Profound motor blockade with epidural ropivacaine. Anaesthesia 2000;55(1):91.

174. Evron S, Krumholtz S, Wiener Y, Brohorov T, Bahar M. Prolonged coma and quadriplegia after accidental subarachnoid injection of a local anesthetic with an opiate. Anesth Analg 2000;90(1):116–8.

175. Taga K, Tomita M, Watanabe I, Sato K, Awamori K, Fujihara H, Shimoji K. Complete recovery of consciousness in a patient with decorticate rigidity following cardiac arrest after thoracic epidural injection. Br J Anaesth 2000;85(4):632–4.

176. Liu M, Kim PS, Chen CK, Smythe WR. Delayed Horner's syndrome as a complication of continuous thoracic epidural analgesia. J Cardiothorac Vasc Anesth 1998;12(2):195–6.

177. Schregel W, Brudny P. Just another explanation for: "Horner's syndrome following low-dose epidural infusion for labour" presented by H. G. W. Paw. Eur J Anaesthesiol 1998;15(5):617–8.

178. Hogagard JT, Djurhuus H. Two cases of reiterated Horner's syndrome after lumbar epidural block. Acta Anaesthesiol Scand 2000;44(8):1021–3.

179. Zahn PK, Van Aken HK, Marcus AE. Horner's syndrome following epidural anesthesia with ropivacaine for cesarean delivery. Reg Anesth Pain Med 2002;27(4):445–6.

180. Chandrasekhar S, Peterfreund RA. Horner's syndrome following very low concentration bupivacaine infusion for labor epidural analgesia. J Clin Anesth 2003;15:217-19.

181. Rajasekaran AK, Kirk P, Varshney S. Transient hearing loss with labour epidural block. Anaesthesia 2003;58:613-14.

182. Hardy PA. Transient hearing loss with labour epidural block. Anaesthesia 2003;58:1041.

183. Kehlet H, Brandt MR, Hansen AP, Alberti KG. Effect of epidural analgesia on metabolic profiles during and after surgery. Br J Surg 1979;66(8):543–6.

184. Lund J, Stjernstrom H, Jorfeldt L, Wiklund L. Effect of extradural analgesia on glucose metabolism and gluconeogenesis. Studies in association with upper abdominal surgery. Br J Anaesth 1986;58(8):851–7.

185. Jacobs JS, Vallejo R, DeSouza GJ, TerRiet MF. Severe hypoglycemia after labor epidural analgesia. Anesth Analg 2000;90(4):892–3.

186. Olofsson CI, Ekblom AO, Ekman-Ordeberg GE, Irestedt LE. Post-partum urinary retention: a comparison between two methods of epidural analgesia. Eur J Obstet Gynecol Reprod Biol 1997;71(1):31–4.

187. Ban M, Hattori M. Delayed hypersensitivity due to epidural block with ropivacaine. BMJ 2005;330(7485):229.

188. Wildsmith JA. Delayed hypersensitivity due to epidural block with ropivacaine: report raises several issues. BMJ 2005;330(7497):966; author reply.

189. Thomson SJ, Lomax DM, Collett BJ. Chemical meningism after lumbar facet joint block with local anaesthetic and steroids. Anaesthesia 1991;46(7):563–4.

190. Reiz S, Nath S. Cardiotoxicity of local anaesthetic agents. Br J Anaesth 1986;58(7):736–46.

191. Meister GC, D'Angelo R, Owen M, Nelson KE, Gaver R. A comparison of epidural analgesia with 0.125% ropivacaine with fentanyl versus 0.125% bupivacaine with fentanyl during labor Anesth Analg 2000;90(3):632–7.

192. Bjornestad E, Smedvig JP, Bjerkreim T, Narverud G, Kolleros D, Bergheim R. Epidural ropivacaine 7.5 mg/ml for elective Caesarean section: a double-blind comparison of efficacy and tolerability with bupivacaine 5 mg/ml Acta Anaesthesiol Scand 1999;43(6):603–8.

193. Dick W. Gefährdung der Mutter durch Allgemeinanaesthesie und Regionalanaesthesie. [Maternal risk from general anaesthesia and regional anaesthesia.] Anaesthesist 1980;29(5):219–25.

194. Douglas MJ. Potential complications of spinal and epidural anesthesia for obstetrics. Semin Perinatol 1991;15(5): 368–374.

195. Knitza R, Sirtl C, Wisser J, Rhein R, Fischer B. Zerebraler Krampfanfall nach Periduralanästhesie mit Bupivacain zur Sectio caesarea. [Cerebral convulsion following peridural anesthesia with bupivacaine in cesarean section.] Geburtshilfe Frauenheilkd 1988;48(1):47–9.

196. Muth H, Schliemann F. Zur Periduralanaesthesie in der Geburthilfe. [Peridural anesthesia during labor. Report on 2726 cases.] Med Welt 1981;32(13):420–1.

197. Bratteby LE. Effects on the infant of obstetric regional analgesia. J Perinat Med 1981;9(Suppl 1):54–6.

198. Morikawa S, Ishikawa J, Kamatsuki H, Shinzato Y, Watanabe A, Ishikawa H, Chihara H, Nagata T, Kometani K. [Neurobehavior and mental development of newborn infants delivered under epidural analgesia with bupivacaine.]Nippon Sanka Fujinka Gakkai Zasshi 1990;42(11):1495–502.

199. Golub MS, Germann SL. Perinatal bupivacaine and infant behavior in rhesus monkeys. Neurotoxicol Teratol 1998;20(1):29–41.

200. Meunier JF, Goujard E, Dubousset AM, Samii K, Mazoit JX. Pharmacokinetics of bupivacaine after continuous epidural infusion in infants with and without biliary atresia. Anesthesiology 2001;95(1):87–95.

201. Oba H. Large-volume tumescent anesthesia for extensive liposuction in oriental patients: lidocaine toxicity and its safe dose level. Plast Reconstr Surg 2003;111:945-6.

202. Brown SL, Morrison AE. Local anesthetic infusion pump systems adverse events reported to the Food and Drug Administration. Anesthesiology 2004;100(5):1305-7.

203. Yang JJ, Wang QP, Wang TY, Sun J, Wang ZY, Zuo D, Xu JG. Marked hypotension induced by adrenaline contained in local anesthetic. Laryngoscope 2005;115(2):348-52.

204. Meyer HJ, Monticelli F, Kiesslich J. Fatal embolism of the anterior spinal artery after local cervical analgetic infiltration. Forensic Sci Int 2005;149(2-3):115-9.

205. Shlizerman L, Ashkenazi D. Peripheral facial nerve paralysis after peritonsillar infiltration of bupivacaine: a case report. Am J Otolaryngol 2005;26(6):406-7.

206. Nordstrom H, Stange K. Plasma lidocaine levels and risks after liposuction with tumescent anaesthesia. Acta Anaesthesiol Scand 2005;49(10):1487-90.

207. Sudhakar S, Kundra P, Madhurima S, Ravishankar M. Unilateral bronchospasm following interpleural analgesia with bupivacaine. Acta Anaesthesiol Scand 2005;49(1):104-5.

208. Parkinson SK, Mueller JB, Rich TJ, Little WL. Unilateral Horner's syndrome associated with interpleural catheter injection of local anesthetic. Anesth Analg 1989;68(1):61–2.

209. Abbott PJ Jr, Sullivan G. Cardiovascular toxicity following preincisional intra-articular injection of bupivacaine. Arthroscopy 1997;13(2):282.

210. Wand A, Junger H. Embolia cutis medicamentosa in atypical localisation. Aktuelle Derm 1990;16:128–9.

211. Nevarre DR, Tzarnas CD. The effects of hyaluronidase on the efficacy and on the pain of administration of 1% lidocaine. Plast Reconstr Surg 1998;101(2):365–9.

212. Bartfield JM, Sokaris SJ, Raccio-Robak N. Local anesthesia for lacerations: pain of infiltration inside vs outside the wound. Acad Emerg Med 1998;5(2):100–4.

213. Bartfield JM, Pauze D, Raccio-Robak N. The effect of order on pain of local anesthetic infiltration. Acad Emerg Med 1998;5(2):105–7.

214. Colaric KB, Overton DT, Moore K. Pain reduction in lidocaine administration through buffering and warming. Am J Emerg Med 1998;16(4):353–6.

215. Ahmed SM, Khan RM, Bano S, Ajmani P, Kumar A. Is spinal anaesthesia safe in pre-eclamptic toxaemia patients? J Indian Med Assoc 1999;97(5):165–8.

216. McDonald SB, Liu SS, Kopacz DJ, Stephenson CA. Hyperbaric spinal ropivacaine: a comparison to bupivacaine in volunteers. Anesthesiology 1999;90(4):971–7.

217. Malinovsky JM, Charles F, Kick O, Lepage JY, Malinge M, Cozian A, Bouchot O, Pinaud M. Intrathecal anesthesia: ropivacaine versus bupivacaine. Anesth Analg 2000;91(6):1457–60.

218. Mollmann M, Cord S, Holst D, Auf der Landwehr U. Continuous spinal anaesthesia or continuous epidural anaesthesia for post-operative pain control after hip replacement? Eur J Anaesthesiol 1999;16(7):454–61.

219. Concepcion MA, Lambert DH, Welch KA, Covino BG. Tourniquet pain during spinal anesthesia: a comparison of plain solutions of tetracaine and bupivacaine. Anesth Analg 1988;67(9):828–32.

220. Karakan M, Tahtaci N, Goksu S. The effects of intrathecal bupivacaine and fentanyl in combined spinal epidural anesthesia. Int Med J 2000;7:145–9.

221. Owen MD, Ozsarac O, Sahin S, Uckunkaya N, Kaplan N, Magunaci I. Low-dose clonidine and neostigmine prolong the duration of intrathecal bupivacaine–fentanyl for labor analgesia. Anesthesiology 2000;92(2):361–6.

222. Kathirvel S, Sadhasivam S, Saxena A, Kannan TR, Ganjoo P. Effects of intrathecal ketamine added to bupivacaine for spinal anaesthesia. Anaesthesia 2000;55(9):899–904.

223. Ben-David B, Miller G, Gavriel R, Gurevitch A. Low-dose bupivacaine-fentanyl spinal anesthesia for cesarean delivery. Reg Anesth Pain Med 2000;25(3):235–9.

224. Tsui BC, Malherbe S, Koller J, Aronyk K. Reversal of an unintentional spinal anesthetic by cerebrospinal lavage. Anesth Analg 2004;98(2):434-6.

225. Whiteside JB, Burke D, Wildsmith JA. Comparison of ropivacaine 0.5% (in glucose 5%) with bupivacaine 0.5% (in glucose 8%) for spinal anaesthesia for elective surgery. Br J Anaesth 2003;90:304-8.

226. Mulroy MF, Greengrass R, Ganapathy S, Chan V, Heierson A. Sameridine is safe and effective for spinal anesthesia: a comparative dose-ranging study with lidocaine for inguinal hernia repair. Anesth Analg 1999;88(4):815–21.

227. Unzueta Merino MC, Escolan Villen F, Aliaga Font L, Cantallops Pericas B, Sabate Pes A, Aguilar JL, Villar Landeira JM. Revision de las complicaciones de la anestesia espinal en un periodo de 8 anos (1977–1984). [Review

of the complications of spinal anesthesia in an 8-year period (1977–1984).] Rev Esp Anestesiol Reanim 1986;33(5):336–41.

228. Holst D, Mollmann M, Karmann S, Wendt M. Kreislaufverhalten unter Spinalanasthesie. Kathetertechnik versus Single-dose-Verfahren. [Circulatory reactions under spinal anesthesia. The catheter technique versus the single dose procedure.] Anaesthesist 1997;46(1):38–42.

229. Puncuh F, Lampugnani E, Kokki H. Use of spinal anaesthesia in paediatric patients: a single centre experience with 1132 cases. Paediatr Anaesth 2004;14(7):564-7.

230. Martyr JW, Stannard KJ, Gillespie G. Spinal-induced hypotension in elderly patients with hip fracture. A comparison of glucose-free bupivacaine with glucose-free bupivacaine and fentanyl. Anaesth Intensive Care 2005;33(1):64-8.

231. Bonnet MP, Larousse E, Asehnoune K, Benhamou D. Spinal anesthesia with bupivacaine decreases cerebral blood flow in former preterm infants. Anesth Analg 2004;98(5):1280-3.

232. Critchley LA, Short TG, Gin T. Hypotension during subarachnoid anaesthesia: haemodynamic analysis of three treatments. Br J Anaesth 1994;72(2):151–5.

233. Mark JB, Steele SM. Cardiovascular effects of spinal anesthesia. Int Anesthesiol Clin 1989;27(1):31–9.

234. Hemmingsen C, Poulsen JA, Risbo A. Prophylactic ephedrine during spinal anaesthesia: double-blind study in patients in ASA groups I–III. Br J Anaesth 1989;63(3):340–2.

235. Critchley LA, Stuart JC, Conway F, Short TG. Hypotension during subarachnoid anaesthesia: haemodynamic effects of ephedrine. Br J Anaesth 1995;74(4):373–8.

236. Critchley LA, Conway F. Hypotension during subarachnoid anaesthesia: haemodynamic effects of colloid and metaraminol. Br J Anaesth 1996;76(5):734–6.

237. Critchley LA, Morley AP, Derrick J. The influence of baricity on the haemodynamic effects of intrathecal bupivacaine 0.5% Anaesthesia 1999;54(5):469–74.

238. Hallworth S, Fernando R. The spread and side-effects of intrathecally administered bupivacaine. Anaesthesia 1999;54(10):1016–7.

239. Bandi E, Weeks S, Carli F. Spinal block levels and cardiovascular changes during post-Cesarean transport. Can J Anaesth 1999;46(8):736–40.

240. Mahe V, Ecoffey C. Spinal anaesthesia with isobaric bupivacaine in infants. Anesthesiology 1988;68(4):601–3.

241. Kiran S, Singal NK. A comparative study of three different doses of 0.5% hyperbaric bupivacaine for spinal anaesthesia in elective caesarean section Int J Obstet Anesth 2002;11(3):185–9.

242. Caplan RA, Ward RJ, Posner K, Cheney FW. Unexpected cardiac arrest during spinal anesthesia: a closed claims analysis of predisposing factors. Anesthesiology 1988;68(1):5–11.

243. Jordi EM, Marsch SC, Strebel S. Third degree heart block and asystole associated with spinal anesthesia. Anesthesiology 1998;89(1):257–60.

244. Coleman MM, Bardwaj A, Chan VV. Back pain and collapse associated with receding subarachnoid blockade. Can J Anaesth 1999;46(5 Pt 1):464–6.

245. Casati A, Fanelli G, Beccaria P, Aldegheri G, Berti M, Senatore R, Torri G. Block distribution and cardiovascular effects of unilateral spinal anaesthesia by 0.5% hyperbaric bupivacaine. A clinical comparison with bilateral spinal block Minerva Anestesiol 1998;64(7–8):307–12.

246. Kuczkowski KM. Respiratory arrest in a parturient following intrathecal administration of fentanyl and bupivacaine

as part of a combined spinal-epidural analgesia for labour. Anaesthesia 2002;57(9):939–40.

247. Sartorelli KH, Abajian JC, Kreutz JM, Vane DW. Improved outcome utilizing spinal anesthesia in high-risk infants. J Pediatr Surg 1992;27(8):1022–5.

248. Tobias JD, Burd RS, Helikson MA. Apnea following spinal anaesthesia in two former pre-term infants. Can J Anaesth 1998;45(10):985–9.

249. Zaric D, Christiansen C, Pace NL, Punjasawadwong Y. Transient neurologic symptoms (TNS) following spinal anaesthesia with lidocaine versus other local anaesthetics. Cochrane Database Syst Rev 2003 (2):CD003006.

250. Piquet CY, Mallaret MP, Lemoigne AH, Barjhoux CE, Danel VC, Vincent FH. Respiratory depression following administration of intrathecal bupivacaine to an opioid-dependent patient. Ann Pharmacother 1998;32(6):653–5.

251. Katsiris S, Williams S, Leighton BL, Halpern S. Respiratory arrest following intrathecal injection of sufentanil and bupivacaine in a parturient. Can J Anaesth 1998;45(9):880–3.

252. Zaric D, Christiansen C, Pace NL, Punjasawadwong Y. Transient neurologic symptoms after spinal anesthesia with lidocaine versus other local anesthetics: a systematic review of randomized, controlled trials. Anesth Analg 2005;100(6):1811-6.

253. Cramer BG, Stienstra R, Dahan A, Arbous MS, Veering BT, Van Kleef JW. Transient neurological symptoms with subarachnoid lidocaine: effect of early mobilization. Eur J Anaesthesiol 2005;22(1):35-9.

254. Zaric D, Christiansen C, Pace NL, Punjasawadwong Y. Transient neurologic symptoms (TNS) following spinal anaesthesia with lidocaine versus other local anaesthetics. Cochrane Database Syst Rev 2003(2):CD003006.

255. YaDeau JT, Liguori GA, Zayas VM. The incidence of transient neurologic symptoms after spinal anesthesia with mepivacaine. Anesth Analg 2005;101(3):661-5.

256. Zeidan A, Samii K. A case of unusually prolonged hyperbaric spinal anesthesia. Acta Anaesthesiol Scand 2005;49(6):885.

257. Aldrete JA. Neurologic deficits and arachnoiditis following neuroaxial anesthesia. Acta Anaesthesiol Scand 2003;47:3-12.

258. Kuczkowski KM, Goldsworthy M. Transient aphonia and aphagia in a parturient after induction of combined spinal-epidural labor analgesia with subarachnoid fentanyl and bupivacaine. Acta Anaesthesiol Belg 2003;54:165-6.

259. McMillan MR, Doud T, Nugent W. Catheter-associated masses in patients receiving intrathecal analgesic therapy. Anesth Analg 2003;96:186-90.

260. Celik Y, Bekir Demirel C, Karaca S, Kose Y. Transient segmental spinal myoclonus due to spinal anaesthesia with bupivacaine. J Postgrad Med 2003;49:286.

261. Perren F, Buchser E, Ch del D, Hirt L, Maeder P, Vingerhoets F. Spinal cord lesion after long-term intrathecal clonidine and bupivacaine treatment for the management of intractable pain. Pain 2004;109(1-2):189-94.

262. Fragneto RY, Fisher A. Mental status change and aphasia after labor analgesia with intrathecal sufentanil/bupivacaine. Anesth Analg 2000;90(5):1175–6.

263. Chan YK, Gopinathan R, Rajendram R. Loss of consciousness following spinal anaesthesia for caesarean section. Br J Anaesth 2000;85(3):474–6.

264. Wajima Z, Shitara T, Inoue T, Ogawa R. Severe lightning pain after subarachnoid block in a patient with neuropathic pain of central origin: which drug is best to treat the pain? Clin J Pain 2000;16(3):265–9.

265. Robles Romero M, Gonzalez Mesa JM, de las Heras Rosas MA, Rojas Caracuel MA, Garcia Perez A, Hurtado Leiva F. Meningitis aseptica tras anestesia intradura. [Aseptic meningitis after intradural anesthesia.] Rev Esp Anestesiol Reanim 2000;47(5):226.

266. Schou H, Hole P. Neurologic deficit following spinal anesthesia. Acta Anaesthesiol Belg 1987;38(3):241–3.

267. Chen IC, Lin CS, Chou HM, Peng TH, Liu CH, Wang CF, Lin IS. Unexpected recurrent seizures following repeated spinal injections of tetracaine—a case report. Acta Anaesthesiol Sin 2000;38(2):103–6.

268. Benson JS. U.S. Food and Drug Administration safety alert: cauda equina syndrome associated with use of small-bore catheters in continuous spinal anesthesia AANA J 1992;60(3):223.

269. Standl T, Eckert S, Schulte am Esch J. Microcatheter continuous spinal anaesthesia in the post-operative period: a prospective study of its effectiveness and complications. Eur J Anaesthesiol 1995;12(3):273–9.

270. Loo CC, Irestedt L. Cauda equina syndrome after spinal anaesthesia with hyperbaric 5% lignocaine: a review of six cases of cauda equina syndrome reported to the Swedish Pharmaceutical Insurance 1993–1997. Acta Anaesthesiol Scand 1999;43(4):371–9.

271. Uefuji T. [Persistent neurological deficit and adhesive arachnoiditis following spinal anesthesia with bupivacaine containing preservatives.]Masui 1999;48(2):176–80.

272. Chabbouh T, Lentschener C, Zuber M, Jude N, Delaitre B, Ozier Y. Persistent cauda equina syndrome with no identifiable facilitating condition after an uneventful single spinal administration of 0.5% hyperbaric bupivacaine. Anesth Analg 2005;101(6):1847-8.

273. Kubina P, Gupta A, Oscarsson A, Axelsson K, Bengtsson M. Two cases of cauda equina syndrome following spinal-epidural anesthesia. Reg Anesth 1997;22(5):447-50.

274. Horlocker TT, McGregor DG, Matsushige DK, Chantigian RC, Schroeder DR, Besse JA. Neurologic complications of 603 consecutive continuous spinal anesthetics using macrocatheter and microcatheter techniques. Perioperative Outcomes Group. Anesth Analg 1997;84(5):1063–70.

275. Tetzlaff JE, Dilger J, Yap E, Smith MP, Schoenwald PK. Cauda equina syndrome after spinal anaesthesia in a patient with severe vascular disease. Can J Anaesth 1998;45(7):667–9.

276. Lee DS, Bui T, Ferrarese J, Richardson PK. Cauda equina syndrome after incidental total spinal anesthesia with 2% lidocaine. J Clin Anesth 1998;10(1):66–9.

277. Kubina P, Gupta A, Oscarsson A, Axelsson K, Bengtsson M. Two cases of cauda equina syndrome following spinal-epidural anaesthesia. Reg Anesth 1997;22(5):447–50.

278. Akioka K, Torigoe K, Maruta H, Shimizu N, Kobayashi Y, Kaneko Y, Shiratori R. A case of cauda equina syndrome following spinal anesthesia with hyperbaric dibucaine. J Anesth 2001;15(2):106–7.

279. Gisvold SE. Lidocaine may still be an excellent drug for spinal anaesthesia. Acta Anaesthesiol Scand 1999;43(4):369–70.

280. Salmela L, Aromaa U. Transient radicular irritation after spinal anesthesia induced with hyperbaric solutions of cerebrospinal fluid-diluted lidocaine 50 mg/ml or mepivacaine 40 mg/ml or bupivacaine 5 mg/ml Acta Anaesthesiol Scand 1998;42(7):765–9.

281. Salazar F, Bogdanovich A, Adalia R, Chabas E, Gomar C. Transient neurologic symptoms after spinal anaesthesia using isobaric 2% mepivacaine and isobaric 2% lidocaine. Acta Anaesthesiol Scand 2001;45(2):240–5.

282. Saito S, Radwan I, Obata H, Takahashi K, Goto F. Direct neurotoxicity of tetracaine on growth cones and neurites of growing neurons in vitro. Anesthesiology 2001;95(3): 726–33.

283. Hampl K, Schneider M, Corbey MP, Bach AB, Dahlgren N. Transient radicular irritation after spinal anaesthesia with Xylocain. Acta Anaesthesiol Scand 1999;43(3):359–65.

284. Neal JM, Pollock JE. Can scapegoats stand on shifting sands? Reg Anesth Pain Med 1998;23(6):533–7.

285. deJong RH. In my opinion: spinal lidocaine: a continuing enigma. J Clin Monit Comput 1998;14(2):147–8.

286. Henderson DJ, Faccenda KA, Morrison LM. Transient radicular irritation with intrathecal plain lignocaine. Acta Anaesthesiol Scand 1998;42(3):376–8.

287. Panadero A, Monedero P, Fernandez-Liesa JI, Percaz J, Olavide I, Iribarren MJ. Repeated transient neurological symptoms after spinal anaesthesia with hyperbaric 5% lidocaine. Br J Anaesth 1998;81(3):471–2.

288. Liguori GA, Zayas VM. Repeated episodes of transient radiating back and leg pain following spinal anesthesia with 1.5% mepivacaine and 2% lidocaine Reg Anesth Pain Med 1998;23(5):511–5.

289. Sia S, Pullano C. Transient radicular irritation after spinal anaesthesia with 2% isobaric mepivacaine. Br J Anaesth 1998;81(4):622–4.

290. Casati A, Fanelli G, Aldegheri G, Berti M, Leoni A, Torri G. A transient neurological deficit following intrathecal injection of 1% hyperbaric bupivacaine for unilateral spinal anaesthesia. Eur J Anaesthesiol 1998;15(1):112–3.

291. Wong CA, Slavenas P. The incidence of transient radicular irritation after spinal anesthesia in obstetric patients. Reg Anesth Pain Med 1999;24(1):55–8.

292. de Weert K, Traksel M, Gielen M, Slappendel R, Weber E, Dirksen R. The incidence of transient neurological symptoms after spinal anaesthesia with lidocaine compared to prilocaine. Anaesthesia 2000;55(10):1020–4.

293. Hodgson PS, Liu SS, Batra MS, Gras TW, Pollock JE, Neal JM. Procaine compared with lidocaine for incidence of transient neurologic symptoms. Reg Anesth Pain Med 2000;25(3):218–22.

294. Ostgaard G, Hallaraker O, Ulveseth OK, Flaatten H. A randomised study of lidocaine and prilocaine for spinal anaesthesia. Acta Anaesthesiol Scand 2000;44(4):436–40.

295. Ben-David B, Maryanovsky M, Gurevitch A, Lucyk C, Solosko D, Frankel R, Volpin G, DeMeo PJ. A comparison of minidose lidocaine–fentanyl and conventional-dose lidocaine spinal anesthesia. Anesth Analg 2000; 91(4):865–70.

296. Morisaki H, Masuda J, Kaneko S, Matsushima M, Takeda J. Transient neurologic syndrome in one thousand forty-five patients after 3% lidocaine spinal anesthesia. Anesth Analg 1998;86(5):1023–6.

297. Corbey MP, Bach AB. Transient radicular irritation (TRI) after spinal anaesthesia in day-care surgery. Acta Anaesthesiol Scand 1998;42(4):425–9.

298. Freedman JM, Li DK, Drasner K, Jaskela MC, Larsen B, Wi S. Transient neurologic symptoms after spinal anesthesia: an epidemiologic study of 1,863 patients. Anesthesiology 1998;89(3):633–41.

299. Liguori GA, Zayas VM, Chisholm MF. Transient neurologic symptoms after spinal anesthesia with mepivacaine and lidocaine. Anesthesiology 1998;88(3):619–23.

300. Hampl KF, Heinzmann-Wiedmer S, Luginbuehl I, Harms C, Seeberger M, Schneider MC, Drasner K. Transient neurologic symptoms after spinal anesthesia: a lower incidence with prilocaine and bupivacaine than with lidocaine. Anesthesiology 1998;88(3):629–33.

301. Martinez-Bourio R, Arzuaga M, Quintana JM, Aguilera L, Aguirre J, Saez-Eguilaz JL, Arizaga A. Incidence of transient neurologic symptoms after hyperbaric subarachnoid anesthesia with 5% lidocaine and 5% prilocaine. Anesthesiology 1998;88(3):624–8.

302. Axelrod EH, Alexander GD, Brown M, Schork MA. Procaine spinal anesthesia: a pilot study of the incidence of transient neurologic symptoms. J Clin Anesth 1998;10(5):404–9.

303. Le Truong HH, Girard M, Drolet P, Grenier Y, Boucher C, Bergeron L. Spinal anesthesia: a comparison of procaine and lidocaine. Can J Anaesth 2001;48(5):470–3.

304. Tsen LC, Schultz R, Martin R, Datta S, Bader AM. Intrathecal low-dose bupivacaine versus lidocaine for in vitro fertilization procedures. Reg Anesth Pain Med 2001;26(1):52–6.

305. Philip J, Sharma SK, Gottumukkala VN, Perez BJ, Slaymaker EA, Wiley J. Transient neurologic symptoms after spinal anesthesia with lidocaine in obstetric patients. Anesth Analg 2001;92(2):405–9.

306. Rorarius M, Suominen P, Haanpaa M, Puura A, Baer G, Pajunen P, Tuimala R. Neurologic sequelae after caesarean section. Acta Anaesthesiol Scand 2001;45(1):34–41.

307. Eberhart LH, Morin AM, Kranke P, Geldner G, Wulf H. Transiente neurologische Symptome nach Spinalanästhesie. Eine quantitative systematische Übersicht (Metaanalyse) randomisierter kontrollierter Studien. [Transient neurologic symptoms after spinal anesthesia. A quantitative systematic overview (meta-analysis) of randomized controlled studies.] Anaesthesist 2002;51(7):539–46.

308. Al-Nasser B, Negre M, Hubert C. Transient neurological manifestations after epidural analgesia with ropivacaine. Anaesthesia 2002;57(3):306–7.

309. Moore DC, Thompson GE. Commentary: neurotoxicity of local anesthetics—an issue or a scapegoat? Reg Anesth Pain Med 1998;23(6):605–10.

310. Youngs EJ. Rate of injection and neurotoxicity of spinal lidocaine. Anesthesiology 1999;90(1):323–6.

311. Hampl KF, Schneider MC, Thorin D, Ummenhofer W, Drewe J. Hyperosmolarity does not contribute to transient radicular irritation after spinal anesthesia with hyperbaric 5% lidocaine. Reg Anesth 1995;20(5):363–8.

312. Hampl KF, Schneider MC, Ummenhofer W, Drewe J. Transient neurologic symptoms after spinal anesthesia. Anesth Analg 1995;81(6):1148–53.

313. Strichartz GR, Lambert DH. Neurotoxicity of 5% lignocaine. Br J Anaesth 1995;75(3):376.

314. Pollock JE, Liu SS, Neal JM, Stephenson CA. Dilution of spinal lidocaine does not alter the incidence of transient neurologic symptoms. Anesthesiology 1999;90(2):445–50.

315. Pollock JE, Burkhead D, Neal JM, Liu SS, Friedman A, Stephenson C, Polissar NL. Spinal nerve function in five volunteers experiencing transient neurologic symptoms after lidocaine subarachnoid anesthesia. Anesth Analg 2000;90(3):658–65.

316. Keld DB, Hein L, Dalgaard M, Krogh L, Rodt SA. The incidence of transient neurologic symptoms (TNS) after spinal anaesthesia in patients undergoing surgery in the supine position. Hyperbaric lidocaine 5% versus hyperbaric bupivacaine 0.5% Acta Anaesthesiol Scand 2000;44(3):285–90.

317. Oka S, Matsumoto M, Ohtake K, Kiyoshima T, Nakakimura K, Sakabe T. The addition of epinephrine to tetracaine injected intrathecally sustains an increase in glutamate concentrations in the cerebrospinal fluid and worsens neuronal injury. Anesth Analg 2001;93(4):1050–7.

318. Ohtake K, Matsumoto M, Wakamatsu H, Kawai K, Nakakimura K, Sakabe T. Glutamate release and neuronal injury after intrathecal injection of local anesthetics. Neuroreport 2000;11(5):1105–9.

319. Mahajan R, Batra YK, Grover VK, Kajal J. A comparative study of caudal bupivacaine and midazolam–bupivacaine mixture for post-operative analgesia in children undergoing genitourinary surgery. Int J Clin Pharmacol Ther 2001;39(3):116–20.

320. Lindh A, Andersson AS, Westman L. Is transient lumbar pain after spinal anaesthesia with lidocaine influenced by early mobilisation? Acta Anaesthesiol Scand 2001;45(3):290–3.

321. Davies MJ, Cook RJ, Quach K. Transient lumbar pain after 5% hyperbaric lignocaine spinal anaesthesia in patients having minor vascular surgery. Anaesth Intensive Care 2002;30(6):782–5.

322. Bang-Vojdanovski B, Hannibal H, Eberhardt M. Vorübergehende neurologische Symptome nach einer Spinalanästhesie mit 4%igem hyperbarem Scandicain (Mepivacain). [Transient neurologic symptoms after spinal anesthesia with 4% hyperbaric mepivacaine.] Anaesthesist 2002;51(12):989–92.

323. Takenami T, Kondou Y, Kimotsuki H, Okamoto H, Hoka S. A case of transient neurologic symptoms following epidural mepivacaine and spinal tetracaine. J Anesth 2002;16(4):336–8.

324. Alley EA, Pollock JE. Transient neurologic syndrome in a patient receiving hypobaric lidocaine in the prone jack-knife position. Anesth Analg 2002;95(3):757–9.

325. Takenami T, Yagishita S, Asato F, Arai M, Hoka S. Intrathecal lidocaine causes posterior root axonal degeneration near entry into the spinal cord in rats. Reg Anesth Pain Med 2002;27(1):58–67.

326. Radwan IA, Saito S, Goto F. The neurotoxicity of local anesthetics on growing neurons: a comparative study of lidocaine, bupivacaine, mepivacaine, and ropivacaine. Anesth Analg 2002;94(2):319–24.

327. Michel O, Brusis T. Hearing loss as a sequel of lumbar puncture. Ann Otol Rhinol Laryngol 1992;101(5):390–4.

328. Fog J, Wang LP, Sundberg A, Mucchiano C. Hearing loss after spinal anesthesia is related to needle size. Anesth Analg 1990;70(5):517–22.

329. Hussain SS, Heard CM, Bembridge JL. Hearing loss following spinal anaesthesia with bupivacaine. Clin Otolaryngol Allied Sci 1996;21(5):449–54.

330. Gultekin S, Yilmaz N, Ceyhan A, Karamustafa I, Kilic R, Unal N. The effect of different anaesthetic agents in hearing loss following spinal anaesthesia. Eur J Anaesthesiol 1998;15(1):61–3.

331. Musch G, Liposky J. Dysphagia following intrathecal local anesthetic-opioid administration. J Clin Anesth 1999;11(5):413–5.

332. Adachi Y, Watanabe K, Uchihashi Y, Sato T. [Urinary retention as a transient neurologic symptom after accidental total spinal anesthesia with mepivacaine hydrochloride.] Masui 1999;48(9):1009–10.

333. Osuga K, Hirabayashi Y, Fukuda H, Shimizu R, Asahara H. [Severe lightning limb pain induced by spinal anesthesia.]Masui 1999;48(1):67–9.

334. Hiller A, Karjalainen K, Balk M, Rosenberg PH. Transient neurological symptoms after spinal anaesthesia with hyperbaric 5% lidocaine or general anaesthesia. Br J Anaesth 1999;82(4):575–9.

335. Kuczkowski KM. Severe persistent fetal bradycardia following subarachnoid administration of fentanyl and bupivacaine for induction of a combined spinal-epidural analgesia for labor pain. J Clin Anesth 2004;16(1):78-9.

336. Bartholomew K, Sloan JP. Prilocaine for Bier's block: how safe is safe? Arch Emerg Med 1990;7(3):189–95.

337. Machado HS, Bastos RS. Inadequate tourniquet inflation associated with a case of prilocaine toxicity. Eur J Anaesthesiol 1998;15(2):234–6.

338. Abdulla W, Kroll S, Eckhardt-Abdulla R. Intravenous regional anaesthesia—a new approach in clinical application. Anasthesiol Intensivmed 2000;41:94–103.

339. Kireker HD, Aynacioglu AS, Goksu S. Determination of 0.5% lidocaine serum concentrations and evaluation for toxicity in intravenous regional anaesthesia Turk Anesteziyol Reanim 2000;28:211–6.

340. Lang SA. Intravenous regional anesthesia. Anesth Analg 1998;86(6):1334–5.

341. Laborde Y, Gimenez V, Besset-Lehmann J. Une complication rare de l'anesthésie locorégionale endoveineuse: le phlébite humérale. [A rare complication of intravenous locoregional anesthesia: branchial phlebitis.] Presse Méd 1989;18(31):1527.

342. Chan VW, Weisbrod MJ, Kaszas Z, Dragomir C. Comparison of ropivacaine and lidocaine for intravenous regional anesthesia in volunteers: a preliminary study on anesthetic efficacy and blood level. Anesthesiology 1999;90(6):1602–8.

343. Cherng CH, Wong CS, Ho ST. Acute aphasia following tourniquet release in intravenous regional anesthesia with 0.75% lidocaine Reg Anesth Pain Med 2000;25(2):211–2.

344. Atanassoff PG, Ocampo CA, Bande MC, Hartmannsgruber MW, Halaszynski TM. Ropivacaine 0.2% and lidocaine 0.5% for intravenous regional anesthesia in outpatient surgery Anesthesiology 2001;95(3):627–31.

345. Ahmed SU, Vallejo R, Hord ED. Seizures after a Bier block with clonidine and lidocaine. Anesth Analg 2004;99(2):593-4.

346. Garg S, Piva A, Sanchez RN, Sadun AA. Death associated with an indwelling orbital catheter. Ophthal Plast Reconstr Surg 2003;19:398-400.

347. Lavin PA, Henderson CL, Vaghadia H. Non-alkalinized and alkalinized 2-chloroprocaine vs lidocaine for intravenous regional anesthesia during outpatient hand surgery. Can J Anaesth 1999;46(10):939–45.

348. Ansari MM, Abraham A. Unusual discoloration of forearm with Bier's block using 0.5% lidocaine. Anesth Analg 2005;100(6):1866-7.

349. Ryder W. Two cautionary tales. Anaesthesia 1994;49(2): 180–1.

350. Hsu CH, Lin TC, Yeh CC, Ho ST, Wong CS. Convulsions during superior laryngeal nerve block—a case report. Acta Anaesthesiol Sin 2000;38(2):93–6.

351. Quinton DN. Local anaesthetic toxicity of haematoma blocks in manipulation of Colles' fractures. Injury 1988;19(4):239–40.

352. Deltombe T, Nisolle JF, De Cloedt P, Hanson P, Gustin T. Tibial nerve block with anesthetics resulting in Achilles tendon avulsion. Am J Phys Med Rehabil 2004;83(4):331-4.

353. Mullanu Ch, Gaillat F, Scemama F, Thibault S, Lavand'homme P, Auffray JP. Acute toxicity of local anesthetic ropivacaine and mepivacaine during a combined lumbar plexus and sciatic block for hip surgery. Acta Anaesthesiol Belg 2002;53(3):221–3.

354. Moorthy SS, Zaffer R, Rodriguez S, Ksiazek S, Yee RD. Apnea and seizures following retrobulbar local anesthetic injection. J Clin Anesth 2003;15:267-70.

355. Stewart D, Simpson GT, Nader ND. Postoperative anisocoria in a patient undergoing endoscopic sinus surgery. Reg Anesth Pain Med 1999;24(5):467–9.

356. Hari CK, Roblin DG, Clayton MI, Nair RG. Acute angle closure glaucoma precipitated by intranasal application of cocaine. J Laryngol Otol 1999;113(3):250–1.

357. Brooker CD, Lawson AD. Convulsions following bupivacaine infiltration for excision of carotid body tumour. Anaesth Intensive Care 1993;21(6):877–8.

358. Menahem S. Neonatal cyanosis, methaemoglobinaemia and haemolytic anaemia. Acta Paediatr Scand 1988;77(5):755–6.

359. Howells RE, Tucker H, Millinship J, Shroff JF, Dhar KK, Jones PW, Redman CW. A comparison of the side effects of prilocaine with felypressin and lignocaine with adrenaline in large loop excision of the transformation zone of the cervix: results of a randomised trial. BJOG 2000;107(1):28–32.

360. Pignotti MS, Indolfi G, Ciuti R, Donzelli G. Perinatal asphyxia and inadvertent neonatal intoxication from local anaesthetics given to the mother during labour. BMJ 2005;330(7481):34-5.

361. Martin G, Grant SA, Macleod DB, Breslin DS, Brewer RP. Severe phantom leg pain in an amputee after lumbar plexus block. Reg Anesth Pain Med 2003;28:475-8.

362. Brown SM, Brooks SE, Mazow ML, Avilla CW, Braverman DE, Greenhaw ST, Green ME, McCartney DL, Tabin GC. Cluster of diplopia cases after periocular anesthesia without hyaluronidase. J Cataract Refract Surg 1999;25(9):1245–9.

363. Hagan JC 3rd, Whittaker TJ, Byars SR. Diplopia cases after periocular anesthesia without hyaluronidase. J Cataract Refract Surg 1999;25(12):1560–1.

364. Troll G, Borodic G. Diplopia after cataract surgery using 4% lidocaine in the absence of Wydase (sodium hyaluronidase). J Clin Anesth 1999;11(7):615–6.

365. Wessels IF, Wessels DA, Zimmerman GJ. The photic sneeze reflex and ocular anesthesia. Ophthalmic Surg Lasers 1999;30(3):208–11.

366. Wessels IF, Najjar MF. Paroxysmal sneezing during local anesthesia for ocular surgery with thiopentone hypnosis. Can J Anaesth 1999;46(6):617.

367. Vishwanath MR, Jain A. Conjunctival inclusion cyst following sub-Tenon's local anaesthetic injection. Br J Anaesth 2005;95(6):825-6.

368. Mukherji S, Esakowitz L. Orbital inflammation after sub-Tenon's anesthesia. J Cataract Refract Surg 2005;31(11):2221-3.

369. Adam F, Jaziri S, Chauvin M. Psoas abscess complicating femoral nerve block catheter. Anesthesiology 2003;99:230-1.

370. Chen HT, Chen KH, Hsu WM. Toxic keratopathy associated with abuse of low-dose anesthetic: a case report. Cornea 2004;23(5):527-9.

371. Kim SK, Andreoli CM, Rizzo JF 3rd, Golden MA, Bradbury MJ. Optic neuropathy secondary to sub-Tenon anesthetic injection in cataract surgery. Arch Ophthalmol 2003;121:907-9.

372. Bullock JD, Warwar RE, Green WR, Cox MS. Ocular explosions from periocular anesthetic injections: a clinical, histopathologic, experimental, and biophysical study. Ophthalmology 1999;106(12):2341–53.

373. Warwar RE, Romriell EK, Pennock EA. Contralateral amaurosis after retrobulbar anesthetic injection. J Neuroophthalmol 2004;24(2):187-8.

374. Han SK, Kim JH, Hwang JM. Persistent diplopia after retrobulbar anesthesia. J Cataract Refract Surg 2004;30(6):1248-53.

375. Khawam E, El-Dairi M, Al-Haddad C, Younis M. Inferior oblique overaction/contracture following retrobulbar anesthesia for cataract extraction with a positive Bielschowsky Head Tilt test to the contralateral shoulder. A report of one case. Binocul Vis Strabismus Q 2004;19(4):247-50.

376. Irving EL, Arshinoff SA, Samis W, Lillakas L, Lui B, Laporte JT, Steinbach MJ. Effect of retrobulbar injection

of lidocaine on saccadic velocities. J Cataract Refract Surg 2004;30(2):350-6.

377. Teichmann KD, Uthoff D. Retrobulbar (intraconal) anesthesia with a curved needle: technique and results. J Cataract Refract Surg 1994;20(1):54–60.

378. Elk JR, Wood J, Holladay JT. Pulmonary edema following retrobulbar block. J Cataract Refract Surg 1988;14(2):216–7.

379. Ruusuvaara P, Setala K, Tarkkanen A. Respiratory arrest after retrobulbar block. Acta Ophthalmol (Copenh) 1988;66(2):223–5.

380. Wittpenn JR, Rapoza P, Sternberg P Jr, Kuwashima L, Saklad J, Patz A. Respiratory arrest following retrobulbar anesthesia. Ophthalmology 1986;93(7):867–70.

381. Pilz J. Headache in ophthalmological local anaesthesia in dependence on the kind of the vasoconstrictor additive. Fol Ophthalmol 1988;13:133–5.

382. Rao VA, Kawatra VK. Ocular myotoxic effects of local anesthetics. Can J Ophthalmol 1988;23(4):171–3.

383. Hunter DG, Lam GC, Guyton DL. Inferior oblique muscle injury from local anesthesia for cataract surgery. Ophthalmology 1995;102(3):501–9.

384. Labelle PF, Lapointe A, Boucher MC. Vitreous hemorrhage following retrobulbar anesthesia. Can J Ophthalmol 1996;31(1):21–4.

385. Lam DS, Tam BS, Chan WM, Bhende P. Combined cataract extraction and submacular blood clot evacuation for globe perforation caused by retrobulbar injection. J Cataract Refract Surg 2000;26(7):1089–91.

386. Olitsky SE, Juneja RG. Orbital hemorrhage after the administration of sub-tenon's infusion anesthesia. Ophthalmic Surg Lasers 1997;28(2):145–6.

387. Cowley M, Campochiaro PA, Newman SA, Fogle JA. Retinal vascular occlusion without retrobulbar or optic nerve sheath hemorrhage after retrobulbar injection of lidocaine. Ophthalmic Surg 1988;19(12):859–61.

388. Wadood AC, Dhillon B, Singh J. Inadvertent ocular perforation and intravitreal injection of an anesthetic agent during retrobulbar injection. J Cataract Refract Surg 2002;28(3):562–5.

389. Liang C, Peyman GA, Sun G. Toxicity of intraocular lidocaine and bupivacaine. Am J Ophthalmol 1998;125(2):191–6.

390. Gills JP, Loyd TL. A technique of retrobulbar block with paralysis of orbicularis oculi. J Am Intraocul Implant Soc 1983;9(3):339–40.

391. el Harrar N, Idali B, el Belhaji M, el Amraoui A, Benaguida M. Arrêt respiratoire après une anesthésie rétrobulbaire. A propos de deux cas. [Respiratory arrest after retrobulbar anesthesia. Apropos of 2 cases.] Cah Anesthesiol 1996;44(4):355–6.

392. Kwinten FA, de Moor GP, Lamers RJ. Acute pulmonary edema and trigeminal nerve blockade after retrobulbar block. Anesth Analg 1996;83(6):1322–4.

393. Rosen WJ. Brainstem anesthesia presenting as dysarthria. J Cataract Refract Surg 1999;25(8):1170–1.

394. Bharti N, Shende D. Transient cardiopulmonary arrest following retrobulbar block with lignocaine. Anaesth Intensive Care 2002;30(3):388–9.

395. Garutti I, Hervias M, Barrio JM, Fortea F, De La Torre J. Subdural spread of local anesthetic agent following thoracic paravertebral block and cannulation. Anesthesiology 2003;98:1005-7.

396. McCombe M, Heriot W. Penetrating ocular injury following local anaesthesia. Aust NZ J Ophthalmol 1995;23(1):33–6.

397. To EW, Chan DT. Arteriovenous fistula induced by a peribulbar nerve block. J Cataract Refract Surg 2000;26(8):1253–5.

398. Kumar CM, Lawler PG. Pulmonary oedema after peribulbar block. Br J Anaesth 1999;82(5):777–9.

399. Wells AP, Maslin K. Diplopia from peribulbar ropivicaine. Clin Experiment Ophthalmol 2000;28(1):32–3.

400. Hamel P, Boghen D. Bilateral amaurosis following peribulbar anesthesia. Can J Ophthalmol 1998;33(4):216–8.

401. Dorey SE, Gillespie IH, Barton F, MacSweeney E. Magnetic resonance image changes following optic nerve trauma from peribulbar anesthetic. Br J Ophthalmol 1998;82(5):586–7.

402. Gioia L, Prandi E, Codenotti M, Casati A, Fanelli G, Torri TM, Azzolini C, Torri G. Peribulbar anesthesia with either 0.75% ropivacaine or a 2% lidocaine and 0.5% bupivacaine mixture for vitreoretinal surgery: a double-blinded study Anesth Analg 1999;89(3):739–42.

403. McLure HA, Rubin AP, Westcott M, Henderson H. A comparison of 1% ropivacaine with a mixture of 0.75% bupivacaine and 2% lignocaine for peribulbar anaesthesia Anaesthesia 1999;54(12):1178–82.

404. Calenda E, Olle P, Muraine M, Brasseur G. Peribulbar anesthesia and sub-tenon injection for vitreoretinal surgery: 300 cases. Acta Ophthalmol Scand 2000;78(2):196–9.

405. Belfort R Jr, Muccioli C. Hyphema after peribulbar anesthesia for cataract surgery in Fuchs' heterochromic iridocyclitis. Ocul Immunol Inflamm 1998;6(1):57–8.

406. Cadera W. Diplopia after peribulbar anesthesia for cataract surgery. J Pediatr Ophthalmol Strabismus 1998;35(4):240–1.

407. Eltzschig H, Rohrbach M, Schroeder TH. Methaemoglobinaemia after peribulbar blockade: an unusual complication in ophthalmic surgery Br J Ophthalmol 2000;84(4):442.

408. Callear AB. The effect of temperature on the discomfort caused by topical local anaesthesia. J R Soc Med 1995;88(12):709p–11p.

409. Rosenwasser GO, Holland S, Pflugfelder SC, Lugo M, Heidemann DG, Culbertson WW, Kattan H. Topical anesthetic abuse. Ophthalmology 1990;97(8):967–72.

410. Lawrenson JG, Edgar DF, Tanna GK, Gudgeon AC. Comparison of the tolerability and efficacy of unit-dose, preservative-free topical ocular anaesthetics. Ophthalmic Physiol Opt 1998;18(5):393–400.

411. Sugar A. Topical anesthetic abuse after radial keratotomy. J Cataract Refract Surg 1998;24(11):1535–7.

412. Pharmakakis NM, Katsimpris JM, Melachrinou MP, Koliopoulos JX. Corneal complications following abuse of topical anesthetics. Eur J Ophthalmol 2002;12(5):373–8.

413. Barequet IS, Soriano ES, Green WR, O'Brien TP. Provision of anesthesia with single application of lidocaine 2% gel. J Cataract Refract Surg 1999;25(5):626–31.

414. Spalton DJ. Problems with unpreserved lignocaine for intraocular use. J Cataract Refract Surg 2000;26(5):633.

415. Masket S, Gokmen F. Efficacy and safety of intracameral lidocaine as a supplement to topical anesthesia. J Cataract Refract Surg 1998;24(7):956–60.

416. Martin RG, Miller JD, Cox CC 3rd, Ferrel SC, Raanan MG. Safety and efficacy of intracameral injections of unpreserved lidocaine to reduce intraocular sensation. J Cataract Refract Surg 1998;24(7):961–3.

417. Wubbolt I, Winter R, Brockmann D, Sistani F. Endotheltoxizität verschiedener Lokalanästhetika. Spektrum Augenheilkd 2002;16:206–10.

418. Adams W, Morgan SJ. Diplopia following sub-tenon's infiltration of local anesthesia. J Cataract Refract Surg 2002;28(9):1694–7.

419. Dahlmann AH, Appaswamy S, Headon MP. Orbital cellulitis following sub-Tenon's anaesthesia. Eye 2002;16(2):200–1.

420. Burton AJ, Backhouse O, Metcalfe TW. Prilocaine versus lignocaine for minor lid procedures. Eye 2000;14(Pt 4): 594–6.

421. Schlote T, Freudenthaler N, von Eicken J, Rohrbach JM. Transiente Erblindung nach subkonjunktivaler Anästhesie

zur Diodenlaser—Zyklophotokoagulation bei fortgeschrittenen Glaukomen. [Transient blindness after subconjunctival anesthesia for diode laser cyclophotocoagulation.] Klin Monatsbl Augenheilkd 2000;217(5):296–8.

422. Mondardini A, Turco D, Garripoli A, Martinoglio P, Ferrari A. Acute bilateral edema of the parotids after topical anesthesia with lidocaine: an uncommon clinical event. G Ital Endosc Dig 1999;22:111–3.

423. Zuberi BF, Shaikh MR, Jatoi NU, Shaikh WM. Lidocaine toxicity in a student undergoing upper gastrointestinal endoscopy. Gut 2000;46(3):435.

424. Lemke T. Vorübergehender Vestibularisausfall als Komplikation der Lokalanästhesie des Ohres. [Temporary vestibular loss following local anaesthesia of the ear.] Laryngol Rhinol Otol (Stuttg) 1977;56(7):623–5.

425. Sharrock NE. Postural headache following thoracic somatic paravertebral nerve block. Anesthesiology 1980;52(4):360–2.

426. Jackson S, Smith D, Durkin A. Hematuria as a complication of lumbar paravertebral sympathetic block. Reg Anesth 1986;11:31.

427. Pusch F, Freitag H, Weinstabl C, Obwegeser R, Huber E, Wildling E. Single-injection paravertebral block compared to general anaesthesia in breast surgery. Acta Anaesthesiol Scand 1999;43(7):770–4.

428. Richardson J, Sabanathan S, Jones J, Shah RD, Cheema S, Mearns AJ. A prospective, randomized comparison of preoperative and continuous balanced epidural or paravertebral bupivacaine on post-thoracotomy pain, pulmonary function and stress responses. Br J Anaesth 1999;83(3):387–92.

429. Pottage A, Scott DB. Safety of "topical" lignocaine. Lancet 1988;1(8592):1003.

430. Alsarraf R, Sie KC. Brain stem stroke associated with bupivacaine injection for adenotonsillectomy. Otolaryngol Head Neck Surg 2000;122(4):572–3.

431. Kang PB, Phuah HK, Zimmerman RA, Handler SD, Dure LS, Ryan SG. Medial medullary injury during adenoidectomy. J Pediatr 2001;138(5):772–4.

432. Sher MH, Laing DI, Brands E. Life-threatening upper airway obstruction after glossopharyngeal nerve block: possibly due to an inappropriately large dose of bupivacaine? Anesth Analg 1998;86(3):678.

433. Beydon L, Lorino AM, Verra F, Labroue M, Catoire P, Lofaso F, Bonnet F. Topical upper airway anaesthesia with lidocaine increases airway resistance by impairing glottic function. Intensive Care Med 1995;21(11):920–6.

434. Farmery AD. Severe unilateral bronchospasm mimicking inadvertent endobronchial intubation: a complication of the use of a topical lidocaine Laryngojet injector. Br J Anaesth 2000;85(6):917–9.

435. Keller C, Sparr HJ, Brimacombe JR. Laryngeal mask lubrication. A comparative study of saline versus 2% lignocaine gel with cuff pressure control. Anaesthesia 1997;52(6):592–7.

436. Avery JK. Routine procedure—bad outcome. Tenn Med 1998;91(7):280–1.

437. Day RO, Chalmers DR, Williams KM, Campbell TJ. The death of a healthy volunteer in a human research project: implications for Australian clinical research. Med J Aust 1998;168(9):449–51.

438. Ruetsch YA, Fattinger KE, Borgeat A. Ropivacaine-induced convulsions and severe cardiac dysrhythmia after sciatic block. Anesthesiology 1999;90(6):1784–6.

439. Bauer A, Geier J, Elsner P. Allergic contact dermatitis in patients with anogenital complaints. J Reprod Med 2000;45(8):649–54.

440. Marren P, Wojnarowska F, Powell S. Allergic contact dermatitis and vulvar dermatoses. Br J Dermatol 1992;126(1):52–6.

441. Goldsmith PC, Rycroft RJ, White IR, Ridley CM, Neill SM, McFadden JP. Contact sensitivity in women with anogenital dermatoses. Contact Dermatitis 1997;36(3):174–5.

442. Brenan JA, Dennerstein GJ, Sfameni SF, Drinkwater P, Marin G, Scurry JP. Evaluation of patch testing in patients with chronic vulvar symptoms. Australas J Dermatol 1996;37(1):40–3.

443. Lewis FM, Harrington CI, Gawkrodger DJ. Contact sensitivity in pruritus vulvae: a common and manageable problem. Contact Dermatitis 1994;31(4):264–5.

444. Wilkinson JD, Andersen KE, Lahti A, Rycroft RJ, Shaw S, White IR. Preliminary patch testing with 25% and 15% "caine"-mixes. The EECDRG. Contact Dermatitis 1990;22(4):244–5.

445. Fisher A. Contact Dermatitis. 3rd ed.. Philadelphia: Lea & Febiger;. 1995.

446. Ismail F, Goldsmith PC. Emla cream-induced allergic contact dermatitis in a child with thalassaemia major. Contact Dermatitis 2005;52(2):111.

447. Neri I, Savoia F, Guareschi E, Medri M, Patrizi A. Purpura after application of EMLA cream in two children. Pediatr Dermatol 2005;22(6):566-8.

448. Ajith C, Somesh G, Kumar B. Iatrogenic swollen penis. Sex Transm Infect 2005;81(1):15-6.

449. Hahn IH, Hoffman RS, Nelson LS. EMLA-induced methemoglobinemia and systemic topical anesthetic toxicity. Hahn IH, Hoffman RS, Nelson LS. J Emerg Med 2004;26(1):85-8.

450. Parker JF, Vats A, Bauer G. EMLA toxicity after application for allergy skin testing. Pediatrics 2004;113(2):410-1.

451. Vallance H, Chaba T, Clarke L, Taylor G. Pseudo-lysosomal storage disease caused by EMLA cream. J Inherit Metab Dis 2004;27(4):507-11.

452. Perrin JH. Hazard of compounded anesthetic gel. Am J Health Syst Pharm 2005;62(14):1445-6.

453. Young D. Student's death sparks concerns about compounded preparations. Am J Health Syst Pharm 2005;62(5):450-2.

454. Goldman RD. ELA-max: A new topical lidocaine formulation. Ann Pharmacother 2004;38(5):892-4.

455. Kapral S, Krafft P, Gosch M, Fridrich P, Weinstabl C. Subdurale, extraarachnoidale Blockade als Komplikation des Ganglion-Stellatum-Blocks: Dokumentation mittels Sonographie. [Subdural, extra-arachnoid block as a complication of stellate ganglion block: documentation with ultrasound.] Anästhesiol Intensivmed Notfallmed Schmerzther 1997;32(10):638–40.

456. Stohr M, Mayer K, Petruch F. Armplexusparesen nach Stellatumblockade und Plexusanästhesie. [Brachial plexus paralysis after stellate blockade and plexus anaesthesia.] Dtsch Med Wochenschr 1978;103(2):68–70.

457. Omote K, Kawamata M, Namiki A. Adverse effects of stellate ganglion block on Raynaud's phenomenon associated with progressive systemic sclerosis. Anesth Analg 1993;77(5):1057–60.

458. Mahli A, Coskun D, Akcali DT. Aetiology of convulsions due to stellate ganglion block: a review and report of two cases. Eur J Anaesthesiol 2002;19(5):376–80.

459. Marica LS, O'Day T, Janosky JE, Nystrom EU. Chloroprocaine is less painful than lidocaine for skin infiltration anesthesia. Anesth Analg 2002;94(2):351–4.

460. Klein JA. Tumescent technique for local anesthesia improves safety in large-volume liposuction. Plast Reconstr Surg 1993;92(6):1085–98.

461. Rao RB, Ely SF, Hoffman RS. Deaths related to liposuction. N Engl J Med 1999;340(19):1471–5.

462. Breuninger H. Slow infusion tumescent anesthesia. Dermatol Surg 1999;25(2):151–2.

463. Matsumae T. [Circulatory disaster following infiltration of epinephrine contained in local anesthetic.]Masui 1999;48(9):1020–3.

464. Linchitz RM, Raheb JC. Subcutaneous infusion of lidocaine provides effective pain relief for CRPS patients. Clin J Pain 1999;15(1):67–72.

465. Imison A, Nunan P. An unusual case of transient paraplegia. Anaesth Intensive Care 2002;30(1):102–3.

466. Grose DJ. Cigarette burn after tumescent anesthesia and intravenous sedation: a case report. Dermatol Surg 2003;29:433-5.

467. Sundaram MB. Seizures after intraurethral instillation of lidocaine. CMAJ 1987;137(3):219–20.

468. Priya V, Dalal K, Sareen R. Convulsions with intraurethral instillation of lignocaine. Acta Anaesthesiol Scand 2005;49(1):124.

469. Pantuck AJ, Goldsmith JW, Kuriyan JB, Weiss RE. Seizures after ureteral stone manipulation with lidocaine. J Urol 1997;157(6):2248.

470. Ho KJ, Thompson TJ, O'Brien A, Young MR, McCleane G. Lignocaine gel: does it cause urethral pain rather than prevent it? Eur Urol 2003;43:194-6.

471. Feldman S, Karalliedde L. Drug interactions with neuromuscular blockers. Drug Saf 1996;15(4):261–73.

472. Ohlgisser M, Adler M, Ben-Dov D, Taitelman U, Birkhan HJ, Bursztein S. Methaemoglobinaemia induced by mafenide acetate in children. A report of two cases. Br J Anaesth 1978;50(3):299–301.

473. Jakobson B, Nilsson A. Methemoglobinemia associated with a prilocaine–lidocaine cream and trimetoprim–sulphamethoxazole. A case report. Acta Anaesthesiol Scand 1985;29(4):453–5.

474. Matsuo S, Rao DB, Chaudry I, Foldes FF. Interaction of muscle relaxants and local anesthetics at the neuromuscular junction. Anesth Analg 1978;57(5):580–7.

475. Usubiaga JE, Wikinski JA, Morales RL, Usubiaga LE. Interaction of intravenously administered procaine, lidocaine and succinylcholine in anesthetized subjects. Anesth Analg 1967;46(1):39–45.

476. Matsuo S, Rao DB, Chaudry I, Foldes FF. Interaction of muscle relaxants and local anesthetics at the neuromuscular junction. Anesth Analg 1978;57(5):580–7.

477. Telivuo L, Katz RL. The effects of modern intravenous local analgesics on respiration during partial neuromuscular block in man. Anaesthesia 1970;25(1):30–5.

478. Davis CO, Wax PM. Prehospital epinephrine overdose in a child resulting in ventricular dysrhythmias and myocardial ischemia. Pediatr Emerg Care 1999;15(2):116–8.

479. Jackman WM, Friday KJ, Anderson JL, Aliot EM, Clark M, Lazzara R. The long QT syndromes: a critical review, new clinical observations and a unifying hypothesis. Prog Cardiovasc Dis 1988;31(2):115–72.

480. Adams MC, McLaughlin KP, Rink RC. Inadvertent concentrated epinephrine injection at newborn circumcision: effect and treatment. J Urol 2000;163(2):592.

481. Galoo E, Godon P, Potier V, Vergeau B. Fibrillation auriculaire compliquant une hémostase endoscopique rectale par injection d' adrénaline. [Atrial fibrillation following a rectal endoscopic injection using epiphedrine solution.] Gastroenterol Clin Biol 2002;26(1):99–100.

482. Chelliah YR, Manninen PH. Hazards of epinephrine in transsphenoidal pituitary surgery. J Neurosurg Anesthesiol 2002;14(1):43–6.

483. Nishina K, Mikawa K, Shiga M, Obara H. Clonidine in paediatric anaesthesia. Paediatr Anaesth 1999;9(3):187–202.

484. Bhushan M, Beck MH. Allergic contact dermatitis from disodium ethylenediamine tetra-acetic acid (EDTA) in a local anaesthetic. Contact Dermatitis 1998;38(3):183.

485. Boada S, Solsona B, Papaceit J, Saludes J, Rull M. Hipotension por bloqueo simpatico refractaria a efedrina en una paciente en tratamiento cronico con antidepresivos triciclicos. [Hypotension refractory to ephedrine after sympathetic blockade in a patient on long-term therapy with tricyclic antidepressants.] Rev Esp Anestesiol Reanim 1999;46(8):364–6.

486. Cagney B, Williams O, Jennings L, Buggy D. Tramadol or fentanyl analgesia for ambulatory knee arthroscopy. Eur J Anaesthesiol 1999;16(3):182–5.

487. Hunt R, Fazekas B, Thorne D, Brooksbank M. A comparison of subcutaneous morphine and fentanyl in hospice cancer patients. J Pain Symptom Manage 1999;18(2):111–9.

488. Fanelli G, Casati A, Magistris L, Berti M, Albertin A, Scarioni M, Torri G. Fentanyl does not improve the nerve block characteristics of axillary brachial plexus anaesthesia performed with ropivacaine. Acta Anaesthesiol Scand 2001;45(5):590–4.

489. Karakaya D, Buyukgoz F, Baris S, Guldogus F, Tur A. Addition of fentanyl to bupivacaine prolongs anesthesia and analgesia in axillary brachial plexus block. Reg Anesth Pain Med 2001;26(5):434–8.

490. Liu SS, Moore JM, Luo AM, Trautman WJ, Carpenter RL. Comparison of three solutions of ropivacaine/fentanyl for postoperative patient-controlled epidural analgesia. Anesthesiology 1999;90(3):727–33.

491. Constant I, Gall O, Gouyet L, Chauvin M, Murat I. Addition of clonidine or fentanyl to local anaesthetics prolongs the duration of surgical analgesia after single shot caudal block in children. Br J Anaesth 1998;80(3):294–8.

492. Niemi G, Breivik H. Epidural fentanyl markedly improves thoracic epidural analgesia in a low-dose infusion of bupivacaine, adrenaline and fentanyl. A randomized, double-blind crossover study with and without fentanyl. Acta Anaesthesiol Scand 2001;45(2):221–32.

493. Wigfull J, Welchew E. Survey of 1057 patients receiving postoperative patient-controlled epidural analgesia. Anaesthesia 2001;56(1):70–5.

494. Lovstad RZ, Stoen R. Postoperative epidural analgesia in children after major orthopaedic surgery. A randomised study of the effect on PONV of two anaesthetic techniques: low and high dose i.v. fentanyl and epidural infusions with and without fentanyl Acta Anaesthesiol Scand 2001;45(4):482–8.

495. Reinoso-Barbero F, Saavedra B, Hervilla S, de Vicente J, Tabares B, Gomez-Criado MS. Lidocaine with fentanyl, compared to morphine, marginally improves postoperative epidural analgesia in children. Can J Anaesth 2002;49(1):67–71.

496. Mendelson JH, Mello NK. Plasma testosterone levels during chronic heroin use and protracted abstinence. A study of Hong Kong addicts. Clin Pharmacol Ther 1975; 17(5):529–33.

497. Coffman JD, Cohen RA. Intra-arterial vasodilator agents to reverse human finger vasoconstriction. Clin Pharmacol Ther 1987;41(5):574–9.

SPECIFIC LOCAL ANESTHETICS

Articaine

General Information

Articaine is an aminoamide that also contains an ester group, which is rapidly hydrolysed by plasma esterases. It is 4-methyl-3([2-(propylamino)propiona-mido)]-2-thiophenecarboxylic acid, methyl ester hydro-chloride. The thiophene group increases its lipid solubility while the ester group enables it to undergo plasma esterase hydrolysis as well as hepatic enzyme metabolism. Articaine is formulated as a 4% solution with adrenaline. It is the most widely used local anesthetic agent in dentistry in some parts of Europe.

The rapid breakdown of articaine to an inactive meta-bolite means that it has low systemic toxicity. However, the risk of intravascular injection is high in dentistry, and articaine can cause central nervous system and cardiovas-cular toxicity. However, articaine is slightly more potent than lidocaine and causes less nervous system toxicity (1).

The safety of articaine has been studied in a series of three randomized trials (2). The adverse effects deemed to be related to articaine were headache, paresthesia/hyperesthesia after injection, infection, and rash. There was one case of mouth ulceration. The overall incidence of adverse effects was comparable to that of lidocaine.

Organs and Systems

Cardiovascular

The incidence of hypotension and headache after spinal anesthesia was similar to that encountered with lidocaine (SED-12, 256) (3).

Nervous system

Four cases of persistent lingual paresthesia or hyperesthe-sia after inferior dental block with articaine have been reported (4). Although resolution of neurological compli-cations usually occurs within 2 weeks, the authors reported that the symptoms in their cases persisted for 6–18 months and noted that they were aware of another four cases of persistent paresthesia with articaine that had not been formally reported.

Metabolism

Articaine has been implicated in an episode of weakness of the limb muscles, fatigue, and anorexia in a patient with a rare respiratory chain disorder due to a genetic defect in mitochondrial DNA (Kearn–Sayre Syndrome).

- A 28 year-old woman with Kearns-Sayre Syndrome, previously exposed multiple times to lidocaine, underwent planned tooth extraction after injection of articaine 1.5 ml (60 mg) with adrenaline (0.009 mg) (5). Within 5 minutes she complained of a feeling of heat, fatigue, weakness, and a desire to sleep. She was unable to walk or stand and had frequent urination. At 20 hours after the injection she had diffuse weakness, reduced tendon and absent patellar reflexes, and sub-clonic Achilles tendon reflexes. She recovered fully 48 hours after the injection.

The authors assumed a direct mitochondrial toxic effect of articaine, although this was disputed by others in cor-respondence (6).

Skin

A fixed drug eruption has been described after the use of articaine (7).

- A 45-year-old woman noted dark red plaques after dental treatment with articaine local anesthesia on seven occasions over 8 years. The lesions developed within 8–12 hours after drug exposure and resolved spontaneously over the next 14 days. Skin prick and patch tests were negative. However, subsequent provo-cation tests and skin biopsies were consistent with a diagnosis of fixed rug eruption.

The authors noted that this was the first documented report of articaine-induced fixed drug eruption; two pre-vious reports had implicated mepivacaine and lidocaine.

- An 11-year-old boy developed severe dermatomyositis only a few days after injection of articaine in the jaw for tooth extraction; cause and effect were not established (SEDA-10, 105).

Immunologic

An immediate skin reaction has been reported after the use of articaine.

- A 51-year-old woman developed immediate erythema and edema of the lips, face, and eyelids without any other symptoms after subcutaneous administration of a combination of articaine and adrenaline (8). The reac-tion resolved with a glucocorticoid in 2 days. Skin prick tests with local anesthetics (lidocaine, bupivacaine, mepivacaine, articaine) were negative except for arti-caine.

The results suggested that there is no cross-reactivity between articaine and other amide local anesthetics. A difference in the chemical structure between articaine, being a tiofen, and the other amide local anesthetics, which have a phenyl-methylated ring, is a possible expla-nation.

References

1. Oertel R, Rahn R, Kirch W. Clinical pharmacokinetics of articaine. Clin Pharmacokinet 1997;33(6):417–25.
2. Malamed SF, Gagnon S, Leblanc D. Articaine hydrochloride: a study of the safety of a new amide local anesthetic. J Am Dent Assoc 2001;132(2):177–85.
3. Kaukinen S, Eerola R, Eerola M, Kaukinen L. A comparison of carticaine and lidocaine in spinal anaesthesia. Ann Clin Res 1978;10(4):191–4.
4. van Eeden SP, Patel MF. Re: prolonged paraesthesia following inferior alveolar nerve block using articaine. Br J Oral Maxillofac Surg 2002;40(6):519–20.
5. Finsterer J, Haberler C, Schmiedel J. Deterioration of Kearns-Sayre syndrome following articaine administration for local anesthesia. Clin Neuropharmacol 2005;28(3):148–9.
6. Stehr SN, Oertel R, Schindler C, Hubler M. Re: deterioration of Kearns-Sayre syndrome following articaine administration for local anesthesia. Clin Neuropharmacol 2005;28(5):253.
7. Kleinhans M, Böer A, Kaufmann R, Boehncke WH. Fixed drug eruption caused by articain. Allergy 2004;59(1):117.
8. El-Qutob D, Morales C, Pelaez A. Allergic reaction caused by articaine. Allergol Immunopathol (Madr) 2005;33(2):115–6.

Benzocaine

General Information

Benzocaine is a poorly soluble local anesthetic, an ester of para-aminobenzoic acid. It is used in many countries as a component of some free-sale formulations for topical use, for example in skin creams, as a dry powder for skin ulcers, as throat lozenges, and as teething formulations for young children. It is also used in aerosol sprays when anesthetizing the oropharynx. Relatively high concentrations of local anesthetic are required to be effective topically, increasing tissue penetration and the risk of subsequent toxicity. Benzocaine formulations are available in concentrations of 1–20%.

Organs and Systems

Cardiovascular

An 11-month-old child consumed about 2 ml of a benzocaine anesthetic gel 20% accidentally (1). He developed a tachycardia (200/minute) which resolved over 24 hours. The author explained that although the cardiotoxicity of benzocaine is milder than that of other local anesthetics, it can cause life-threatening effects and so pediatricians should counsel parents about the potential hazard of anesthetic teething gels; formulations that contain benzocaine should be in a childproof container.

Hematologic

Cases of methemoglobinemia have been reported after the use of benzocaine in many different settings, including endoscopy (2), transesophageal echocardiography (3) (4),

percutaneous gastrostomy tube placement (5), and intubation (6,7,8). There were no deaths and all the patients recovered fully when treated with methylthioninium chloride (methylene blue) 1–2 mg/kg. The problem arises in both adults and children (9–12), and the risk has led to criticism of its free availability. It has, amongst other things, been suggested that it should be eliminated from products for use in children, that concentrations in over-the-counter products should be limited, and that there should be explicit label warnings of the hematological risk (SED-12, 256) (SEDA-17, 135) (9). Early diagnosis and treatment are crucial, as the condition is potentially fatal, particularly in neonates.

Five cases of benzocaine-induced methemoglobinemia were reported in 1998, following its use for transesophageal echocardiography (13–16). Methemoglobin concentrations over 15% can lead to cyanosis, whilst concentrations over 70% lead to circulatory collapse and death (15,16). The degree of methemoglobinemia depends on the total dose of drug and any factors that enhance systemic absorption. The elderly and neonates are particularly susceptible to methemoglobinemia, as are those with inherited methemoglobin reductase deficiency or the abnormal hemoglobin M. Adequate monitoring and observation of patients both during and after transesophageal echocardiography is essential, as this rare complication of benzocaine and other local anesthetics, such as prilocaine, is both potentially fatal and eminently treatable.

- Severe methemoglobinemia was suspected in a 1-year-old infant after topical application of 10% benzocaine ointment around an enterostomy; on postoperative day 3 the SpO_2 was 90% and arterial blood was dark red in color (17).

The authors pointed out the serious potential for toxicity in infants of a local anesthetic that is commonly used for this purpose in adults.

However, adult cases have been reported with Cetacaine (a proprietary mixture of 14% benzocaine, 2% tetracaine, and 2% butylaminobenzoate) (18–20) and with benzocaine alone (21).

Cetacaine spray used to anesthetize the oropharynx before endoscopy led to dyspnea, central cyanosis, and an oxygen saturation of 80%; methemoglobinemia was diagnosed, and the patient recovered rapidly with methylthioninium chloride 1 mg/kg over 5 minutes. There have been reports of methemoglobinemia after topical use of cetacaine (22,23).

- A 77-year-old woman received two sprays of Cetacaine for an attempted emergency nasotracheal intubation. After intubation she became cyanosed. The arterial blood was chocolate-brown in color and the SaO_2 by CO oximetry was 54–58%, despite a high PaO_2. The methemoglobin concentration was 39% and she was treated with methylthioninium chloride. Three weeks later Cetacaine again caused cyanosis with a drop in SpO_2 to 76% and a methemoglobin concentration of 24%, which resolved spontaneously.
- A 74-year-old man received Cetacaine spray to his oropharynx for transesophageal echocardiography. His

SpO$_2$ fell to 85%. He became drowsy, then unresponsive, cyanotic, and apneic, and required intubation. His PaO$_2$ was 37 kPa (280 mmHg), SaO$_2$ 40%, and methemoglobin concentration 60%. Intravenous methylthioninium chloride produced an immediate improvement in the cyanosis and the methemoglobin concentration fell to 0.6%.

- A 71-year-old man received 20% benzocaine spray to the upper airway for bronchoscopy. His SpO$_2$ gradually fell to under 85% and he required intubation. His methemoglobin concentration was 19%, SaO$_2$ 75%, and PaO$_2$ 44 kPa (329 mmHg). After intravenous methylthioninium chloride the methemoglobin concentration fell to 1.8%.

Several other cases of methemoglobinemia after the administration of topical benzocaine formulations have been reported (24–29). All recovered completely without sequelae after the intravenous administration of methylthioninium chloride 1–2 mg/kg.

- A 69-year-old man developed methemoglobinemia (68%) after pharyngeal anesthesia using 20% benzocaine 15 ml (swish and swallow) for transesophageal echocardiography (30). He responded to intravenous methylthioninium chloride, but a diagnosis of non-Q wave myocardial infarction was made on the basis of raised cardiac enzymes and a normal electrocardiogram.

In one case there was rebound methemoglobinemia after treatment with methylthioninium chloride (31). The authors pointed out that clinicians have to be aware that a falling methemoglobin concentration does not necessarily indicate successful treatment. High doses of benzocaine or later release from fat tissue can cause life-threatening rebound effects after the initial dose of methylthioninium chloride, and continuing monitoring is required until methemoglobin concentrations have returned to normal.

In one case, oral application of 20% benzocaine resulted in acute respiratory failure requiring mechanical ventilation of 2 days, although methemoglobin concentrations returned to normal 13 hours after treatment with methylthioninium chloride (32).

Whether benzocaine-induced methemoglobinemia is a hypersusceptibility or collateral reaction is controversial. There has been a retrospective review of 188 benzocaine exposures in children under 18 years of age, reported to four regional poison information centers, in 1993–96 (33). Mean and median ingested dosages were 87 and 50 mg/kg respectively and 55% patients had an exposure over 40 mg/kg. In all, 92% patients were asymptomatic. Reported symptoms included oral numbness ($n = 8$), vomiting ($n = 3$), and oral irritation, dizziness, and nausea ($n = 1$ each). Methemoglobin concentrations were measured in eight patients, seven of whom had concentrations over 1%. A child, who had had 5–10 applications of over-the-counter teething gel applied in 24 hours, had a methemoglobin concentration of 19% and was the only patient to have cyanosis. The authors concluded that accidental ingestion of over-the-counter benzocaine-containing products rarely causes cyanosis. The lack of

dose dependence suggests that this reaction is a hypersusceptibility reaction.

Four cases of methemoglobinemia have been described after the use of benzocaine spray for topical anesthesia of the airways.

- A 42-year-old woman had a superior laryngeal nerve block with lidocaine, topical anesthesia with benzocaine spray, and intravenous midazolam for awake fiberoptic intubation (34). Her SpO$_2$ fell from about 85% to about 30%, and despite high-frequency jet ventilation with 100% oxygen she had persistent SpO$_2$ readings in the low 80s. Her arterial blood was chocolate-brown in color, with a PaO$_2$ of 44 kPa (330 mmHg) and an oxyhemoglobin saturation (SaO$_2$) of 51%. This discrepancy between PaO$_2$ and SaO$_2$ suggested methemoglobinemia, and co-oximetry showed a concentration of 51%. Methylthioninium chloride 140 mg produced an immediate improvement in her color, and her SaO$_2$ improved over the next 10 minutes.

- An elderly man received benzocaine 20% spray to the throat in preparation for transesophageal echocardiography. He became unwell 1 hour later, with lethargy, central cyanosis, hypoxia, dyspnea, tachypnea, and tachycardia (35). His arterial blood was burgundy-colored and the methemoglobin concentration was 41%. He was treated with two doses of methylthioninium chloride 2 mg/kg and was weaned from oxygen within 10 hours.

- Significant methemoglobinemia occurred in a 65-year-old man on re-exposure to topical 20% benzocaine spray for anesthesia of the airways in preparation for awake fiberoptic intubation (36). This occurred despite exposure 3 days before to 14% benzocaine for the same procedure. During attempted intubation, he suddenly desaturated to 80% and had significant hypotension and bradycardia, necessitating external cardiac massage and cricothyroid puncture. His SaO$_2$ did not improve significantly, despite seemingly adequate resuscitation with 100% oxygen and intravenous adrenaline. His arterial methemoglobin concentration was 55%. Methylthioninium chloride 100 mg intravenously led to rapid improvement in the SaO$_2$, allowing surgery to continue.

- A 57-year-old man developed severe methemoglobinemia after receiving topical benzocaine spray and lidocaine jelly during awake fiberoptic intubation (37). After intubation, his oxygen saturation fell to 65% on 100% oxygen. He was cyanosed and had dark arterial blood sample with normal gas tensions. His methemoglobin concentration was 60% and treatment with methylthioninium chloride was successful.

These cases illustrate the importance of co-oximetry on grounds of clinical suspicion. Methemoglobin concentrations of 10–15% can cause dark-colored blood and cyanosis. Concentrations of 20–45% can cause lethargy, dizziness, headache, and collapse. Higher concentrations (50–70%) can cause seizures, dysrhythmias, coma, and death.

Methemoglobinemia followed the use of topical benzocaine for transesophageal echocardiography in three cases and fiberoptic intubation in one case (38) (39) (40). All the patients were successfully treated with methylthioninium chloride (methylene blue) 1–2 mg/kg. Another case occurred with use of benzocaine to treat throat ache after intubation (41).

In a cohort study of this problem, two out of more than 1000 gastric bypass patients who underwent endoscopy developed methemoglobinemia (42). In both cases benzocaine spray 20% had been used and the patients developed cyanosis, dyspnea, and tachycardia within 7 and 13 minutes. The methemoglobin concentrations were 19% and 36%. Both were resuscitated successfully with methylthioninium chloride and one with added ascorbic acid 1 g orally. The authors suggested that benzocaine spray should be limited and pointed out that pulse oximetry underestimates the degree of hypoxia. Prompt diagnosis and treatment with methylthioninium chloride can be life-saving. In subsequent correspondence others acknowledged the difficulty in determining the dose in a spray and suggest nebulized lidocaine as an alternative (43).

Two other cases of methemoglobinemia in morbidly obese patients who underwent bariatric surgery have been reported (44). Blood gas analysis was the only clue that led to the diagnosis in both these patients, in whom pulmonary compromise would have otherwise been blamed on obesity. Both recovered well with methylthioninium chloride.

In a review of 198 reports to the FDA of adverse events related to benzocaine, 67% involved methemoglobinemia; 101 were serious and two were fatal (45). Benzocaine spray was most commonly involved.

The FDA has issued a Public Health Advisory warning to highlight the fact that the use of benzocaine sprays in the mouth and throat has occasionally been linked with methemoglobinemia (46). The agency has also advised that the Veterans Health Administration has announced its decision to cease using benzocaine spray for local numbing of the mouth and throat mucous membranes for minor surgical procedures or tube insertion. It has further warned that methemoglobinemia has occurred when benzocaine spray was used for a longer duration or more often than recommended. The agency has suggested the following points for consideration when using benzocaine in the mouth or throat:

- Patients with breathing problems, or who smoke, are at greater risk of methemoglobinemia.
- The use of products with different active ingredients (for example lidocaine) may be beneficial in patients who are more likely to develop methemoglobinemia, such as children aged less than 4 months and older patients with certain inborn defects.
- Patients should receive the minimum dosage required to reduce the risk of methemoglobinemia.
- Patients who receive benzocaine should be carefully monitored for methemoglobinemia.
- Blood analysis for methemoglobinemia should be done using co-oximetry.
- A change in the color of the blood to chocolate-brown may be a danger sign.
- Patients with suspected methemoglobinemia should be promptly treated.

Skin

Granuloma gluteale adultorum is a rare skin condition of unknown etiology, characterized by reddish purple granulomatous nodules on the gluteal surfaces and groin areas.

- Granuloma gluteale adultorum occurred in a 40-year-old woman who presented with a 3-year history of the condition associated with the use of topical benzocaine (47).

Immunologic

Benzocaine can cause sensitization, and being a para-aminobenzoic acid derivative it can cross-react with para-phenylenediamine, sulfonamides, aniline dyes, and related local anesthetics. However, in a recent retrospective study of 5464 patients it was concluded that benzocaine allergy is not common in the UK, confirming earlier reports that benzocaine should not be used as a single screening agent for local anesthetic allergy (48).

Allergic contact dermatitis has been attributed to local benzocaine (49).

- A 72-year-old woman was treated for thoracic *Herpes zoster* with oral aciclovir and topical benzocaine 20% ointment. She subsequently developed painful pruritic erythematous dermatitis in the area of the lesions, spreading to her arm. The dermatitis was initially misdiagnosed as aciclovir resistance, but on patch testing she had a positive reaction to benzocaine.

The authors highlighted the problem in diagnosing allergic contact dermatitis in patients who have other skin lesions in that area. They emphasized the importance of patch testing to identify the causative agent.

References

1. Calello DP, Muller AA, Henretig FM, Osterhoudt KC. Benzocaine: not dangerous enough? Pediatrics. 115(5):1452.
2. Bayard M, Farrow J, Tudiver F. Acute methemoglobinemia after endoscopy. J Am Board Fam Pract 2004;17(3):227–9.
3. Vidyarthi V, Manda R, Ahmed A, Khosla S, Lubell DL. Severe methemoglobinemia after transesophageal echocardiography. Am J Ther 2003;10:225–7.
4. Aepfelbacher FC, Breen P, Manning WJ. Methemoglobinemia and topical pharyngeal anesthesia. New Engl J Med 2003;348:85–6.
5. Patel PB, Logan GW, Karnad AB, Byrd RP Jr, Roy TM. Acquired methemoglobinemia: a rare but serious complication. Tenn Med 2003;96:373–6.
6. Gray TA, Hawkins S. A PACU crisis: a case study on the development and management of methemoglobinemia. J Perianesth Nurs 2004;19(4):242–53.
7. Rinehart RS, Norman D. Suspected methemoglobinemia following awake intubation: one possible effect of benzocaine topical anesthesia-a case report. AANA J 2003;71:117–18.
8. Henry LR, Pizzini M, Delarso B, Ridge JA. Methemoglobinemia: early intraoperative detection by clinical observation. Laryngoscope 2004;114(11):2025–6.
9. Gentile DA. Severe methemoglobinemia induced by a topical teething preparation. Pediatr Emerg Care 1987;3(3):176–8.

10. Cooper HA. Methemoglobinemia caused by benzocaine topical spray. South Med J 1997;90(9):946-8.

11. Gilman CS, Veser FH, Randall D. Methemoglobinemia from a topical oral anesthetic. Acad Emerg Med 1997;4(10):1011-3.

12. Guerriero SE. Methemoglobinemia caused by topical benzocaine. Pharmacotherapy 1997;17(5):1038-40.

13. McGrath PD, Moloney JF, Riker RR. Benzocaine-induced methemoglobinemia complicating transesophageal echocardiography: a case report. Echocardiography 1998;15(4):389-92.

14. Malhotra S, Kolda M, Nanda NC. Local anesthetic-induced methemoglobinemia during transesophageal echocardiography. Echocardiography 1998;15(2):165-8.

15. Ho RT, Nanevicz T, Yee R, Figueredo VM. Benzocaine-induced methemoglobinemia—two case reports related to transesophageal echocardiography premedication. Cardiovasc Drugs Ther 1998;12(3):311-2.

16. Fisher MA, Henry D, Gillam L, Chen C. Toxic methemoglobinemia: a rare but serious complication of transesophageal echocardiography. Can J Cardiol 1998;14(9):1157-60.

17. Adachi T, Fukumoto M, Uetsuki N, Yasui O, Hayashi M. Suspected severe methemoglobinemia caused by topical application of an ointment containing benzocaine around the enterostomy. Anesth Analg 1999;88(5):1190-1.

18. Maher P. Methemoglobinemia: an unusual complication of topical anesthesia. Gastroenterol Nurs 1998;21(4):173-5.

19. Khan NA, Kruse JA. Methemoglobinemia induced by topical anesthesia: a case report and review. Am J Med Sci 1999;318(6):415-8.

20. Stoiber TR. Toxic Methemoglobinemia complicating transesophageal echocardiography. Echocardiography 1999;16(4):383-5.

21. Lunenfeld E, Kane GC. Methemoglobinemia: sudden dyspnea and oxyhemoglobin desaturation after esophagoduodenoscopy. Respir Care 2004;49(8):940-2.

22. Slaughter MS, Gordon PJ, Roberts JC, Pappas PS. An unusual case of hypoxia from benzocaine-induced methemoglobinemia. Ann Thorac Surg 1999;67(6):1776-8.

23. Maimo G, Redick E. Recognizing and treating methemoglobinemia: a rare but dangerous complication of topical anesthetic or nitrate overdose. Dimens Crit Care Nurs 2004;23(3):116-8.

24. Haynes JM. Acquired methemoglobinemia following benzocaine anesthesia of the pharynx. Am J Crit Care 2000;9(3):199-201.

25. Gregory PJ, Matsuda K. Cetacaine spray-induced methemoglobinemia after transesophageal echocardiography. Ann Pharmacother 2000;34(9):1077.

26. Nguyen ST, Cabrales RE, Bashour CA, Rosenberger TE Jr, Michener JA, Yared JP, Starr NJ. Benzocaine-induced methemoglobinemia. Anesth Analg 2000;90(2):369-71.

27. Kern K, Langevin PB, Dunn BM. Methemoglobinemia after topical anesthesia with lidocaine and benzocaine for a difficult intubation. J Clin Anesth 2000;12(2):167-72.

28. Gupta PM, Lala DS, Arsura EL. Benzocaine-induced methemoglobinemia. South Med J 2000;93(1):83-6.

29. Gunaratnam NT, Vazquez-Sequeiros E, Gostout CJ, Alexander GL. Methemoglobinemia related to topical benzocaine use: is it time to reconsider the empiric use of topical anesthesia before sedated EGD? Gastrointest Endosc 2000;52(5):692-3.

30. Wurdeman RL, Mohiuddin SM, Holmberg MJ, Shalaby A. Benzocaine-induced methemoglobinemia during an outpatient procedure. Pharmacotherapy 2000;20(6):735-8.

31. Fitzsimons MG, Gaudette RR, Hurford WE. Critical rebound methemoglobinemia after methylene blue treatment: case report. Pharmacotherapy 2004;24(4):538-40.

32. Khalife WI, Wang R, Khalil J. Respiratory failure secondary to methemoglobinemia induced by benzocaine: a case report. S D J Med 2004;57(4):145-7.

33. Spiller HA, Revolinski DH, Winter ML, Weber JA, Gorman SE. Multi-center retrospective evaluation of oral benzocaine exposure in children. Vet Hum Toxicol 2000;42(4):228-31.

34. Singh RK, Kambe JC, Andrews LK, Russell JC. Benzocaine-induced methemoglobinemia accompanying adult respiratory distress syndrome and sepsis syndrome: case report. J Trauma 2001;50(6):1153-7.

35. Ramsakal A, Lezama JL, Adelman HM. A potentially fatal effect of topical anesthesia. Hosp Pract (Off Ed) 2001;36(6):13-4.

36. Udeh C, Bittikofer J, Sum-Ping ST. Severe methemoglobinemia on reexposure to benzocaine. J Clin Anesth 2001; 13(2):128-30.

37. Keld DB, Hein L, Dalgaard M, Krogh L, Rodt SA. The incidence of transient neurologic symptoms (TNS) after spinal anaesthesia in patients undergoing surgery in the supine position. Hyperbaric lidocaine 5% versus hyperbaric bupivacaine 0.5% Acta Anaesthesiol Scand 2000;44(3):285-90.

38. Hegedus F, Herb K. Benzocaine-induced methemoglobinemia. Anesth Prog 2005;52(4):136-9.

39. Alonso GF. A wild reaction to a topical anesthetic. RN 2005;68(10):57-60.

40. Birchem SK. Benzocaine-induced methemoglobinemia during transesophageal echocardiography. J Am Osteopath Assoc 2005;105(8):381-4.

41. LeClaire AC, Mullett TW, Jahania MS, Flynn JD. Methemoglobinemia secondary to topical benzocaine use in a lung transplant patient. Ann Pharmacother 2005;39(2):373-6.

42. Srikanth MS, Kahlstrom R, Oh KH, Fox SR, Fox ER, Fox KM. Topical benzocaine (Hurricaine) induced methemoglobinemia during endoscopic procedures in gastric bypass patients. Obes Surg 2005;15(4):584-90.

43. Wong DH, Wilson SE. Avoiding topical anesthesia-induced methemoglobinemia. Obes Surg 2005;15(7):1088.

44. Carrodeguas L, Szomstein S, Jacobs J, Arias F, Antozzi P, Soto F, Zundel N, Whipple O, Simpfendorfer C, Gordon R, Villares A, Rosenthal RJ. Topical anesthesia-induced methemoglobinemia in bariatric surgery patients. Obes Surg 2005;15(2):282-5.

45. Moore TJ, Walsh CS, Cohen MR. Reported adverse event cases of methemoglobinemia associated with benzocaine products. Arch Intern Med 2004;164(11):1192-6.

46. Anonymous Benzocaine. Mouth and throat use linked with methaemoglobinaemia. WHO Newslett 2006;2:4.

47. Dytoc MT, Fiorillo L, Liao J, Krol AL. Granuloma gluteale adultorum associated with use of topical benzocaine preparations: case report and literature review. J Cutan Med Surg 2002;6(3):221-5.

48. Sidhu SK, Shaw S, Wilkinson JD. A 10-year retrospective study on benzocaine allergy in the United Kingdom. Am J Contact Dermat 1999;10(2):57-61.

49. Roos TC, Merk HF. Allergic contact dermatitis from benzocaine ointment during treatment of *Herpes zoster*. Contact Dermatitis 2001;44(2):104.

Bucricaine

General Information

Bucricaine (centbucridine) is a quinolone derivative with local anesthetic activity.

Nausea, vomiting, bradycardia, backache, shivering, and hypotension can occur with a similar incidence to that of lidocaine (SED-12, 256) (1). It has been suggested that bucricaine is more potent than lidocaine and has few cardiovascular and nervous system adverse effects in animals, at high doses. One study in humans suggested that bucricaine may be associated with fewer cardiovascular adverse effects than lidocaine, but there are insufficient data to confirm this impression (2).

References

1. Dasgupta D, Garasia M, Gupta KC, Satoskar RS. Randomised double-blind study of centbucridine and lignocaine for subarachnoid block. Indian J Med Res 1983; 77:512–6.
2. Samsi AB, Bhalerao RA, Shah SC, Mody BB, Paul T, Satoskar RS. Evaluation of centbucridine as a local anesthetic. Anesth Analg 1983;62(1):109–11.

Bupivacaine

General Information

Bupivacaine is a long-acting aminoamide local anesthetic with significantly more systemic toxicity than lidocaine.

In a randomized controlled study after total knee arthroplasty in 14 patients the effects of a continuous infusion of intra-articular bupivacaine were examined (1). The patients were randomized to three groups who received 4ml/hour of isotonic saline, bupivacaine 0.25%, and bupivacaine 0.5%. Opioid-sparing effects and patient satisfaction were the primary observations, and serum bupivacaine was also measured in two patients who received bupivacaine 0.5%. The study was halted because of a serum bupivacaine concentration of 1.2 µg/ml in one of these patients, close to presumed toxic concentrations.

Organs and Systems

Cardiovascular

Bupivacaine-induced cardiotoxicity, notably after epidural use, is a matter of concern and controversy (2–4). The risk can be greatly reduced or eliminated by careful dosage and/or the use of lower concentrations (SEDA-12, 108) (2).

All studies of the cardiotoxic effects of local anesthetics on the isolated heart published from 1981 to 2001 have been reviewed (5). Thirteen studies were identified, all of which studied bupivacaine, either alone or compared with other local anesthetics. The general conclusions were:

- Highly lipid-soluble, extensively protein-bound, highly potent local anesthetics, such as tetracaine, bupivacaine, and etidocaine, are much more cardiotoxic than less lipid-soluble, protein-bound, and potent local anesthetics, such as lidocaine and prilocaine.
- Bupivacaine has a potent depressant effect on electrical conduction in the heart, primarily via an action on voltage-gated sodium channels that govern the initial rapid depolarization of the cardiac action potential.
- The $S(-)$ isomer of bupivacaine is less cardiotoxic than the $R(+)$ form.
- Bupivacaine predisposes the heart to re-entrant dysrhythmias.
- The actions of bupivacaine on channels other than voltage-gated sodium channels probably contribute to the dose-dependent cardiotoxic effects of bupivacaine.

The recommended safe upper dose limit for bupivacaine is commonly 2–2.5 mg/kg. However, some authors recommend a lower dose of 1.25 mg/kg as the safe upper limit in dental practice (SEDA-20, 128) (6).

Hyperkalemia, acidosis, severe hypoxia, and myocardial ischemia increase the cardiovascular depressive effects of bupivacaine.

There has been a report of T wave changes on the electrocardiogram during caudal administration of local anesthetics (7).

- A 4.2 kg 2-month-old baby was given a caudal injection under general anesthesia for an inguinal hernia repair. A mixture of 1% lidocaine 2 ml and 0.25% bupivacaine 2 ml was injected. Every 1 ml was preceded by an aspiration test and followed by observation for 20 seconds for electrocardiographic changes. On administration of the third 1 ml dose, there was a significant increase in T wave amplitude. The aspiration test was repeated and was positive for blood. The caudal injection was stopped and the electrocardiogram returned to normal after 35 seconds. The patient remained cardiovascularly stable with no postoperative sequelae.

Previous reports have suggested that an increase in T wave amplitude could result from inadvertent intravascular administration of adrenaline-containing local anesthetics. This is the first case report of local anesthetics alone causing significant T wave changes.

Bradycardia has been reported very occasionally (8).

Bupivacaine can cause ventricular extra beats (9). Ventricular dysrhythmias and seizures were reported in a patient who received 0.5% bupivacaine 30 ml with adrenaline 5 micrograms/ml for lumbar plexus block, after a negative aspiration test (10). The patient developed ventricular fibrillation and required advanced cardiac life support for 1 hour, including 15 defibrillations, and adrenaline 40 mg before sinus rhythm could be restored. There were no neurological sequelae.

Infusions of 0.25% bupivacaine into pig coronary arteries caused ventricular fibrillation at lower rates of infusion than 0.25% bupivacaine with 1% lidocaine (11). The lidocaine/bupivacaine mixture did not have a greater myocardial depressant effect than bupivacaine alone. The authors suggested that when regional anesthesia requires high doses of local anesthetics, bupivacaine should not be used alone but in a mixture with lidocaine, and that lidocaine should be useful in the management of bupivacaine-induced ventricular fibrillation.

An animal study of the mechanism of bupivacaine-induced dysrhythmias has shown that bupivacaine facilitates early after-depolarization in rabbit sinoatrial nodal cells by blocking the delayed rectifier potassium current (12).

Inadvertent administration of bupivacaine can lead to fatal cardiovascular collapse that may be refractory to conventional resuscitation. A study in rats has suggested that in addition to its direct cardiotoxic effect, bupivacaine may have a toxic action on the brainstem, and that cardiovascular collapse may result from dysfunction of vital cardiorespiratory control systems (13).

Conduction disturbances have been attributed to bupivacaine.

- A 60-year-old woman with pre-existing heart failure awaiting surgery for a fractured humerus was accidentally given a mixture of bupivacaine 75 mg and clonidine 15 micrograms intravenously (14). She developed a nodal rhythm with extreme bradycardia, severe shock, and convulsions. Seizures were controlled with thiopental, and suxamethonium and adrenaline partially restored the blood pressure to 50/30 mmHg and the heart rate to 60/minute (nodal rhythm). After clonidine 75 micrograms intravenously, her blood pressure rose to 90/70 mmHg and her heart rate to 70/minute. Her cardiac rhythm reverted to sinus rhythm with first degree atrioventricular block.

The authors concluded that clonidine had reversed bupivacaine-induced conduction disturbances.

The effect of a lipid emulsion infusion on bupivacaine-induced cardiac toxicity has been studied in dogs (15). Bupivacaine 10 mg/kg was given intravenously over 10 minutes to fasted dogs under general anesthesia. Resuscitation included 10 minutes of internal cardiac massage followed by either saline or 20% lipid infusion, as a 4 mg/kg bolus followed by a continuous infusion of 0.5 ml/kg/minute for 10 minutes. Electrocardiography, arterial blood pressure, myocardial pH, and myocardial PO_2 were continuously monitored. All six lipid treated dogs survived after 10 minutes of cardiac massage, but there were no survivors among the six dogs who were given saline. Hemodynamics, PO_2, and myocardial pH were also improved in the treatment group. This study supports the need for further investigation of lipid-based resuscitation to treat bupivacaine toxicity in order to determine the optimum dosage regimen.

The longer-acting, more lipophilic agents, such as bupivacaine, can cause cardiovascular toxicity at serum concentrations that are not much greater than those required to cause nervous system toxicity.

- A 65-year-old man had 15 ml of plain bupivacaine 0.5% infiltrated before a planned radiofrequency ablation of a lumbar sympathetic ganglion (16). He immediately developed respiratory arrest with bradycardia and hypotension (54/40 mmHg). Asystolic cardiac arrest was treated successfully but he subsequently developed pulmonary edema after a hypotensive episode. Angiography showed left anterior descending artery ischemia and his electrocardiographic T waves normalized 7 months later.

The authors report this case as bupivacaine-induced cardiovascular collapse with several novel features. Firstly, it developed after the administration of a relatively low dose of bupivacaine, less than 1.1 mg/kg. Secondly, the presentation was that of mixed cardiogenic and vasomotor shock. Finally, he developed an unexplained delayed cardiographic finding of symmetrically inverted anterior T waves. The authors thought that drug-drug interactions may also have contributed; since he was taking amitriptyline and carbamazepine, each of which is potentially cardiotoxic and may have lowered the threshold for bupivacaine toxicity.

Cardiopulmonary bypass has been used to successfully treat bupivacaine-induced cardiovascular collapse (17).

- A 39-year-old woman (72 kg, 165 cm) with congenital clubfoot presented for total right ankle arthroplasty. She had no history of syncope, seizures, coronary artery disease, or congenital heart disease. After induction of anesthesia she received a popliteal nerve block with 30 ml of 0.5% bupivacaine using a nerve stimulator device. Communication was maintained with the patient throughout the injection, and she denied any neurological symptoms suggestive of intravascular injection. About 30 seconds after the block, she had a generalized tonic–clonic seizure and soon afterwards developed ventricular fibrillation. Advanced cardiac life support was begun. She was given adrenaline 2 mg and bretylium 1000 mg intravenously, as well as six attempts at electrical defibrillation. Bupivacaine cardiotoxicity because of inadvertent intravascular injection was suspected and cardiopulmonary bypass was begun and continued for 30 minutes. She was extubated on the second postoperative day and discharged home on postoperative day 10 with no neurological sequelae.

The prolonged duration of cardiac support needed after refractory drug-induced cardiotoxicity may make cardiopulmonary bypass, although invasive, the best option for successful resuscitation of such patients. Notwithstanding the practical and technical limitations of staff and equipment availability, the authors argued that cardiopulmonary bypass should become first-line therapy after unsuccessful basic resuscitation in such cases.

Methods of mitigating bupivacaine cardiotoxicity have been investigated in animals. Insulin–dextrose–potassium infusion was extremely successful in the treatment of bupivacaine-induced cardiotoxicity in dogs—all those who were treated survived, while the controls all developed irreversible cardiac arrest (18). In contrast, clonidine pretreatment did not alter bupivacaine cardiotoxicity or resuscitability in rats (19).

Death

Fatal bupivacaine toxicity occurred after recreational use by injection into the external genitalia for autoerotic purposes (20).

Nervous system

Neurological symptoms subsequent to unrecognized intravascular injection are the major complications of bupivacaine: tinnitus, muscle twitching, nystagmus, and convulsions can occur. The use of vasoconstrictors is probably not advisable, as they prolong the duration of action of local anesthetics. Whether the addition of hyperbaric glucose to 0.5% bupivacaine for spinal anesthesia alters the incidence of pain from an orthopedic tourniquet is disputed; some findings suggest that it aggravates the problem (SED-12, 256) (21).

- A 13-year-old girl developed tonic-clonic seizures followed by ventricular fibrillation after subcutaneous infiltration of extensive skin abrasions with 30 mg (0.5 mg/kg) of bupivacaine over about 1 hour. She was successfully resuscitated with cardiopulmonary resuscitation and intubation, intravenous diazepam, adrenaline, and sodium bicarbonate (22).

The authors noted that although the anticonvulsant effect of diazepam is significant, some animal studies have shown that diazepam can prolong the half-life of bupivacaine. They stressed the difficulty in treating bupivacaine-induced dysrhythmias and suggested the use of phenytoin as a first-line agent in their management. However, this advice is based on only two case reports.

In seven children (aged 36–52 weeks) given caudal anesthesia with bupivacaine 3.1 mg/kg + adrenaline 5 micrograms/ml, there were significant electroencephalographic signs of central nervous system toxicity in six, and two had clinical signs of possible epileptic activity. The authors stopped the study early because of the high incidence of adverse effects. They felt that these were due to the fact that no sedative or anesthetic drugs that could have masked or alleviated local anesthetic toxicity were given, and also that infants have low concentrations of alpha$_1$ acid glycoprotein, leading to increased unbound plasma concentrations (23). However, it should be noted that 2 mg/kg is the usual upper dose limit recommended for bupivacaine. It is hardly surprising that such a high proportion of those studied showed evidence of systemic toxicity after the administration of a much higher dose of bupivacaine to such small children by a route that is known to result in rapid absorption of local anesthetic into the systemic circulation.

Reactions to local anesthetics often occur as a result of inadvertent overdose or accidental intravenous injection.

- A 53-year-old woman received postoperative epidural analgesia by nurse-administered bolus doses after a total knee replacement (24). She received her first

epidural bolus of 0.25% bupivacaine 6 ml with morphine 2 mg 2 hours after the operation, with good effect. Six hours later she was accidentally given a second top-up dose intravenously. She became distressed and complained of tinnitus, palpitation, and dizziness. She was able to cooperate and was in sinus rhythm with a tachycardia of 120/minute. She was observed overnight on ICU and made a full recovery.

Despite correct epidural placement, this complication arose as a result of human error, and the authors believed that the low concentration and volume of the top-up had protected the patient from more serious sequelae.

Musculoskeletal

Muscular atrophy after intramuscular injection has been documented (25).

Immunologic

A non-IgE-mediated allergic reaction to bupivacaine has been reported (SEDA-21, 136).

- A 69-year-old woman with a history of bronchospasm after NSAID administration had heavy feelings in her arms and itchy eyes, without any change in hemodynamics, 30 minutes after an intradermal injection of bupivacaine. The same symptoms occurred during subsequent retesting 1 month later, with the addition of coughing and sneezing.

Second-Generation Effects

Pregnancy

Cardiotoxicity due to bupivacaine is more likely in pregnancy (26).

When epidural anesthesia was used for cesarean section, bupivacaine (with oxytocin) produced a higher frequency of neonatal jaundice than similar treatment using lidocaine (SEDA-14, 111).

Fetotoxicity

Adverse effects of bupivacaine on the fetus are uncommon (27), but fetal bradycardia has very occasionally been reported (28).

Susceptibility Factors

Genetic factors

Isovaleric acidemia (an autosomal recessive disorder of leucine metabolism causing episodes of acidosis during catabolic stress) and carnitine deficiency have been associated with a lowered threshold for bupivacaine-induced dysrhythmias (SEDA-22, 142).

Age

In the elderly, some local anesthetics (including lidocaine and bupivacaine) have longer durations of action (26).

Drug Administration

Drug formulations

A formulation of bupivacaine called Regibloc (bupivacaine HCl; Intramed, South Africa) was the only common factor in a series of serious complications after regional anesthesia (29).

- Three consecutive patients had prolonged blockade after retrobulbar block. One had not resolved after 3 months and three others had prolonged mydriasis for 2 weeks.
- Severe neuralgia developed in eight patients after interscalene blocks lasting 6–12 weeks.
- A 36-year-old woman developed supraclavicular skin necrosis, followed by sloughing of subcutaneous tissue down to the first rib, including the dorsal roots of the brachial plexus, after receiving an interscalene block followed by an infusion; 5 months later she still had complete sensory and motor paralysis of the C5 nerve root requiring nerve grafting.
- Skin sloughing after a penile ring-block required plastic reconstruction.
- A 16-year-old girl had a median nerve block followed by an area of skin and fat necrosis at the site of injection and a middle-aged patient received an interscalene block resulting in subsequent fat necrosis at the injection site.

No further complications were encountered after the authors changed to another formulation of bupivacaine and stopped using Regibloc.

Drug–Drug Interactions

Calcium channel blockers

Calcium channel blockers in combination with bupivacaine produce significant negative inotropic effects on the heart in animals, possibly due to reduced protein binding of the local anesthetic, as well as a generalized myocardial depressant effect (30,31).

However, bupivacaine cardiotoxicity was reduced in rats by pretreatment with low doses of calcium channel blockers (32). In vivo, the LD_{50} for bupivacaine was increased from 3.08 to 3.58 mg/kg after pretreatment with verapamil 150 micrograms/kg, and to 3.50 mg/kg after nimodipine 200 micrograms/kg. Of the rats that died, only one developed cardiac arrest first, whilst the majority developed respiratory arrest. In vitro, bupivacaine alone dose-dependently reduced heart rate, contractile force, and coronary perfusion pressure. Dysrhythmias were also noted: bradycardias, ventricular extra beats, and ventricular tachycardia were the most common. Verapamil made no difference to these adverse effects, but nimodipine significantly reduced the negative chronotropic and dysrhythmogenic effects of bupivacaine. These results, although interesting, cannot be used to reach any clinical conclusions, particularly as the mechanism of interaction between bupivacaine and calcium channel blockers has yet to be elucidated.

Clonidine

The analgesic efficacy of the addition of clonidine to an epidural solution of bupivacaine plus fentanyl has been subjected to a randomized, double-blind study in 61 parturients who received bupivacaine plus fentanyl with or without clonidine (median dose 28 micrograms/hour). There was no difference between the groups in pruritus or nausea score, but those given clonidine had less shivering and better analgesia (33).

In another randomized, double-blind study, a combination of clonidine and neostigmine was added to intrathecal bupivacaine plus fentanyl in 45 parturients (34). The combination increased the duration of labor analgesia by 83%, but was associated with significantly more nausea. However, the results were equivocal, and larger studies are needed.

Clonidine inhibits the hepatic metabolism of bupivacaine in mice (35).

Desipramine

Desipramine displaces bupivacaine from plasma proteins (36).

Diazepam

Animal studies have shown that diazepam can prolong the half-life of bupivacaine (39).

Fentanyl

Bupivacaine is increasingly being used in combination with fentanyl for obstetric analgesia and has been reported to reduce the incidence of pruritus. In a prospective study, 65 parturients in labor were randomly assigned to receive intrathecal fentanyl (25 μg), intrathecal bupivacaine (2.5 mg), or both as part of epidural anesthesia (40). The group that received both drugs had more prolonged analgesia and significantly less pruritus than those who received fentanyl alone (36 versus 95%). However, the incidence of facial pruritus was not significantly different. The type of analgesia did not affect the outcome of labor, although one patient in the combined treatment group required ephedrine for reduced blood pressure. It was proposed that pruritus is the result of stimulation of mu receptors supraspinally and in the dorsal horn of the spinal cord, and that facial itching is associated with mu receptor activation in the medullary dorsal horn, affecting the trigeminal nerve. Local anesthetics may alter this adverse effect by local neuronal blockade or by direct modulation of mu-opioid receptors. Bupivacaine also promotes opioid binding to kappa-opioid receptors, which reduce pruritus. The failure to relieve facial pruritus suggests a direct effect of fentanyl in the brain stem.

Itraconazole

The interaction of itraconazole 200 mg orally od for 4 days with a single intravenous dose of racemic bupivacaine (0.3 mg /kg given over 60 minutes) has been examined in a placebo-controlled crossover study in 10 healthy volunteers (41). Itraconazole reduced the clearance of R-bupivacaine by 21% and that of S-bupivacaine by

25%, but had no other significant effects on the pharmacokinetics of the enantiomers. Reduction of bupivacaine clearance by itraconazole is likely to increase steady-state concentrations of bupivacaine enantiomers by 20–25%, and this should be taken into account in the concomitant use of itraconazole and bupivacaine.

Mepivacaine

Bupivacaine displaces mepivacaine from protein binding sites on alpha$_1$ acid glycoprotein in vitro (37).

Pethidine

Pethidine displaces bupivacaine from plasma proteins (36). However, this interaction is probably not of clinical importance (38).

Phenytoin

Phenytoin displaces bupivacaine from plasma proteins (36).

Quinidine

Quinidine displaces bupivacaine from plasma proteins (36).

References

1. Hoeft MA, Rathmell JP, Dayton MR, Lee P, Howe JG, Incavo SJ, Lawlis JF. Continuous, intra-articular infusion of bupivacaine after total-knee arthroplasty may lead to potentially toxic serum levels of local anesthetic. Reg Anesth Pain Med 2005;30(4):414–5.
2. Nolte H. Zur Problematik der Cardiotoxizität von Bupivacain 0.75%. [The problem of the cardiotoxicity of bupivacaine 0.75%.] Reg Anaesth 1986;9(3):57–9.
3. Marx GF. Bupivacaine cardiotoxicity-concentration or dose? Anesthesiology 1986;65(1):116.
4. Hurley R, Feldman H. Toxicity of local anesthetics in obstetrics. I. Bupivacaine. Clin Anaesthesiol 1986;4:93.
5. Heavner JE. Cardiac toxicity of local anesthetics in the intact isolated heart model: a review. Reg Anesth Pain Med 2002;27(6):545–55.
6. Bacsik CJ, Swift JQ, Hargreaves KM. Toxic systemic reactions of bupivacaine and etidocaine. Oral Surg Oral Med Oral Pathol Oral Radiol Endod 1995;79(1):18–23.
7. Tanaka M, Nitta R, Nishikawa T. Increased T-wave amplitude after accidental intravascular injection of lidocaine plus bupivacaine without epinephrine in sevoflurane-anesthetized child. Anesth Analg 2001;92(4):915–7.
8. Exler U, Nolte H, Milatz W. Die Überwachung der Herzleitung bei Anwendung von Bupivacain 0.75% mit Hilfe der Ventrikulographie (^{99m}Tc). [Monitoring of cardiac output during use of bupivacaine 0.75% by ventriculography (^{99m}Tc).] Reg Anaesth 1986;9(3):68–73.
9. Pape R, Ammer W. Holter-EKG-Überwachung bei Periduralanaesthesie mit Bupivacain 0.75%. [Holter ECG monitoring during peridural anesthesia with bupivacaine 0.75%.] Reg Anaesth 1986;9(3):74–8.
10. Pham-Dang C, Beaumont S, Floch H, Bodin J, Winer A, Pinaud M. Accident aign toxique après bloc du plexus lombaire à la bupivacaine. [Acute toxic accident following lumbar plexus block with bupivacaine.] Ann Fr Anesth Reanim 2000;19(5):356–9.
11. Fujita Y, Endoh S, Yasukawa T, Sari A. Lidocaine increases the ventricular fibrillation threshold during bupivacaine-induced cardiotoxicity in pigs. Br J Anaesth 1998;80(2):218–22.
12. Matsuda T, Kurata Y. Effects of nicardipine and bupivacaine on early after depolarization in rabbit sinoatrial node cells: a possible mechanism of bupivacaine-induced arrhythmias. Gen Pharmacol 1999;33(2):115–25.
13. Pickering AE, Waki H, Headley PM, Paton JF. Investigation of systemic bupivacaine toxicity using the in situ perfused working heart-brainstem preparation of the rat. Anesthesiology 2002;97(6):1550–6.
14. Favier JC, Da Conceicao M, Fassassi M, Allanic L, Steiner T, Pitti R. Successful resuscitation of serious bupivacaine intoxication in a patient with pre-existing heart failure. Can J Anaesth 2003;50:62–6.
15. Weinberg G, Ripper R, Feinstein DL, Hoffman W. Lipid emulsion infusion rescues dogs from bupivacaine-induced cardiac toxicity. Reg Anesth Pain Med 2003;28:198–202.
16. Levsky ME, Miller MA. Cardiovascular collapse from low dose bupivacaine. Can J Clin Pharmacol 2005;12(3):e240–5.
17. Soltesz EG, van Pelt F, Byrne JG. Emergent cardiopulmonary bypass for bupivacaine cardiotoxicity. J Cardiothorac Vasc Anesth 2003;17:357–8.
18. Kim JT, Jung CW, Lee KH. The effect of insulin on the resuscitation of bupivacaine-induced severe cardiovascular toxicity in dogs. Anesth Analg 2004;99(3):728–33.
19. Gulec S, Aydin Y, Uzuner K, Yelken B, Senturk Y. Effects of clonidine pre-treatment on bupivacaine and ropivacaine cardiotoxicity in rats. Eur J Anaesthesiol 2004;21(3):205–9.
20. Yazzie J, Kelly SC, Zumwalt RE, Kerrigan S. Fatal bupivacaine intoxication following unusual erotic practices. J Forensic Sci 2004;49(2):351–3.
21. Bridenbaugh PO, Hagenouw RR, Gielen MJ, Edstrom HH. Addition of glucose to bupivacaine in spinal anesthesia increases incidence of tourniquet pain. Anesth Analg 1986;65(11):1181–5.
22. Yan AC, Newman RD. Bupivacaine-induced seizures and ventricular fibrillation in a 13-year-old girl undergoing wound debridement. Pediatr Emerg Care 1998;14(5):354–5.
23. Breschan C, Hellstrand E, Likar R, Lonnquist PA. Toxizität und "subtoxische" Fruhzeich in Wachzustand bei Sauglingen. Bupivacain plasspiegel nach Kaudalanästhesist. [Early signs of toxicity and "subtoxic" conditions in infant monitoring. Bupivacaine plasma levels following caudal anesthesia.] Anaesthesist 1998;47(4):290–4.
24. Karaca S, Unlusoy EO. Accidental injection of intravenous bupivacaine. Eur J Anaesthesiol 2002;19(8):616–7.
25. Parris WCV, Dettbarn WD. Muscle atrophy following bupivacaine trigger point injection. Anesthesiol Rev 1989;16:50–4.
26. Chauvin M. Toxicité aiguë des anesthésiques locaux en fonction du terrain. [Acute toxicity of local anesthetics as a function of the patient's condition.] Ann Fr Anesth Reanim 1988;7(3):216–23.
27. Seebacher J, Chareire F, Galli-Douant P, Viars P. L'utilisation de la Marcaine en analgésie obstétricale. [The use of Marcaine in obstetrical analgesia.] Ann Anesthesiol Fr 1978;19(4):247–53.
28. Kuczkowski KM. Severe persistent fetal bradycardia following subarachnoid administration of fentanyl and bupivacaine for induction of a combined spinal-epidural analgesia for labor pain. J Clin Anesth 2004;16(1):78–9.
29. Boezaart AP, du Toit JC, van Lill G, Donald R, van der Spuy G, Bolus M. Urgent local anaesthetic drug alarm. S Afr Med J 1999;89(6):570–2.
30. Wulf H, Godicke J, Herzig S. Functional interaction between local anaesthetics and calcium antagonists in

guineapig myocardium: 2. Electrophysiological studies with bupivacaine and nifedipine. Br J Anaesth 1994;73(3): 364–70.

31. Herzig S, Ruhnke L, Wulf H. Functional interaction between local anaesthetics and calcium antagonists in guineapig myocardium: 1. Cardiodepressant effects in isolated organs. Br J Anaesth 1994;73(3):357–63.

32. Adsan H, Tulunay M, Onaran O. The effects of verapamil and nimodipine on bupivacaine-induced cardiotoxicity in rats: an in vivo and in vitro study. Anesth Analg 1998;86(4):818–24.

33. Paech MJ, Pavy TJ, Orlikowski CE, Evans SF. Patient-controlled epidural analgesia in labor: the addition of clonidine to bupivacaine–fentanyl. Reg Anesth Pain Med 2000;25(1):34–40.

34. Owen MD, Ozsarac O, Sahin S, Uckunkaya N, Kaplan N, Magunaci I. Low-dose clonidine and neostigmine prolong the duration of intrathecal bupivacaine-fentanyl for labor analgesia. Anesthesiology 2000;92(2):361–2.

35. Naguib M, Magboul MM, Samarkandi AH, Attia M. Adverse effects and drug interactions associated with local and regional anaesthesia. Drug Saf 1998;18(4):221–50.

36. Ghoneim MM, Pandya H. Plasma protein binding of bupivacaine and its interaction with other drugs in man. Br J Anaesth 1974;46(6):435–8.

37. Hartrick CT, Dirkes WE, Coyle DE, Raj PP, Denson DD. Influence of bupivacaine on mepivacaine protein binding. Clin Pharmacol Ther 1984;36(4):546–50.

38. Denson DD, Myers JA, Coyle DE. The clinical relevance of the drug displacement interaction between meperidine and bupivacaine. Res Commun Chem Pathol Pharmacol 1984;45(3):323–30.

39. Yan AC, Newman RD. Bupivacaine-induced seizures and ventricular fibrillation in a 13-year-old girl undergoing wound debridement. Pediatr Emerg Care 1998;14(5):354–5.

40. Asokumar B, Newman LM, McCarthy RJ, Ivankovich AD, Tuman KJ. Intrathecal bupivacaine reduces pruritus and prolongs duration of fentanyl analgesia during labor: a prospective, randomized controlled trial. Anesth Analg 1998;87(6):1309–15.

41. Palkama VJ, Neuvonen PJ, Olkkola KT. Effect of itraconazole on the pharmacokinetics of bupivacaine enantiomers in healthy volunteers. Br J Anaesth 1999;83(4):659–61.

Chloroprocaine

General Information

Chloroprocaine is a local anesthetic, an aminoester of para-aminobenzoic acid. Its systemic toxicity is low, owing to rapid hydrolysis by plasma pseudocholinesterases (1).

Comparative studies

Chloroprocaine was compared with lidocaine in a double-blind, randomized, crossover study (2). Eight healthy volunteers each received two spinal anesthetics, one with 2% lidocaine (40 mg) and the other with 2% chloroprocaine (40 mg). Chloroprocaine produced an anesthetic effect similar to that of lidocaine, but with significantly faster resolution of the block. In seven of the eight subjects lidocaine produced mild transient neurological symptoms, whereas in the chloroprocaine group there were no such complaints.

Organs and Systems

Cardiovascular

Of 25 patients who received epidural chloroprocaine for various day procedures, 23 had a fall in arterial blood pressure of 15%, and in two it fell by 25% (3).

Cardiotoxicity occurred in a 2-month-old child after accidental intravenous injection of chloroprocaine via an epidural catheter (4).

- A 2-month-old child (4 kg) was given 4 ml of chloroprocaine 3% via an epidural catheter, which had been placed via the caudal position with a negative aspiration test. The child immediately developed a broad-complex bradycardia, which terminated spontaneously after 30 seconds. The catheter was left in situ and intravenous placement was confirmed by contrast dye injection.

Rapid metabolism of ester local anesthetics by plasma cholinesterase would be expected to protect against toxicity, and the authors noted that this was the first published report of cardiotoxicity after inadvertent intravenous injection of such an anesthetic. Consistent with established practice, they recommended using a test dose to rule out intravascular placement of an epidural catheter and giving the local anesthetic slowly and incrementally.

Neuromuscular function

Prolonged neuromuscular blockade has been reported after epidural chloroprocaine (5).

- A 29-year-old woman in labor was given an epidural infusion of bupivacaine 0.04% plus fentanyl 1.66 micrograms/ml, running at 15 ml/hour for 7 hours. She then required an urgent cesarean section and 15 ml of chloroprocaine 3% was given, followed 20 minutes later by 12 ml of 2% lidocaine. Half an hour later she showed signs of high epidural blockade with dyspnea followed by unresponsiveness, and required immediate intubation with suxamethonium. She then developed prolonged neuromuscular blockade with a first-twitch response occurring after 1.75 hours. It took 3.75 hours before she could be extubated. Her plasma cholinesterase activity was low immediately postpartum, with a concentration of 1.3 U/ml (reference range 2.8–11), returning to normal within 7 weeks.

The authors believed that the high epidural blockade and the prolonged neuromuscular block had resulted from reduced pseudocholinesterase activity.

Second-Generation Effects

Pregnancy

Reduced pseudocholinesterase activity has been described both in pregnancy and with magnesium therapy. As most ester local anesthetics (with the exception of cocaine) are metabolized by this enzyme, caution should be exercised when using ester local anesthetics in pregnancy, especially with the increasing use of magnesium sulfate in this field.

Susceptibility Factors

Genetic factors

When there is an atypical pseudocholinesterase, complications can occur, notably convulsions (1).

Drug Administration

Drug formulations

Chloroprocaine does not itself appear to be neurotoxic at clinical concentrations. However, formulations that contain EDTA can cause burning back pain when used in epidurals (SEDA-22, 142).

Local neural irritation can occur when large doses of formulations containing sodium bisulfate as a preservative are used epidurally or intrathecally, probably because of the low pH and the sodium bisulfate content rather than the local anesthetic (SEDA-14, 111). Prolonged neural deficits have been described, the pathophysiology of which is controversial (SEDA-10, 105).

A preservative-free formulation of chloroprocaine may be a serious contender for drug of choice in short-acting spinal anesthesia and might even replace lidocaine.

In a dose-ranging, randomized, crossover study, three different doses of chloroprocaine (30, 45, and 60 mg) were compared in health volunteers (6). The authors estimated that the appropriate dose range of preservative- and antioxidant-free chloroprocaine for spinal anesthesia is 30–60 mg. Eleven of 18 administrations of chloroprocaine with adrenaline led to flu-like symptoms, while there were no such complaints with chloroprocaine alone; the authors advised against using adrenaline.

In a randomized, double-blind, crossover study, chloroprocaine spinal anesthesia was performed with or without dextrose in eight healthy volunteers (7). Each received two spinal anesthetics using 2 ml of chloroprocaine 2% (40 mg) with 0.25 ml of saline or 0.25 ml of dextrose 10%. Spinal anesthesia was successful in all subjects. The addition of dextrose did not significantly change the characteristics of the spinal block, but increased bladder dysfunction.

Drug–Drug Interactions

Suxamethonium

Because it is hydrolysed by plasma cholinesterase, chloroprocaine may competitively enhance the action of suxamethonium (8).

References

1. Smith AR, Hur D, Resano F. Grand mal seizures after 2-chloroprocaine epidural anesthesia in a patient with plasma cholinesterase deficiency. Anesth Analg 1987;66(7):677–8.
2. Kouri ME, Kopacz DJ. Spinal 2-chloroprocaine: a comparison with lidocaine in volunteers. Anesth Analg 2004;98(1):75–80.
3. Allen RW, Fee JP, Moore J. A preliminary assessment of epidural chloroprocaine for day procedures. Anaesthesia 1993;48(9):773–5.
4. Cladis FP, Litman RS. Transient cardiovascular toxicity with unintentional intravascular injection of 3% 2-chloroprocaine in a 2-month-old infant. Anesthesiology 2004;100(1):181–3.
5. Monedero P, Hess P. High epidural block with chloroprocaine in a parturient with low pseudocholinesterase activity. Can J Anaesth 2001;48(3):318–9.
6. Smith KN, Kopacz DJ, McDonald SB. Spinal 2-chloroprocaine: a dose-ranging study and the effect of added epinephrine. Anesth Analg 2004;98(1):81–8.
7. Warren DT, Kopacz DJ. Spinal 2-chloroprocaine: the effect of added dextrose. Anesth Analg 2004;98(1):95–101.
8. Matsuo S, Rao DB, Chaudry I, Foldes FF. Interaction of muscle relaxants and local anesthetics at the neuromuscular junction. Anesth Analg 1978;57(5):580–7.

Cinchocaine

General Information

Cinchocaine (dibucaine) is an aminoamide local anesthetic. It is ten times more potent than lidocaine and potentially very toxic. It is available in a number of over-the-counter topical formulations, such as antihemorrhoidal drugs.

Organs and Systems

Nervous system

Low concentrations of cinchocaine (0.003 and 0.03% respectively) caused irreversible neurotoxicity in A_β and C rabbit vagus nerve preparations (1). Cinchocaine had the greatest neurotoxic effect and the lowest safety margin compared with tetracaine and bupivacaine.

Cauda equina syndrome has been reported after a spinal anesthetic using cinchocaine (2).

- A 64-year-old man with a history of borderline diabetes who had undergone two previous operations uneventfully under spinal anesthetic received a spinal anesthetic with hyperbaric 0.24% dibucaine 2.2 ml and then a general anesthetic because of unilateral block. The next day he complained of difficulty in defecation and urination, with abnormal anal sensation. A diagnosis of cauda equina syndrome was made. He made a gradual recovery, but mild hypesthesia remained after 4 months.

A possible cause for this adverse event may have been maldistribution in the intrathecal space of the high concentration of cinchocaine, affecting the cauda equina and resulting in nerve damage; the incomplete block achieved in this case is suggestive of this. Elderly patients undergoing urological surgery often have risk factors for cauda equina syndrome, such as intraoperative lithotomy position, frequent spinal anesthetics, old age, and diabetes mellitus. The authors suggested that cinchocaine should be avoided for spinal anesthesia in these patients, because of its high neurotoxicity compared with other local anesthetics.

Hematologic

Cinchocaine inhibits ADP-mediated platelet aggregation (3); it is not known whether this has any clinical significance.

Skin

Two cases of contact dermatitis have been reported after the use of Proctosedyl and Ruscens Llorens, both of which contain cinchocaine. After patch testing, the first case was found to be allergic in origin and the second was due to photosensitivity. Neither showed cross-sensitivity to other local anesthetics (4).

Two cases of allergic contact dermatitis have been described after the use of cinchocaine formulations.

- A 71-year-old Japanese man, who was using an over-the-counter formulation, Makiron, for minor wounds, developed an itchy rash with seropapules and erosions on his right leg at the site of application (5). Makiron contains 0.1% cinchocaine hydrochloride and chlorphenamine maleate as well as naphazoline hydrochloride and benzethonium chloride. On patch testing, he was positive to both chlorphenamine and cinchocaine.
- A 79-year-old man presented with a 10-day history of weeping dermatitis affecting the perianal skin, buttocks, and proximal thighs (6). He had used Proctosedyl ointment topically for the preceding 3 weeks. Proctosedyl is an over-the-counter topical formulation for use as an antihemorrhoidal agent. It contains cinchocaine 5%, hydrocortisone, and lanolin. Patch testing was strongly positive to cinchocaine.

The authors highlighted the potential limitations of the International Contact Dermatitis Research Group (ICDRG) standard series for topical anesthetics. Benzocaine is the only topical anesthetic in the series and it will not detect contact allergy to amide agents; cross-sensitivity can also exist. They suggested that patch testing should include agents from both groups.

DoloPosterine N is an ointment for topical application in the treatment of hemorrhoids. Its active ingredient is cinchocaine. Although cinchocaine is a known contact sensitizer, as described above, systemic contact dermatitis is rare.

- A 62-year-old woman, who had applied DoloPosterine N ointment topically to the perianal skin and rectal mucosa for several days, developed erythematous vesicular lesions in the perianal area and an erythematous edematous rash of the face, axillae, elbow flexures, and inner thighs (7). This abated on withdrawal of the drug and the administration of oral prednisolone for 10 days. Patch testing was positive with cinchocaine.

Immunologic

An anaphylactic reaction to cinchocaine has been described.

- A 71-year-old man received intrathecal anesthesia using 0.3% cinchocaine 2 ml for a transurethral prostatectomy (8). He had a history of allergic rhinitis, and 2 months before had had an uneventful prostate biopsy and cystoscopy, also under spinal anesthesia with isobaric bupivacaine. Within 45 minutes of the spinal injection he complained of periorbital itching, started to shake, and developed muscle rigidity. He rapidly became unconscious, with a systolic blood pressure of 40 mmHg and widespread erythema. He was treated with hydrocortisone and antihistamines and required an infusion of adrenaline. Intradermal testing after full recovery was positive with cinchocaine.

Death

Three deaths after seizures and cardiac arrest have been reported in toddlers who accidentally ingested small amounts of cinchocaine (SEDA-21, 135).

References

1. Ogawa S, Mikuni E, Nakamura T, Noda K, Ito S. [Neurotoxicity of dibucaine on the isolated rabbit cervical vagus nerve.] Masui 1998;47(4):439–46.
2. Yorozu T, Matsumoto M, Hayashi S, Yamada T, Nakaohji T, Nakatsuka I. [Dibucaine for spinal anesthesia is a probable risk for cauda equina syndrome.] Masui 2002;51(10):1151–4.
3. Peerschke EI. Platelet membrane alterations induced by the local anesthetic dibucaine. Blood 1986;68(2):463–71.
4. Lee AY. Allergic contact dermatitis from dibucaine in Proctosedyl ointment without cross-sensitivity. Contact Dermatitis 1998;39(5):261.
5. Hayashi K, Kawachi S, Saida T. Allergic contact dermatitis due to both chlorpheniramine maleate and dibucaine hydrochloride in an over-the-counter medicament. Contact Dermatitis 2001;44(1):38–9.
6. Kearney CR, Fewings J. Allergic contact dermatitis to cinchocaine. Australas J Dermatol 2001;42(2):118–9.
7. Erdmann SM, Sachs B, Merk HF. Systemic contact dermatitis from cinchocaine. Contact Dermatitis 2001;44(4):260–1.
8. Mizuno Y, Esaki Y, Kato H. [Anaphylactoid reaction to dibucaine during spinal anesthesia.] Masui 2002;51(11):1254–6.

Cocaine

General Information

Cocaine was the first aminoester local anesthetic, and its adverse effects differ from those of other local anesthetics. Owing to its rapid absorption by mucous membranes, cocaine applied topically can cause systemic toxic effects. There is a wide variation in the rate and amount of cocaine that is systemically absorbed. This variability can be affected by the type and concentration of vasoconstrictor used with cocaine and also accounts for the differences in cocaine pharmacokinetics in cocaine abusers (SEDA-20, 128).

As a recreational drug cocaine can be snorted (sniffed), swallowed, injected, or smoked. The street drug comes in the form of a white powder, cocaine hydrochloride. The hydrochloride salt and the cutting agents are removed to create the free base, which is smoked. The inexpensive widely available crack formulation is prepared by alkalinizing cocaine hydrochloride and precipitating the resultant alkaloidal free-base cocaine, which, unlike the hydrochloride, is not destroyed by heat when smoked. Smoking crack provides a rapid effect, comparable to that of intravenous injection. Intense euphoria, followed within minutes by dysphoria, leads to frequent dosing and a greater potential for rapid addiction (1). As with amphetamines, the euphoric effect can enhance craving, and repeated reinforcement can lead to conditioned drug responses, which facilitate dependence. Facilitated conditioned effects with cocaine may be due to its rapid elimination and the development of acute tolerance. Frequent repeated dosing becomes necessary to sustain euphoria, thereby promoting a tight temporal juxtaposition of euphoria with recent drug-taking (2).

Rapid intravenous or inhalational administration of cocaine can cause very high concentrations in areas of high vascular perfusion, for example the heart and brain, before eventual distribution to other tissues. Under these conditions there is a catecholaminergic storm in the heart and a local anesthetic effect, with prolongation of conduction. Once beyond the immediate period of vulnerability, accumulation (for example through frequent overdosing or accidents from body packing of condom-filled stimulants to avoid detection) leads to a different cascade of events over a period of hours, leading to death. This cascade includes a catecholaminergic hypermetabolic state, with hyperpyrexia and acidosis, anorexia, and repeated seizures, usually ending in cardiac collapse (3,4). On the other hand, chronic dosing can cause catecholaminergic cardiomyopathy, for example contraction bands, cardiomegaly (5,6), and repeated vasospastic insults to cerebral and coronary arteries (7). Whether these chronic effects predispose to increased sensitivity to acute toxicity has not been systematically explored, but autopsy studies suggest that they do.

In addition to other chronic changes in abusers, personality deterioration carries a significant association with high-risk behaviors, which are a source of physical and psychiatric morbidity and mortality. These include suicide, violent trauma and aggressive behavior, high-risk methods of drug use (for example needle sharing), and high-risk sexual behavior, with increased risks of HIV, hepatitis B, and other infections.

The stimulant properties of cocaine are similar to those of amphetamines, although the differences are notable, in part because of the very short half-life of cocaine. However, cocaine has the same problem of abuse potential as other stimulants, and at high doses causes stimulant psychosis (8). In addition, even when it is used as a local nasopharyngeal anesthetic, it has toxic, even fatal, effects in high doses.

Death from cocaine often occurs within 2–3 minutes, suggesting direct cardiac toxicity, fatal dysrhythmias, and depression of medullary respiratory centers as common causes of death (9,10). Thus, cocaine's local anesthetic properties can contribute additional hazards when high doses are used, reminiscent of deaths reported in the era when it was used as a mucous membrane paste for nasopharyngeal surgery (11).

Periods of increased cocaine use, especially intravenous administration, inhalation of the free base, and high-dose use, are associated with cocaine-related deaths. For example, according to the Drug Abuse Warning Network, there was a three-fold increase in such deaths from 195 to 580 per year in the USA between 1981 and 1985. Despite the importance of these mortality data, relatively little is known of the types of pathophysiological sequences involved in the cascade of events leading to death. More important, there is a paucity of guidelines to appropriate diagnostic and treatment strategies for the various prefatal conditions.

As a general rule, mortality is higher when cocaine is used intravenously or as smoked free base than if taken nasally or orally (12). The symptoms of acute cocaine poisoning include agitation, sweating, tachycardia, tonic-clonic seizures, severe respiratory and metabolic acidosis, apnea, and ventricular dysrhythmias. Seizures occur at high doses, and may be a major determinant of fatal outcomes; their control with sedatives is important to reduce lethality (13). Associated hyperthermia can contribute as a primary cause in cases of fatal hyperpyrexia, and can potentiate the hypoxic cardiovascular events in cardiac deaths in those who survive the initial acute dose (14,15). A study of a very large number of cocaine deaths showed that the morbidity rate increased by four times on days on which the ambient temperature rose above 31.1°C (16). The final agonal events in cocaine deaths involve the combination of sympathomimetic myocardial responses and/or cardiac conduction slowing, secondary to cocaine's local anesthetic effect, leading to dysrhythmias (17). In reported fatal overdoses, convulsions and death have usually occurred within minutes. Most patients who have survived for the first 3 hours after an initial acute overdose have been likely to recover. Treatment includes respiratory and cardiovascular resuscitative measures. Short-acting barbiturates, benzodiazepines, beta-blockers, and phentolamine have all been used with some success (28,18). Because of a possible risk of coronary vasodilatation with the use of propranolol to manage dysrhythmias in cocaine overdose, the use of labetalol for this indication is recommended, if a beta-blocker is required (19,20). In one study of 60 cocaine-related deaths, autopsy findings were non-specific but typical of those found in respiratory depression of central origin (21).

Cardiovascular

Cardiovascular effects include tachycardia, hypertension, and increased cardiac irritability; large intravenous doses can cause cardiac failure. Cardiac dysrhythmias have been ascribed to a direct toxic effect of cocaine and a secondary sensitization of ventricular tissue to catecholamines (22), along with slowed cardiac conduction secondary to local anesthetic effects. Myocardial infarction has increased as a complication of cocaine abuse (5,6). Dilated cardiomyopathies, with subsequent recurrent myocardial infarction, have been associated with long-term use of cocaine, raising the possibility of chronic effects on the heart (23). Many victims have evidence of pre-existing fixed coronary artery disease precipitated by cocaine (SEDA-9, 35) (24–26). However, myocardial infarction has been noted even in young intranasal users with no evidence of coronary disease (27), defined by autopsy or angiography (28,29). If applied to mucous membranes, cocaine causes local vasoconstriction, and, with chronic use, necrosis.

Cardiovascular effects due to enhanced sympathetic activity include tachycardia, increased cardiac output, vasoconstriction, and increased arterial pressure. Myocardial infarction is the most common adverse cardiac effect (30), and there is an increased risk of myocardial depression when amide-type local anesthetics, such as bupivacaine, levobupivacaine, lidocaine, or ropivacaine are administered with antidysrhythmic drugs.

- A woman who inappropriately used cocaine on the nasal mucosa to treat epistaxis had a myocardial infarction (31).
- A patient who was treated with intranasal cocaine and phenylephrine during a general anesthetic had a myocardial infarction and a cardiac arrest due to ventricular fibrillation (SEDA-20, 128).
- Myocardial ischemia was reported in a fit 29-year-old patient after the nasal application of cocaine for surgery. No relief was gained from vasodilators or intracoronary verapamil, and there were no other signs of cocaine toxicity. Although coronary vasoconstriction and platelet activation are systemic effects of cocaine, pre-existing thrombus may also have played a part (SEDA-22, 142).

Previous cocaine abuse has also been implicated in increasing the risk of myocardial ischemia when other local anesthetics are used.

Cardiac dysrhythmias have also been described in patients after the use of topical cocaine for nasal surgery (SEDA-20, 128).

- A patient who was treated with intranasal cocaine and submucosal lidocaine during general anesthesia developed ventricular fibrillation (SEDA-17, 142).

These events do not appear to have been related to the concomitant use of a vasoconstrictor, but more to excessive doses of cocaine.

Substantial systemic absorption of cocaine can cause severe cardiovascular complications (32).

- An 18-year-old man had both nasal cavities prepared with a pack soaked in 3–5 ml of Brompton solution (3% cocaine, about 3 mg/kg, plus adrenaline 1:4000) 2 hours preoperatively. In the anesthetic room he was anxious and withdrawn, with a mild tachycardia. Ten minutes later the nasal pack was removed and polypectomy was begun, with immediate sinus tachycardia and marked ST depression on lead II of the electrocardiogram. Increasing the depth of anesthesia and giving fentanyl had little effect, and the procedure was terminated. After extubation a further electrocardiogram showed T wave flattening in leads II, III, aVF, and aVL. Further cardiac investigations ruled out a myocardial infarction, an anatomical defect, or other pathological or metabolic processes. On day 4 a stress electrocardiogram showed no ischemic changes.

Absorption of cocaine from the nasal mucosa in eight patients using cotton pledglets soaked in 4 ml of 4% cocaine and applied for 10 or 20 minutes resulted in an absorption rate four times higher than expected, but was not associated with any cardiovascular disturbance; however, one of four patients who received 4 ml of 10% cocaine for 20 minutes developed intraoperative hypertension and another transient ventricular tachycardia (33). The authors advised against topical use of 10% cocaine.

Nervous system

Genitoperineal numbness has been described after recreational use of cocaine per rectum (34).

- A 42-year-old man developed numbness of the penis and scrotum, with altered anal sphincter sensation, 2 hours after using cocaine per rectum. His symptoms resolved spontaneously within 4 hours.

The authors suggested that the per rectum route had resulted in anesthesia of the pudendal nerve, and that circulatory vasoconstriction may also have played a part in causing these symptoms.

Sexual function

Superficial penile necrosis has been reported after topical application of cocaine (35).

- A 32-year-old man developed black painful lesions over his penis after applying cocaine to the glans penis 5 days before. He was given antibiotics and the lesions healed completely.

The authors suggested that the necrotic lesions had been secondary to dermal vasoconstriction caused by cocaine.

For a complete review of the adverse effects of cocaine as a drug of abuse, see SED-15, pp. 848–79.

References

1 Gawin FH, Ellinwood EH Jr. Cocaine and other stimulants. Actions, Abuse, Treatment. N Engl J Med 1988;318(18):1173–82.

2 Clayton RR. Cocaine use in the United States: in a blizzard or just being snowed? NIDA Res Monogr 1985;61:8–34.

3 Stein R, Ellinwood EH Jr. Medical complication of cocaine abuse. Drug Ther 1990;10:40.

4 Lathers CM, Tyau LS, Spino MM, Agarwal I. Cocaine-induced seizures, arrhythmias and sudden death. J Clin Pharmacol 1988;28(7):584–93.

5 Karch SB, Billingham ME. The pathology and etiology of cocaine-induced heart disease. Arch Pathol Lab Med 1988;112(3):225–30.

6 Jiang JP, Downing SE. Catecholamine cardiomyopathy: review and analysis of pathogenetic mechanisms. Yale J Biol Med 1990;63(6):581–91.

7 Hong R, Matsuyama E, Nur K. Cardiomyopathy associated with the smoking of crystal methamphetamine. JAMA 1991;265(9):1152–4.

8 Ellinwood EH Jr, Petrie WM. Dependence on amphetamine, cocaine, and other stimulants. In: Pradhan SN, editor. Drug Abuse: Clinical and Basic Aspects. New York: CV: Mosby, 1977:248.

9 Barinerd H, Krupp M, Chatton J, et al. Current Medical Diagnosis and Treatment. Los Altos CA: Lange. Medical Publishers;. 1970.

10 Moe GK, Akildskov JA. Antiarrhythmic drugs. In: Gilman AG, Goodman LS, editors. The Pharmacological Basis of Therapeutics. New York: MacMillan, 1970:43.

11 Ellinwood EH Jr, Petrie WM. Drug induced psychoses. In: Pickens RW, Heston LL, editors. Psychiatric Factors in Drug Abuse. New York: Grune & Stratton, 1979:301.

12 Stark TW, Pruet CW, Stark DU. Cocaine toxicity. Ear Nose Throat J 1983;62(3):155–8.

13 Jonsson S, O'Meara M, Young JB. Acute cocaine poisoning. Importance of treating seizures and acidosis. Am J Med 1983;75(6):1061–4.

14 Catravas JD, Waters IW. Acute cocaine intoxication in the conscious dog: studies on the mechanism of lethality. J Pharmacol Exp Ther 1981;217(2):350–6.

15 Covino BG, Vasalla HG. In: Local Anesthetics: Mechanism of Action and Clinical Use. New York: Grune and Stratton, 1976:127.

16 Marzuk PM, Tardiff K, Leon AC, Hirsch CS, Portera L, Iqbal MI, Nock MK, Hartwell N. Ambient temperature and mortality from unintentional cocaine overdose. JAMA 1998;279(22):1795–800.

17 Jaffe JH. Drug Addiction and Drug Abuse. In: Gilman AG, Goodman LS, Rall TW, Murad F, editors. The Pharmacological Basis of Therapeutics. 7th edn.. New York: McMillan, 1985:54.

18 Hollander JE, Carter WA, Hoffman RS. Use of phentolamine for cocaine-induced myocardial ischemia. N Engl J Med 1992;327(5):361.

19 Lange RA, Cigarroa RG, Flores ED, McBride W, Kim AS, Wells PJ, Bedotto JB, Danziger RS, Hillis LD. Potentiation of cocaine-induced coronary vasoconstriction by beta-adrenergic blockade. Ann Intern Med 1990;112(12):897–903.

20 Boehrer JD, Moliterno DJ, Willard JE, Hillis LD, Lange RA. Influence of labetalol on cocaine-induced coronary vasoconstriction in humans. Am J Med 1993;94(6):608–10.

21 Mittleman RE, Wetli CV. Death caused by recreational cocaine use. An update. JAMA 1984;252(14):1889–93.

22 Nanji AA, Filipenko JD. Asystole and ventricular fibrillation associated with cocaine intoxication. Chest 1984;85(1):132–3.

23 Wiener RS, Lockhart JT, Schwartz RG. Dilated cardiomyopathy and cocaine abuse. Report of two cases. Am J Med 1986;81(4):699–701.

24 Wodarz N, Boning J. "Ecstasy"-induziertes psychotisches Depersonalisationssyndrom. ["Ecstasy"-induced psychotic depersonalization syndrome.] Nervenarzt 1993;64(7):478–80.

25 McCann UD, Ricaurte GA. MDMA ("ecstasy") and panic disorder: induction by a single dose. Biol Psychiatry 1992;32(10):950–3.

26 Williams H, Meagher D, Galligan P. MDMA. ("Ecstasy"); a case of possible drug-induced psychosis. Ir J Med Sci 1993;162(2):43–4.

27 Isner JM, Estes NA 3rd, Thompson PD, Costanzo-Nordin MR, Subramanian R, Miller G, Katsas GSweeney K, Sturner WQ. Acute cardiac events temporally related to cocaine abuse. N Engl J Med 1986;315(23): 1438–43.

28 Minor RL Jr, Scott BD, Brown DD, Winniford MD. Cocaine-induced myocardial infarction in patients with normal coronary arteries. Ann Intern Med 1991;115(10):797–806.

29 Virmani R. Cocaine-associated cardiovascular disease: clinical and pathological aspects. NIDA Res Monogr 1991;108:220–9.

30 Sofuoglu M, Nelson D, Dudish-Poulsen S, Lexau B, Pentel PR, Hatsukami DK. Predictors of cardiovascular response to smoked cocaine in humans. Drug Alcohol Depend 2000;57(3):239–45.

31 Tanenbaum JH, Miller F. Electrocardiographic evidence of myocardial injury in psychiatrically hospitalized cocaine abusers. Gen Hosp Psychiatry 1992;14(3):201–3.

32 Laffey JG, Neligan P, Ormonde G. Prolonged perioperative myocardial ischemia in a young male: due to topical intranasal cocaine? J Clin Anesth 1999;11(5):419–24.

33 Liao BS, Hilsinger RL Jr, Rasgon BM, Matsuoka K, Adour KK. A preliminary study of cocaine absorption from the nasal mucosa. Laryngoscope 1999;109(1):98–102.

34 Davidson JA, Isaacs RA. A novel case of numb bum. Eur J Emerg Med 2004;11(5):285–6.

35 Carey F, Dinsmore WW. Cocaine-induced penile necrosis. Int J STD AIDS 2004;15(6):424–5.

Etidocaine

General Information

Etidocaine is a highly lipid-soluble, long-acting aminoamide. It has a similar toxicity profile to that of bupivacaine and there is an increased risk of life-threatening cardiac events compared with lidocaine (1).

Reference

1. Bacsik CJ, Swift JQ, Havgreaves KM. Toxic systemic reactions of bupivacaine and etidocaine. Oral Surg Oral Med Oral Pathol Oral Radiol Endod 1995;79(1):18–23.

Levobupivacaine

General Information

Levobupivacaine is the levorotatory isomer, $S(-)$-bupivacaine, of bupivacaine, an amide local anesthetic.

In a comparison of the clinical efficacy of epidural $S(-)$-bupivacaine with standard racemic RS-bupivacaine in 88 patients $S(-)$-bupivacaine was clinically indistinguishable from RS-bupivacaine in the three groups studied (0.75% or 0.5% $S(-)$-bupivacaine and 0.5% RS-bupivacaine). Hypotension was distributed evenly across the groups and five patients complained of minor neurological abnormalities (hypesthesia and paresthesia), which resolved quickly after the operation (1).

Organs and Systems

Cardiovascular

Levobupivacaine is less cardiotoxic than racemic bupivacaine (2). In seven sheep, racemic bupivacaine caused mild cardiac depression, which was superseded by central nervous system toxicity and then proceeded to severe ventricular dysrhythmias, which were fatal in three sheep, at doses of 125, 150, and 200 mg (3). Levobupivacaine was consistently less toxic than bupivacaine, and higher doses were needed to produce adverse effects. Convulsions were less severe and of shorter duration, and although levobupivacaine produced QRS prolongation and ventricular dysrhythmias, there were no deaths.

Several animal studies have shown that levobupivacaine on an equivalent dose basis is safer than bupivacaine; 32–57% more levobupivacaine is required to cause death (4). In sheep, the mean lethal dose of levobupivacaine was 78% higher than that of bupivacaine; the author suggested that there may be a similar trend in humans and concluded that levobupivacaine should be used in preference to bupivacaine, based on safety data alone.

Nervous system

Tonic-clonic seizures have been attributed to levobupivacaine.

- A 60-year-old 70 kg woman with a fractured radius had an axillary brachial plexus block for postoperative analgesia after uneventful general anesthesia (5). A 50 mm insulated regional block needle attached to a nerve stimulator was used to locate the brachial plexus, and after negative aspiration, levobupivacaine 125 mg was injected with intermittent aspiration. Within 30 seconds the patient had a generalized tonic-clonic seizure which lasted about 30 seconds and self-terminated. She remained cardiovascularly stable and made an uneventful recovery.

The authors proposed that some or all of the local anesthetic had been inadvertently injected intravascularly, despite negative aspiration tests. There were no cardiovascular complications, underlining the proposed greater cardiovascular safety of levobupivacaine over bupivacaine. The authors accepted that if the patient had been awake during the procedure, earlier detection of neurological symptoms might have been possible.

- A 71-year-old woman presented for elective total knee arthroplasty under combined lumbar plexus and sciatic nerve block. After midazolam and fentanyl sedation a lumbar plexus block was performed with 30 ml of levobupivacaine 0.5% and adrenaline 2.5 micrograms/ml. Slow injection of levobupivacaine with repeated negative aspiration of blood was performed over 90 seconds. She had a tonic–clonic seizure within 1 minute of injection. She was given thiopental, midazolam, and suxamethonium and was intubated and ventilated. There were no cardiovascular problems, surgery was completed, and she made a full recovery.

Postoperatively she had sensory and motor blockade in the distribution of the lumbar plexus.

- A 66-year-old man scheduled for total hip arthroplasty under general anesthesia had a lumbar plexus block performed after sedation with midazolam and fentanyl. He was in the lateral position and received 35 ml of levobupivacaine 0.5% with adrenaline 2 micrograms/ml over 90 seconds with aspiration every 5 ml. Immediately after the end of the injection he had a tonic–clonic seizure, which was terminated by intravenous thiopental 75 mg. There were no further adverse events and he underwent the planned procedure under general anesthesia and had an unremarkable postoperative course. Postoperatively he had a motor and sensory block in the distribution of the lumbar plexus.

In a similar report tonic–clonic seizures after interscalene brachial plexus block have been described (6).

- A 27-year-old woman was given 30 ml of levobupivacaine for shoulder surgery, with no evidence of blood or CSF aspiration at any time during the injection. Her seizure activity ended after 2 minutes and after the administration of midazolam 2 mg. She remained cardiovascularly stable throughout the procedure with no electrocardiographic disturbance. Despite signs of pulmonary edema postoperatively, she made a full recovery and was discharged the following morning.

Although it is well-known that tonic–clonic seizures can occur as a result of toxic effects of other local anesthetics, including bupivacaine and ropivacaine, these are the first reports of seizures after levobupivacaine. The authors concluded that in view of the rapid onset of seizure activity there was probably inadvertent intravascular injection of local anesthetic in all three cases. This was despite slow injection, careful attention to aspiration, and the addition of adrenaline as a marker of intravascular injection. None of the patients developed any dysrhythmias or cardiovascular changes attributable to local anesthetic toxicity.

These case reports are in line with previous descriptions of toxic effects of single enantiomers of local anesthetics, in which nervous system manifestations are predominant and cardiovascular collapse is rare. In a volunteer study ropivacaine and levobupivacaine had similar nervous system and cardiovascular effects after deliberate intravenous infusion (7).

Hematologic

The effects of the low molecular weight heparin enoxaparin in combination with levobupivacaine on coagulation have been studied in vitro (8). Whole blood from 10 patients treated with enoxaparin was mixed with levobupivacaine to concentrations of 2.5 µg/ml and 2.5 mg/ml, followed by thromboelastography. Levobupivacaine produced a dose-dependent reduction in clotting. The clinical implications of these findings are yet to be acknowledged; larger, in vivo studies are required.

Drug Administration

Drug overdose

Successful resuscitation after accidental intravenous infusion of levobupivacaine has been described.

- A 63-year-old man with localized prostate cancer scheduled for brachytherapy received an infusion of levobupivacaine 100 ml (125 mg) instead of an antibiotic after intravenous induction (9). He developed severe hypotension and bradycardia without a recordable blood pressure and was treated with boluses of adrenaline. Later he developed a supraventricular tachycardia, nodal rhythm, and ST changes. He was extubated uneventfully and his postoperative electrocardiogram and troponin were normal. The arterial levobupivacaine concentrations were 1.74 µg/ml after 40 minutes of infusion, 0.81 µg/ml at 100 minutes, and 0.61 µg/ml at 160 minutes.

The packaging of the intended antibiotic and L-bupivacaine were similar. This illustrates the value of having clearly identifiable packaging and color coding of giving sets and pumps.

References

1. Cox CR, Faccenda KA, Gilhooly C, Bannister J, Scott NB, Morrison LM. Extradural S(−)-bupivacaine: comparison with racemic RS-bupivacaine. Br J Anaesth 1998;80(3):289–93.
2. Thomas JM, Schug SA. Recent advances in the pharmacokinetics of local anaesthetics. Long-acting amide enantiomers and continuous infusions. Clin Pharmacokinet 1999;36(1):67–83.
3. Huang YF, Pryor ME, Mather LE, Veering BT. Cardiovascular and central nervous system effects of intravenous levobupivacaine and bupivacaine in sheep. Anesth Analg 1998;86(4):797–804.
4. Gristwood RW. Cardiac and CNS toxicity of levobupivacaine: strengths of evidence for advantage over bupivacaine. Drug Saf 2002;25(3):153–63.
5. Pirotta D, Sprigge J. Convulsions following axillary brachial plexus blockade with levobupivacaine. Anaesthesia 2002;57(12):1187–9.
6. Crews JC, Rothman TE. Seizure after levobupivacaine for interscalene brachial plexus block. Anesth Analg 2003;96:1188–90.
7. Stewart J, Kellett N, Castro D. The central nervous system and cardiovascular effects of levobupivacaine and ropivacaine in healthy volunteers. Anesth Analg 2003;97:412–16.
8. Leonard SA, Lydon A, Walsh M, Fleming C, Boylan J, Shorten GD. Does prior administration of enoxaparin influence the effects of levobupivacaine on blood clotting? Assessment using the Thrombelastograph. Br J Anaesth 2001;86(6):808–13.
9. Salomaki TE, Laurila PA, Ville J. Successful resuscitation after cardiovascular collapse following accidental intravenous infusion of levobupivacaine during general anesthesia. Anesthesiology 2005;103(5):1095–6.

Lidocaine

General Information

Lidocaine is the most widely used aminoamide local anesthetic agent, with a low toxic potential; its effects are mostly typical for this class of drug. It can be given by injection or topically and is also combined with prilocaine in Emla for topical administration. It is also used as an antidysrhythmic drug and has occasionally been used in other conditions, such as multiple sclerosis, chronic daily headache, migraine and cluster headaches, and neuropathic pain, such as postherpetic neuralgia.

Local anesthetic gels and creams used liberally on traumatized epithelium can be rapidly absorbed, resulting in systemic effects, such as convulsions, particularly if excessive quantities are used. This has been highlighted in the case of a 40-year-old woman who developed seizures after lidocaine gel 40 ml was injected into the ureter during an attempt to remove a stone (1). Site of administration is also important, as local conditions, particularly vascularity, affect the rate of absorption. Adverse effects of lidocaine when it is used as a local anesthetic can also occur after inadvertent intravascular injection.

The incidence of adverse effects to lidocaine in antidysrhythmic dosages is low. In one series of 750 patients given lidocaine intravenously for cardiac dysrhythmias, adverse reactions occurred in only 47 (6.3%) and were thought to have been life-threatening in 12 (1.6%) (2). However, the risk of adverse effects is dose-related and increases at intravenous infusion rates of around 3 mg/minute (3). Most of the adverse effects are on the cardiovascular and central nervous systems. Nervous system toxicity is directly related to blood concentrations, with symptoms that include lightheadedness, headache, dizziness, tremor, confusion, tinnitus, dysarthria, paresthesia, alterations in the level of consciousness from drowsiness to coma, respiratory depression, and convulsions. Cardiovascular effects, including dysrhythmias and very rarely worsening of cardiac function, only occur at very high blood concentrations. The intravenous dose of lidocaine required to produce cardiovascular collapse is seven times that which causes seizures. Risks of serious systemic effects do not increase with age. Deaths have occurred with voluntary intoxication, primarily because of the cardiac effects.

The active metabolites of lidocaine, glycinexylidide and monoethylglycinexylidide, are toxic and intravenous infusion should not continue for more than 24–48 hours.

Hypersensitivity reactions are rare, and not all reports are clear, but cases do occur and are usually mild (SED-12, 255) (4). Some patients are highly sensitive to lidocaine, yet insensitive to other aminoamide local anesthetics (5), and the reverse has also been found (SEDA-14, 109). True anaphylaxis with rechallenge has been documented (6). A few cases of contact dermatitis have been reported.

Even topical administration of lidocaine continues to generate reports with tragic outcomes, as absorption from mucosal surfaces is underestimated.

- A patient due to have a bronchoscopy was given an overdose of lidocaine to anesthetize the airway by an inexperienced health worker. He was then left unobserved and subsequently developed convulsions and cardiopulmonary arrest (7). He survived with severe cerebral damage.

His lidocaine concentration was 24 μg/ml about 1 hour after initial administration (a blood concentration over 6 μg/ml is considered to be toxic).

Drug studies

Lidocaine has been used to treat some of the symptoms of multiple sclerosis in 30 patients with painful tonic seizures, attacks of neuralgia, paroxysmal itching, and Lhermitte's sign (8). Lidocaine was given by intravenous infusion for 5.5 hours in a maintenance dose of 2.0–2.8 mg/kg/hour after a loading dose, and the mean steady-state concentration was 2.4 μg/ml. Lidocaine almost completely abolished the paroxysmal symptoms and markedly alleviated the persistent symptoms of multiple sclerosis. Adverse effects were not specifically mentioned, but in one case, when the plasma concentration of lidocaine rose above 3.5 μg/ml, weakness of the left leg became marked and was associated with an extensor plantar response; this disappeared when the lidocaine was replaced by saline single-blind, but subsequently the positive symptoms recurred.

Intravenous lidocaine has been used to treat severe chronic daily headache in 19 patients (three men, median age 37 years) (9). There were adverse effects during four infusions of lidocaine: hyperkalemia (6.4 mmol/l), which did not resolve after withdrawal of lidocaine; transient hypotension (75/50 mmHg), which was attributed to concomitant droperidol; an unspecified abnormality of cardiac rhythm and on another occasion a transient bradycardia; and chest pain with a normal electrocardiogram, fever, and intractable nausea. The study was neither randomized nor placebo-controlled, and in no case was the adverse event strongly associated with the administration of lidocaine.

In a double-blind, placebo-controlled study of the use of intravenous lidocaine for neuropathic pain, 16 patients were given 5 ml/kg intravenously over 30 minutes (10). Lidocaine was better than placebo in relieving pain. The major adverse effect was light-headedness, which occurred in seven patients given lidocaine and none given saline. Other adverse effects included somnolence, nausea and vomiting, dysarthria or garbled speech, blurred vision, and malaise. In two patients the rate of infusion had to be reduced because of adverse effects.

Organs and Systems

Cardiovascular

Lidocaine can cause dysrhythmias and hypotension. The dysrhythmias that have been reported include sinus bradycardia, supraventricular tachycardia (11), and rarely torsade de pointes (12). There have also been rare reports of cardiac arrest (2) and worsening heart failure (13). Lidocaine can also cause an increased risk of asystole after repeated attempts at defibrillation (14). Lidocaine may increase mortality after acute myocardial infarction, and it should be used only in patients with specific so-called warning dysrhythmias (that is frequent or multifocal ventricular extra beats, or salvos) (15).

Sinus bradycardia has been seen after a bolus injection of 50 mg, atrioventricular block after a dose of 800 mg given over 12 hours, and left bundle branch block after a mere subconjunctival injection of 2% lidocaine.

- High-grade atrioventricular block has been reported in a 14-day-old infant who was given lidocaine 2 mg/kg intravenously (SED-12, 255) (16).

A death due to ventricular fibrillation after 50 mg and another due to sinus arrest after 100 mg have been reported (SED-12, 255) (17). Two cases of ventricular fibrillation and cardiopulmonary arrest occurred after local infiltration of lidocaine for cardiac catheterization (SEDA-21, 136).

Lidocaine does not usually cause conduction disturbances, but two cases have been reported in the presence of hyperkalemia (18).

- A 57-year-old man with a wide-complex tachycardia was given lidocaine 100 mg intravenously and immediately became asystolic. Resuscitation was unsuccessful.
- A 31-year-old woman had a cardiac arrest and was resuscitated to a wide-complex tachycardia, which was treated with intravenous lidocaine 100 mg. She immediately became asystolic but responded to calcium chloride.

In both cases there was severe hyperkalemia, and the authors suggested that hyperkalemia-induced resting membrane depolarization had increased the number of inactivated sodium channels, thus increasing the binding of lidocaine and potentiating its effects.

The degree of hypotension occurring after epidural anesthesia with alkalinized lidocaine (with adrenaline) was greater than with a standard commercial solution (SED-12, 255) (19).

In 23 patients there was a significant dose-dependent reduction in blood pressure following submucosal infiltration of lidocaine plus adrenaline compared with saline plus adrenaline for orthognathic surgery (20). The study was randomized but small; larger studies are needed to confirm effects that could easily have been due to multifactorial causes in patients undergoing general anesthesia.

There have been two reports of lidocaine-induced vasospasm after intra-arterial injection to overcome constriction of a brachial artery after vascular surgical repair and after digital nerve block for hand surgery (21). While this sounds paradoxical, the authors pointed out that local anesthetics regulate vascular tension in a biphasic manner, and that lower concentrations cause vasoconstriction.

Respiratory

Topical anesthesia of the airways is commonly used to facilitate endoscopy and sometimes manipulation of the airways. This can result in an increase in airway flow resistance, possibly due to laryngeal dysfunction (22). Lidocaine spray 10%, used for upper airways anesthesia for fiberoptic intubation in a grossly obese patient, caused acute airway obstruction. The patient went on to have a percutaneous tracheotomy, and it was postulated that the local anesthetic had abolished laryngeal receptors responsible for airway maintenance, or that laryngospasm and reduced muscle tone due to the lidocaine might have been the cause (SEDA-22, 140).

Life-threatening bronchospasm can occur after either spinal or topical use of lidocaine. In one series of patients being treated with lidocaine spray 40 mg for persistent cough, there was an increase of airway resistance (SED-12, 255) (23).

Ear, nose, throat

Local anesthesia to the larynx, for example with 4% lidocaine, is generally safe. Laryngeal edema has been reported in a few cases and could be due to the propellant rather than to lidocaine itself (24).

Intranasal 4% lidocaine has been used for migraine and cluster headaches with success and few serious adverse effects: a bitter taste was common and some patients complained of nasal burning and oropharyngeal numbness (SEDA-20, 127).

Lidocaine gel is not recommended for lubrication of laryngeal masks. It confers no benefits and increases the incidence of adverse effects such as intraoperative hiccups, postoperative hoarseness, nausea, vomiting, and tongue paresthesia (25).

Nervous system

Nervous system toxicity is most often seen with rapid intravenous infusion (3,26,27). The effects include headache, dizziness, tremor, confusion, tinnitus, dysarthria,

paresthesia, respiratory depression, altered level of consciousness (from drowsiness to coma), and convulsions.

Two cases have illustrated the effects of lidocaine in precipitating partial seizures in patients with a previous history of epilepsy (28).

- A 36-year-old woman developed chest pain and ventricular tachycardia. She had a 14-year history ofsided focal motor seizures controlled with phenytoin. After receiving intravenous lidocaine 100 mg to treat the dysrhythmias, she developed a typical seizure involving the right side of her face and arm. She was given a loading dose of phenytoin and the seizure abated. However, the ventricular tachycardia persisted and was treated with additional lidocaine 50 mg followed by an infusion of 3.3 mg/minute; 6 hours later she had a generalized seizure with a venous blood lidocaine concentration of 21 µg/ml. The infusion was stopped and the seizure was treated with intravenous diazepam 10 mg.
- A 41-year-old woman with a long-standing history of focal and secondarily generalized seizures controlled with carbamazepine underwent cerebral arteriography, during which she was inadvertently given lidocaine 20 mg via an intra-arterial catheter in the right internal carotid artery; within 20 seconds she had a focal seizure.

These two patients had their typical partial seizures triggered by high doses of lidocaine. In both cases the serum concentrations of their usual anticonvulsants were initially low. The first patient received a loading dose of phenytoin after the partial seizure, was then given a second bolus of lidocaine and an infusion, and then had a second seizure, which was generalized. There was no evidence that this second seizure evolved from the left seizure focus. The authors concluded that lidocaine can activate seizure foci in patients with a history of partial seizures and that this may be more likely if the serum concentrations of anticonvulsants are low. However, therapeutic concentrations of antiepileptic drugs may not prevent generalized seizures that result from the widespread lowering of seizure threshold caused by high concentrations of lidocaine.

A tonic-clonic seizure occurred after the application of 400 mg of lidocaine jelly to traumatized ureteric mucosa (SEDA-22, 142).

- A 54-year-old woman who was given lidocaine, 200 mg intravenously, for ventricular fibrillation during cardiopulmonary bypass, had a tonic-clonic seizure (29). The seizure occurred immediately after the administration of lidocaine and was relieved by the intravenous administration of thiopental and midazolam. Her ventricular fibrillation responded to procainamide 1 g intravenously over 10 minutes.

The pharmacokinetics of lidocaine are altered by cardiopulmonary bypass, because of hemodilution, changed protein binding, the exclusion of the lungs as an organ for first-pass elimination, altered acid-base balance, and sometimes drug interactions. In particular, reduced protein binding may have contributed in this case to the risk of seizure, but plasma lidocaine concentrations were not measured.

- A 30-year-old woman received two 5 g applications of 40% lidocaine cream with occlusion by plastic wrap during and after laser therapy to areas of her skin (30). She developed dizziness and headache postoperatively, followed 45 minutes later by light-headedness, increasing dizziness, and confusion. The dressings were removed. The lidocaine concentration was 2.7 µg/ml 7 hours later.

It is recommended that repeat applications of lidocaine, especially in high-concentration formulations, be avoided and the area of application limited.

- A 16-year-old woman had had an adverse reaction after administration of an unknown local anesthetic agent for a dental procedure. Patch testing had elicited similar symptoms with lidocaine only, and 20 minutes after subcutaneous lidocaine 0.05 mg she developed perioral paresthesia, nausea, vomiting, vertigo, dizziness, mild agitation, drowsiness, and euphoria. Hemodynamic parameters remained stable but her symptoms were thought to be part of a genuine non-allergic, neuropsychiatric reaction, as the patch testing was double-blind and placebo-controlled (31).

Transient and permanent nerve damage can occur after regional anesthesia, particularly neuraxial anesthesia. The mechanism of this nerve damage is unclear. Some studies have shown an indirect effect. However, in crayfish giant axon, lidocaine had a dose- and time-dependent effect on isolated nerve function in vitro (32). At high concentrations lidocaine caused irreversible conduction block and total loss of resting membrane potential. These results in an isolated nerve suggest a direct neurotoxic effect of lidocaine.

Two cases of toxicity associated with excessive lidocaine concentrations during low-dose treatment in terminally ill patients have been reported (33).

- An 82-year-old woman with mucinous adenocarcinoma received intravenous lidocaine 300 mg/day for neuropathic pain. Her renal function and liver function were normal. After 2 days her pain was controlled, but 1 week later she developed severe somnolence. Her serum lidocaine concentration was 8.4 µg/ml. The symptoms were attributed to lidocaine, which was withdrawn. She improved the next day and was given an intravenous infusion of lidocaine 100 mg/day and achieved adequate pain control without any adverse effects.
- A 70-year-old woman with ovarian cancer was given a neurolytic mesenteric plexus block, NSAIDs, transdermal fentanyl 75 micrograms/hour, and intravenous morphine 80 mg/day. On day 100 intravenous lidocaine 200 mg/day was added for new neuropathic pain in the legs secondary to progressive intrapelvic tumor. One week later she became somnolent. Her serum lidocaine concentration was 8.4 µg/ml. Her renal and liver tests were normal. Lidocaine was withdrawn and 2 days later the somnolence disappeared without an increase in pain.

The authors suggested that measuring lidocaine concentrations helps to avoid toxicity in terminally ill patients, who seem to tolerate much lower daily doses.

A generalized seizure occurred after a 4.5 kg infant was given excess lidocaine 1% for dorsal penile nerve block performed for circumcision (34). The authors remarked on the extra care required when administering local anesthetics to infants, as the maximum safe doses are readily attained.

Euphoria in two cases was an early sign of lidocaine toxicity and preceded the development of classical early signs of local anesthetic neurotoxicity, such as tinnitus, diplopia, and tongue numbness (35).

Sensory systems

Tinnitus and visual disturbances are early components of a systemic toxic reaction to lidocaine.

Eyes

A potentially beneficial effect of lidocaine has been studied in a randomized, double-blind, placebo-controlled study of the effects of preinstillation of lidocaine on tropicamide-induced mydriasis (36). Pupillary diameter was significantly increased by the instillation of lidocaine before tropicamide. It was thought that lidocaine can enhance intraocular penetration and hence potentiate the effect of tropicamide.

Double vision and difficulty in focusing have been attributed to lidocaine applied to the tongue (37).

- A 22-year-old man developed double vision and difficulty in focusing after using 2% viscous lidocaine for a painful tongue ulcer. He used viscous 2% lidocaine 10 ml hourly and developed symptoms when the daily dose exceeded 240 ml (4800 mg of lidocaine hydrochloride) after 10 days of use. At that time his serum lidocaine concentration was 6.7 µg/ml. His symptoms persisted when the serum concentration of lidocaine fell to below toxic concentrations, implying that metabolites of lidocaine had contributed.

Temporary blindness, an unusual feature of lidocaine toxicity, has been reported in an otherwise healthy young woman (38).

- A 21-year-old 50 kg woman, previously fit, was to have an open reduction and fixation of a fractured proximal phalanx with intravenous regional anesthesia. As a result of misreading the vial label, 30 ml (600 mg) of 2% lidocaine was injected, and this inadvertent error was immediately recognized. The decision was made to continue with the procedure, which was uneventful, with a tourniquet time of 45 minutes. At this point the patient complained of severe tourniquet pain, and without the anesthesiologist's knowledge the cuff was deflated. Immediately she developed a tachycardia, complained of visual disturbances, and became unconscious. She had a seizure, which lasted 30 seconds and resolved with midazolam. She became more alert, but complained of reduced vision. Neurological examination was normal, apart from temporary blindness; this fully resolved within 10 minutes. There were no long-term neurological or visual sequelae.

The authors suggested that the visual symptoms could have occurred as a result of occipital lobe seizure activity or subcortical stimulation, due to the acute high cerebral concentration of lidocaine. The speed of spontaneous resolution was consistent with the pharmacokinetics of lidocaine.

Pupillary mydriasis occurred in a neonate who was given intravenous lidocaine 3 mg/kg/hour as an anticonvulsant (39).

Taste

Taste disturbance has been reported with lidocaine (40).

- A 73-year-old woman was given a Nadbath Rehman block behind the left pinna to provide motor blockade of cranial nerve VII, before retrobulbar block for cataract surgery. Several minutes later she complained of a metallic taste in her mouth. After surgery she had altered taste sensation on the anterior left side of the tongue, with recovery a day later.

The author postulated this to be due to block of the chorda tympani, which runs with cranial nerve VII close to the site of the Nadbath Rehman block.

Metabolism

High systemic doses of lidocaine can cause transient hypoglycemia (SED-12, 255) (41).

Electrolyte balance

There has been one report of hypokalemia (2.2 mmol/l), probably due to potassium channel blockade, after administration of high-dose intravenous lidocaine (8 mg/l) for raised intracranial pressure (SEDA-21, 136).

Hematologic

Severe thrombocytopenic purpura with a lidocaine-mediated antiplatelet IgM antibody has been reported (SED-12, 255) (42).

Three cases of lidocaine-induced methemoglobinemia have been reported in patients undergoing topical anesthesia of the airway and oropharynx (43).

- A 26-year-old woman undergoing bronchoscopy received lidocaine jelly 2% to each nostril, lidocaine solution 2% sprayed on the throat, and 10 ml of lidocaine solution 2% into the trachea. She was also given intravenous diazepam 5 mg and pethidine 75 mg and intramuscular atropine 0.6 mg. She developed dyspnea and cyanosis after the procedure and despite 100% oxygen, her SpO$_2$ was 85%. Her methemoglobin concentration was 14%.
- A 61-year-old woman was given 15 ml of lidocaine solution 2% and lidocaine spray 4% for topical anesthesia of the throat and oropharynx before upper gastrointestinal endoscopy. She was also sedated with intravenous midazolam 2 mg and pethidine 75 mg. She became cyanosed and desaturated (SpO$_2$ 78%)

immediately after the procedure. Her SpO$_2$ did not recover, despite 100% oxygen. Her methemoglobin concentration was 37%.
- In preparation for transesophageal echocardiogram, a 73-year-old woman was given 15 ml of lidocaine solution 2% and lidocaine spray 4% to anesthetize the oropharynx, plus intravenous midazolam 1 mg and pethidine 12.5 mg. She very rapidly became cyanosed, but remained asymptomatic. Her SpO$_2$ was 85% on oxygen 2 l/minute and her methemoglobin concentration was 25%.

Liver

Liver damage due to lidocaine has rarely been reported. However, severe liver damage has been reported shortly after the withdrawal of mexiletine 300 mg/day and the introduction of lidocaine 1000 mg/day, although lidocaine in the same dose had been used during the previous week (44). The lidocaine was withdrawn and the liver enzymes normalized after treatment with prednisolone.

Skin

Topical 5% lidocaine to 33 patients with postherpetic neuralgia in a crossover trial provided significantly more pain relief than a vehicle patch placebo (45). There was no difference in reported adverse effects: skin redness or rash was reported by 9 in the lidocaine patch phase and 11 in the placebo phase. One patient stopped using the placebo patch owing to red irritated skin, which resolved after the application of lidocaine patches.

Treatment of 27 HIV-infected patients with distal sensory polyneuropathy (the most common neurological disorder associated with HIV) with 5% lidocaine gel resulted in effective analgesia in 75% of patients; three had dry skin and one had blisters (46).

In a phase IV trial, 66% patients with postherpetic neuralgia gained relief from a 5% lidocaine patch applied to the most painful area of the body (47). The lidocaine patch was well tolerated, a rash being the most common adverse effect, in 14% of patients.

Several cases of contact dermatitis have been reported with lidocaine. Generalized exfoliative dermatitis has also been noted once. Local inflammation and necrosis, possibly due to mechanical pressure, are both complications at the injection site.

- A 60-year-old woman was given infiltration anesthesia with lidocaine hydrochloride for removal of a melanoma (48). She developed an itchy dermatitis over the area 36 hours later. Conventional patch testing was negative at 48 and 72 hours to lidocaine and mepivacaine (both amides), as was intracutaneous testing with lidocaine 2%, mepivacaine 2%, and bupivacaine 0.5%. However, intradermal testing at 1/100 dilutions was positive, with itching and erythema at 48 hours with lidocaine and mepivacaine, suggesting delayed hypersensitivity to these drugs, but not with bupivacaine.

It has previously been reported that lidocaine and mepivacaine have a high degree of cross-reactivity not seen with bupivacaine.

Sexual function

Two cases of impotence after anesthesia for elective circumcision in adults have been described (SED-12, 256) (49), but it is very doubtful whether this was a pharmacological and not merely a psychological effect.

Immunologic

There were 62 reports of allergic contact dermatitis to lidocaine worldwide between 1972 and 1996; 49 were in Australia and several showed cross-reactivity with other amide local anesthetics, such as bupivacaine, mepivacaine, and prilocaine (50).

Delayed-type hypersensitivity to lidocaine is rare; of 1883 patients patch tested for suspected contact type IV sensitivity, only four had positive reactions (51).

The predictability of allergy to local anesthetics still remains elusive, owing to its rarity. Hypersensitivity due to local anesthetics and its additives continues to be reported.

- A 63-year-old man without any known allergies developed pruritus, generalized urticaria, and dyspnea and collapsed after application of topical lidocaine gel in a dental clinic (52). After treatment a prick test, performed with various agents and components, turned positive for guar gum, which is included as a gelling agent in lidocaine gel. Total serum immunoglobulin E (IgE) was raised to 99.0 Ku/l but specific IgE to guar gum was negative.

This case highlights the importance of meticulous investigation and testing of all components of local anesthetics. The authors suggested that a possible explanation of the negative guar-specific IgE could have been a varying degree of contamination in guar products not detected by commercial highly purified assays.

Body temperature

There is no reliable evidence to support reports of malignant hyperthermia due to local anesthetic agents. In 307 dental patients susceptible to malignant hyperthermia who received local anesthesia, only one had ever developed symptoms suggestive of malignant hyperthermia, after mepivacaine and on another occasion lidocaine (53). Both reactions resolved without specific therapy. There has been one case report of cyanosis, muscle rigidity, tachycardia, tachypnea, a temperature of 41.5°C, and loss of consciousness in a patient who received epidural lidocaine and bupivacaine (54). However, perioperative stress may itself be a potential trigger of malignant hyperthermia.

Death

In New York City, five of 50 000 deaths over a 5-year period were associated with tumescent liposuction; all had received lidocaine in doses of 10–40 mg/kg in association with general anesthesia and/or intravenous sedation and analgesia (55). Three patients died as a result of severe acute intraoperative hypotension and bradycardia with no identified cause, one died of fluid overload, and another died of pulmonary embolism. The authors speculated that lidocaine toxicity or lidocaine-related drug interactions could have contributed to some of the deaths, but other causes could not be ruled out.

In California, six cases of cardiac arrest or severe hypoxemia associated with outpatient liposuction resulted in four deaths over a 3.5-year period, all in women aged 38–62 years; one had a cardiac arrest after sedation and the administration of local anesthetic but before liposuction was started, four had respiratory difficulties and cardiac arrest after liposuction, and one had respiratory difficulties during liposuction (56). Whether the cause of morbidity and mortality in any of these cases was related to local anesthetic toxicity was not mentioned.

A weak solution of lidocaine has sometimes been injected into excess fat before liposuction, so that the procedure can be carried out without general anesthesia. The technique is generally regarded as safe (57). However, deaths are increasingly reported, associated with local anesthetic toxicity or drug interactions (55).

A 19-year-old healthy volunteer undergoing bronchoscopy was given about 1200 mg of lidocaine to anesthetize the airway and was sent home after the procedure, despite complaining of chest pain. Shortly afterwards she had a tonic-clonic seizure and cardiopulmonary arrest and died 2 days later. The research protocol had failed to specify an upper dose limit for lidocaine (58).

Second-Generation Effects

Fetotoxicity

Because of rapid transfer across the placenta and the prolonged half-life of lidocaine in neonates, lidocaine can cause fetal acidosis (SEDA-8, 127). Fetal bradycardia is usually observed only in those fetuses with pre-existing heart rate deceleration. Despite massive intoxication at birth, one child had normal behavioral development at 7 months of age (SED-12, 256) (59).

Lactation

Low concentrations of lidocaine and its metabolite monoethylglycinexylidide (MEGX) have been found in breast milk after a dental procedure, but no risk seems to be involved (60).

Susceptibility Factors

Age

Children
Two reports have illustrated the need for particular care when using local anesthetics in neonates and small children. A 2-year-old child died from the combined effects of chloral hydrate, lidocaine, and nitrous oxide for a dental procedure (61). The doses used were not clarified, but in postmortem blood the plasma concentration of lidocaine was 12 μg/ml. The level and adequacy of perioperative monitoring was also not clear.

A neonate who needed a tracheostomy 10 days after a tracheoesophageal fistula repair was given intravenous lidocaine, 1 mg/kg followed 15–20 minutes later by 0.7 mg/kg. Immediately after, tonic-clonic seizures developed. The child recovered, with no observable ill effects at 6 months.

The authors pointed out that the dose of lidocaine used was well within recommended dosage limits. However, they stressed that a more appropriate dosing schedule should be worked out for neonates.

Lidocaine pharmacokinetics tend to follow a single compartment model in neonates, with an increased half-life, and substantially reduced protein binding, leading to a much larger volume of distribution than in adults, but an increased proportion of unbound drug (62).

Elderly people
In the elderly, some local anesthetics (including lidocaine and bupivacaine) have longer durations of action (63).

Sex

That sex differences can affect lidocaine pharmacokinetics is suggested by a report of higher blood concentrations in men than in women after administration of the same dose (SED-12, 256) (64).

Hepatic disease

In patients with heart and liver disease, the dosage requirement of lidocaine is reduced; the half-life of lidocaine is substantially longer in patients with liver disease (65).

Other features of the patient

The adverse effects of lidocaine are dose-related, and are more common in people of light weight and in patients with acute myocardial infarction or congestive cardiac failure. There is also an increased risk of central nervous system effects during cardiopulmonary bypass (66). In cardiac failure, shock, and postoperatively, there are reductions in both the metabolism and the apparent volume of distribution of lidocaine; dosages should be altered accordingly (67).

Drug Administration

Drug additives

The addition of dextran to a lidocaine + adrenaline solution used for infiltration reduced the absorption of both (68).

Alkalinization of local anesthetic solutions should theoretically lead to a faster onset of effect and prolonged anesthesia. However, raising the pH of the solution can cause the local anesthetic to precipitate out of solution, and one study with 2% lidocaine has shown no difference in quality or onset of anesthesia (SEDA-20, 129).

Adrenaline 1:100 000, added to lidocaine 2%, has caused full-thickness skin necrosis when used for ambulatory phlebectomy for varicose veins (SEDA-21, 136).

Drug administration route

Creams and gels
Cutaneous absorption of lidocaine is negligible through normal skin after short-term application. However, when applied to erosive lesions over large body areas, significant absorption may occur. When the drug is applied to mucous membranes, blood levels simulate those resulting from intravenous injection. Local anesthetic creams and gels used liberally on traumatized epithelium can be rapidly absorbed, resulting in systemic effects, such as convulsions, particularly if excessive quantities are used. This has been highlighted in the case of a 40-year-old woman who developed seizures after lidocaine gel 40 ml was injected into the ureter during an attempt to remove a stone (1).

Topical administration of lidocaine to the nasal mucosa occasionally causes severe methemoglobinemia in patients who have the heterozygous form of NADH methemoglobin reductase deficiency (69).

Subcutaneously in liposuction
Some have suggested that lidocaine is unnecessary and potentially toxic in liposuction, and that it provides no postoperative pain relief (70). Others think that lidocaine toxicity is not a major cause of death during liposuction, stating that all reported deaths after liposuction have been associated with general anesthesia or sedation, including the five in New York, and that doses of lidocaine higher than those used in these cases (10–40 mg/kg) are routinely used in tumescent liposuction, no deaths having been reported (56,71). It is possible that adrenaline, high pressure injection, removal of lidocaine by liposuction, and the development of tolerance all contribute to delay in absorption and lack of toxic symptoms at higher than expected plasma concentrations (72).

Patches
Lidocaine is available as a topical analgesic in an adhesive patch formulation for the pain of postherpetic neuralgia. The pharmacokinetics and safety of the 5% lidocaine patches have been studied in 20 healthy volunteers, who applied four patches to the skin either every 24 hours or every 12 hours for 3 days (73). Mean steady-state plasma concentrations were 186 and 225 ng/ml respectively, well below those required for an antidysrhythmic effect (1500 ng/ml) or a risk of toxicity (5000 ng/ml). The patches were well tolerated, with no major cutaneous adverse effects. This is in line with data from postmarketing surveillance studies, which have shown that since the availability of lidocaine patches in 1999, no adverse cardiac or other serious adverse events have been reported (74).

The pharmacokinetics of lidocaine in patches have been investigated in two studies. In 20 healthy volunteers, 5% lidocaine patches were applied for 18 hours/day on 3 consecutive days (75). The mean peak concentrations on days 1, 2, and 3 were 145, 153, and 154 ng/ml respectively; the median values of t_{max} were 18.0, 16.5, and 16.5 hours; and the mean trough concentrations were 83, 86, and 77 ng/ml. The patches were well tolerated; local skin reactions were generally minimal and self-limiting. In 20 healthy volunteers, 4 lidocaine patches were applied every 12 or 24 hours on 3 consecutive days (73). The mean maximum-plasma lidocaine concentrations at steady state were 225 and 186 ng/ml respectively. There was no loss of sensation at the site of application. No patient had edema and most cases of erythema were very slight. No systemic adverse events were judged to be related to the patches.

Drug overdose

Inadvertent intravenous injection of lidocaine 1 g resulted in asystole, apnea, and tonic-clonic seizures, with full recovery after 6 hours of intensive resuscitation (SED-12, 256) (76).

Fatal accidental overdose has been reported in a child (77).

- An 18-month-old infant died after swallowing an unknown amount of 2% viscous lidocaine. He rapidly became unwell at home, with convulsions, followed by an asystolic cardiorespiratory arrest. He was intubated and resuscitated by paramedics, but continued to have seizures. He was given anticonvulsants and cardiorespiratory resuscitation was unsuccessful. Toxicological tests identified high concentrations of lidocaine and its metabolites.

Owing to the rare but serious poisonings reported to date, 2% viscous lidocaine should not be prescribed for children under 6 years of age.

An unusual case of homicide using an overdose of intravenous lidocaine has been described (78).

- A 32-year-old man, who had been in hospital for several months because of acute intermittent porphyria and chronic pancreatitis, had a seizure and an asystolic cardiac arrest. Resuscitation was unsuccessful. There was a suspicion of patient mistreatment by one of the attending nurses, and toxicological analyses showed high blood concentrations of lidocaine, diazepam, phenytoin, and promethazine. Diazepam and phenytoin had been administered during resuscitation but lidocaine had not.

The cause of death was given as a ventricular dysrhythmia caused by a lidocaine overdose (total dose about 1500 mg); a nurse was later arrested and tried for murder.

Drug–Drug Interactions

Argatroban

The thrombin inhibitor argatroban had no effect on the pharmacokinetics of intravenous lidocaine 1.5 mg/kg for 10 minutes followed by 2 mg/kg/hour for 16 hours in 12 healthy volunteers; the argatroban was given as an intravenous infusion of 2 µg/kg/minute for 16 hours (79).

Beta-adrenoceptor antagonists

The combination of lidocaine with beta-adrenoceptor antagonists is associated with a slightly increased risk of some minor non-cardiac adverse events (dizziness,

numbness, somnolence, confusion, slurred speech, and nausea and vomiting) (80). The combination is not associated with an increased risk of dysrhythmias.

Some beta-blockers reduce hepatic blood flow and inhibit microsomal enzymes, reducing the clearance of lidocaine; there is a clinically significant increase in the plasma concentration of lidocaine during concomitant propranolol therapy (81).

Cimetidine

Cimetidine inhibits the metabolism of lidocaine (82,83) and reduces protein binding, increasing toxicity.

Erythromycin

The effects of erythromycin, an inhibitor of CYP3A4, on the pharmacokinetics of lidocaine have been studied in nine healthy volunteers. Steady-state oral erythromycin had no effect on the plasma concentration versus time curve of lidocaine after intravenous administration, but erythromycin increased the plasma concentrations of the major metabolite of lidocaine, MEGX (84). It is not clear what the interpretation of these results is, particularly since the authors did not study enough subjects to detect what might have been small but significant changes in various disposition parameters of lidocaine and did not report unbound concentrations of lidocaine or its metabolites. However, whatever the pharmacokinetic explanation, the clinical relevance is that one would expect that erythromycin would potentiate the toxic effects of lidocaine that are mediated by MEGX.

Erythromycin can increase the plasma concentration and toxicity of oral lidocaine, as shown in a crossover study in nine volunteers who took erythromycin orally (500 mg tds) for 4 days and 1 mg/kg of oral lidocaine on day 4 (85).

Itraconazole

The effects of itraconazole, an inhibitor of CYP3A4, on the pharmacokinetics of lidocaine have been studied in nine healthy volunteers. Steady-state oral itraconazole had no effect on the plasma concentration versus time curve of lidocaine after intravenous administration nor on the plasma concentrations of the major metabolite of lidocaine, MEGX (84).

Mexiletine

An interaction of lidocaine with mexiletine, which resulted in toxic concentrations of lidocaine, has been reported (86).

- An 80-year-old man with a dilated cardiomyopathy was given a lidocaine infusion started at 90 mg/hour for a ventricular tachycardia. He was already taking mexiletine 400 mg/day, and the plasma concentration was within the usual target range; however, the dose was reduced to 200 mg/day to avoid possible adverse effects. Intermittent ventricular tachycardia persisted, and so the lidocaine infusion was increased to 120 mg/day, but adverse effects (involuntary movements, muscle rigidity) were observed. The lidocaine infusion was stopped and within 20 minutes the adverse effects abated; the lidocaine concentration was 6.84 µg/ml. The ventricular tachycardia persisted, lidocaine was restarted at a lower rate, and the oral dose of mexiletine was increased to 450 mg/day. This resulted in an unexpectedly high concentration of lidocaine and the lidocaine concentration was significantly higher while the mexiletine dose was high.

Further studies suggested that mexiletine had displaced lidocaine from tissue binding sites. The authors suggested that this finding has implications for loading doses and acute effects of lidocaine in the concurrent therapy of lidocaine and mexiletine and highlighted the importance of close monitoring of lidocaine concentrations in this setting.

Nitrates, organic

Complete atrioventricular block has been reported after the use of sublingual nitrates in patients receiving lidocaine by infusion (87,88) and can result in asystole.

Opioid analgesics

A synergistic interaction of intrathecal fentanyl 100 µg and morphine 0.5 mg, given before induction, with systemically administered lidocaine 200 mg 4 hours later for ventricular tachycardia, resulted in potentiation of opioid effects in a 74-year-old man with major heart disease after coronary artery bypass grafting; during the 5 minutes after lidocaine he had a respiratory arrest with loss of consciousness and miotic pupils, all reversed by naloxone (89). The proposed mechanism was thought to be a reduction in calcium ion concentrations in opioid-sensitive CNS sites.

Propafenone

The CNS toxicity of lidocaine was increased in 11 healthy volunteers who simultaneously received propafenone, which reduced the metabolism of lidocaine (90).

Propofol

Propofol dose-dependently reduced the threshold for lidocaine-induced convulsions in rats (91). Higher doses of propofol completely abolished convulsions. However, there was no difference in the dose of lidocaine that caused cardiac arrest and death, when it was given with three different propofol infusions and placebo.

Ranitidine

Ranitidine inhibits the clearance of lidocaine (83).

Suxamethonium

Procaine and cocaine are esters that are hydrolysed by plasma cholinesterase and may therefore competitively enhance the action of suxamethonium (92). Chloroprocaine may have a similar action. Lidocaine also interacts, although the mechanism is not clear unless very high doses are used (93).

References

1. Pantuck AJ, Goldsmith JW, Kuriyan JB, Weiss RE. Seizures after ureteral stone manipulation with lidocaine. J Urol 1997;157(6):2248.
2. Pfeifer HJ, Greenblatt DJ, Koch-Weser J. Clinical use and toxicity of intravenous lidocaine. A report from the Boston Collaborative Drug Surveillance Program. Am Heart J 1976;92(2):168–73.
3. Greenspon AJ, Mohiuddin S, Saksena S, Lengerich R, Snapinn S, Holmes G, Irvin J, Sappington E, et al. Comparison of intravenous tocainide with intravenous lidocaine for treating ventricular arrhythmias. Cardiovasc Rev Rep 1989;10:55–9.
4. Adriani J, Coffman VD, Naraghi M. The allergenicity of lidocaine and other amide and related local anesthetics. Anesthesiol Rev 1986;13:30–6.
5. Bonnet MC, du Cailar G, Deschodt J. Anaphylaxie à la lidocaine. [Anaphylaxis caused by lidocaine.] Ann Fr Anesth Reanim 1989;8(2):127–9.
6. Kennedy KS, Cave RH. Anaphylactic reaction to lidocaine. Arch Otolaryngol Head Neck Surg 1986;112(6):671–3.
7. Avery JK. Routine procedure—bad outcome. Tenn Med 1998;91(7):280–1.
8. Sakurai M, Kanazawa I. Positive symptoms in multiple sclerosis: their treatment with sodium channel blockers, lidocaine and mexiletine. J Neurol Sci 1999;162(2):162–8.
9. Hand PJ, Stark RJ. Intravenous lignocaine infusions for severe chronic daily headache. Med J Aust 2000;172(4):157–9.
10. Attal N, Gaude V, Brasseur L, Dupuy M, Guirimand F, Parker F, Bouhassira D. Intravenous lidocaine in central pain: a double-blind, placebo-controlled, psychophysical study. Neurology 2000;54(3):564–74.
11. Ziegelbaum M, Lever H. Acute urinary retention associated with flecainide. Cleve Clin J Med 1990;57(1):86–7.
12. Krikler DM, Curry PV. Torsade de pointes, an atypical ventricular tachycardia. Br Heart J 1976;38(2):117–20.
13. Gottlieb SS, Packer M. Deleterious hemodynamic effects of lidocaine in severe congestive heart failure. Am Heart J 1989;118(3):611–2.
14. Weaver WD, Fahrenbruch CE, Johnson DD, Hallstrom AP, Cobb LA, Copass MK. Effect of epinephrine and lidocaine therapy on outcome after cardiac arrest due to ventricular fibrillation. Circulation 1990;82(6):2027–34.
15. Tisdale JE. Lidocaine prophylaxis in acute myocardial infarction. Henry Ford Hosp Med J 1991;39(3–4):217–25.
16. Garner L, Stirt JA, Finholt DA. Heart block after intravenous lidocaine in an infant. Can Anaesth Soc J 1985;32(4):425–8.
17. Hansoti RC, Ashar PN. Atrioventricular block and ventricular fibrillation due to lidocaine therapy. Bombay Hosp J 1975;17:26.
18. McLean SA, Paul ID, Spector PS. Lidocaine-induced conduction disturbance in patients with systemic hyperkalemia. Ann Emerg Med 2000;36(6):615–8.
19. Parnass SM, Curran MJ, Becker GL. Incidence of hypotension associated with epidural anesthesia using alkalinized and nonalkalinized lidocaine for cesarean section. Anesth Analg 1987;66(11):1148–50.
20. Enlund M, Mentell O, Krekmanov L. Unintentional hypotension from lidocaine infiltration during orthognathic surgery and general anaesthesia. Acta Anaesthesiol Scand 2001;45(3):294–7.
21. Azma T, Okida M. Does lidocaine provoke clinically significant vasospasm? Acta Anaesthesiol Scand 2003;47:1174–5.
22. Beydon L, Lorino AM, Verra F, Labroue M, Catoire P, Lofaso F, Bonnet F. Topical upper airway anaesthesia

with lidocaine increases airway resistance by impairing glottic function. Intensive Care Med 1995;21(11):920–6.

23. Howard P, Cayton RM, Brennan SR, Anderson PB. Lignocaine aerosol and persistent cough. Br J Dis Chest 1977;71(1):19–24.

24. Ryder W. Two cautionary tales. Anaesthesia 1994;49(2): 180–1.

25. Keller C, Sparr HJ, Brimacombe JR. Laryngeal mask lubrication. A comparative study of saline versus 2% lignocaine gel with cuff pressure control. Anaesthesia 1997;52(6):592–7.

26. Stargel WW, Shand DG, Routledge PA, Barchowsky A, Wagner GS. Clinical comparison of rapid infusion and multiple injection methods for lidocaine loading. Am Heart J 1981;102(5):872–6.

27. Olthoff D, Vetter B, Deutrich C, Burkhardt U. Pharmakokinetische Untersuchungen zu den Ursachen der erhohten Neurotoxizität des Lidokains während kardiochirurgischer Operationen. [Pharmacokinetic studies on the causes of increased neurotoxicity of lidocaine during heart surgery.] Anaesthesiol Reanim 1989;14(4):207–14.

28. DeToledo JC, Minagar A, Lowe MR. Lidocaine-induced seizures in patients with history of epilepsy: effect of antiepileptic drugs. Anesthesiology 2002;97(3):737–9.

29. Lee DL, Ayoub C, Shaw RK, Fontes ML. Grand mal seizure during cardiopulmonary bypass: probable lidocaine toxicity. J Cardiothorac Vasc Anesth 1999;13(2):200–2.

30. Goodwin DP, McMeekin TO. A case of lidocaine absorption from topical administration of 40% lidocaine cream. J Am Acad Dermatol 1999;41(2 Pt 1):280–1.

31. Anibarro B, Seoane FJ. Adverse reaction to lidocaine. Allergy 1998;53(7):717–8.

32. Kanai Y, Katsuki H, Takasaki M. Graded, irreversible changes in crayfish giant axon as manifestations of lidocaine neurotoxicity in vitro. Anesth Analg 1998;86(3):569–73.

33. Tei Y, Morita T, Shishido H, Inoue S. Lidocaine intoxication at very small doses in terminally ill cancer patients. J Pain Symptom Manage 2005;30(1):6–7.

34. Donald MJ, Derbyshire S. Lignocaine toxicity; a complication of local anaesthesia administered in the community. Emerg Med J 2004;21(2):249–50.

35. Zeidan A, Baraka A. Is euphoria a side-effect of lidocaine? Anaesthesia 2004;59(12):1253–4.

36. Ghose S, Garodia VK, Sachdev MS, Kumar H, Biswas NR, Pandey RM. Evaluation of potentiating effect of a drop of lignocaine on tropicamide-induced mydriasis. Invest Ophthalmol Vis Sci 2001;42(7):1581–5.

37. Yamashita S, Sato S, Kakiuchi Y, Miyabe M, Yamaguchi H. Lidocaine toxicity during frequent viscous lidocaine use for painful tongue ulcer. J Pain Symptom Manage 2002;24(5):543–5.

38. Sawyer RJ, von Schroeder H. Temporary bilateral blindness after acute lidocaine toxicity. Anesth Analg 2002;95(1):224–6.

39. Berger I, Steinberg A, Schlesinger Y, Seelenfreund M, Schimmel MS. Neonatal mydriasis: intravenous lidocaine adverse reaction. J Child Neurol 2002;17(5):400–1.

40. Bigeleisen PE. An unusual presentation of metallic taste after lidocaine injections. Anesth Analg 1999;89(5):1239–40.

41. Janda A, Salem C. Hypoglykämie durch Lidocain-Überdosierung. [Hypoglycemia caused by lidocaine overdosage.] Reg Anaesth 1986;9(3):88–90.

42. Stefanini M, Hoffman MN. Studies on platelets: XXVIII: acute thrombocytopenic purpura due to lidocaine (Xylocaine)-mediated antibody. Report of a case. Am J Med Sci 1978;275(3):365–71.

43. Karim A, Ahmed S, Siddiqui R, Mattana J. Methemoglobinemia complicating topical lidocaine used during endoscopic procedures. Am J Med 2001;111(2):150–3.

44. Kakinoki K, Tachibana Y, Yonejima H, Ogino H, Satomura Y, Unoura M. A case of mexiletine and lidocaine induced severe liver injury Acta Hepatol Jpn 2000;41: 812–6.

45. Galer BS, Rowbotham MC, Perander J, Friedman E. Topical lidocaine patch relieves postherpetic neuralgia more effectively than a vehicle topical patch: results of an enriched enrollment study. Pain 1999;80(3):533–8.

46. Dorfman D, Dalton A, Khan A, Markarian Y, Scarano A, Cansino M, Wulff E, Simpson D. Treatment of painful distal sensory polyneuropathy in HIV-infected patients with a topical agent: results of an open-label trial of 5% lidocaine gel. AIDS 1999;13(12):1589–90.

47. Anonymous. Lidocaine patch shown to relieve postherpetic neuralgia. J Pharm Technol 2001;17:154.

48. Scala E, Giani M, Pirrotta L, Guerra EC, Girardelli CR, De Pita O, Puddu P. Simultaneous allergy to ampicillin and local anesthetics. Allergy 2001;56(5):454–5.

49. Palmer JM, Link D. Impotence following anesthesia for elective circumcision. JAMA 1979;241(24):2635–6.

50. Weightman W, Turner T. Allergic contact dermatitis from lignocaine: report of 29 cases and review of the literature. Contact Dermatitis 1998;39(5):265–6.

51. Mackley CL, Marks JG Jr, Anderson BE. Delayed-type hypersensitivity to lidocaine. Arch Dermatol 2003;139:343–6.

52. Roesch A, Haegele T, Vogt T, Babilas P, Landthaler M, Szeimies RM. Severe contact urticaria to guar gum included as gelling agent in a local anaesthetic. Contact Dermatitis 2005;52(6):307–8.

53. Minasian A, Yagiela JA. The use of amide local anesthetics in patients susceptible to malignant hyperthermia. Oral Surg Oral Med Oral Pathol 1988;66(4):405–15.

54. Klimanek J, Majewski W, Walencik K. A case of malignant hyperthermia during epidural analgesia. Anaesth Resusc Intensive Ther 1976;4(2):143–5.

55. Rao RB, Ely SF, Hoffman RS. Deaths related to liposuction. N Engl J Med 1999;340(19):1471–5.

56. Ginsberg MM, Gresham L, Vermeulen C, Serra M, Roujeau JC, Talmor M, Barie PS, Klein JA, Rigel DS, Wheeland RG, Schnur P, Penn J, Fodor PB. Deaths related to liposuction. N Engl J Med 1999;341(13):1000–3.

57. Klein JA. Tumescent technique for local anesthesia improves safety in large-volume liposuction. Plast Reconstr Surg 1993;92(6):1085–100.

58. Day RO, Chalmers DR, Williams KM, Campbell TJ. The death of a healthy volunteer in a human research project: implications for Australian clinical research. Med J Aust 1998;168(9):449–51.

59. Kim WY, Pomerance JJ, Miller AA. Lidocaine intoxication in a newborn following local anesthesia for episiotomy. Pediatrics 1979;64(5):643–5.

60. Lebedevs TH, Wojnar-Horton RE, Yapp P, Roberts MJ, Dusci LJ, Hackett LP, Ilett K. Excretion of lignocaine and its metabolite monoethylglycinexylidide in breast milk following its use in a dental procedure. A case report. J Clin Periodontol 1993;20(8):606–8.

61. Engelhart DA, Lavins ES, Hazenstab CB, Sutheimer CA. Unusual death attributed to the combined effects of chloral hydrate, lidocaine, and nitrous oxide. J Anal Toxicol 1998;22(3):246–7.

62. Resar LM, Helfaer MA. Recurrent seizures in a neoate after lidocaine administration. J Perinatol 1998;18(3):193–5.

63. Chauvin M. Toxicité aiguë des anesthésiques locaux en fonction du terrain. [Acute toxicity of local anesthetics as a function of the patient's condition.] Ann Fr Anesth Reanim 1988;7(3):216–23.

64. Bruguerolle B, Isnardon R, Valli M, Vadot G. Influence du sexe sur les taux plasmatiques de lidocaine en anesthésie dentaire. Thérapie (Paris) 1982;37:593.

65. Thomson PD, Rowland M, Melmon KL. The influence of heart failure, liver disease, and renal failure on the disposition of lidocaine in man. Am Heart J 1971;82(3):417–21.

66. Bauer LA, Brown T, Gibaldi M, Hudson L, Nelson S, Raisys V, Shea JP. Influence of long-term infusions on lidocaine kinetics. Clin Pharmacol Ther 1982;31(4):433–7.

67. Kumana CR. Therapeutic drug monitoring—antidysrhythmic drugs. In: Richens A, Marks V, editors. Therapeutic Drug Monitoring. London, Edinburgh: Churchill-Livingstone, 1981:370 Ch 16A.

68. Adams HA, Biscoping J, Kafurke H, Muller H, Hoffmann B, Boerner U, Hempelmann G. Influence of dextran on the absorption of adrenaline-containing lignocaine solutions: a protective mechanism in local anaesthesia. Br J Anaesth 1988;60(6):645–50.

69. Kotler RL, Hansen-Flaschen J, Casey MP. Severe methaemoglobinaemia after flexible fibreoptic bronchoscopy. Thorax 1989;44(3):234–5.

70. Perry AW, Petti C, Rankin M. Lidocaine is not necessary in liposuction. Plast Reconstr Surg 1999;104(6):1900–2.

71. Klein JA. Lidocaine is not necessary in liposuction: discussion. Plast Reconstr Surg 1999;104:1903–6.

72. Rubin JP, Bierman C, Rosow CE, Arthur GR, Chang Y, Courtiss EH, May JW Jr. The tumescent technique: the effect of high tissue pressure and dilute epinephrine on absorption of lidocaine. Plast Reconstr Surg 1999;103(3):990–1002.

73. Gammaitoni AR, Alvarez NA, Galer BS. Pharmacokinetics and safety of continuously applied lidocaine patches 5%. Am J Health Syst Pharm 2002;59(22):2215–20.

74. Galer BS. Effectiveness and safety of lidocaine patch 5%. J Fam Pract 2002;51(10):867–8.

75. Gammaitoni AR, Davis MW. Pharmacokinetics and tolerability of lidocaine patch 5% with extended dosing. Ann Pharmacother 2002;36(2):236–40.

76. Finkelstein F, Kreeft J. Massive lidocaine poisoning. N Engl J Med 1979;301(1):50.

77. Nisse P, Lhermitte M, Dherbecourt V, Fourier C, Leclerc F, Houdret N, Mathieu-Nolf M. Intoxication mortelle après ingestion accidentelle de Xylocaine visqueuse a 2% chez une jeune enfant. [Fatal intoxication after accidental ingestion of viscous 2% lidocaine in a young child.] Acta Clin Belg Suppl 2002;(1):51–3.

78. Kalin JR, Brissie RM. A case of homicide by lethal injection with lidocaine. J Forensic Sci 2002;47(5):1135–8.

79. Inglis AM, Sheth SB, Hursting MJ, Tenero DM, Graham AM, DiCicco RA. Investigation of the interaction between argatroban and acetaminophen, lidocaine, or digoxin. Am J Health Syst Pharm 2002;59(13):1258–66.

80. Wyse DG, Kellen J, Tam Y, Rademaker AW. Increased efficacy and toxicity of lidocaine in patients on beta-blockers. Int J Cardiol 1988;21(1):59–70.

81. Naguib M, Magboul MM, Samarkandi AH, Attia M. Adverse effects and drug interactions associated with local and regional anaesthesia. Drug Saf 1998;18(4):221–50.

82. Jackson JE, Bentley JB, Glass SJ, Fukui T, Gandolfi AJ, Plachetka JR. Effects of histamine-2 receptor blockade on lidocaine kinetics. Clin Pharmacol Ther 1985;37(5):544–8.

83. Kowalsky SF. Lidocaine interaction with cimetidine and ranitidine: a critical analysis of the literature. Adv Ther 1988;5:229–44.

84. Isohanni MH, Neuvonen PJ, Palkama VJ, Olkkola KT. Effect of erythromycin and itraconazole on the pharmacokinetics of intravenous lignocaine. Eur J Clin Pharmacol 1998;54(7):561–5.

85. Isohanni MH, Neuvonen PJ, Olkkola KT. Effect of erythromycin and itraconazole on the pharmacokinetics of oral lignocaine. Pharmacol Toxicol 1999;84(3):143–6.

86. Maeda Y, Funakoshi S, Nakamura M, Fukuzawa M, Kugaya Y, Yamasaki M, Tsukiai S, Murakami T, Takano M. Possible mechanism for pharmacokinetic interaction between lidocaine and mexiletine. Clin Pharmacol Ther 2002;71(5):389–97.

87. Lancaster L, Fenster PE. Complete heart block after sublingual nitroglycerin. Chest 1983;84(1):111–2.

88. Antonelli D, Barzilay J. Complete atrioventricular block after sublingual isosorbide dinitrate. Int J Cardiol 1986;10(1):71–3.

89. Jensen E, Nader ND. Potentiation of narcosis after intravenous lidocaine in a patient given spinal opioids. Anesth Analg 1999;89(3):758–9.

90. Ujhelyi MR, O'Rangers EA, Fan C, Kluger J, Pharand C, Chow MS. The pharmacokinetic and pharmacodynamic interaction between propafenone and lidocaine. Clin Pharmacol Ther 1993;53(1):38–48.

91. Lee VC, Moscicki JC, DiFazio CA. Propofol sedation produces dose-dependent suppression of lidocaine-induced seizures in rats. Anesth Analg 1998;86(3):652–7.

92. Matsuo S, Rao DB, Chaudry I, Foldes FF. Interaction of muscle relaxants and local anesthetics at the neuromuscular junction. Anesth Analg 1978;57(5):580–7.

93. Usubiaga JE, Wikinski JA, Morales RL, Usubiaga LE. Interaction of intravenously administered procaine, lidocaine and succinylcholine in anesthetized subjects. Anesth Analg 1967;46(1):39–45.

Mepivacaine

General Information

Mepivacaine is an aminoamide local anesthetic. Systemic toxicity is its major complication and can prove fatal. Vasoconstrictors are not warranted, as they do not alter the rate of systemic reactions.

Organs and Systems

Cardiovascular

Severe bradypnea and bradycardia requiring external ventricular pacing occurred in a previously asymptomatic 30-year-old woman with a known cardiac conduction defect 85 minutes after a paracervical block with mepivacaine 400 mg (1). First-degree atrioventricular block has been reported (2).

Nervous system

Hyperbaric mepivacaine has also been implicated in causing transient radicular irritation after spinal anesthesia, of the same order of magnitude as lidocaine

(3,4). Three cases of transient radicular irritation have been reported after spinal anesthesia with isobaric 2% mepivacaine (5).

Skin

Allergic skin reactions to amide local anesthetics are uncommon and little is known about cross-reactivity among these drugs. Two cases of cross-reactivity of mepivacaine with ropivacaine and lidocaine have been reported.

- A 35-year-old woman with no previous history of allergy developed urticaria on her face, neck, and legs 15 minutes after receiving mepivacaine for extirpation of a nevus (6). She was treated with an oral antihistamine, and the rash completely resolved in 1 hour. Prick and intradermal tests with undiluted mepivacaine 1% were negative. A single-blind, placebo-controlled, subcutaneous challenge test and an intradermal test with mepivacaine were positive. A latex-prick test was negative. In order to evaluate cross-reactivity among different amides, prick and intradermal tests were carried out with undiluted lidocaine 1%, bupivacaine 0.5%, and ropivacaine 1%. The tests were negative with lidocaine and bupivacaine, but positive with ropivacaine. An intradermal test with ropivacaine was also positive.
- A 54-year-old woman with no history of atopy or allergy developed a maculopapular rash and pruritus in the injection area 2 days after surgery (7). The skin lesions resolved in 7 days without treatment. Skin prick and intradermal tests for cross-reactivity to various dilutions of lidocaine, mepivacaine, bupivacaine, and articaine were performed. Patch tests at 2 and 4 days with lidocaine and mepivacaine were positive.

Amide local anesthetics rarely cause allergic reactions. Formerly, cross-reactivity among them was considered non-existent, but these cases demonstrate that that is not necessarily so.

Immunologic

An allergic reaction has been described in a patient given mepivacaine (8).

Susceptibility Factors

Renal disease

Mepivacaine toxicity has been studied in 10 patients with end-stage chronic renal insufficiency undergoing vascular access surgery (9). These patients represent a high-risk group for general anesthesia, as they often have concomitant coronary artery disease, hypertension, and diabetes. Brachial plexus block is often used: as well as avoiding systemic effects, it enhances regional blood flow.

References

1. Ayestaran C, Matorras R, Gomez S, Arce D, Rodriguez-Escudero F. Severe bradycardia and bradypnea following vaginal oocyte retrieval: a possible toxic effect of paracervical mepivacaine. Eur J Obstet Gynecol Reprod Biol 2000;91(1):71–3.
2. Griebenow R, Saborouski F, Matthes H, Wald-Oloumier H. EKG-Veränderungen bein Infiltrationsanesthesie mit Mepivacain. [ECG changes after spinal anesthesia using mepivacaine.] Intensivmed 1979;16:163.
3. Salmela L, Aromaa U. Transient radicular irritation after spinal anesthesia induced with hyperbaric solutions of cerebrospinal fluid-diluted lidocaine 50 mg/ml or mepivacaine 40 mg/ml or bupivacaine 5 mg/ml Acta Anaesthesiol Scand 1998;42(7):765–9.
4. Hiller A, Rosenberg PH. Transient neurological symptoms after spinal anaesthesia with 4% mepivacaine and 0.5% bupivacaine Br J Anaesth 1997;79(3):301–5.
5. Sia S, Pullano C. Transient radicular irritation after spinal anaesthesia with 2% isobaric mepivacaine. Br J Anaesth 1998;81(4):622–4.
6. Prieto A, Herrero T, Rubio M, Tornero P, Baeza ML, Velloso A, Perez C, De Barrio M. Urticaria due to mepivacaine with tolerance to lidocaine and bupivacaine. Allergy 2005;60(2):261–2.
7. Sanchez-Morillas L, Martinez JJ, Martos MR, Gomez-Tembleque P, Andres ER. Delayed-type hypersensitivity to mepivacaine with cross-reaction to lidocaine. Contact Dermatitis 2005;53(6):352–3.
8. Hiyoshi K, Iwanaga Y, Kado K, Takeda K. [Allergic reactions caused by mepivacaine ECG changes after spinal anesthesia using mepivacaino.]Masui 1978;27(2):177–80.
9. Rodriguez J, Quintela O, Lopez-Rivadulla M, Barcena M, Diz C, Alvarez J. High doses of mepivacaine for brachial plexus block in patients with end-stage chronic renal failure. A pilot study. Eur J Anaesthesiol 2001;18(3):171–6.

Oxybuprocaine

General Information

Oxybuprocaine is an ester of para-aminobenzoic acid. It is a popular local anesthetic for use in ophthalmology.

Organs and Systems

Cardiovascular

An episode of severe bradycardia, with no perceptible cardiac output, was reported in a previously healthy patient after one drop of 0.4% oxybuprocaine was applied to each eye (1).

Sensory systems

When used in the eye, oxybuprocaine can enter the anterior chamber, and fibrinous iritis and moderate corneal swelling have been described (SED-12, 257) (2). Abuse has often been reported and can lead to keratopathy, severe visual impairment, and even enucleation (3).

Skin

There have been two reports of patients scheduled for tonometry who developed periorbital dermatitis following the topical instillation of local anesthetic eye drops (4). The first patient reacted strongly positive on patch testing to Thilorbin AT (oxybuprocaine, fluorescein, phenylmercuric borate, polysorbate 20, mannitol) and also to oxybuprocaine alone. The second reacted to Conjucain EDO (oxybuprocaine, sorbitol, sodium hydroxide) and to oxybuprocaine alone. The authors believed these to be the only described cases of a delayed hypersensitivity reaction to oxybuprocaine, an ester local anesthetic commonly used for topical anesthesia in the eye.

References

1. Christensen C. Bradycardia as a side-effect to oxybuprocaine. Acta Anaesthesiol Scand 1990;34(2):165–6.
2. Haddad R. Fibrinous iritis due to oxybuprocaine. Br J Ophthalmol 1989;73(1):76–7.
3. Rosenwasser GO, Holland S, Pflugfelder SC, Lugo M, Heidemann DG, Culbertson WW, Kattan H. Topical anesthetic abuse. Ophthalmology 1990;97(8):967–72.
4. Blaschke V, Fuchs T. Periorbital allergic contact dermatitis from oxybuprocaine. Contact Dermatitis 2001;44(3):198.

Prilocaine and Emla

General Information

Prilocaine is an aminoamide local anesthetic. It can be used on its own, but it is also included in Emla in a eutectic combination with lidocaine (25 mg/ml each), which is widely used as a local anesthetic in topical administration for, for example, superficial surgery and venepuncture.

Emla cream causes minor local adverse effects, such as itch, burning, and localized purpura (SEDA-19, 131) (SEDA-20, 127) (SEDA-22, 140). A meta-analysis of the use of Emla cream in the elderly (over 65) showed that the technique is generally safe, with only mild transient effects (pallor, redness, and edema) at the application site; there were no systemic effects (1).

However, if large amounts are applied, particularly under occlusion, it can be sufficiently well absorbed to cause systemic effects. Three of 1648 children who received measles vaccination with Emla 1 g had adverse reactions 10–20 minutes later; all required adrenaline for similar symptoms of weakness and dizziness with a cold clammy skin and no pulse or a weak pulse (2). One went on to wheeze markedly and had peripheral cyanosis and shivering, improving with hydrocortisone. The authors proposed that these unusual reactions could have been due to a biphasic local reaction to Emla, with vasodilatation leading to increased absorption and further toxicity.

Organs and Systems

Nervous system

Particular care must be taken with Emla in children, since seizures can occur.

- A 5-year-old child had 35 g of Emla applied under an occlusive dressing to eczematous skin in preparation for cryotherapy for molluscum contagiosum (3). Within 1 hour, the child had a generalized seizure that lasted 10 minutes. The plasma concentrations of lidocaine and prilocaine 30 minutes later were 5.5 and 2.0 µg/ml, respectively, and 6 hours later, the methemoglobin concentration was 19%. The child was given vitamin C 500 mg intravenously, and 2 days later had a methemoglobin concentration of 0.3%.

Errors by pharmacists or parents continue to contribute to severe complications, such as seizures, after overdose of Emla cream in children (4).

- A 21-month-old girl had four generalized tonic-clonic seizures after inadvertent overuse of Emla before curettage of skin lesions of molluscum contagiosum. Because of a pharmacy error, 30 g tubes of Emla were dispensed instead of 5 g tubes. The toddler's mother applied 75 g under occlusive dressing, covering about 350 cm^2 of the child's surface area. This dose significantly exceeds the recommendations for a 14 kg child—maximum 10 g on a maximum area of 100 cm^2. Two doses of intravenous lorazepam (0.1 mg/kg) did not control the seizures, which stopped only after phenobarbital (20 mg/kg) was given. The child then required intubation and ventilation for respiratory depression. The lidocaine concentration 4 hours after the first application of Emla was 2.5 µg/ml and the methemoglobin concentration was 8%.

Seizures have also been reported in adults.

- An 84-year-old woman had three generalized tonic-clonic seizures after repeated applications of Emla (17 applications of 10 g over 23 weeks) (5,6).

Sensory systems

Emla cream can cause severe eye irritation (7).

- Emla cream 30 g was applied to both periorbital and proximal nasal sidewall areas for laser treatment in a 20-year-old woman. Despite the use of a right eye shield for corneal protection, the next day she developed right eye pain and blurred vision and remembered that Emla cream had accidentally entered her right eye before treatment. This caused immediate discomfort, which subsided and then recurred several hours later. She had severe conjunctival injection with loss of epithelium from over 90% of the surface of her cornea, in a pattern more suggestive of chemical than mechanical damage. Treatment with a bandage contact lens and prophylactic antibiotics was effective and her visual acuity returned to baseline.

Hematologic

Methemoglobinemia as an adverse effect of prilocaine (8) has been reported more often than with any other local anesthetic. It is caused by a metabolite and is a particular problem in neonates, who have an immature methemoglobin reductase system and residual fetal hemoglobin, increasing the risk of symptomatic methemoglobinemia.

Neonates and small children who have penile block with prilocaine, for circumcision can develop severe methemoglobinemia (9,10). A report has emphasized the severity of methemoglobinemia in infants especially if premature, when even a small dose of prilocaine is used for infiltration (11).

- A 1.3 kg premature neonate of 30-week gestation, having required ventilation over the first 3 days for respiratory distress syndrome, required reintubation on day 12 of life for recurrent apnea. He developed a pneumothorax requiring an intercostal drain; 0.5 ml of 1% prilocaine was used for infiltration, after which his oxygen requirements overnight went from 28 to 100%; his SpO_2 was 90% and he turned pale gray. His PaO_2 was 23 kPa (170 mmHg) and his methemoglobin concentration was 15%. He was given methylthioninium chloride, and within 8 hours, his methemoglobin concentration was 0.5% and his SpO_2 96%.

Methemoglobinemia can occur with overdosage of prilocaine (SEDA-20, 129) and after inadvertent intravenous administration, particularly in neonates and children (SEDA-11, 221) (12).

- In a 6-year-old boy, 10 ml of a 2% solution given for bilateral percutaneous nephrostomy produced a degree of cyanosis that demanded methylthioninium chloride treatment (13).

In adults, even those with anemia, the shift in methemoglobin concentrations from prilocaine, while measurable, is not of clinical significance (SEDA-12, 257) (14).

Despite concerns that Emla cream can cause methemoglobinemia in neonates and preterm babies, a French study of 116 infants in neonatal intensive care, who were treated with small amounts of Emla once a day before skin puncture, showed that methemoglobin concentrations never exceeded 5% and were not related to gestational age or duration of application (SEDA-20, 127). Two other studies on the use of Emla as analgesia for neonates and low birth weight infants showed localized pallor, but no evidence of methemoglobinemia (SEDA-22, 140).

However, high doses of Emla have been responsible for two cases of methemoglobinemia in neonates. In one, 3.5 g of Emla was used before circumcision, and in the other 25 g of cream had been applied to a buttock hemangioma by the parents before laser therapy (SEDA-22, 140).

- A 3-year-old girl with multiple lesions of molluscum contagiosum had Emla applied to the lesions before curettage (15). She became lethargic and hypoactive 2 hours later, with periorbital discoloration and cyanosed lips. Her SaO_2 was 85%, systolic blood pressure 185 mmHg, pulse 144/minute, and her methemoglobin concentration 21%. Her

caregiver had applied about 25 g of cream to her entire torso, a massive dose of prilocaine (about 625 mg).

This report reinforces previously described problems arising from carers' lack of understanding of instructions when using Emla in children or babies.

- A 4-day-old boy developed methemoglobinemia (16%) after the application of Emla cream to his penis before circumcision (16).
- A 7-month-old girl was ventilated with inhaled nitric oxide 40 ppm and developed methemoglobinemia after the application of Emla to an 8 cm^2 area of skin for 5 hours (17). Shortly after removal she developed cyanosis, with a methemoglobin concentration of 16%, which resolved with two doses of methylthioninium chloride.

In these cases, the prolonged duration of Emla application was thought to be the cause, but concomitant use of inhaled nitric oxide may have contributed.

Skin

The adverse effects of Emla include localized blanching or erythema, burning or itching sensations, irritant and allergic reactions, and purpura (18).

In 29 children with atopic dermatitis who were given Emla cream before curettage of molluscum contagiosum, there were no adverse reactions, apart from mild transient application site reactions, such as pallor, redness, and edema. No systemic reactions were reported, but the authors emphasized that Emla can be rapidly absorbed through atopic skin, and they therefore recommended that when Emla is applied under occlusive dressing, the maximum dose should be 10 g for 30 minutes (19).

The analgesic effects of single and repeated applications of Emla over six consecutive days have been studied in 11 patients with post-herpetic neuralgia (20). There was no evidence of systemic adverse effects, but four patients developed mild erythema at 30 minutes, which may have been due to the occlusive dressing, and one patient had pruritus on day 7.

Two children developed petechial eruptions after the application of Emla for treatment curettage of molluscum contagiosum (21). Neither became systemically unwell, and subsequent reapplication of Emla in one child did not elicit a petechial eruption.

There has been a report of hyperpigmentation following the use of Emla cream (22).

- A 12-year-old black child developed a patch of hyperpigmentation on his forehead where Emla cream had been used for cutaneous anesthesia before local infiltration with lidocaine for removal of a nevus. This persisted, although fading, for at least 4 months. No other cause could be found.

Hypopigmentation has also been reported with Emla (23).

Contact dermatitis was reported in three hemodialysis patients who used Emla cream repeatedly as analgesia for AV fistula cannulation (SEDA-21, 136).

- A 6-year-old boy developed contact dermatitis following the application of Emla for a skin biopsy to diagnose graft-versus-host disease (24). The histopathological features of the contact dermatitis were similar to graft-versus-host disease.

The use of Emla to provide topical anesthesia should be documented in order to avoid misdiagnosis.

References

1. Wahlgren CF, Lillieborg S. Split-skin grafting with lidocaine–prilocaine cream: a meta-analysis of efficacy and safety in geriatric versus nongeriatric patients. Plast Reconstr Surg 2001;107(3):750–6.
2. Dilraj A, Cutts FT, Bennett JV, Coovadia HM, Hopkinson C. Adverse reactions possibly associated with the use of Emla cream. S Afr Med J 1999;89(4):419–20.
3. Capron F, Perry D, Capolaghi B. Crise convulsive et méthémoglobinémie après application de crème anèsthesique. [Convulsive crisis and methemoglobinemia after the application of anesthetic cream.] Arch Pediatr 1998;5(7):812.
4. Rincon E, Baker RL, Iglesias AJ, Duarte AM. CNS toxicity after topical application of EMLA cream on a toddler with molluscum contagiosum. Pediatr Emerg Care 2000;16(4):252–4.
5. Boulinguez S, Sparsa A, Bouyssou-Gauthier ML, Bedane C, Bonnetblanc JM. Adverse effects associated with EMLA cream used as topical anesthetic for the mechanical debridement of leg ulcers. J Am Acad Dermatol 2000;42(1 Pt 1):146–8.
6. Lok C. Adverse effects associated with EMLA cream used as topical anesthetic for the mechanical debridement of leg ulcers. Reply. J Am Acad Dermatol 2000;42(1 Pt 1):147–8.
7. McKinlay JR, Hofmeister E, Ross EV, MacAllister W. EMLA cream-induced eye injury. Arch Dermatol 1999;135(7):855–6.
8. Elsner P, Dummer R. Signs of methaemoglobinaemia after topical application of EMLA cream in an infant with haemangioma. Dermatology 1997;195(2):153–4.
9. Prineas S, Wilkins BH, Halliday RJ. Circumcision blues. Med J Aust 1997;166(11):615.
10. Tse S, Barrington K, Byrne P. Methemoglobinemia associated with prilocaine use in neonatal circumcision. Am J Perinatol 1995;12(5):331–2.
11. Ergenekon E, Atalay Y, Koc E, Turkyilmaz C. Methaemoglobinaemia in a premature infant secondary to prilocaine. Acta Paediatr 1999;88(2):236.
12. Menahem S. Neonatal cyanosis, methaemoglobinaemia and haemolytic anaemia. Acta Paediatr Scand 1988;77(5):755–6.
13. Kilic I, Kalayci O. Methemoglobinemia due to prilocain local anesthesia. Doga Turk J Med Sci 1993;19:.
14. Bardoczky GI, Wathieu M, D'Hollander A. Prilocaine-induced methemoglobinemia evidenced by pulse oximetry. Acta Anaesthesiol Scand 1990;34(2):162–4.
15. Touma S, Jackson JB. Lidocaine and prilocaine toxicity in a patient receiving treatment for mollusca contagiosa. J Am Acad Dermatol 2001;44(Suppl 2):399–400.
16. Couper RT. Methaemoglobinaemia secondary to topical lignocaine/prilocaine in a circumcised neonate. J Paediatr Child Health 2000;36(4):406–7.
17. Sinisterra S, Miravet E, Alfonso I, Soliz A, Papazian O. Methemoglobinemia in an infant receiving nitric oxide after the use of eutectic mixture of local anesthetic. J Pediatr 2002;141(2):285–6.
18. de Waard-van der Spek FB, Oranje AP. Purpura caused by Emla is of toxic origin. Contact Dermatitis 1997;36(1):11–3.
19. Ronnerfalt L, Fransson J, Wahlgren CF. EMLA cream provides rapid pain relief for the curettage of molluscum contagiosum in children with atopic dermatitis without causing serious application-site reactions. Pediatr Dermatol 1998;15(4):309–12.
20. Attal N, Brasseur L, Chauvin M, Bouhassira D. Effects of single and repeated applications of a eutectic mixture of local anaesthetics (EMLA) cream on spontaneous and evoked pain in post-herpetic neuralgia. Pain 1999;81(1–2):203–9.
21. Calobrisi SD, Drolet BA, Esterly NB. Petechial eruption after the application of EMLA cream. Pediatrics 1998;101(3 Pt 1):471–3.
22. Godwin Y, Brotherston M. Hyperpigmentation following the use of Emla cream. Br J Plast Surg 2001;54(1):82–3.
23. Santacana E, Aliaga L, Bayo M, Vilanova F, Villar-Landeira JM. Emla cream for 15 or 30 min before venopuncture. Reg Anaesth 1994;19:24.
24. Dong H, Kerl H, Cerroni L. EMLA cream-induced irritant contact dermatitis. J Cutan Pathol 2002;29(3):190–2.

Procaine

General Information

Procaine is an aminoester local anesthetic. It is most widely used as a component of procaine penicillin.

Organs and Systems

Nervous system

Rare cases of tonic seizures have been reliably attributed to the presence of procaine in procaine penicillin (1).

Skin

The incidence of pruritus has been evaluated in a retrospective study of patients receiving procaine, lidocaine, or bupivacaine in combination with fentanyl for spinal anesthesia for a variety of different surgical procedures (2). Procaine plus fentanyl and bupivacaine plus fentanyl produced a higher incidence of pruritus than lidocaine plus fentanyl. The severity of pruritus was also greater in those given procaine plus fentanyl. The incidence and severity of pruritus was not related to the dose of fentanyl. Although this may represent an interaction between fentanyl and ester local anesthetics that differs from the synergy occurring between fentanyl and amide local anesthetics, this was an observational study and was neither randomized nor blinded. Furthermore, the doses of local anesthetic or fentanyl were not standardized. Further prospective randomized studies are therefore required to confirm or refute these claims.

Drug–Drug Interactions

Acetylcholinesterase inhibitors

Acetylcholinesterase inhibitors inhibit the hydrolysis of procaine and concomitant use can cause procaine toxicity (3).

Suxamethonium

Procaine is hydrolysed by plasma cholinesterase and may therefore competitively enhance the action of suxamethonium (4).

References

1. Malone JD, Lebar RD, Hilder R. Procaine-induced seizures after intramuscular procaine penicillin G. Mil Med 1988;153(4):191–2.
2. Morikawa S, Ishikawa J, Kamatsuki H, Shinzato Y, Watanabe A, Ishikawa H, Chihara H, Nagata T, Kometani K. [Neurobehavior and mental development of newborn infants delivered under epidural analgesia with bupivacaine.] Nippon Sanka Fujinka Gakkai Zasshi 1990; 42(11):1495–502.
3. Ellis PP, Littlejohn K. Effects of topical anticholinesterases on procaine hydrolysis. Am J Ophthalmol 1974;77(1):71–5.
4. Matsuo S, Rao DB, Chaudry I, Foldes FF. Interaction of muscle relaxants and local anesthetics at the neuromuscular junction. Anesth Analg 1978;57(5):580–7.

Proxymetacaine

General Information

Proxymetacaine is an ester of meta-aminobenzoic acid. It is often used in ophthalmology.

Organs and Systems

Skin

Proparacaine has been reported to cause contact dermatitis.

- A 49-year-old ophthalmologist developed fissuring and bleeding of his finger-tips (1). Skin patch tests using a series of standard and preservative allergens showed only mild reactions to some. Various treatments were attempted, with minimal success, and skin patch testing was repeated using 32 specific formulations that he had contact with in his practice; he had a severe reaction to proxymetacaine hydrochloride 0.5%. Subsequent removal of proparacaine from his practice resulted in resolution over 6 months.
- An ophthalmologist developed chronic finger pad dermatitis with fissuring and scaling, which mainly affected his thumbs for 3 years (2). Patch testing confirmed that "ophthetic solution" (proxymetacaine hydrochloride 0.5%, glycerine, and benzalkonium chloride 0.01%)

was the sensitizing agent. He was instructed to change to tetracaine, to which he had had a negative patch test. However, 2 years later his symptoms recurred and a repeat patch testing was carried out. This was now positive to both tetracaine 1% and proxymetacaine 0.5%.

Cross-sensitization between proxymetacaine and tetracaine is thought to be rare. Moreover, the chemical structure of proxymetacaine is sufficiently different from tetracaine to make cross-reactivity unlikely. This case suggests, however, that some degree of cross-sensitization can occur.

References

1. Liesegang TJ, Perniciaro C. Fingertip dermatitis in an ophthalmologist caused by proparacaine. Am J Ophthalmol 1999;127(2):240–1.
2. Dannaker CJ, Maibach HI, Austin E. Allergic contact dermatitis to proparacaine with subsequent cross-sensitization to tetracaine from ophthalmic preparations. Am J Contact Dermatitis 2001;12(3):177–9.

Ropivacaine

General Information

Ropivacaine is an enantiomeric aminoamide local anesthetic, structurally related to bupivacaine but with a wider margin of safety between concentrations that cause nervous system and cardiovascular effects (1). It is mainly metabolized by CYP1A2.

The safety, pharmacokinetics and efficacy of two doses of ropivacaine (300 and 375 mg) for wound infiltration after surgical incision have been studied in an open nonrandomized study of 20 men undergoing elective hernia repair (2). Efficacy was similar. There were wide variations in mean plasma concentrations of ropivacaine, the highest individual plasma concentration of total drug being 3.0 µg/ml for the 375 mg dose. One patient in the low-dose group had two episodes of bradycardia at 2 and 12 hours after drug administration. The first episode corresponded to a total plasma drug concentration of 1.3 mg/ml. Three patients in the high-dose group had several recorded episodes of sinus bradycardia. Two of these were within the first hour of ropivacaine administration and corresponded to plasma concentrations of 2.5 and 2.9 µg/ml. One patient in the 300 mg group complained of dizziness at 12 and 21 hours and of nausea at 12 hours. Another patient in the same group vomited 4 hours after the injection of ropivacaine. Two patients had transient hypesthesia in the leg on the operated side, thought to be due to partial block of the femoral nerve. The authors felt that systemic toxicity due to ropivacaine was unlikely to be a cause of any of these adverse effects and they concluded that high-dose ropivacaine is safe for wound infiltration.

Organs and Systems

Cardiovascular

The effects on the cardiovascular system of ropivacaine are similar to those of bupivacaine, although direct cardiotoxicity is less severe with ropivacaine than bupivacaine in both man and animals (SEDA-22, 143). Hypotension and bradycardia are prominent adverse effects when ropivacaine is used epidurally, particularly with concentrations of ropivacaine over 0.5% (SEDA-20, 129) (SEDA-22, 143); in one series, hypotension was observed in 30% of patients who received ropivacaine, but in only 13% of those given an equivalent dose of bupivacaine (3).

Cardiac arrest due to ropivacaine toxicity has been reported; in three cases it was related to lower limb block.

- A 76-year-old woman underwent foot osteotomy under combined femoral and sciatic nerve block (4). A femoral nerve block using 20 ml of mepivacaine 1.5% with 1: 400 000 adrenaline was followed by sciatic nerve block with 32 ml of ropivacaine 0.5% and 1: 400 000 adrenaline. The injection was stopped as the patient became less responsive, developed twitching of the hand and face, and had a tonic–clonic seizure, which was terminated with intravenous propofol. She was intubated, developed a bradycardia with wide QRS complexes, and subsequently developed ventricular fibrillation. She was given adrenaline and sinus rhythm returned. She made a complete recovery and was discharged on the next day. The total ropivacaine concentration was 3.2 µg/ml, the unbound ropivacaine concentration 0.5 µg/ml, and the mepivacaine concentration 0.22 µg/ml 5 minutes after the injection.
- A 66-year-old woman was admitted for foot surgery and underwent sciatic nerve block with 25 ml of ropivacaine 0.75% (5). The block was deemed inadequate for surgery and a further 15 ml of ropivacaine 0.75% was used to block the tibial and peroneal nerves at the ankle, resulting in a total ropivacaine dose of 300 mg (6.7 mg/kg). After 1 hour she became agitated and confused and then unresponsive with abnormal oculogyric movements. An electrocardiogram showed wide QRS complexes with worsening bradycardia, despite treatment with atropine and ephedrine. She then had an asystolic cardiac arrest and cardiopulmonary resuscitation was started. More ephedrine was given intravenously. Sinus rhythm was rapidly restored and return of cardiac output was accompanied by return of spontaneous respiration. The ropivacaine concentration was 1.88 µg/ml 70 minutes after the adverse event. She made a full recovery.
- A 66-year-old man scheduled for hip arthroplasty received a lumbar plexus block with 25 ml of ropivacaine 0.75% (total dose 187.5 mg, 1.88 mg/kg) (6). Two minutes after the injection he had a tonic–clonic seizure, for which diazepam was given. He became asystolic and cardiopulmonary resuscitation was begun. After 5 minutes of cardiopulmonary resuscitation and intravenous adrenaline, cardiac activity was restored. An electrocardiogram showed sinus bradycardia with wide QRS complexes, but this normalized after a

further 10 minutes. He was extubated 2 hours later and made a full recovery. The ropivacaine concentration 55 minutes after the episode was 5.61 µg/ml.

In two of these cases the onset of adverse effects was within moments of injection of ropivacaine; the authors concluded that inadvertent intravascular injection was likely to have occurred, despite negative aspiration of blood. In the other case there was a delay of 1 hour between nerve block and cardiac arrest, implying ropivacaine toxicity due to absorption, and the authors acknowledged that the dose of ropivacaine had been excessive.

While cardiac arrest after administration of other local anesthetic agents, such as bupivacaine, is often reported, these are the first cases associated with the use of ropivacaine. In the first case a combination of mepivacaine and ropivacaine was used; however, it is reasonable to conclude that cardiac arrest was due to inadvertent intravascular administration of ropivacaine, as ropivacaine concentrations were high after the episode.

On all three occasions cardiac arrest was immediately preceded by loss of consciousness and a seizure or seizure-like activity. All cases were also associated with bradycardia and wide QRS complexes. On all three occasions cardiac massage was rapidly successful and sinus rhythm was restored without defibrillation or antidysrhythmic drugs. These findings are in stark contrast to cardiac arrest associated with bupivacaine toxicity, which is particularly refractory to treatment and often requires prolonged resuscitation. This suggests that cardiac arrest in the context of ropivacaine toxicity may not only be less likely than with equal doses of bupivacaine, but also more easily treated. Ropivacaine also had significantly less myotoxic potential than bupivacaine in experimental minipigs, when it was injected through femoral nerve catheters (7).

However, ropivacaine-induced cardiac toxicity is not nearly as troublesome as bupivacaine toxicity (8).

Successful resuscitation after systemic ropivacaine toxicity during peripheral nerve block has been described.

- A 15-year-old girl was given 18 ml of ropivacaine 0.75% to the sciatic nerve after negative aspiration, and developed convulsions, immediately followed by ventricular fibrillation (9). Oxygen was delivered by face mask and she received two DC shocks of 200 J. The convulsions stopped and sinus rhythm returned. Postoperatively, there was no evidence of sciatic block. She did not remember the episode and was discharged the next day.

The authors emphasized the importance of electrocardiographic monitoring during nerve block for early identification of complications, the effectiveness of appropriate resuscitation measures in ropivacaine toxicity, and the potential usefulness of low-dose adrenaline in the test dose to detect inadvertent intravascular injection.

Nervous system

Convulsions have occurred after inadvertent intravenous injection of ropivacaine during regional anesthesia

(10,11). CNS adverse effects from ropivacaine occur before or without severe cardiovascular toxicity, as there have been several similar reports of CNS toxicity, but not yet one with severe or fatal cardiotoxicity. This reinforces the claim of increased safety from cardiovascular toxicity with this enantiomeric local anesthetic compared with racemic bupivacaine.

Two episodes of central nervous system toxicity without significant cardiovascular toxicity have been described in a patient who had brachial plexus blocks with excessively high doses of ropivacaine 6 weeks apart (12).

- A 45-year-old woman with rheumatoid arthritis asked for regional anesthesia for arthrodesis of her wrist. An interscalene block was performed with ropivacaine 300 mg (6 mg/kg). After 3 minutes she complained of circumoral numbness and twitching in her throat. She developed irrational speech and perioral twitching and 15 minutes after injection developed involuntary clonic twitching in her left upper arm. She was anesthetized with thiopental and ventilated with 100% oxygen via a bag and mask. She regained consciousness within 20 minutes and at 135 minutes was fully conscious, with complete sensorimotor block of her left upper limb. Six weeks later she had an axillary nerve block with ropivacaine 225 mg (4.5 mg/kg) and lidocaine 200 mg (4 mg/kg) with adrenaline. After 25 minutes she complained of a strange feeling in her tongue and became dysarthric and unresponsive to voice. She was anesthetized with propofol and the arthrodesis was performed under general anesthetic. Postoperatively she had a complete brachial plexus block, which resolved after 6 hours. In both instances the only cardiovascular effect noted was sinus tachycardia (150–170/minute).

Seizure after epidural ropivacaine have been reported.

- A 26-year-old primigravid woman in labor had an epidural anesthetic with ropivacaine (a background infusion of 18 mg/hour and three bolus doses totalling 44 mg, followed by an infusion of 24 mg/hour) (13). She failed to progress and another three boluses totalling 150 mg were given. She received a total of 279 mg of ropivacaine over 5 hours. Immediately after the final bolus she developed oculogyric movements and slurred speech and then twitching of her face and arms. The seizure ceased with thiopental and the operation was carried out uneventfully under general anesthesia. Her serum ropivacaine concentration 1 hour later was 3.5 mg/l check units; in previous studies, symptoms of toxicity during intravenous infusions occurred at plasma concentrations of 1–2 µg/ml.

This shows that it is important to leave adequate time between bolus doses to detect adverse effects.

- A 48-year-old woman scheduled for abdominal total hysterectomy had an uneventful lumbar epidural insertion for postoperative pain relief (14). She was asymptomatic after a test dose of 2 ml of lidocaine 1%. To begin epidural anesthesia, ropivacaine 1% was injected epidurally at a rate of about 12 ml/minute. She became confused and had a classical tonic–clonic seizure after injection of 8 ml of ropivacaine. The convulsions ceased with intravenous midazolam 5 mg. Aspiration was negative for blood before the catheter was removed.

The arterial plasma concentration of ropivacaine 2 minutes after the start of the seizure was 1.5 µg/ml. Although tachycardia occurred at this time, the effect on the cardiovascular system was minimal. The authors repeated the suggestion that adding adrenaline to the test dose could have predicted intravascular injection.

Inadvertent intravenous injection of ropivacaine resulted in systemic toxicity in two cases (11–15).

- A 13-year-old boy weighing 44 kg was given a bolus of 20 mg of ropivacaine through an 18 G Tuohy needle. No cerebrospinal fluid or blood had been aspirated. However, he immediately complained that his face "felt different," and within 1 minute developed a tonic-clonic seizure and a tachycardia of 160/minute. In a blood sample taken about 35 minutes later the plasma concentration of ropivacaine was 1.4 mg/ml, consistent with intravascular injection. In humans, symptoms of toxicity occur at plasma concentrations of 1–2 mg/ml. The authors thought that the rate of injection of epidural local anesthetic should be slower, which would give a greater safety margin between the onset of facial numbness and seizures.

- A ropivacaine-induced seizure occurred in a 23-year-old woman undergoing postpartum tubal ligation. An epidural that had been inserted for labor the evening before the procedure was used to give ropivacaine 120 mg in increments over 11 minutes. She complained of nervousness and within a few seconds had a generalized tonic-clonic seizure and a sinus tachycardia of 120/minute.

In both of these cases reasonable precautions had been taken to ensure correct catheter placement, but nevertheless systemic toxicity occurred. However, neither patient had any serious cardiotoxicity. However, it is worth emphasizing that large doses of local anesthetics should be given slowly and in divided doses and that lidocaine, one of the least toxic of the commonly used local anesthetics, has more obvious prodromal symptoms than ropivacaine, and could be a useful marker for intravenous injection (16).

Three patients suffered convulsions as a result of inadvertent intravascular injection of ropivacaine during placement of local blocks.

- A 75-year-old woman received ropivacaine 160 mg intravenously through an epidural catheter (17). After completion of the injection, she suddenly became unresponsive and had a generalized tonic-clonic convulsion accompanied by a sinus tachycardia of 120/minute but no other cardiac dysrhythmias.

- A 56-year-old 70 kg woman with a Colles fracture received a brachial plexus block at the humeral canal with 0.75% ropivacaine 40 ml using a nerve stimulator (18). The local anesthetic was administered slowly with negative intermittent aspiration. However, 15 minutes later she had two generalized convulsions, which were treated with diazepam. The total venous ropivacaine concentration measured 2 hours after the block was 2.3 µg/ml.

- A 25-year-old man received ropivacaine 75 mg intravenously during sciatic nerve block (19). The nerve was located using a nerve stimulator and the injection was performed after elicitation of a distal extensor response. Numerous aspirations were performed during the procedure, but 1 minute after injection he suddenly became unresponsive and developed a tonic-clonic seizure, which resolved after treatment with midazolam and propofol. The only cardiovascular effect was a sinus tachycardia of 130/minute.

In the last case, the authors noted that the motor response to stimulation was maintained throughout the injection; it is generally felt that the motor response to stimulation should disappear after the injection of the first milliliters of local anesthetic; if the response does not disappear the injection should be stopped. In all three cases nervous system toxicity occurred with minimal or no cardiovascular toxicity, which is in keeping with previous reports, confirming the relative safety of ropivacaine; there has still not been one single fatal outcome reported with this agent.

Drug Administration

Drug administration route

There have been two reports of patients who accidentally received ropivacaine intravenously from a bag of ropivacaine intended for postoperative epidural use.

- A 36-year-old man, ASA grade I, received 200 ml of ropivacaine 0.15% (300 mg = 4.6 mg/kg) after hip arthroplasty (20). He developed tonic–clonic convulsions, hypotension, and respiratory arrest; 20 minutes later the plasma ropivacaine concentration was 3.1 mg/l. There were no dysrhythmias. Recovery was uneventful.

This was the first report in which ropivacaine was given directly through an intravenous line. The authors used a pharmacokinetic model to estimate the plasma ropivacaine concentration at the time of the seizure to have been 17 mg/l, which is above the experimental human threshold for nervous system toxicity.

- In an incident based on a similar error, an 84-year-old woman received ropivacaine 380 mg inadvertently by intravenous infusion over 1.75 hours (21). Despite serum concentrations in the lower toxic range she had no signs of nervous system or cardiovascular toxicity, confirming the assumed wide therapeutic range for ropivacaine.

References

1. Markham A, Faulds D. Ropivacaine. A review of its pharmacology and therapeutic use in regional anaesthesia. Drugs 1996;52(3):429–49.
2. Pettersson N, Emanuelsson BM, Reventlid H, Hahn RG. High-dose ropivacaine wound infiltration for pain relief after inguinal hernia repair: a clinical and pharmacokinetic evaluation. Reg Anesth Pain Med 1998;23(2):189–96.
3. Morrison LM, Emanuelsson BM, McClure JH, Pollok AJ, McKeown DW, Brockway M, Jozwiak H, Wildsmith JA. Efficacy and kinetics of extradural ropivacaine: comparison with bupivacaine. Br J Anaesth 1994;72(2):164–9.
4. Bisschop DY, Alardo JP, Razgallah B, Just BY, Germain ML, Millart HG, Trenque TC. Seizure induced by ropivacaine. Ann Pharmacother 2001;35(3):311–3.
5. Iwama H. A case of normal ropivacaine concentration causing grand mal seizure after epidural injection. Eur J Anaesthesiol 2005;22(4):322–3.
6. Plowman AN, Bolsin S, Mather LE. Central nervous system toxicity attributable to epidural ropivacaine hydrochloride. Anaesth Intensive Care 1998;26(2):204–6.
7. Checketts MR, Wildsmith JA. Accidental i.v. injection of local anaesthetics: an avoidable event? Br J Anaesth 1998;80(6):710–1.
8. Cherng CH, Wong CS, Ho ST. Ropivacaine-induced convulsion immediately after epidural administration—a case report. Acta Anaesthesiol Sin 2002;40(1):43–5.
9. Ould-Ahmed M, Drouillard I, Fourel D, Roussaly P, Almanza L, Segalen F. Convulsions induites par la ropivacaine lors d'un bloc au canal humeral. [Convulsions induced by ropivacaine after midhumeral block.] Ann Fr Anesth Réanim 2002;21(8):681–4.
10. Klein SM, Pierce T, Rubin Y, Nielsen KC, Steele SM. Successful resuscitation after ropivacaine-induced ventricular fibrillation. Anesth Analg 2003;97:901–3.
11. Chazalon P, Tourtier JP, Villevielle T, Giraud D, Saissy JM, Mion G, Benhamou D. Ropivacaine-induced cardiac arrest after peripheral nerve block: successful resuscitation. Anesthesiology 2003;99:1449–51.
12. Huet O, Eyrolle LJ, Mazoit JX, Ozier YM. Cardiac arrest after injection of ropivacaine for posterior lumbar plexus blockade. Anesthesiology 2003;99:1451–3.
13. Zink W, Seif C, Bohl JRE, Hacke N, Braun PM, Sinner B, Martin E, Fink RH, Graf BM. The acute myotoxic effects of bupivacaine and ropivacaine after continuous peripheral nerve blockades. Anesth Analg 2003;97:1173–9.
14. Petitjeans F, Mion G, Puidupin M, Tourtier JP, Hutson C, Saissy JM. Tachycardia and convulsions induced by accidental intravascular ropivacaine injection during sciatic block. Acta Anaesthesiol Scand 2002;46(5):616–7.
15. Finucane BT. Ropivacaine cardiac toxicity-not as troublesome as bupivacaine. Can J Anaesth 2005;52(5):449–53.
16. Gielen M, Slappendel R, Jack N. Successful defibrillation immediately after the intravascular injection of ropivacaine. Can J Anaesth 2005;52(5):490–2.
17. Korman B, Riley RH. Convulsions induced by ropivacaine during interscalene brachial plexus block. Anesth Analg 1997;85(5):1128–9.
18. Abouleish EI, Elias M, Nelson C. Ropivacaine-induced seizure after extradural anaesthesia. Br J Anaesth 1998;80(6):843–4.
19. Ala-Kokko TI, Lopponen A, Alahuhta S. Two instances of central nervous system toxicity in the same patient following repeated ropivacaine-induced brachial plexus block. Acta Anaesthesiol Scand 2000;44(5):623–6.
20. Dernedde M, Furlan D, Verbesselt R, Gepts E, Boogaerts JG. Grand mal convulsion after an accidental intravenous injection of ropivacaine. Anesth Analg 2004;98(2):521–3.
21. Pfeiffer G, Bör K, Neubauer P, H—hne M. Versehentliche intraven—se Infusion von 380 mg Naropin (Ropivacain). [Inadvertent intravenous infusion of 380 mg ropivacaine.] Anaesthesist 2004;53(7):633–6.

Tetracaine

General Information

Tetracaine is a highly lipid-soluble, potent aminoester. It is primarily used as a constituent of many different topical formulations and for spinal anesthesia. It is four times as potent as lidocaine, and unless great caution is taken in dosage, serious systemic adverse effects can develop, owing to rapid absorption after topical use (for example in a 0.5% gargle) (1) or use in endoscopy. It is more effective than Emla in reducing the pain of venous cannulation in children.

Tetracaine can cause local reactions when applied to the skin, but because it is rapidly metabolized by plasma cholinesterase systemic reactions are unlikely (2).

Organs and Systems

Cardiovascular

- An 18-month-old child undergoing cardiac surgery developed discoloration of the hand, consistent with severe bruising, after application of 4% tetracaine gel, which was inadvertently left under an occlusive dressing for about 24 hours (3). There were no long-term sequelae and no treatment was required.

The authors blamed a combination of the vasodilatory properties of tetracaine and the fact that the child was heparinized for surgery, causing capillary leak at the area of application.

Hematologic

Adult cases of methemoglobinemia have been reported with Cetacaine (a proprietary mixture of 14% benzocaine, 2% tetracaine, and 2% butylaminobenzoate) (4–6).

Cetacaine spray used to anesthetize the oropharynx before endoscopy led to dyspnea, central cyanosis, and an oxygen saturation of 80%; methemoglobinemia was diagnosed, and the patient recovered rapidly with methylthioninium chloride 1 mg/kg over 5 minutes.

- A 77-year-old woman received two sprays of Cetacaine for an attempted emergency nasotracheal intubation. After intubation, she became cyanosed. The arterial blood was chocolate brown and the SaO_2 by CO oximetry was 54–58%, despite a high PaO_2. The methemoglobin concentration was 39% and she was treated with methylthioninium chloride. Three weeks later, Cetacaine again caused cyanosis with a drop in SpO_2 to 76% and a methemoglobin concentration of 24%, which resolved spontaneously.
- A 74-year-old man received Cetacaine spray to his oropharynx for transesophageal echocardiography. His SpO_2 fell to 85%, he became drowsy, then unresponsive, cyanotic, and apneic, and required intubation. His PaO_2 was 37 kPa (280 mmHg), SaO_2 40%, and methemoglobin concentration 60%. Intravenous methylthioninium

chloride produced an immediate improvement in the cyanosis and the methemoglobin concentration fell to 0.6%.

Skin

Reported local adverse effects of tetracaine include itch and a high incidence of erythema as a consequence of vasodilatation, which may actually be an advantage. There was no evidence of dermatitis (SEDA-20, 127) (7).

In 272 children who required topical local anesthesia for venepuncture, there was no association between the duration of application of 4% tetracaine gel and the development of adverse skin reactions (8). However, two reports discussed by the same authors highlighted rare adverse reactions.

- A 4-year-old child with no previous exposure complained of severe pain, erythema, and blistering 5 minutes after the application of 4% tetracaine gel.
- An anesthetist who was suspected of occupational exposure developed redness and blistering after applying a test dose of tetracaine.

The authors recommended minimizing occupational contact and quickly removing the cream in patients who report pain after application of tetracaine.

- A 71-year-old man developed severe contact dermatitis in the groin area after transurethral resection of prostate, during which a probe lubricated with an ointment containing tetracaine was used (9). Biopsy and patch testing showed a positive reaction to tetracaine. The dermatitis resolved with topical glucocorticoids and antihistamines.

There may be a higher incidence of skin sensitization from tetracaine gel than Emla. At one hospital, in a 3-month period, there were seven site reactions to tetracaine (10). While the Summary of Product Characteristics says that significant skin reactions are rare, the authors estimated that seven reactions in their hospital represented a higher rate than 0.01–0.1% (usually regarded as the frequency of rare events). Indeed, the reported incidence of moderate to severe local skin reactions in clinical trials is 0.6–8.8%, compared with 0–1.7% with Emla. According to the Summary of Product Characteristics there is also a risk of sensitization with repeated exposure (four of the seven children who had reactions to tetracaine had had prior exposure to it), which is not known to happen with Emla.

Immunologic

Anaphylactic shock has been reported after spinal anesthesia (SED-12, 257) (11).

Allergic dermatitis has been reported after repeated contact with tetracaine in the beauty industry (12). This highlights the importance of educating employees in the health and beauty industry to increase their awareness of potential sensitizing agents, including local anesthetics The authors mentioned the lack of data on the penetration rates of some topical formulations through gloves.

References

1. Patel D, Chopra S, Berman MD. Serious systemic toxicity resulting from use of tetracaine for pharyngeal anesthesia in upper endoscopic procedures. Dig Dis Sci 1989;34(6):882–4.
2. Geraint M. Check long contact with Ametop. Pharm Pract 1998;8:208.
3. Hewitt T, Eadon H. Check long contact with Ametop. Pharm Pract 1998;8:47–8.
4. Maher P. Methemoglobinemia: an unusual complication of topical anesthesia. Gastroenterol Nurs 1998;21(4):173–5.
5. Khan NA, Kruse JA. Methemoglobinemia induced by topical anesthesia: a case report and review. Am J Med Sci 1999;318(6):415–8.
6. Stoiber TR. Toxic methemoglobinemia complicating transesophageal echocardiography. Echocardiography 1999;16(4):383–5.
7. Lawson RA, Smart NG, Gudgeon AC, Morton NS. Evaluation of an amethocaine gel preparation for percutaneous analgesia before venous cannulation in children. Br J Anaesth 1995;75(3):282–5.
8. Wongprasartsuk P, Main BJ. Adverse local reactions to amethocaine cream—audit and case reports. Anaesth Intensive Care 1998;26(3):312–4.
9. Huerta Brogeras M, Aviles JA, Gonzalez-Carrascosa M, de la Cueva P, Suarez R, Lazaro P. Dermatitis sistemica de contacto por tetracainas. Allergol Immunopathol (Madr) 2005;33(2):112–4.
10. Clarkson A, Choonara I, O'Donnell K. Localized adverse skin reactions to topical anaesthetics. Paediatr Anaesth 1999;9(6):553–5.
11. Moriwaki K, Higaki A, Sasaki H, Murata K, Sumida T, Baba I. [A case report of anaphylactic shock induced by tetracaine used for spinal anesthesia.] Masui; 35(8):1279–84.
12. Connolly M, Mehta A, Sansom JE, Dunnill MG. Allergic contact dermatitis from tetracaine in the beauty industry. Contact Dermatitis 2004;51(2):95–6.

NEUROMUSCULAR BLOCKING DRUGS AND MUSCLE RELAXANTS

General Information

There are two broad classes of neuromuscular blocking drugs: non-depolarizing agents, of which the prototype is curare (for example, d-tubocurarine, atracurium, metocurine, mivacurium, pancuronium, rocuronium, vecuronium) and depolarizing blockers, such as suxamethonium. This monograph is largely concerned with the former; suxamethonium is the subject of a separate monograph.

Non-depolarizing neuromuscular blocking agents compete with acetylcholine for receptors at the neuromuscular junction and clinical relaxation begins when 80–85% of the receptors on the motor end-plate are blocked. They do not produce depolarization themselves and, by blocking access to the receptors, prevent the normal acetylcholine-induced depolarization. Flaccid paralysis ensues. Their action terminates when acetylcholine again gains access to the receptors, due to diffusion of the relaxant molecules away from the neuromuscular junction. This may be hastened by greatly increasing the number of acetylcholine molecules at the motor end-plate by giving an anticholinesterase such as neostigmine. In contrast, the depolarizing blockers first depolarize the motor end-plate and then prevent further depolarization.

Combining different non-depolarizing neuromuscular blocking agents can result in additive or synergistic effects. When pancuronium is given together with D-tubocurarine or metocurine, the resulting block is greater than would be expected if the effects were purely additive. This potentiation is not seen with the metocurine D-tubocurarine combination (1). Synergism resulting from such combinations is thought to be a postsynaptic effect (2). When different non-depolarizing agents are given consecutively, the neuromuscular blocking action of the second may be considerably modified by the first; the action of vecuronium, for example, lasts longer than expected if pancuronium has been given first (SEDA-11, 124) (3). Caution should therefore be exercised when giving a small dose of a normally short-acting non-depolarizer near the end of an operation when another long-acting agent has been given earlier. The resulting block can be greater than expected and last much longer than desired. Reversal with anticholinesterases can be difficult at the end of surgery if the block is still greater than 90%.

Specialized accounts of adverse effects and interactions in this field are available (4–7), including a review of the older literature (8).

Organs and Systems

Ear, nose, throat

Endotracheal intubation is less traumatic when it is facilitated by a muscle relaxant. Vocal cord hematoma after intubation occurred in six of 36 patients when only fentanyl plus propofol was used, compared with one of 37 when atracurium was added (9).

Nervous system

Drug accumulation will result in paralysis lasting from hours to days. Occasionally, however, paralysis can persist for weeks or even months because of relaxant-associated myopathy (10). Muscle weakness, causing difficulties in the subsequent weaning of such patients from artificial ventilation, has often been described (11–15). This condition has been observed most often after concomitant administration of muscle relaxants and high-dose glucocorticoids, typically in patients with exacerbated asthma requiring mechanical ventilation (16–21). It is not known how these factors combine to produce myopathy; myopathic changes can also occur after either high-dose glucocorticoid therapy or long-term muscle relaxant administration alone. Serial electrophysiological testing, and eventually muscle biopsy, is necessary to diagnose myopathy accurately and to avoid useless trials of weaning the patient from the ventilator. Within some weeks, muscle weakness will resolve sufficiently to allow successful weaning, but extensive rehabilitative measures are required for several months until the patient is independent. In view of the multitude of potential mechanisms of muscle weakness in critically ill patients, it is advisable always to monitor neuromuscular function and to avoid complete paralysis for any length of time in intensive care patients who are treated with muscle relaxants.

Musculoskeletal

Several authors have described heterotopic ossification or myositis ossificans after long-term administration of neuromuscular blocking agents to ICU patients (22–25). However, the causative role of muscle relaxants in the development of this phenomenon has been questioned (26), because of the observation that heterotopic ossification also occurred in critically ill patients not treated with such agents (27). It was suggested that prolonged immobilization is an important factor in the pathogenesis of heterotopic ossification, and that both deep sedation and neuromuscular blockade, by producing complete immobilization, might contribute to the pathophysiology of this severe complication in critical illness, which may require prolonged rehabilitation and surgical removal of ectopic bone to allow the patient to be ambulatory and self-sufficient.

Residual paralysis

Residual paralysis after the use of long-acting muscle relaxants, such as pancuronium, is not uncommon and can result in significant pulmonary complications (28). Many anesthetists have assumed that this was less of a problem with agents of intermediate duration. However, a surprisingly high incidence of residual neuromuscular impairment has been reported after a single intubating dose of muscle relaxants of intermediate duration as well (29). Two hours after either rocuronium, vecuronium, or atracurium, the train-of-four ratio was still below 0.7 in 10% of patients and below 0.9 in 37%, which was not reliably detected by clinical evaluation (head lift, tongue depressor test) or qualitative measurements (repetitive nerve stimulation with tactile evaluation of fade). Similar results have been reported by others (30–33). Pharyngeal dysfunction with a risk of aspiration has been observed in partially paralysed awake volunteers at train-of-four ratios below 0.9 (34–35). Therefore, patients with a train-of-four ratio below 0.9 at the end of the operation should receive a cholinesterase inhibitor, such as neostigmine, in order to reduce the impact of residual paralysis. This obviously implies that quantitative monitoring of neuromuscular transmission should be used routinely. Only if this is not possible should a cholinesterase inhibitor be given blindly. This represents a change in our opinion: we had previously stated that anticholinesterase drugs should be used to reverse residual neuromuscular block detected by monitoring of neuromuscular transmission or producing clinical symptoms (SEDA-24, 157). Now we acknowledge that a reversal agent is justified, even in asymptomatic patients, because residual dysfunction of certain muscle groups may still be present. For the time being, there is nothing to support the routine use of an anticholinesterase drug if spontaneous recovery with a train-of-four ratio of 0.9 or above can be demonstrated. We should like to stress that attempts to reverse intense neuromuscular blockade must be avoided. Therefore, some evidence of recovery of neuromuscular transmission (for example spontaneous ventilation, voluntary movements, twitch response to nerve stimulation) should be observed before any anticholinesterase is given. In addition, it should be mentioned that large doses of cholinesterase inhibitors can cause deterioration rather than improvement of neuromuscular function (36,37). It is unnecessary to use more than 2.5 mg of neostigmine or equivalent (38). Neostigmine 1.25 mg or equivalent can be as effective (39) and is associated with a reduced incidence of postoperative nausea and vomiting (40).

Immunologic

Hypersensitivity reactions can occur with all neuromuscular blocking agents, including the newer agents (41–43). Allergic reactions during anesthesia have been reviewed (44).

Frequency

The incidence of life-threatening anaphylactic or anaphylactoid reactions occurring during anesthesia is variably reported as being between one in 1000 and one in 10 000 anesthetics (45,46), and in one survey was one in 6500 (47). The frequency quoted depends on the criteria used. An epidemiological study (48) has suggested that the incidence is somewhat greater than one in 5000 anesthetics. The mortality from such serious reactions is reported to be in the range of 3.4–6% (46–48). Minor systemic reactions attributable to histamine release probably occur in more than 1% of anesthesia (49). Neuromuscular blocking drugs are the triggering agents in 50% or more of these reactions (50–52), and of them D-tubocurarine is the most potent histamine liberator. During the last two decades, however, several large series of patients have been investigated, and the data suggest that suxamethonium is the relaxant most likely to produce

life-threatening reactions, if allowances are made for the frequency of usage of the different agents (SEDA-17, 12) (48,50,52–56). Pancuronium has repeatedly been shown to be the relaxant least often associated with anaphylactoid reactions major or minor.

The incidence of allergic reactions to several muscle relaxants has been assessed in relation to the number of vials sold in France (57). In line with a previous publication (58), the proportion of reported reactions to rocuronium was higher than its corresponding market share. Based on that, the authors suggested classifying the risk of allergic reactions to neuromuscular blocking agents as high (suxamethonium, rocuronium), intermediate (pancuronium, vecuronium, mivacurium), and low (atracurium, cisatracurium). This classification is based on the assumption that the ratio of used/sold vials is similar for each agent, which may or may not be true. The authors themselves insisted that they did not recommend one muscle relaxant over another on the basis of their allergic potential (59). As highlighted before (SEDA-26, 150), there are significant methodological and statistical problems when such rare events are compared. What we need is an international network of clinics specialized in investigating patients after suspected intraoperative allergic reactions, and the French GERAP centers are an excellent example of this.

Regional variations

A few years ago the Norwegian Medicines Authority responded to 29 reports of anaphylaxis to rocuronium among 150 000 patients exposed by recommending restricted use of this agent. However, Norway's Scandinavian neighbors, Finland, Sweden, and Denmark, had observed only eight cases among 800 000 patients exposed, and it was not clear if this difference was entirely due to reporting bias (60).

The presence of IgE antibodies to suxamethonium (succinylcholine) and morphine is much more common in Norway than in Sweden (61). A total of 800 blood samples from Norway were tested for IgE antibodies to morphine or suxamethonium; the results were compared with those of 800 blood samples from Sweden. Among 500 samples from blood donors in Norway, 5% had antibodies to morphine and 0.4% to suxamethonium. Among 300 patients with a history of allergy, 10% had IgE to morphine and 0.7% had IgE to suxamethonium. In contrast, no positive samples were found in Sweden. The authors also investigated a variety of other substances as possible sensitizers by using an IgE antibody inhibition assay. Several agents inhibited the antibody reaction to suxamethonium and/or morphine, for example skin care ointments, hair-care products, cough syrups, cleansers, toothpastes, and lozenges. The only chemicals available in Norway but not in Sweden were cough syrups containing pholcodine. The authors detected IgE to pholcodine in 6% of Norwegian blood donors and in none of the Swedish samples. Pholcodine is an opioid contained in over-the-counter cough syrups, which seems to be widely used in Norway. Based on the observation that the presence of antibodies to morphine and pholcodine was closely correlated in cross-inhibition studies, the authors suggested that exposure of the population in Norway to pholcodine could have resulted in sensitization not just to this substance but also to morphine. Morphine, on the other hand, has some structural similarities to the quaternary ammonium groups in muscle relaxants. So could exposure to pholcodine also have resulted in sensitization to neuromuscular blocking agents? Altogether 42 of 65 patients (65%) with confirmed anaphylaxis to neuromuscular blocking agents had antibodies to pholcodine. Pholcodine is used as an antitussive agent in Australia, Belgium, Finland, France, Ireland, New Zealand, Norway, and the UK, all of which have reported several cases of anaphylaxis to rocuronium as well as other neuromuscular blocking agents. In contrast, pholcodine is not used in Denmark, Germany, Sweden, and the USA, where anaphylaxis to rocuronium is thought to be extremely rare. However, many of the patients tested in Norway had antibodies to morphine but not to suxamethonium. The authors therefore concluded that further studies are needed to identify agents that could result in sensitization to neuromuscular blocking agents.

In this context it should be noted that rocuronium was actually confirmed as the causative agent in several cases of suspected anaphylaxis in Norway (62). From 1996 to 2001, 83 patients with suspected intraoperative anaphylaxis were investigated by the Allergy Investigation Unit in Bergen; 55 (66%) were allergic to NMBA, 40 (36%) to suxamethonium, and 17 (21%) to rocuronium. Referring to statistical problems, the authors refrained from relating these figures to the number of ampoules sold and did not answer the question whether the incidence of anaphylaxis to rocuronium is higher in Norway than in other countries. However, 93% of their confirmed cases were related to neuromuscular blocking agents. Compared with other countries this is a high proportion. Of course, this does not prove that anaphylaxis to neuromuscular blocking agents is more common in Norway, but it is still worth noting. Even if the incidence of anaphylaxis to rocuronium in Norway is not known, anesthetists seem to be cautious, and sales figures of rocuronium in Norway have fallen markedly. The same has apparently happened in France. We shall therefore probably not see much more information related to this matter from these countries. One can only hope that the mystery surrounding anaphylaxis to rocuronium will prompt more research into sensitizing substances as well as geographical, racial, and other differences in sensitization to anesthetics, with a view to improving patient safety.

Mechanisms

Much controversy still surrounds the issue of the possible mechanisms by which a neuromuscular blocking agent produces the clinical picture of an anaphylactoid reaction, but new insight into the matter has been gathered (63). In most cases (that is the mechanism is a Type I hypersensitivity reaction) (50,52,56,64,65), even though the frequent lack of previous exposure to relaxants seems to exclude this. Direct histamine release and several other mechanisms have also been postulated (66,67). Non-specific histamine release probably is dose dependent (63).

Drug-specific IgE antibodies to suxamethonium and other neuromuscular blocking agents have been demonstrated (52,68,69). It has been hypothesized that such antibodies are directed against quaternary and tertiary ammonium ion determinants (68,69). This would help to explain the phenomenon of cross-reactivity with different relaxants and also suggests that prior sensitization could occur via other quaternary or tertiary ammonium-ion-containing compounds in drugs, cosmetics, disinfectants, and the like (50,64). Two quaternary ammonium groups may be necessary for histamine release by neuromuscular blocking agents (65,66). Quaternary an as benzalkonium, in cosmeti role in sensitization ((70)).

Diagnosis

Anaphylactoid reactions are easily misdiagnosed during anesthesia (71), since circulatory collapse accompanied by sinus tachycardia may be the only signs (49). These are the presenting features in 70–90% of cases. Mucocutaneous manifestations (erythema, urticaria, angioedema) are reported in 60–80% of reactions, but are often only noticed much later when the acute phase is over. Bronchospasm is present in about 40% of cases. Reactions are more common in women (up to 80%), in atopic patients, and in those who have a history of asthma (who are particularly prone to develop bronchospasm) or allergy, and in patients who have had a previous reaction to anesthetic drugs (50,53); they also seem to be more common in patients under 40 years of age (54).

The diagnosis of an allergic reaction to a muscle relaxant is based on clinical features, measurement of histamine and tryptase concentrations in the plasma during the reaction, and subsequent skin testing a few weeks later. However, during general anesthesia isolated symptoms can occur, most often hypotension or bronchospasm. Therefore, the clinical features of anaphylaxis may not be recognized as such.

The investigation of a reaction during anesthesia requires serial blood samples during the first 24–72 hours and further laboratory tests, such as basophil histamine release, and intradermal skin testing 4–8 weeks later (45,52,53,67,72). Plasma tryptase concentration, measured 30 and 120 minutes after the shock, is a sensitive and relatively specific marker of anaphylaxis (63,73). The possibilities of postmortem diagnosis have now been extended to the use of blood samples taken up to 3 hours after a patient's death and subjected to radioimmunoassay for mast cell tryptase activity and drug-specific IgEantibodies (74). However, histamine and tryptase concentrations may be ambiguous.

Radioallergosorbent tests (RAST) which detect IgE antibodies to specific muscle relaxants have been developed (68,69) and are commercially available for some anesthetic drugs (67,75). However, the sensitivity of IgE testing is variable and reached 90–97% in selected specialized centers only (76).

Skin testing has been used to confirm the diagnosis and to identify the causative agent (77). The sensitivity of skin testing for reactions to muscle relaxants is thought to be greater than 95% (77), although significantly lower for opioids, barbiturates, and synthetic colloids (44). However, opinions differ as to the value and the reliability of intradermal skin testing. The proponents of skin testing emphasize that strict criteria must be used in performing and interpreting the tests (78).

Additional biological tests have been suggested to improve the accuracy further. The leukocyte histamine release test has been found helpful (79) but it is expensive and time-consuming. Several surface molecules have been studied as markers, for example CD63. IgE-mediated degranulation of basophils after incubation of the patient's serum with a neuromuscular blocking agent can be detected by flow cytometry if a relevant proportion of basophils express the surface marker CD63 (80–81). An assay for CD63 and CCR3 was reported to have a sensitivity of 54% compared with 63% for the detection of specific IgE (82). Combined, these tests had a sensitivity of 80% and a specificity of 100%. The authors regarded this as a promising approach to the diagnosis of muscle relaxant allergy in cases where discrepancies between the clinical presentation and the laboratory result.

Morphine, which has a single substituted quaternary ammonium ion group, binds to antibodies that react with neuromuscular blocking drugs. Morphine radioimmunoassay was more sensitive in detecting IgE antibodies to neuromuscular blocking agents than assays specific for the various agents (83). Consequently, morphine radioimmunoassay was suggested as a diagnostic tool in cases of suspected anaphylaxis to neuromuscular blocking agents. In addition, IgE-mediated degranulation of basophils after incubation of the patient's serum with a neuromuscular blocking agent may be detected by flow cytometry if a relevant proportion of basophils express the surface marker CD63 (80,81).

Flow cytometry as an additional tool has received considerable attention over the last few years. Detection of the basophil surface marker CD63 after incubation with the suspected agent has a higher sensitivity (79%) than skin prick testing (64%) (84). This is higher than the sensitivity of CD63 in a previous study (54%) (85), but the authors did not discuss this difference. Even so, basophil activation testing by flow cytometry is a very interesting and promising tool for the workup of suspected anaphylaxis. New developments, such as the use of anti-CRTH2/DP2 antibodies for basophil recognition, might further improve its value (86).

Prevention and treatment
Measures for the prevention and treatment of hypersensitivity reactions have been reviewed (53,54,87,89).

The possibility of cross-reactivity with different relaxants (87,90,91) should also be investigated and the patient issued with an appropriate warning-card. After an anaphylactic reaction during anesthesia, the drug responsible is usually determined by skin testing. Most often in such cases, a neuromuscular blocking drug is found to be the triggering substance, and since cross-sensitivity between neuromuscular blocking agents can occur, a variety of these drugs should be tested. Neuromuscular blocking agents that produce negative skin results are considered

safe for future anesthesia. However, there have been descriptions of several patients with previous anaphylactic reactions to neuromuscular blocking agents who had a second severe anaphylactic reaction when skin-test negative agents were used (92,93). The authors assumed that the skin tests had been falsely negative in these patients, but they conceded that newly acquired sensitivity might also have been an explanation. They concluded that all neuromuscular blocking agents should be avoided in patients with previous anaphylaxis to one of these drugs. If that is not possible the patient should be given antiallergic pretreatment and the anesthetic team should be prepared for resuscitation. In addition to standard pretreatment with both H1 and H2 histamine receptor antagonists, monovalent haptens might prove effective in blocking anaphylaxis to neuromuscular blocking agents (87).

Second-Generation Effects

Pregnancy

The pharmacokinetics of neuromuscular blocking agents in pregnancy and the impact on anesthesia for cesarean section have been reviewed (94). Key statements are:

(1) The umbilical/maternal vein concentration ratio of non-depolarizing neuromuscular relaxants varies from 7 to 26%. Clinical doses of these drugs can induce partial curarization in neonates.
(2) Despite reduced plasma cholinesterase activity, the duration of effect of suxamethonium 1 mg/kg is usually not significantly increased in pregnant women.
(3) At clinical doses, transplacental passage of suxamethonium is insufficient to produce paralysis of the neonate.

However, inadequate muscular activity requiring ventilatory support has been reported in babies born to mothers with atypical plasma cholinesterase.

Susceptibility Factors

Age

Children
Neonates are said to be more sensitive to non-depolarizing neuromuscular blocking drugs. Neonates have a lower muscle mass per kilogram body weight, maturation of neuromuscular transmission occurs in the 2 months after full-term birth (95,96), and the "margin of safety" for neuromuscular transmission (that is the fraction of receptors that must be occupied before neuromuscular block can be detected) is reduced in infants under 12 weeks of age (97). Thus, smaller doses should be used in the very young. The greater body water content of neonates, however, tends to mitigate the increased sensitivity, so that several authors recommend similar doses to adults (calculated on a body weight basis). Owing to longer elimination half-lives, recovery is slower in neonates and maintenance doses are needed at longer intervals (98),

certainly where most of the older, long-acting relaxants are concerned. There are conflicting data about whether the actions of vecuronium and atracurium (and even pancuronium) are prolonged or not (99).

Most investigators concur that neonates and infants require a larger dose per kilogram of suxamethonium (2–4 mg/kg) to achieve an equivalent effect to that seen in adults. In young children the plasma clearance of non-depolarizing relaxants is quicker and their duration of action shorter (100,101), so that doses may have to be given more often.

Interindividual variation in dose requirements is even more marked in neonates and infants than in adults, so that monitoring of neuromuscular function is essential. Small dysmature babies, especially with temperatures below 36°C, are notoriously unpredictable in their response to relaxants.

Elderly people

In elderly people there is much slower recovery from non-depolarizing relaxants (about 60% in patients over 75 years of age given pancuronium), associated with a decreased rate of elimination (probably through reduced glomerular clearance and, to a lesser extent, reduced hepatic blood flow). The potency of relaxants is not altered. While the initial dose required to produce full relaxation is the same as in young adults, smaller maintenance doses are required at much longer intervals (102,103). The duration of action of atracurium is not increased, since termination of its action does not depend on renal or hepatic function.

Other features of the patient

Acid–base and electrolyte changes

It has long been accepted that respiratory acidosis tends to potentiate the blockade produced by non-depolarizing relaxants and respiratory alkalosis produces resistance to their action. This is true for the monoquaternary agents D-tubocurarine, vecuronium, and rocuronium (possibly by increased conversion to the bisquaternary forms at lower pH), but it may not hold for the bisquaternary relaxants metocurine, pancuronium, and alcuronium (104–106).

Protein binding of muscle relaxants is maximal between pH 8 and 9 and this may account for increased dose requirements in alkalosis.

Alkalosis is often associated with hypokalemia, in which the actions of non-depolarizing agents may be increased and those of depolarizing agents reduced. Hyperkalemia has the opposite effects, probably by lowering muscle transmembrane potential.

Variations in serum sodium affect neuromuscular blocking agents in a similar manner to potassium changes. However, serum concentrations of electrolytes do not always reflect intracellular concentrations or, perhaps more important, the intra/extracellular concentration ratios; in addition, changes in pH and the concentrations of potassium, sodium and other electrolytes are linked and have opposing influences at several sites in the processes of neuromuscular function, so that the expected effect of a change, taken in isolation, may not be found. Nevertheless, it is of practical importance that respiratory acidosis may enhance non-depolarizing block and makes its reversal by neostigmine more difficult. Such a vicious circle in the recovery room is best broken by ventilating the patient until the cause of the respiratory depression is removed or corrected.

Hypermagnesemia enhances the actions of both depolarizing and non-depolarizing neuromuscular blocking agents. Lithium may also do this. Hypercalcemia may be associated with prolongation of suxamethonium blockade and reduced potency of non-depolarizing agents.

Body temperature

In hypothermia, a reduction in blood flow to muscle increases the time to onset of neuromuscular blockade. The actions (depth of block and duration) of depolarizing relaxants are increased. The potency of non-depolarizing neuromuscular blocking agents is reduced according to some investigators, while others maintain that potency is increased and the duration of action prolonged (107–109). Hypothermia produces different changes in the twitch (110) and electromyographic (111) responses to nerve stimulation in the absence of relaxants. The excretion and the metabolism of relaxants are reduced by hypothermia.

Hemodilution

Hemodilution (for example the replacement of 1 liter of blood by dextran-40) increased the potencies and prolonged the actions of suxamethonium, pancuronium, D-tubocurarine, and vecuronium (SEDA-17, 151) (112). To avoid this, blood collection should be carried out before the administration of anesthetic drugs.

Muscle diseases

The neuromuscular blocking effects of muscle relaxants in patients with neuromuscular disorders can differ significantly from those in healthy individuals. This can result in overdose and residual curarization on the one hand or in inadequate muscle relaxation on the other. Patients with Duchenne muscular dystrophy often require surgery for contractures and kyphoscoliosis. The neuromuscular blocking effects of vecuronium in eight children with Duchenne muscular dystrophy (11–15 years old) have been compared with those in eight children (8–18 years old) without this disease (113). After vecuronium 50 microgram/kg, the median train-of-four ratio was 0.14 in the patients versus 0.86 in the controls. The median time for recovery of the train-of-four ratio from 0.1 to 0.25 was 36 minutes in the patients versus 6 minutes in the controls. The authors concluded that patients with Duchenne muscular dystrophy need smaller initial doses of vecuronium. Because of the increased recovery time, patients should be closely observed for signs of residual curarization. Monitoring of neuromuscular transmission is strongly recommended in all patients with neuromuscular disorders who are given neuromuscular blocking agents.

Organ failure

Long-term administration of non-depolarizing muscle relaxants can result in prolonged paralysis, owing to accumulation of the drug itself or of pharmacologically active metabolites (114,115). Patients with renal or hepatic insufficiency are prone to this complication, but prolonged paralysis also has been noted in patients without these risk factors. The incidence of prolonged paralysis can probably be reduced if neuromuscular transmission monitoring is used to guide relaxant administration (116,117). In addition, agents with non-organ-dependent metabolic pathways may be of advantage (118). Residual curarization is only one of the potential reasons for prolonged paralysis after long-term neuromuscular blockade in severely ill patients. The interaction of different agents with other neuromuscular abnormalities, such as relaxant-associated myopathy, critical illness polyneuropathy, or other myopathic changes in the critically ill, still have to be evaluated.

Use in the intensive care unit

In the intensive care unit muscle relaxants are used to facilitate airway management and mechanical ventilation. The duration of administration can range from a single dose to continuous infusions for up to several weeks. Patients in ICU are more likely to have abnormalities of acid–base balance, electrolyte balance, body temperature, and liver and kidney function, predisposing them to the adverse effects of neuromuscular blocking drugs.

The most dangerous adverse effect of muscle relaxants in the ICU is suxamethonium-induced hyperkalemic cardiac arrest (119–124). Prolonged immobilization is believed to result in a spread of immature acetylcholine receptors on the muscle surface, which may mediate massive long-lasting potassium release if suxamethonium is given (125). By this mechanism, cardiac arrest can occur within minutes after suxamethonium administration. Standard resuscitative techniques have often failed, and several patients have died of this complication. Suxamethonium should therefore not be used in patients who are immobilized in the ICU for more than a few days. The shortest period of immobilization reported to be associated with fatal hyperkalemic cardiac arrest after suxamethonium administration was 4 days in a previously healthy young woman with bacterial meningitis (124).

Drug–Drug Interactions

Antibiotics

In very high doses or in sensitive patients (for example in myasthenia), antibiotics can produce paralysis and act additively or synergistically with neuromuscular blocking drugs.

If it is suspected that an antibiotic is contributing to prolonged neuromuscular blockade, the patient should be monitored and the effect of calcium (up to 1 g of calcium chloride slowly) should be observed. If this is unsuccessful, neostigmine (maximum dose 5 mg for an adult) or edrophonium (0.5 mg/kg) can be tried, but these agents may intensify a block due to colistin, lincomycin, or polymyxin B. If the other remedies fail, 4-aminopyridine (maximum dose 0.3 mg/kg) can be successful. Artificial ventilation should be continued until adequate spontaneous efforts are achieved and other possible factors, such as acidosis or electrolyte disturbances, are corrected.

This subject has been reviewed (126,127,128).

Aminoglycosides

The aminoglycosides have a magnesium-like effect, acting prejunctionally to reduce transmitter release and postjunctionally to increase transmitter release; they also reduce postjunctional sensitivity to acetylcholine. In most cases their effects can be reversed, partly at least by calcium or 4-aminopyridine. Tobramycin is thought also to have a direct effect on muscle.

The aminoglycosides have a curare-like action, which can be antagonized by calcium ions and acetylcholinesterase inhibitors (129). In patients who require general anesthesia, the effect of muscle relaxants, such as D-tubocurarine, pancuronium, and suxamethonium, can be potentiated by aminoglycosides (130).

Amphotericin

Hypokalemia due to amphotericin can enhance the curariform effect of neuromuscular blocking agents (131,132,133).

Beta-lactam antibiotics

Penicillins G and V (126) have been reported to cause neuromuscular block in animal preparations, but only at exceptionally high doses. Calcium is effective in reversal. The acylaminopenicillins augment vecuronium-induced blockade (134). Possible "re-curarization" with piperacillin was successfully reversed by neostigmine (135).

Lincosamides

The lincosamides have prejunctional and postjunctional effects, the principal action probably being on the muscle. This blockade is difficult to reverse with cholinesterase inhibitors or calcium.

Clindamycin and lincomycin potentiate the action of non-depolarizing neuromuscular blocking drugs, such as pancuronium and D-tubocurarine. The lincosamide-induced block cannot be reliably reversed pharmacologically (136).

Peptide antibiotics

An unusually high dose of vancomycin augmented vecuronium-induced block during recovery, thus delaying the detubation of the patient for about 30 minutes (SEDA-16, 7). In another patient vancomycin prolonged the recovery from blockade induced by a suxamethonium infusion for some hours (SEDA-18, 14).

Polymixins

The polymyxins probably produce a predominantly postjunctional effect (via ion channel block) and reduce muscle contractility. The block is difficult to reverse, calcium being only partly successful. Neostigmine has been reported to increase blockade produced by polymyxin B and colistin; in such cases 4-aminopyridine might be helpful.

There may be difficulty in reversing neuromuscular blockade if polymyxin is given in combination with neuromuscular blocking drugs (137).

Tetracyclines

The tetracyclines produce a small effect, partly by calcium chelation, thus reducing transmitter release. Reversal is usually, but inconsistently, obtained with calcium or neostigmine.

Vancomycin

Some authors stress the fact that vancomycin can interact with anesthetic drugs, particularly muscle relaxants. In the reported cases anaphylactoid reactions were seen, with intense erythema and marked permeability changes (138).

Botulinum toxin

As botulinum toxin inhibits acetylcholine release it can interfere with neuromuscular blocking agents (139). It has been suggested that each dose of botulinum toxin may have two effects: first, a direct increase in sensitivity to neuromuscular blocking agents; second, compensatory synaptic remodeling resulting in reduced sensitivity (139). Thus, the effects of neuromuscular blocking agents on neuromuscular transmission cannot be predicted in patients receiving botulinum toxin.

Lithium

A few cases of potentiation of the neuromuscular blocking effects of suxamethonium and pancuronium were reported about 30 years ago (140,141) and have been reviewed (142).

Quinidine

Quinidine is a non-depolarizing muscle blocker and potentiates the effects of neuromuscular blocking drugs (143).

General anesthetics

Inhalational anesthetics

The volatile inhalational anesthetic agents and cyclopropane potentiate the actions of neuromuscular blocking drugs. The extent depends on the particular relaxant and inhalational agent used and the concentration of the latter. In comparative studies, isoflurane was the most potent in this respect, enflurane almost as potent, and both were 2–3 times more potent than halothane, which was in turn twice as potent as nitrous oxide, the volatile agents being administered at concentrations of 1.25 MAC (mean alveolar concentration) and the relaxant studied being D-tubocurarine (144). Concerning the older agents, the relaxant dose can be reduced by half with ether anesthesia and by one-fifth or more when cyclopropane is used. The degrees of potentiation by ether and cyclopropane probably lie between those of enflurane and halothane.

The higher the anesthetic concentration, the greater the degree of potentiation and the smaller the dose of relaxant needed (145). The full potentiating effect will only be seen when the tissues are saturated by the inhalational agent. Reducing the concentration of the inhalational agent generally reduces the degree of neuromuscular blockade (146), a desirable feature at the end of an operation. However, this maneuver can take some time to be effective (about half-an-hour for enflurane) and will only diminish the "volatile" contribution to the total block. Nevertheless, there may be occasions, such as in patients with myasthenia or renal or hepatic disease, when the advantages of using higher concentrations of inhalational anesthetic and lower doses of relaxants may outweigh the disadvantages (147).

The potentiation of D-tubocurarine block produced by enflurane slowly continues to increase with time, even after the usual equilibration period has passed (SEDA-5, 132) (148). This does not occur with halothane, and the discrepancy is said to mean that more D-tubocurarine will be required in the first hour of enflurane anesthesia than during equipotent halothane anesthesia, but that thereafter less will be required during enflurane anesthesia. It has been suggested that enflurane, unlike halothane, may produce an effect on muscle that takes time to develop. This may also be part of the mechanism, in addition to the greater potentiating action of enflurane, that explains the report that there is slower spontaneous recovery from pancuronium and a greatly impaired antagonistic effect of neostigmine in patients anesthetized with enflurane 1.3–1.4% compared with halothane 0.55–0.65% (end-tidal, in 70% nitrous oxide) (149). The experimental conditions in this last study, however, were somewhat different from usual clinical practice (150).

It is unfortunately not possible to come to a categorical conclusion on precisely how great the potentiation of a given relaxant will be by a particular inhalational anesthetic, because the effects of inhalational agents are multifactorial and diverse, and the numerous studies done have involved different methods (145,146,151–154). Very approximately, isoflurane and enflurane potentiate the longer-acting relaxants, such as D-tubocurarine and pancuronium, by 50–70% and the shorter-acting agents, vecuronium, atracurium, and mivacurium, by 20–25%. However, the degree of potentiation reported for the shorter-acting relaxants varies greatly (from 0 to 70% for vecuronium), depending on the duration of exposure of the skeletal muscles to the inhalational agent, the mode of nerve stimulation, whether the relaxant is given as a single bolus or by cumulative bolus doses or by infusion (steady-state or not), and the nature of the circulatory changes produced. The potentiation produced by halothane is much less than for isoflurane and enflurane.

Muscle relaxants may also contribute to anesthesia. Pancuronium 0.1 mg/kg has been reported to lower the MAC for halothane by 25% (155). It was conjectured that this could be due to a central effect or peripheral effect, through reduction of afferent input from muscle spindles to the reticular activating system. Recently, however, a similar though not identical study (SEDA-15, 124) (156) failed to confirm that pancuronium, vecuronium, or atracurium lowers the MAC for halothane.

Intravenous anesthetics

Intravenous anesthetic agents have much less influence on the neuromuscular blocking effects of relaxants and most have no clinically significant effect. However, ketamine (SEDA-14, 113) has been reported to significantly potentiate atracurium (157), and also D-tubocurarine but not pancuronium (158) in man. Animal studies suggest that all relaxants will be potentiated by ketamine in a dose-dependent manner (159,160). It has been suggested that had Johnston et al. (158) used a higher dose of ketamine (than 75 mg/m^2), they would have seen potentiation of pancuronium. The main effect of ketamine appears to be a reduction in the sensitivity of the postjunctional membrane to acetylcholine, possibly by ion-channel blockade. Propofol has been reported to potentiate vecuronium-induced and atracurium-induced blocks (161).

Laboratory investigations have shown that some benzodiazepines can produce biphasic effects (162,163), higher doses potentiating neuromuscular blocking agents (162,164); however, several human investigations have failed to show a significant effect (165–167). It has been suggested that agents that are added to commercial formulations of some benzodiazepines to render them more water-soluble may mask the benzodiazepine effect (167).

References

1. Lebowitz PW, Ramsey FM, Savarese JJ, Ali HH. Potentiation of neuromuscular blockade in man produced by combinations of pancuronium and metocurine or pancuronium and d-tubocurarine. Anesth Analg 1980;59(8):604–9.
2. Waud BE, Waud DR. Interaction among agents that block end-plate depolarization competitively. Anesthesiology 1985;63(1):4–15.
3. Rashkovsky OM, Agoston S, Ket JM. Interaction between pancuronium bromide and vecuronium bromide. Br J Anaesth 1985;57(11):1063–6.
4. Bowman WC. Pharmacology of Neuromuscular Function. 2nd ed.. London/Boston/Singapore/Sydney/Toronto/Wellington: Wright;. 1990.
5. Muscle Relaxants. In: Agoston S, Bowman WC, editors. Monographs in Anaesthesiology. Amsterdam: Elsevier Science Publishers BV, 1990:19.
6. Lingle CJ, Steinbach JH. Neuromuscular blocking agents. Int Anesthesiol Clin 1988;26(4):288–301.
7. Bowman WC. Non-relaxant properties of neuromuscular blocking drugs. Br J Anaesth 1982;54(2):147–60.
8. Walts LF. Complications of muscle relaxants. In: Katz RL, editor. Muscle Relaxants. Amsterdam: Excerpta Medica, 1975:209.
9. Mencke T, Echternach M, Kleinschmidt S, Lux P, Barth V, Plinkert PK, Fuchs-Buder T. Laryngeal morbidity and quality of tracheal intubation: a randomized controlled trial. Anesthesiology 2003;98(5):1049–56.
10. Gooch JL. Prolonged paralysis after neuromuscular blockade. J Toxicol Clin Toxicol 1995;33(5):419–26.
11. Smith CL, Hunter JM, Jones RS. Vecuronium infusions in patients with renal failure in an ITU. Anaesthesia 1987;42(4):387–93.
12. Op de Coul AA, Lambregts PC, Koeman J, van Puyenbroek MJ, Ter Laak HJ, Gabreels-Festen AA. Neuromuscular complications in patients given Pavulon (pancuronium bromide) during artificial ventilation. Clin Neurol Neurosurg 1985;87(1):17–22.
13. Yate PM, Flynn PJ, Arnold RW, Weatherly BC, Simmonds RJ, Dopson T. Clinical experience and plasma laudanosine concentrations during the infusion of atracurium in the intensive therapy unit. Br J Anaesth 1987;59(2):211–7.
14. Rutledge ML, Hawkins EP, Langston C. Skeletal muscle growth failure induced in premature newborn infants by prolonged pancuronium treatment. J Pediatr 1986;109(5):883–6.
15. Torres CF, Maniscalco WM, Agostinelli T. Muscle weakness and atrophy following prolonged paralysis with pancuronium bromide in neonates. Ann Neurol 1985;18:403.
16. Barohn RJ, Jackson CE, Rogers SJ, Ridings LW, McVey AL. Prolonged paralysis due to nondepolarizing neuromuscular blocking agents and corticosteroids. Muscle Nerve 1994;17(6):647–54.
17. Hirano M, Ott BR, Raps EC, Minetti C, Lennihan L, Libbey NP, Bonilla E, Hays AP. Acute quadriplegic myopathy: a complication of treatment with steroids, nondepolarizing blocking agents, or both. Neurology 1992;42(11):2082–7.
18. Leatherman JW, Fluegel WL, David WS, Davies SF, Iber C. Muscle weakness in mechanically ventilated patients with severe asthma. Am J Respir Crit Care Med 1996;153(5):1686–90.
19. Subramony SH, Carpenter DE, Raju S, Pride M, Evans OB. Myopathy and prolonged neuromuscular blockade after lung transplant. Crit Care Med 1991; 19(12):1580–2.
20. Giostra E, Magistris MR, Pizzolato G, Cox J, Chevrolet JC. Neuromuscular disorder in intensive care unit patients treated with pancuronium bromide. Occurrence in a cluster group of seven patients and two sporadic cases, with electrophysiologic and histologic examination. Chest 1994;106(1):210–20.
21. Margolis BD, Khachikian D, Friedman Y, Garrard C. Prolonged reversible quadriparesis in mechanically ventilated patients who received long-term infusions of vecuronium. Chest 1991;100(3):877–8.
22. Ackman JB, Rosenthal DI. Generalized periarticular myositis ossificans as a complication of pharmacologically induced paralysis. Skeletal Radiol 1995;24(5):395–7.
23. Clements NC Jr, Camilli AE. Heterotopic ossification complicating critical illness. Chest 1993;104(5):1526–8.
24. Ray TD, Lowe WD, Anderson LD, Muller AL, Brogdon BG. Periarticular heterotopic ossification following pharmacologically induced paralysis. Skeletal Radiol 1995;24(8):609–12.
25. Goodman TA, Merkel PA, Perlmutter G, Doyle MK, Krane SM, Polisson RP. Heterotopic ossification in the setting of neuromuscular blockade. Arthritis Rheum 1997;40(9):1619–27.
26. Dellestable F, Gaucher A, Voltz C. Heterotopic ossification in critically ill patients: comment on the article by Goodman et al. Arthritis Rheum 1998;41(7):1329–30.
27. Dellestable F, Voltz C, Mariot J, Perrier JF, Gaucher A. Heterotopic ossification complicating long-term sedation. Br J Rheumatol 1996;35(7):700–1.
28. Berg H, Roed J, Viby-Mogensen J, Mortensen CR, Engbaek J, Skovgaard LT, Krintel JJ. Residual neuromuscular block is a risk factor for postoperative pulmonary complications. A prospective, randomised, and blinded study of postoperative pulmonary complications after atracurium, vecuronium and pancuronium. Acta Anaesthesiol Scand 1997;41(9):1095–103.
29. Debaene B, Plaud B, Dilly MP, Donati F. Residual paralysis in the PACU after a single intubating dose of nondepolarizing muscle relaxant with an intermediate duration of action. Anesthesiology 2003;98(5):1042–8.
30. Appelboam R, Mulder R, Saddler J. Atracurium associated with postoperative residual curarization. Br J Anaesth 2003;90(4):523.

31. Hayes AH, Mirakhur RK, Breslin DS, Reid JE, McCourt KC. Postoperative residual block after intermediate-acting neuromuscular blocking drugs. Anaesthesia 2001;56(4):312–8.

32. Baillard C, Gehan G, Reboul-Marty J, Larmignat P, Samama CM, Cupa M. Residual curarization in the recovery room after vecuronium. Br J Anaesth 2000;84(3):394–5.

33. Fawcett WJ, Dash A, Francis GA, Liban JB, Cashman JN. Recovery from neuromuscular blockade: residual curarisation following atracurium or vecuronium by bolus dosing or infusions. Acta Anaesthesiol Scand 1995;39(3):288–93.

34. Eriksson LI, Sundman E, Olsson R, Nilsson L, Witt H, Ekberg O, Kuylenstierna R. Functional assessment of the pharynx at rest and during swallowing in partially paralyzed humans: simultaneous videomanometry and mechanomyography of awake human volunteers. Anesthesiology 1997;87(5):1035–43.

35. Sundman E, Witt H, Olsson R, Ekberg O, Kuylenstierna R, Eriksson LI. The incidence and mechanisms of pharyngeal and upper esophageal dysfunction in partially paralyzed humans: pharyngeal videoradiography and simultaneous manometry after atracurium. Anesthesiology 2000;92(4):977–84.

36. Payne JP, Hughes R, Al Azawi S. Neuromuscular blockade by neostigmine in anaesthetized man. Br J Anaesth 1980;52(1):69–76.

37. Goldhill DR, Wainwright AP, Stuart CS, Flynn PJ. Neostigmine after spontaneous recovery from neuromuscular blockade. Effect on depth of blockade monitored with train-of-four and tetanic stimuli. Anaesthesia 1989;44(4):293–9.

38. Jones JE, Hunter JM, Utting JE. Use of neostigmine in the antagonism of residual neuromuscular blockade produced by vecuronium. Br J Anaesth 1987;59(11):1454–8.

39. Jones JE, Parker CJ, Hunter JM. Antagonism of blockade produced by atracurium or vecuronium with low doses of neostigmine. Br J Anaesth 1988;61(5):560–4.

40. Tramer MR, Fuchs-Buder T. Omitting antagonism of neuromuscular block: effect on postoperative nausea and vomiting and risk of residual paralysis. A systematic review. Br J Anaesth 1999;82(3):379–86.

41. Krombach J, Hunzelmann N, Koster F, Bischoff A, Hoffmann-Menzel H, Buzello W. Anaphylactoid reactions after cisatracurium administration in six patients. Anesth Analg 2001;93(5):1257–9.

42. Legros CB, Orliaguet GA, Mayer MN, Labbez F, Carli PA. Severe anaphylactic reaction to cisatracurium in a child. Anesth Analg 2001;92(3):648–9.

43. Briassoulis G, Hatzis T, Mammi P, Alikatora A. Persistent anaphylactic reaction after induction with thiopentone and cisatracurium. Paediatr Anaesth 2000;10(4):429–34.

44. Mertes PM, Laxenaire MC. Allergic reactions occuring during anaesthesia. Eur J Anaesthesiol 2002;19(4):240–62.

45. Laxenaire MC, Moneret-Vautrin DA, Watkins J. Diagnosis of the causes of anaphylactoid anaesthetic reactions. A report of the recommendations of the joint Anaesthetic and Immuno-allergological Workshop, Nancy, France: 19 March 1982. Anaesthesia 1983;38(2):147–8.

46. Fisher MM, More DG. The epidemiology and clinical features of anaphylactic reactions in anaesthesia. Anaesth Intensive Care 1981;9(3):226–34.

47. Laxenaire MC. Epidémiologie des réactions anaphylactoïdes peranesthésiques. Quatrième enquête multicentrique (juillet 1994–décembre 1996). [Epidemiology of anesthetic anaphylactoid reactions. Fourth multicenter survey (July 1994–December 1996).] Ann Fr Anesth Reanim 1999;18(7):796–809.

48. Hatton F, Tiret L, Maujol L, N'Doye P, Vourc'h G, Desmonts JM, Otteni JC, Scherpereel P. INSERM. Enquête épidémiologique sur les anesthésies. Premiers résultats. [INSERM. Epidemiological survey of anesthesia. Initial results.] Ann Fr Anesth Reanim 1983;2(5):331–86.

49. Thornton JA, Lorenz W. Histamine and antihistamine in anaesthesia and surgery: report of a symposium. Anaesthesia 1983;38:373.

50. Fisher MM, Munro I. Life-threatening anaphylactoid reactions to muscle relaxants. Anesth Analg 1983;62(6):559–64.

51. Boileau S, Hummer-Sigiel M, Moeller R, Drouet N. Réévaluation des risques respectifs d'anaphylaxie et d'histaminoblitération avec les substances anesthésiologiques. [Reassessment of the respective risks of anaphylaxis and histamine liberation with anesthetic substances.] Ann Fr Anesth Reanim 1985;4(2):195–204.

52. Laxenaire MC. Substances responsables des chocs anaphylactiques peranesthésiques. Troisième enquête multicentrique française (1992–1994). [Substances responsible for peranesthetic anaphylactic shock. A third French multicenter study (1992–94).] Ann Fr Anesth Reanim 1996;15(8):1211–8.

53. Laxenaire MC, Moneret-Vautrin DA, Vervloet D, Alazia M, Francois G. Accidents anaphylactoïdes graves peranesthésiques. [Severe perianesthetic anaphylactic accidents.] Ann Fr Anesth Reanim 1985;4(1):30–46.

54. Laxenaire MC, Moneret-Vautrin DA, Vervloet D. The French experience of anaphylactoid reactions. Int Anesthesiol Clin 1985;23(3):145–60.

55. Galletly DC, Treuren BC. Anaphylactoid reactions during anaesthesia. Seven years' experience of intradermal testing. Anaesthesia 1985;40(4):329–33.

56. Pepys J, Pepys EO, Baldo BA, Whitwam JG. Anaphylactic/anaphylactoid reactions to anaesthetic and associated agents. Skin prick tests in aetiological diagnosis. Anaesthesia 1994;49(6):470–5.

57. Mertes PM, Laxenaire MC, Alla F. Groupe d'Etudes des Réactions Anaphylactoïdes Peranesthésiques. Anaphylactic and anaphylactoid reactions occurring during anesthesia in France in 1999–2000. Anesthesiology 2003;99(3):536–45.

58. Laxenaire MC, Mertes PM. Groupe d'Etudes des Réactions Anaphylactoïdes Peranesthésiques. Anaphylaxis during anaesthesia. Results of a two-year survey in France. Br J Anaesth 2001;87(4):549–58.

59. Laxenaire M, Mertes P. Anaphylaxis during anaesthesia. Br J Anaesth 2002;88:605–6.

60. Laake J, Rottingen J. Rocuronium and anaphylaxis—a statistical challenge. Acta Anaesthesiol Scand 2001;45: 1196–203.

61. Florvaag E, Johansson SG, Oman H, Venemalm L, Degerbeck F, Dybendal T, Lundberg M. Prevalence of IgE antibodies to morphine. Relation to the high and low incidences of NMBA anaphylaxis in Norway and Sweden, respectively. Acta Anaesthesiol Scand 2005;49:437–44.

62. Harboe T, Guttormsen AB, Irgens A, Dybendal T, Florvaag E. Anaphylaxis during anesthesia in Norway: a 6-year single-center follow-up study. Anesthesiology 2005;102:897–903.

63. Aimone-Gastin I, Gueant JL, Laxenaire MC, Moneret-Vautrin DA. Pathogenesis of allergic reactions to anaesthetic drugs. Int J Immunopathol Pharmacol 1997;10:193–6.

64. Vervloet D, Nizankowska E, Arnaud M, Senft M, Alazia M, Charpin J. Adverse reactions to suxamethonium and other muscle relaxants under general anesthesia. J Allergy Clin Immunol 1983;71(6):552–9.

65. Vervloet D. Allergy to muscle relaxants and related compounds. Clin Allergy 1985;15(6):501–8.

66. Assem ES. Characteristics of basophil histamine release by neuromuscular blocking drugs in patients with anaphylactoid reactions. Agents Actions 1984;14(3–4):435–40.

67. Watkins J. Heuristic decision-making in diagnosis and management of adverse drug reactions in anaesthesia and surgery: the case of muscle relaxants. Theor Surg 1989;4:212.

68. Harle DG, Baldo BA, Fisher MM. Detection of IgE antibodies to suxamethonium after anaphylactoid reactions during anaesthesia. Lancet 1984;1(8383):930–2.

69. Baldo BA, Harle DG, Fisher MM. In vitro diagnosis and studies on the mechanism(s) of anaphylactoid reactions to muscle relaxant drugs. Ann Fr Anesth Reanim 1985;4(2):139–45.

70. Weston A, Assem ES. Possible link between anaphylactoid reactions to anaesthetics and chemicals in cosmetics and biocides. Agents Actions 1994;41(Spec No):C138–9.

71. Youngman PR, Taylor KM, Wilson JD. Anaphylactoid reactions to neuromuscular blocking agents: a commonly undiagnosed condition? Lancet 1983;2(8350):597–9.

72. Bird AG. 'Allergic' drug reactions during anaesthesia. Adverse Drug React Bull 1985;110:408.

73. Gueant JL, Aimone-Gastin I, Laroche D, Pitiot V, Gerard P, Moneret-Vautrin DA, Bricard H, Laxenaire MC. Prospective evaluation of cell mediator release in anaphylaxis to anesthetic drugs. Allergy Clin Immunol Int 1996;8:120.

74. Fisher MM, Baldo BA. The diagnosis of fatal anaphylactic reactions during anaesthesia: employment of immunoassays for mast cell tryptase and drug-reactive IgE antibodies. Anaesth Intensive Care 1993;21(3):353–7.

75. Assem ES. Anaphylactic anaesthetic reactions. The value of paper radioallergosorbent tests for IgE antibodies to muscle relaxants and thiopentone. Anaesthesia 1990;45(12):1032–8.

76. Guilloux L, Ricard-Blum S, Ville G, Motin J. A new radioimmunoassay using a commercially available solid support for the detection of IgE antibodies against muscle relaxants. J Allergy Clin Immunol 1992;90(2):153–9.

77. Moneret-Vautrin DA, Kanny G. Anaphylaxis to muscle relaxants: rational for skin tests. Allerg Immunol (Paris) 2002;34(7):233–40.

78. Fisher M. Intradermal testing after anaphylactoid reaction to anaesthetic drugs: practical aspects of performance and interpretation. Anaesth Intensive Care 1984;12(2):115–20.

79. Mata E, Gueant JL, Moneret-Vautrin DA, Bermejo N, Gerard P, Nicolas JP, Laxenaire MC. Clinical evaluation of in vitro leukocyte histamine release in allergy to muscle relaxant drugs. Allergy 1992;47(5):471–6.

80. Abuaf N, Rajoely B, Ghazouani E, Levy DA, Pecquet C, Chabane H, Leynadier F. Validation of a flow cytometric assay detecting in vitro basophil activation for the diagnosis of muscle relaxant allergy. J Allergy Clin Immunol 1999;104(2 Pt 1):411–8.

81. Monneret G, Benoit Y, Gutowski MC, Bienvenu J. Detection of basophil activation by flow cytometry in patients with allergy to muscle-relaxant drugs. Anesthesiology 2000;92(1):275–7.

82. Monneret G, Benoit Y, Debard AL, Gutowski MC, Topenot I, Bienvenu J. Monitoring of basophil activation using CD63 and CCR3 in allergy to muscle relaxant drugs. Clin Immunol 2002;102(2):192–9.

83. Fisher MM, Baldo BA. Immunoassays in the diagnosis of anaphylaxis to neuromuscular blocking drugs: the value of morphine for the detection of IgE antibodies in allergic subjects. Anaesth Intensive Care 2000;28(2):167–70.

84. Sudheer PS, Hall JE, Read GF, Rowbottom AW, Williams PE. Flow cytometric investigation of peri-anaesthetic anaphylaxis using CD63 and CD203c. Anaesthesia 2005;60:251–6.

85. Monneret G, Benoit Y, Debard AL, Gutowski MC, Topenot I, Bienvenu J. Monitoring of basophil activation using CD63 and CCR3 in allergy to muscle relaxant drugs. Clin Immunol 2002;102:192–9.

86. Boumiza R, Debard AL, Monneret G. The basophil activation test by flow cytometry: recent developments in clinical studies, standardization and emerging perspectives. Clin Mol Allergy 2005;3:9.

87. Moneret-Vautrin DA, Kanny G, Gueant JL, Widmer S, Laxenaire MC. Prevention by monovalent haptens of IgE-dependent leucocyte histamine release to muscle relaxants. Int Arch Allergy Immunol 1995;107(1–3):172–5.

88. Sage DJ. Management of acute anaphylactoid reactions. Int Anesthesiol Clin 1985;23(3):175–86.

89. Fisher MM. Clinical observations on the pathophysiology and treatment of anaphylactic cardiovascular collapse. Anaesth Intensive Care 1986;14(1):17–21.

90. Harle DG, Baldo BA, Fisher MM. Cross-reactivity of metocurine, atracurium, vecuronium and fazadinium with IgE antibodies from patients unexposed to these drugs but allergic to other myoneural blocking drugs. Br J Anaesth 1985;57(11):1073–6.

91. Leynadier F, Dry J. Anaphylaxis to muscle-relaxant drugs: study of cross-reactivity by skin tests. Int Arch Allergy Appl Immunol 1991;94(1–4):349–53.

92. Fisher MM, Merefield D, Baldo B. Failure to prevent an anaphylactic reaction to a second neuromuscular blocking drug during anaesthesia. Br J Anaesth 1999;82(5):770–3.

93. Thacker MA, Davis FM. Subsequent general anaesthesia in patients with a history of previous anaphylactoid/anaphylactic reaction to muscle relaxant. Anaesth Intensive Care 1999;27(2):190–3.

94. Guay J, Grenier Y, Varin F. Clinical pharmacokinetics of neuromuscular relaxants in pregnancy. Clin Pharmacokinet 1998;34(6):483.

95. Goudsouzian NG. Maturation of neuromuscular transmission in the infant. Br J Anaesth 1980;52(2):205–14.

96. Goudsouzian NG, Standaert FG. The infant and the myoneural junction. Anesth Analg 1986;65(11):1208–17.

97. Crumrine RS, Yodlowski EH. Assessment of neuromuscular function in infants. Anesthesiology 1981;54(1):29–32.

98. Fisher DM, O'Keeffe C, Stanski DR, Cronnelly R, Miller RD, Gregory GA. Pharmacokinetics and pharmacodynamics of d-tubocurarine in infants, children, and adults. Anesthesiology 1982;57(3):203–8.

99. Goudsouzian NG. Muscle relaxants in paediatric anaesthesia. In: Agoston S, Bowman WC, editors. Monographs in Anaesthesiology 19. Amsterdam: Elsevier Science Publishers BV, 1990:285.

100. O'Keeffe C, Gregory GA, Stanski DR, et al. d-Tubocurarine: pharmacodynamics and kinetics in children. Anesthesiology 1979;51:S270.

101. Goudsouzian NG, Liu LM, Cote CJ. Comparison of equipotent doses of non-depolarizing muscle relaxants in children. Anesth Analg 1981;60(12):862–6.

102. Duvaldestin P, Saada J, Berger JL, D'Hollander A, Desmonts JM. Pharmacokinetics, pharmacodynamics, and dose-response relationships of pancuronium in control and elderly subjects. Anesthesiology 1982;56(1):36–40.

103. d'Hollander A, Massaux F, Nevelsteen M, Agoston S. Age-dependent dose-response relationship of ORG NC 45 in anaesthetized patients. Br J Anaesth 1982;54(6):653–7.

104. Ono K, Ohta Y, Morita K, Kosaka F. The influence of respiratory-induced acid-base changes on the action of non-depolarizing muscle relaxants in rats. Anesthesiology 1988;68(3):357–62.

105. Aziz L, Ono K, Ohta Y, Morita K, Hirakawa M. The effect of CO_2-induced acid-base changes on the potencies of muscle relaxants and antagonism of neuromuscular block by neostigmine in rat in vitro. Anesth Analg 1994; 78(2):322–7.

106. Ono K, Nagano O, Ohta Y, Kosaka F. Neuromuscular effects of respiratory and metabolic acid-base changes in vitro with and without nondepolarizing muscle relaxants. Anesthesiology 1990;73(4):710–6.

107. Ham J, Stanski DR, Newfield P, Miller RD. Pharmacokinetics and dynamics of d-tubocurarine during hypothermia in humans. Anesthesiology 1981;55:631.

108. Buzello W, Schluermann D, Schindler M, Spillner G. Hypothermic cardiopulmonary bypass and neuromuscular blockade by pancuronium and vecuronium. Anesthesiology 1985;62(2):201–4.

109. Buzello W, Schluermann D, Pollmaecher T, Spillner G. Unequal effects of cardiopulmonary bypass-induced hypothermia on neuromuscular blockade from constant infusion of alcuronium, d-tubocurarine, pancuronium, and vecuronium. Anesthesiology 1987;66(6):842–6.

110. Heier T, Caldwell JE, Sessler DI, Miller RD. The effect of local surface and central cooling on adductor pollicis twitch tension during nitrous oxide/isoflurane and nitrous oxide/fentanyl anesthesia in humans. Anesthesiology 1990;72(5):807–11.

111. Engbaek J, Skovgaard LT, Friis B, Kann T. The effect of temperature on the evoked EMG response. Anesthesiology 1989;72:A810.

112. Schuh FT. Influence off haemodilution on the potency of neuromuscular blocking drugs. Br J Anaesth 1981;53(3):263–5.

113. Ririe DG, Shapiro F, Sethna NF. The response of patients with Duchenne's muscular dystrophy to neuromuscular blockade with vecuronium. Anesthesiology 1998;88(2):351–4.

114. Segredo V, Caldwell JE, Matthay MA, Sharma ML, Gruenke LD, Miller RD. Persistent paralysis in critically ill patients after long-term administration of vecuronium. N Engl J Med 1992;327(8):524–8.

115. Vandenbrom RH, Wierda JM. Pancuronium bromide in the intensive care unit: a case of overdose. Anesthesiology 1988;69(6):996–7.

116. Frankel H, Jeng J, Tilly E, St Andre A, Champion H. The impact of implementation of neuromuscular blockade monitoring standards in a surgical intensive care unit. Am Surg 1996;62(6):503–6.

117. Rudis MI, Sikora CA, Angus E, Peterson E, Popovich J Jr, Hyzy R, Zarowitz BJ. A prospective, randomized, controlled evaluation of peripheral nerve stimulation versus standard clinical dosing of neuromuscular blocking agents in critically ill patients. Crit Care Med 1997;25(4):575–83.

118. Prielipp RC, Coursin DB, Scuderi PE, Bowton DL, Ford SR, Cardenas VJ Jr, Vender J, Howard D, Casale EJ, Murray MJ. Comparison of the infusion requirements and recovery profiles of vecuronium and cisatracurium 51W89 in intensive care unit patients. Anesth Analg 1995;81(1):3–12.

119. Horton WA, Fergusson NV. Hyperkalaemia and cardiac arrest after the use of suxamethonium in intensive care. Anaesthesia 1988;43(10):890–1.

120. Hemming AE, Charlton S, Kelly P. Hyperkalaemia, cardiac arrest, suxamethonium and intensive care. Anaesthesia 1990;45(11):990–1.

121. Markewitz BA, Elstad MR. Succinylcholine-induced hyperkalemia following prolonged pharmacologic neuromuscular blockade. Chest 1997;111(1):248–50.

122. Berkahn JM, Sleigh JW. Hyperkalaemic cardiac arrest following succinylcholine in a longterm intensive care patient. Anaesth Intensive Care 1997;25(5):588–9.

123. Lee YM, Fountain SW. Suxamethonium and cardiac arrest. Singapore Med J 1997;38(7):300–1.

124. Hansen D. Suxamethonium-induced cardiac arrest and death following 5 days of immobilization. Eur J Anaesthesiol 1998;15(2):240–1.

125. Martyn JA, White DA, Gronert GA, Jaffe RS, Ward JM. Up-and-down regulation of skeletal muscle acetylcholine receptors. Effects on neuromuscular blockers. Anesthesiology 1992;76(5):822–43.

126. Sokoll MD, Gergis SD. Antibiotics and neuromuscular function. Anesthesiology 1981;55(2):148–59.

127. Singh YN, Marshall IG, Harvey AL. The mechanisms of the muscle paralysing actions of antibiotics and their interaction with neuromuscular blocking agents. Rev Drug Metab Drug Interact 1980;3:129.

128. Pittinger C, Adamson R. Antibiotic blockade of neuromuscular function. Annu Rev Pharmacol 1972;12:169–84.

129 Adams HR, Mathew BP, Teske RH, Mercer HD. Neuromuscular blocking effects of aminoglycoside antibiotics on fast- and slow-contracting muscles of the cat. Anesth Analg 1976;55(4):500–7.

130 Burkett L, Bikhazi GB, Thomas KC Jr, Rosenthal DA, Wirta MG, Foldes FF. Mutual potentiation of the neuromuscular effects of antibiotics and relaxants. Anesth Analg 1979;58(2):107–15.

131 Lyman CA, Walsh TJ. Systemically administered antifungal agents. A review of their clinical pharmacology and therapeutic applications. Drugs 1992;44(1):9–35.

132 Bernardo JF, Murakami S, Branch RA, Sabra R. Potassium depletion potentiates amphotericin-B-induced toxicity to renal tubules. Nephron 1995;70(2):235–41.

133 Bickers DR. Antifungal therapy: potential interactions with other classes of drugs. J Am Acad Dermatol 1994;31(3 Pt 2): S87–90.

134. Tryba M. Wirkungsverstärkung nicht-depolarisierender Muskelrelaxantien durch Acylaminopenicilline. [Potentiation of the effect of non-depolarizing muscle relaxants by acylaminopenicillins. Studies on the example of vecuronium.] Anaesthesist 1985;34(12):651–5.

135. Mackie K, Pavlin EG. Recurrent paralysis following piperacillin administration. Anesthesiology 1990;72(3):561–3.

136 Marshall IG, Henderson F. Drug interactions at the neuromuscular junction. Clin Anaesthesiol 1985;3:261.

137 Cammu G. Interactions of neuromuscular blocking drugs. Acta Anaesthesiol Belg 2001;52(4):357–63.

138 Symons NL, Hobbes AF, Leaver HK. Anaphylactoid reactions to vancomycin during anaesthesia: two clinical reports. Can Anaesth Soc J 1985;32(2):178–81.

139 Fiacchino F, Grandi L, Soliveri P, Carella F, Bricchi M. Sensitivity to vecuronium after botulinum toxin administration. J Neurosurg Anesthesiol 1997;9(2):149–53.

140 Hill GE, Wong KC, Hodges MR. Potentiation of succinylcholine neuromuscular blockade by lithium carbonate. Anesthesiology 1976;44(5):439–42.

141 Hill GE, Wong KC, Hodges MR. Lithium carbonate and neuromuscular blocking agents. Anesthesiology 1977; 46(2):122–6.

142 Naguib M, Koorn R. Interactions between psychotropics, anaesthetics and electroconvulsive therapy: implications for drug choice and patient management. CNS Drugs 2002;16(4):229–47.

143 Hartshorn EA. Interactions of cardiac drugs. Drug Intell Clin Pharm 1970;4:272.

144. Ali HH, Savarese JJ. Monitoring of neuromuscular function. Anesthesiology 1976;45(2):216–49.

145. Miller RD, Way WL, Dolan WM, Stevens WC, Eger EI 2nd. The dependence of pancuronium- and d-tubocurarine-induced neuromuscular blockades on alveolar concentrations of halothane and forane. Anesthesiology 1972;37(6):573–81.

146. Gencarelli PJ, Miller RD, Eger EI 2nd, Newfield P. Decreasing enflurane concentrations and d-tubocurarine neuromuscular blockade. Anesthesiology 1982;56(3):192–4.

147. Eger EI 2nd. Isoflurane: a review. Anesthesiology 1981;55(5):559–76.

148. Stanski DR, Ham J, Miller RD, Sheiner LB. Time-dependent increase in sensitivity to d-tubocurarine during enflurane anesthesia in man. Anesthesiology 1980;52(6):483–7.

149. Delisle S, Bevan DR. Impaired neostigmine antagonism of pancuronium during enflurane anaesthesia in man. Br J Anaesth 1982;54(4):441–5.

150. Hodges RJ, Harkness J. Suxamethonium sensitivity in health and disease; a clinical evaluation of pseudo-cholinesterase levels. BMJ 1954;4878:18–22.

151. Waud BE. Decrease in dose requirement of d-tubocurarine by volatile anesthetics. Anesthesiology 1979;51(4): 298–302.

152. Rupp SM, Miller RD, Gencarelli PJ. Vecuronium-induced neuromuscular blockade during enflurane, isoflurane, and halothane anesthesia in humans. Anesthesiology 1984; 60(2):102–5.

153. Cannon JE, Fahey MR, Castagnoli KP, Furuta T, Canfell PC, Sharma M, Miller RD. Continuous infusion of vecuronium: the effect of anesthetic agents. Anesthesiology 1987;67(4):503–6.

154. Swen J, Rashkovsky OM, Ket JM, Koot HW, Hermans J, Agoston S. Interaction between nondepolarizing neuromuscular blocking agents and inhalational anesthetics. Anesth Analg 1989;69(6):752–5.

155. Forbes AR, Cohen NH, Eger EI 2nd. Pancuronium reduces halothane requirement in man. Anesth Analg 1979;58(6):497–9.

156. Fahey MR, Sessler DI, Cannon JE, Brady K, Stoen R, Miller RD. Atracurium, vecuronium, and pancuronium do not alter the minimum alveolar concentration of halothane in humans. Anesthesiology 1989;71(1):53–6.

157. Toft P, Helbo-Hansen S. Interaction of ketamine with atracurium. Br J Anaesth 1989;62(3):319–20.

158. Johnston RR, Miller RD, Way WL. The interaction of ketamine with d-tubocurarine, pancuronium, and succinylcholine in man. Anesth Analg 1974;53(4):496–501.

159. Tsai SK, Lee CM, Tran B. Ketamine enhances phase I and phase II neuromuscular block of succinylcholine. Can J Anaesth 1989;36(2):120–3.

160. Amaki Y, Nagashima H, Radnay PA, Foldes FF. Ketamine interaction with neuromuscular blocking agents in the phrenic nerve-hemidiaphragm preparation of the rat. Anesth Analg 1978;57(2):238–43.

161. Robertson EN, Fragen RJ, Booij LH, van Egmond J, Crul JF. Some effects of diisopropyl phenol (ICI 35 868) on the pharmacodynamics of atracurium and vecuronium in anaesthetized man. Br J Anaesth 1983; 55(8):723–8.

162. Driessen JJ, Vree TB, van Egmond J, Booij LH, Crul JF. In vitro interaction of diazepam and oxazepam with pancuronium and suxamethonium. Br J Anaesth 1984; 56(10): 1131–8.

163. Wali FA. Myorelaxant effect of diazepam. Interactions with neuromuscular blocking agents and cholinergic drugs. Acta Anaesthesiol Scand 1985;29(8):785–9.

164. Driessen JJ, Vree TB, van Egmond J, Booij LH, Crul JF. Interaction of midazolam with two non-depolarizing neuromuscular blocking drugs in the rat in vivo sciatic nerve-tibialis anterior muscle preparation. Br J Anaesth 1985;57(11):1089–94.

165. Asbury AJ, Henderson PD, Brown BH, Turner DJ, Linkens DA. Effect of diazepam on pancuronium-induced neuromuscular blockade maintained by a feedback system. Br J Anaesth 1981;53(8):859–63.

166. Cronnelly R, Morris RB, Miller RD. Comparison of thiopental and midazolam on the neuromuscular responses to succinylcholine or pancuronium in humans. Anesth Analg 1983;62(1):75–7.

167. Driessen JJ, Crul JF, Vree TB, van Egmond J, Booij LH. Benzodiazepines and neuromuscular blocking drugs in patients. Acta Anaesthesiol Scand 1986;30(8):642–6.

NEUROMUSCULAR BLOCKING DRUGS

Alcuronium

General Information

Alcuronium is a synthetic derivative of toxiferine, an alkaloid of calabash curare, and is a non-depolarizing relaxant with properties and adverse effects similar to those of D-tubocurarine. It is about twice as potent as D-tubocurarine, 0.15–0.25 mg/kg usually being adequate for abdominal relaxation, and has a similar onset time and a slightly shorter duration of action. It is bound to albumin (40%), and requirements for alcuronium are less if the plasma albumin levels are low, as may occur in hepatic disease.

Like D-tubocurarine, alcuronium does not undergo biotransformation. Excretion occurs mainly in the urine (80–85%), but, as with D-tubocurarine, some is also excreted in the bile (15–20%) (1). Persistent relaxation has been reported in renal insufficiency (2) and the drug is relatively contraindicated in this condition.

Organs and Systems

Cardiovascular

Tachycardia, hypotension, and a fall in total peripheral resistance all occur to an extent similar to that seen with D-tubocurarine, according to most studies (3–6). Others have reported that these effects are short-lived (7). Doses of 0.2 mg/kg or more may be associated with the more extreme cardiovascular effects. Blockade of cardiac muscarinic receptors (8), histamine release, and, possibly, some ganglionic blockade (although it has a very low ganglion-blocking activity in animals) (8) may all play a role in the production of the cardiovascular effects of alcuronium.

Nervous system

Two patients in intensive care treated with infusions of large amounts of alcuronium developed fixed dilated pupils. Within 6–24 hours after stopping the infusion the pupils became normally reactive again (9).

This is a very important and dangerous adverse effect, since the presence of fixed dilated pupils may lead to the mistaken diagnosis of brain death in coma patients if other neurological diagnostic procedures are not carried out.

Immunologic

Histamine release and anaphylactoid reactions occur with alcuronium (10–12). The precise incidence is not clear. Erythema is said to occur much less frequently than after D-tubocurarine (3). A retrospective study in Australia (13) showed that 37% of serious anaphylactoid reactions reported there were associated with alcuronium; alcuronium, however, at that time accounted for almost 50% of the total muscle relaxant consumption in Australia, and if this is taken into account the likelihood of a serious reaction is less than with D-tubocurarine, as others have also concluded (14). Clinical features reported range from erythema to severe hypotension and tachycardia (15) and bronchospasm (16,17). In a large prospective surveillance study (SEDA-15, 125) (SED-12, 473) involving over 1400 patients given alcuronium (initial dose 0.25 + 0.09 mg/kg), there were adverse reactions in almost 18% of the patients, with moderate hypotension (20–50% fall) in 13%, severe hypotension in 0.8%, and bronchospasm in 0.1%.

Second-Generation Effects

Fetotoxicity

Placental transfer (SEDA-6, 130) (18), occurs and is increased if alcuronium is rapidly injected (19). No complications attributable to neuromuscular block were seen in the newborn.

Susceptibility Factors

Hepatic disease

In liver cancer in children, resistance to alcuronium has been reported (SEDA-13, 104) (20).

Other features of the patient

In patients with burns, dosage requirements are increased (21).

Drug–Drug Interactions

Penicillamine

Penicillamine-induced myasthenia gravis (SED-10, 415) was probably the cause of extremely prolonged apnea occurring in two patients given alcuronium (SEDA-12, 111) (22,23). Patients receiving penicillamine should be treated as if they had no myasthenia; if a muscle relaxant is required, they should be given a test dose (of about one-tenth the usual dose), with monitoring of the response, before a full dose is administered.

References

1. Raaflaub J, Frey P. Pharmakokinetik von Diallylnortoxiferin beim Menschen. [Pharmacokinetics of diallyl-nor-toxiferine in man.] Arzneimittelforschung 1972;22(1):73–8.
2. Havill JH, Mee AD, Wallace MR, Chin LS, Rothwell RP. Prolonged curarisation in the presence of renal impairment. Anaesth Intensive Care 1978;6(3):234–8.

3. Pandit SK, Dundee JW, Stevenson HM. A clinical comparison of pancuronium with tubocurarine and alcuronium in major cardiothoracic surgery. Anesth Analg 1971;50(6):926–35.

4. Coleman AJ, Downing JW, Leary WP, Moyes DG, Styles M. The immediate cardiovascular effects of pancuronium, alcuronium and tubocurarine in man. Anaesthesia 1972;27(4):415–22.

5. Baraka A. A comparative study between diallylnortoxiferine and tubocurarine. Br J Anaesth 1967;39(8):624–8.

6. Brandli FR. Pancuronium und Alcuronium: Ein klinischer Vergleich. [Pancuronium and alcuronium: a clinical comparison.] Prakt Anaesth 1976;11:239.

7. Tammisto T, Welling I. The effect of alcuronium and tubocurarine on blood pressure and heart rate: a clinical comparison. Br J Anaesth 1969;41(4):317–22.

8. Hughes R, Chapple DJ. Effects on non-depolarizing neuromuscular blocking agents on peripheral autonomic mechanisms in cats. Br J Anaesth 1976;48(2):59–68.

9. Rao U, Milligan KR. Fixed dilated pupils associated with alcuronium infusions. Anaesthesia 1993;48(10):917.

10. Chan CS, Yeung ML. Anaphylactic reaction to alcuronium. Case report. Br J Anaesth 1972;44(1):103–5.

11. Rowley RW. Hypersensitivity reaction to diallyl nortoxiferine (Alloferine). Anaesth Intensive Care 1975;3:74.

12. Fisher MM, Hallowes RC, Wilson RM. Anaphylaxis to alcuronium. Anaesth Intensive Care 1978;6(2):125–8.

13. Fisher MM, Munro I. Life-threatening anaphylactoid reactions to muscle relaxants. Anesth Analg 1983;62(6):559–64.

14. Galletly DC, Treuren BC. Anaphylactoid reactions during anaesthesia. Seven years' experience of intradermal testing. Anaesthesia 1985;40(4):329–33.

15. Panning B, Peest D, Kirchner E, Schedel I. Anaphylaktoider Schock nach Alloferin. [Anaphylactoid shock following Alloferin.] Anaesthesist 1985;34(4):211–2.

16. Fadel R, Herpin-Richard N, Rassemont R, Salomon J, David B, Laurent M, Henocq E. Choc anaphylactique à la diallylnortoxiferine: étude clinique et immunologique. [Anaphylactic shock from diallylnortoxiferine. Clinical and immunological studies.] Ann Fr Anesth Réanim 1982;1(5):531–4.

17. Plotz J, Schreiber W. Vergleichende Untersuchung von Atracurium und Alcuronium zur Intubation älterer Patienten in Halothannarkose. [Comparative study of atracurium and alcuronium for the intubation of older patients in halothane anesthesia.] Anaesthesist 1984;33(11):548–51.

18. Ho PC, Stephens ID, Triggs EJ. Caesarean section and placental transfer of alcuronium. Anaesth Intensive Care 1981;9(2):113–8.

19. Thomas J, Climie CR, Mather LE. The placental transfer of alcuronium. A preliminary report. Br J Anaesth 1969;41(4):297–302.

20. Brown TC, Gregory M, Bell B, Campbell PC. Liver tumours and muscle relaxants. Electromyographic studies in children. Anaesthesia 1987;42(12):1284–6.

21. Sarubin J. Erhöhter Bedarf an Alloferin bei Verbrennungspatienten. [Increased requirement of alcuronium in burned patients.] Anaesthesist 1982;31(8):392–5.

22. Fried MJ, Protheroe DT. D-penicillamine induced myasthenia gravis. Its relevance for the anaesthetist. Br J Anaesth 1986;58(10):1191–3.

23. Blanloeil Y, Baron D, Gazeau MF, Nicolas F. Curarisation prolongée au cours d'un syndrôme myasthénique induit par la D-pénicillamine. [Prolonged neuromuscular blockade during D-penicillamine-induced myasthenia.] Anesth Analg (Paris) 1980;37(7–8):441–3.

Atracurium dibesilate

General Information

Atracurium is a muscle relaxant with approximately one-fifth the potency of pancuronium (initial doses of 0.3–0.6 mg/kg and maintenance doses of 0.2 mg/kg being commonly used), an onset of action of 1.2–4 minutes (depending on the dose and the investigator), a medium duration of effect similar to (or slightly longer than) vecuronium, a rapid spontaneous recovery (slightly longer than vecuronium), and a virtual lack of accumulation. Atracurium-induced neuromuscular block is easily reversed by neostigmine.

In contrast to other non-depolarizing drugs, atracurium is completely broken down at normal blood pH and temperature by Hofmann elimination, principally (although to disputed degrees) by nucleophilic substitution and enzymatic ester hydrolysis (1–4). Four metabolites are known, laudanosine being the main biotransformation product. Of the other metabolites, the acrylate esters might possibly give rise to adverse effects. Acrylates are highly reactive pharmacologically and are potentially toxic, theoretically having the capacity to form immunogens and to alkylate cellular nucleophils (3), but so far no effects have been reported (5,6).

In animal experiments, atracurium in large concentrations, many times those providing complete neuromuscular blockade, causes vagal blockade and changes attributed to histamine release; at high dosages some hypotension is seen, possibly because of histamine release; alkalosis diminishes the neuromuscular block, and acidosis prolongs it (7). In cats, high doses of some of the breakdown products of atracurium produced dose-dependent neuromuscular blockade, hypotension, and autonomic effects (5). However, it was considered that these effects were of no pharmacological significance, in view of the low potencies of these substances and the quantities likely to be found in man. From interaction studies in cats (8) it was concluded that the action of atracurium is enhanced by D-tubocurarine, halothane, gentamicin, neomycin, and polymyxin, and antagonized by adrenaline and transiently by suxamethonium. Pretreatment with suxamethonium did not affect the subsequent block by atracurium in cats. Ciclosporin has also been reported to potentiate atracurium in cats (SEDA-12, 118) (9).

In man, histamine release by atracurium is common. The clinical significance of this is disputed, but it can cause minor transient skin reactions. Systemic effects of histamine release are much rarer than cutaneous manifestations.

Organs and Systems

Cardiovascular

There have been reports of hypotension (SEDA-15, 125) (10–12), attributed to histamine release by atracurium. A large prospective surveillance study involving more than 1800 patients given atracurium showed a 10% incidence of adverse reactions, with moderate hypotension (20–50% decrease) in 3.5% of patients (13). In one study cardiovascular stability was maintained with atracurium up to doses of 0.4 mg/kg (14). However, at higher doses (0.5 and 0.6 mg/kg) arterial pressure fell by 13 and 20% and heart rate increased by 5 and 8% respectively. These effects were maximal at 1–1.5 minutes. Since these cardiovascular effects were associated with facial flushing, it was suggested that they might have resulted from histamine release. In a subsequent study the same investigators linked significant cardiovascular changes to increased plasma histamine concentrations at a dose of atracurium of 0.6 mg/kg (15). Injecting this dose slowly over 75 seconds caused less histamine release and adverse hemodynamic effects (16). However, other investigators found no correlation between histamine plasma concentrations and hemodynamic reactions after atracurium administration (17).

Cardiovascular effects, apart from those resulting from histamine release, appear to be almost entirely limited to bradycardia. From animal studies, vagolytic (7) and ganglion-blocking (18) effects are very unlikely to occur at neuromuscular blocking doses, and these predictions appear to be borne out by investigations in man, cardiovascular effects being reported only at high dosages associated with signs suggestive of histamine release (14,15,19). The bradycardia (20–22) is occasionally severe, but, as with vecuronium, the explanation seems to be that the bradycardic effects of other agents used during anesthesia are not attenuated by atracurium as they are by alcuronium, gallamine, or pancuronium, which have vagolytic (or sympathomimetic) effects. The possibility that bradycardia can be caused by one of the metabolites, such as laudanosine (SEDA-12, 115), which is structurally similar to apomorphine, has yet to be excluded. An animal study has suggested that noradrenaline release from sympathetic nerve terminals can be increased by very large doses of atracurium, probably because of high concentrations of laudanosine (SEDA-14, 117) (23). Clinically, cardiovascular effects from this source would only be expected in circumstances that produced much higher than usual laudanosine concentrations.

Hypoxemia has been incidentally reported (SEDA-15, 125) (24), and most probably resulted from an increase ino-left cardiac shunting (in a patient with a ventricular septal defect and pulmonary atresia). Atracurium (0.2 mg/kg) may have produced a fall in systemic vascular resistance, perhaps from histamine release; pancuronium was subsequently given without incident.

Nervous system

The major metabolite of atracurium, laudanosine, can cross the blood–brain barrier (CSF/plasma ratios of 0.3–0.6 are found in dogs) (25) and produce strychnine-like nervous system stimulation, which at high plasma concentrations (around 17 ng/ml) leads to convulsions in dogs (25–27). CSF/plasma ratios of laudanosine in man have been reported to be between 0.01 and 0.14 after a 0.5 mg/kg dose of atracurium in a study in which the highest laudanosine concentration was 14 ng/ml (28). Much higher CSF laudanosine

concentrations (mean 202 ng/ml, highest 570 ng/ml) were measured after larger atracurium doses (0.5 mg/kg/hour) during intracranial surgery (SEDA-15, 126) (29).

Patients in whom the blood–brain barrier is not intact, such as during neurosurgical procedures, may be at risk from exposure of the brain to unpredictable concentrations of laudanosine (and other drugs). Two patients had fits but these were not thought to be related to laudanosine (29). Under normal circumstances plasma concentrations in man will be far below those required for significant central nervous stimulation. However, the half-life of laudanosine (25) is considerably longer than that of atracurium (30), so that there is a possibility of laudanosine accumulation if many repeated doses or prolonged infusions of atracurium are given.

Skin

Minor skin reactions lasting 5–30 minutes occur in 10–50% of patients according to various studies and are not usually associated with obvious systemic effects (10,31–34). They are probably due to histamine release. A 42% incidence of cutaneous flushing has been reported in 200 patients; the effect was dose-dependent, being 18% at 0.4 mg/kg, 33% at 0.5 and 0.6 mg/kg, and 73% at 1 mg/kg (35). One patient in this study, in the 1 mg/kg group, developed generalized erythema, hypotension, tachycardia, and bronchospasm.

Immunologic

There have been reports of angioedema (10) and bronchospasm (11,36), attributed to histamine release. A large prospective surveillance study involving more than 1800 patients given atracurium showed a 10% incidence of adverse reactions, with bronchospasm in 0.2% of patients (13).

Extreme sensitivity to an intradermal skin test (0.003 mg), some 24 hours after a severe skin reaction to the intravenous administration of atracurium, has been described (37).

Severe systemic reactions after atracurium administration may be due to antibody-mediated anaphylaxis (38) rather than non-specific histamine liberation. It has been suggested that systemic effects from non-specific histamine release are dose-dependent.

Second-Generation Effects

Fetotoxicity

Placental transfer of atracurium occurs (39). In 46 patients undergoing cesarean section (SEDA-17, 18), while the Apgar scores did not differ between neonates whose mothers had received atracurium (0.3 mg/kg) or tubocurarine (0.3 mg/kg), the neurological and adaptive capacity scores (NACS) at 15 minutes (but not at 2 and 24 hours) after birth were lower after atracurium. The NACS values were normal in 83% of the babies in the tubocurarine group and in 55% of those in the atracurium group. The difference was primarily due to lower scores for active contraction of the neck extensor and flexor muscles. These results cannot be satisfactorily explained by partial curarization in some neonates of the atracurium group because the placental transfer of atracurium was lower in the atracurium group; the umbilical vein concentrations of atracurium after clamping of the umbilical cord being approximately one-tenth of the EC_{50} for block of neuromuscular transmission in neonates.

Susceptibility Factors

Age

It has been recommended that doses also be reduced in small neonates less than 3 days old, particularly if their core temperatures are less than 36°C (40), since the breakdown of atracurium is pH- and temperature-dependent.

In elderly patients atracurium infusion requirements appear not to be reduced and its effects are not prolonged (41), probably because the action of atracurium is independent of routes of elimination that are affected by age.

Other features of the patient

Temperature and pH
The breakdown of atracurium is pH-dependent and temperature-dependent. Alkalosis reduces neuromuscular blockade by atracurium, and acidosis prolongs it.

Hypothermia, during cardiopulmonary bypass, has been reported as reducing atracurium requirements by half (42); pH changes may also have occurred.

Burns
Burns are associated with resistance to atracurium (43), as for several other non-depolarizing neuromuscular blocking agents. The EC_{50} is increased and dose requirements may be increased by up to 2–3 times. The resistance varies with the burn area and the time from injury (SEDA-12, 116), being maximal at 15–40 days in patients repeatedly anesthetized.

Dystrophia myotonica
Patients with dystrophia myotonica may be extremely sensitive to atracurium according to a case report (SEDA-10, 110) (44). Resistance to atracurium and higher than normal concentrations of acetylcholine receptors in muscle biopsies have been reported in a patient with multiple sclerosis (SEDA-13, 105) (45).

Pheochromocytoma
It has been suggested (46) that atracurium is unsuitable for use in patients with a pheochromocytoma, since increases in catecholamine concentrations, which are associated with hypertension and other unwanted cardiovascular effects, occur after the injection of relatively large doses (0.6–0.7 mg/kg). However, in an earlier report catecholamine concentrations did not increase and there were no untoward cardiovascular effects after atracurium (47). Nevertheless, considering atracurium's potential for histamine release (which can secondarily lead to increases in circulating catecholamines), vecuronium or pipecuronium are probably better choices in this condition.

Renal and hepatic insufficiency
Renal and liver dysfunction appear to have little effect on the neuromuscular blocking action of atracurium (30,48,49), although resistance has been reported in end-stage renal insufficiency (37% greater ED_{50} values and shorter duration of bolus doses) (SEDA-13, 103) (50,51).

Laudanosine metabolism may be reduced in liver disease (52), and in renal insufficiency higher plasma concentrations and an apparently delayed elimination of laudanosine have been reported (53). Prolonged infusion of atracurium in intensive care (for 38–219 hours) led to slowly increasing plasma laudanosine concentrations, which appeared to plateau after 2–3 days (54). The maximum plasma laudanosine concentrations in six patients were 1.9–5 µg/ml. There was no evidence of cerebral excitation. Nevertheless, caution is urged in patients with severe hepatic dysfunction (55,56), particularly if associated with renal insufficiency, when repeated bolus doses or an infusion of atracurium are given over a prolonged period.

Drug–Drug Interactions

Aminoglycoside antibiotics

Another interaction that has been reported not to occur in man is potentiation by the aminoglycoside antibiotics, gentamicin and tobramycin (57). In animals, however, gentamicin was found to enhance atracurium blockade (8), so further investigation is required to clarify this point.

Azathioprine

Azathioprine has been reported to reduce atracurium blockade transiently and to a clinically insignificant extent (50).

Carbamazepine

In contrast to reports on other non-depolarizing neuromuscular blocking agents, resistance to atracurium has not been found in patients taking long-term carbamazepine (SEDA-13, 104) (58).

Diisopropylphenol

The intravenous anesthetic agent, diisopropylphenol, is said to potentiate atracurium (59).

Halothane

From animal experiments (8) it seems likely that drug interactions with atracurium will be similar to those for other non-depolarizing neuromuscular blocking agents. Laudanosine has been reported to increase the MAC for halothane in animals (60).

In man, potentiation and prolongation of the action of atracurium by halothane (61–63) have been reported, as has potentiation after 30 minutes of isoflurane anesthesia (64). Whether the dose of atracurium should be reduced from that used during balanced anesthesia by 20, 30, or 50% when patients are anesthetized with inhalational anesthetics can only be decided in the case of an individual patient if neuromuscular monitoring is available, since many other variables, such as the tissue concentrations of the volatile anesthetic and the response of the individual patient to the neuromuscular blocking drug, will influence the overall blocking effect.

Isoflurane

A synergistic interaction between isoflurane and atracurium (high doses) has been incriminated in the causation of an increased incidence of generalized tonic-clonic seizures after neurosurgical operations (SEDA-15, 125) (65).

Ketamine

Ketamine has been shown to prolong the action of atracurium slightly (66).

Pancuronium

Small doses of pancuronium (0.5 or 1 mg) administered 3 minutes before atracurium potentiated its action synergistically (SEDA-12, 117) (67).

Phenytoin

In contrast to reports about other non-depolarizing neuromuscular blocking agents, resistance to atracurium has not been found in patients taking long-term phenytoin (SEDA-13, 104) (68).

Suxamethonium

Prior administration of suxamethonium potentiates the action of atracurium by about 30% (69).

Tamoxifen

Tamoxifen has been associated with prolonged atracurium block in a patient with breast cancer (SEDA-12, 117) (70).

Tubocurarine

Small doses of D-tubocurarine (0.05 or 0.1 mg/kg) administered 3 minutes before atracurium potentiated its action synergistically (SEDA-12, 117) (67).

References

1. Nigrovic V, Auen M, Wajskol A. Enzymatic hydrolysis of atracurium in vivo. Anesthesiology 1985;62(5):606–9.
2. Stiller RL, Cook DR, Chakravorti S. In vitro degradation of atracurium in human plasma. Br J Anaesth 1985;57(11):1085–8.
3. Nigrovic V. New insights into the toxicity of neuromuscular-blocking drugs and their metabolites. Curr Opin Anaesthesiol 1991;4:603.
4. Miller RD, Rupp SM, Fisher DM, Cronnelly R, Fahey MR, Sohn YJ. Clinical pharmacology of vecuronium and atracurium. Anesthesiology 1984;61(4):444–53.
5. Chapple DJ, Clark JS. Pharmacological action of breakdown products of atracurium and related substances. Br J Anaesth 1983;55(Suppl 1):S11–5.
6. Cato AE, Lineberry CG, Macklin AW. Concerning toxicity testing of atracurium. Anesthesiology 1985;62(1):94–5.
7. Hughes R, Chapple DJ. The pharmacology of atracurium: a new competitive neuromuscular blocking agent. Br J Anaesth 1981;53(1):31–44.
8. Chapple DJ, Clark JS, Hughes R. Interaction between atracurium and drugs used in anaesthesia. Br J Anaesth 1983;55(Suppl 1):S17–22.
9. Gramstad L, Gjerlow JA, Hysing ES, Rugstad HE. Interaction of cyclosporin and its solvent, Cremophor, with atracurium and vecuronium. Studies in the cat. Br J Anaesth 1986;58(10):1149–55.
10. Srivastava S. Angioneurotic oedema following atracurium. Br J Anaesth 1984;56(8):932–3.
11. Siler JN, Mager JG Jr, Wyche MQ Jr. Atracurium: hypotension, tachycardia and bronchospasm. Anesthesiology 1985;62(5):645–6.
12. Lynas AG, Clarke RS, Fee JP, Reid JE. Factors that influence cutaneous reactions following administration of thiopentone and atracurium. Anaesthesia 1988;43(10):825–8.
13. Beemer GH, Dennis WL, Platt PR, Bjorksten AR, Carr AB. Adverse reactions to atracurium and alcuronium. A prospective surveillance study. Br J Anaesth 1988;61(6):680–4.
14. Basta SJ, Ali HH, Savarese JJ, Sunder N, Gionfriddo M, Cloutier G, Lineberry C, Cato AE. Clinical pharmacology of atracurium besylate (BW 33A): a new non-depolarizing muscle relaxant. Anesth Analg 1982;61(9):723–9.
15. Basta SJ, Savarese JJ, Ali HH, Moss J, Gionfriddo M. Histamine-releasing potencies of atracurium, dimethyl tubocurarine and tubocurarine. Br J Anaesth 1983;55(Suppl 1):S105–6.
16. Scott RP, Savarese JJ, Ali HH, et al. Atracurium: clinical strategies for preventing histamine release and attenuating the hemodynamic response. Anesthesiology 1984;61:A287.
17. Shorten GD, Goudsouzian NG, Ali HH. Histamine release following atracurium in the elderly. Anaesthesia 1993;48(7):568–71.
18. Healy TE, Palmer JP. In vitro comparison between the neuromuscular and ganglion blocking potency ratios of atracurium and tubocurarine. Br J Anaesth 1982;54(12):1307–11.
19. Guggiari M, Gallais S, Bianchi A, Guillaume A, Viars P. Effets hémodynamiques de l'atracurium chez l'homme. [Hemodynamic effects of atracurium in man.] Ann Fr Anesth Reanim 1985;4(6):484–8.
20. Carter ML. Bradycardia after the use of atracurium. BMJ (Clin Res Ed) 1983;287(6387):247–8.
21. McHutchon A, Lawler PG. Bradycardia following atracurium. Anaesthesia 1983;38(6):597–8.
22. Woolner DF, Gibbs JM, Smeele PQ. Clinical comparison of atracurium and alcuronium in gynaecological surgery. Anaesth Intensive Care 1985;13(1):33–7.
23. Kinjo M, Nagashima H, Vizi ES. Effect of atracurium and laudanosine on the release of ^{3}H-noradrenaline. Br J Anaesth 1989;62(6):683–90.
24. Sudhaman DA. Atracurium and hypoxaemic episodes. Anaesthesia 1990;45(2):166.
25. Hennis PJ, Fahey MR, Canfell PC, Shi WZ, Miller RD. Pharmacology of laudanosine in dogs. Anesthesiology 1984;61:A305.
26. Babel A. Etude comparative de la laudanosine et de la papavérine au point de vue pharmacodynamique. Rev Méd Suisse Romande 1989;19:657.
27. Mercier J, Mercier E. Action de quelques alcaloïdes secondaires de l'opium sur l'électrocorticogramme du chien. [Effect of certain opium alkaloids on electrocorticography in dogs.] C R Seances Soc Biol Fil 1955;149(7-8):760–2.
28. Fahey MR, Canfell PC, Taboada T, Hosobuchi Y, Miller RD. Cerebrospinal fluid concentrations of laudanosine after administration of atracurium. Br J Anaesth 1990;64(1):105–6.

29. Eddleston JM, Harper NJ, Pollard BJ, Edwards D, Gwinnutt CL. Concentrations of atracurium and laudanosine in cerebrospinal fluid and plasma during intracranial surgery. Br J Anaesth 1989;63(5):525–30.

30. Fahey MR, Rupp SM, Fisher DM, Miller RD, Sharma M, Canfell C, Castagnoli K, Hennis PJ. The pharmacokinetics and pharmacodynamics of atracurium in patients with and without renal failure. Anesthesiology 1984;61(6):699–702.

31. Lavery GG, Mirakhur RK. Atracurium besylate in paediatric anaesthesia. Anaesthesia 1984;39(12):1243–6.

32. Mirakhur RK, Lyons SM, Carson IW, Clarke RS, Ferres CJ, Dundee JW. Cutaneous reaction after atracurium. Anaesthesia 1983;38(8):818–9.

33. Watkins J. Histamine release and atracurium. Br J Anaesth 1986;58(Suppl 1):S19–22.

34. Doenicke A, Moss J, Lorenz W, Hoernecke R, Gottardis M. Are hypotension and rash after atracurium really caused by histamine release? Anesth Analg 1994;78(5):967–72.

35. Mirakhur RK, Lavery GG, Clarke RS, Gibson FM, McAteer E. Atracurium in clinical anaesthesia: effect of dosage on onset, duration and conditions for tracheal intubation. Anaesthesia 1985;40(8):801–5.

36. Sale JP. Bronchospasm following the use of atracurium. Anaesthesia 1983;38(5):511–2.

37. Aldrete JA. Allergic reaction after atracurium. Br J Anaesth 1985;57(9):929–30.

38. Kumar AA, Thys J, Van Aken HK, Stevens E, Crul JF. Severe anaphylactic shock after atracurium. Anesth Analg 1993;76(2):423–5.

39. Flynn PJ, Frank M, Hughes R. Use of atracurium in caesarean section. Br J Anaesth 1984;56(6):599–605.

40. Nightingale DA. Use of atracurium in neonatal anaesthesia. Br J Anaesth 1986;58(Suppl 1):S32–6.

41. d'Hollander AA, Luyckx C, Barvais L, De Ville A. Clinical evaluation of atracurium besylate requirement for a stable muscle relaxation during surgery: lack of age-related effects. Anesthesiology 1983;59(3):237–40.

42. Flynn PJ, Hughes R, Walton B. Use of atracurium in cardiac surgery involving cardiopulmonary bypass with induced hypothermia. Br J Anaesth 1984;56(9):967–72.

43. Dwersteg JF, Pavlin EG, Heimbach DM. Patients with burns are resistant to atracurium. Anesthesiology 1986;65(5):517–20.

44. Stirt JA, Stone DJ, Weinberg G, Willson DF, Sternick CS, Sussman MD. Atracurium in a child with myotonic dystrophy. Anesth Analg 1985;64(3):369–70.

45. Brett RS, Schmidt JH, Gage JS, Schartel SA, Poppers PJ. Measurement of acetylcholine receptor concentration in skeletal muscle from a patient with multiple sclerosis and resistance to atracurium. Anesthesiology 1987;66(6):837–9.

46. Amaranath L, Zanettin GG, Bravo EL, Barnes A, Estafanous FG. Atracurium and pheochromocytoma: a report of three cases. Anesth Analg 1988;67(11):1127–30.

47. Stirt JA, Brown RE Jr, Ross TW Jr, Althaus JS. Atracurium in a patient with pheochromocytoma. Anesth Analg 1985;64(5):547–50.

48. Ward S, Neill EA. Pharmacokinetics of atracurium in acute hepatic failure (with acute renal failure). Br J Anaesth 1983;55(12):1169–72.

49. Hunter JM, Jones RS, Utting JE. Use of atracurium in patients with no renal function. Br J Anaesth 1982;54(12):1251–8.

50. Gramstad L. Atracurium, vecuronium and pancuronium in end-stage renal failure. Dose-response properties and interactions with azathioprine. Br J Anaesth 1987;59(8):995–1003.

51. Vandenbrom RH, Wierda JM, Agoston S. Pharmacokinetics of atracurium and metabolites in normal and renal failure patients. Anesthesiology 1987;67:A606.

52. Sharma M, Fahey MR, Castagnoli K, et al. In vitro metabolic studies of atracurium with rabbit liver preparations. Anesthesiology 1984;61:A304.

53. Fahey MR, Rupp SM, Canfell C, Fisher DM, Miller RD, Sharma M, Castagnoli K, Hennis PJ. Effect of renal failure on laudanosine excretion in man. Br J Anaesth 1985;57(11):1049–51.

54. Yate PM, Flynn PJ, Arnold RW, Weatherly BC, Simmonds RJ, Dopson T. Clinical experience and plasma laudanosine concentrations during the infusion of atracurium in the intensive therapy unit. Br J Anaesth 1987;59(2):211–7.

55. Ward S, Weatherley BC. Pharmacokinetics of atracurium and its metabolites. Br J Anaesth 1986;58(Suppl 1):S6–S10.

56. Hughes R. Atracurium: an overview. Br J Anaesth 1986;58(Suppl 1):S2–5.

57. Dupuis JY, Martin R, Tetrault JP. Atracurium and vecuronium interaction with gentamicin and tobramycin. Can J Anaesth 1989;36(4):407–11.

58. Ebrahim Z, Bulkley R, Roth S. Carbamazepine therapy and neuromuscular blockade with atracurium and vecuronium. Anesth Analg 1988;67:555.

59. Robertson EN, Fragen RJ, Booij LH, van Egmond J, Crul JF. Some effects of diisopropyl phenol (ICI 35 868) on the pharmacodynamics of atracurium and vecuronium in anaesthetized man. Br J Anaesth 1983;55(8):723–8.

60. Shi WZ, Fahey MR, Fisher DM, Miller RD, Canfell C, Eger EI 2nd. Laudanosine (a metabolite of atracurium) increases the minimum alveolar concentration of halothane in rabbits. Anesthesiology 1985;63(6):584–8.

61. Payne JP, Hughes R. Evaluation of atracurium in anaesthetized man. Br J Anaesth 1981;53(1):45–54.

62. Katz RL, Stirt J, Murray AL, Lee C. Neuromuscular effects of atracurium in man. Anesth Analg 1982;61(9):730–4.

63. Stirt JA, Murray AL, Katz RL, Schehl DL, Lee C. Atracurium during halothane anesthesia in humans. Anesth Analg 1983;62(2):207–10.

64. Rupp SM, Fahey MR, Miller RD. Neuromuscular and cardiovascular effects of atracurium during nitrous oxide-fentanyl and nitrous oxide–isoflurane anaesthesia. Br J Anaesth 1983;55(Suppl 1):S67–70.

65. Beemer GH, Dawson PJ, Bjorksten AR, Edwards NE. Early postoperative seizures in neurosurgical patients administered atracurium and isoflurane. Anaesth Intensive Care 1989;17(4):504–9.

66. Toft P, Helbo-Hansen S. Interaction of ketamine with atracurium. Br J Anaesth 1989;62(3):319–20.

67. Gerber HR, Romppainen J, Schwinn W. Potentiation of atracurium by pancuronium and D-tubocurarine. Can Anaesth Soc J 1986;33(5):563–70.

68. Ornstein E, Matteo RS, Schwartz AE, Silverberg PA, Young WL, Diaz J. The effect of phenytoin on the magnitude and duration of neuromuscular block following atracurium or vecuronium. Anesthesiology 1987;67(2):191–6.

69. Stirt JA, Katz RL, Murray AL, Schehl DL, Lee C. Modification of atracurium blockade by halothane and by suxamethonium. A review of clinical experience. Br J Anaesth 1983;55(Suppl 1):S71–5.

70. Naguib M, Gyasi HK. Antiestrogenic drugs and atracurium a possible interaction? Can Anaesth Soc J 1986;33(5):682–3.

Cisatracurium besilate

General Information

Cisatracurium is one of the ten isomers of atracurium. With an ED_{95} of 0.05 mg/kg it is about three times more potent than atracurium (1–3). The duration of action of cisatracurium tends to be slightly longer than that of atracurium. Less cisatracurium is required to achieve a given degree of neuromuscular blockade and so less laudanosine is produced.

Cisatracurium and atracurium share the same metabolic pathways, but Hofmann elimination may have a greater role in the elimination of cisatracurium than in atracurium (2,4–7). Spontaneous in vivo degradation accounts for 77% of total body clearance of cisatracurium (6). Organ clearance is 23% of total body clearance. Major metabolites of cisatracurium are laudanosine and a monoquaternary acrylate.

Clinical problems due to histamine release after bolus administration of cisatracurium have not been observed, even with very large doses up to 0.4 mg/kg (3,8), but in some patients there were considerable increases in plasma histamine concentrations (8–10).

Organs and Systems

Cardiovascular

With doses up to eight times the ED_{95} no cardiovascular adverse effects were observed (8) and in other studies cisatracurium had only minor cardiovascular adverse effects (9,11,12). Patients with coronary artery disease undergoing myocardial revascularization tolerated cisatracurium doses up to several fold the ED_{95} well; hemodynamic changes from pre- to postinjection were minimal (13,14).

Neuromuscular

Another example of flaccid paralysis after long-term use of a non-depolarizing muscle relaxant has been published, in this instance related to cisatracurium (15). While prolonged paralysis after the use of cisatracurium in intensive care had been described before (16), the authors of the recent report provided additional information related to the pathophysiology of neuromuscular function in their patient. Based on some previous studies, paralysis after neuromuscular blockers and glucocorticoids was thought to represent an intramuscular problem. However, electrophysiological studies in this case yielded a diagnosis of axonal neuropathy. This points to a critical illness polyneuropathy rather than an effect of cisatracurium.

Immunologic

Anaphylactic reactions have been reported (17–19).

Susceptibility Factors

Age

In line with its non-organ-dependent elimination pathways, neither the plasma clearance nor the duration of action of cisatracurium differed between young and elderly patients (20).

Renal disease

In patients with or without renal failure, there was no difference in the duration of action of cisatracurium (21).

Hepatic disease

In patients with hepatic failure neither the half-life nor the duration of action of cisatracurium was prolonged when compared with controls (22). In another study, however, the volume of distribution was increased and the plasma clearance reduced in patients with end-stage liver disease (23). Recovery times were not statistically different but the variability was greater in patients with liver disease (23).

Drug–Drug Interactions

General anesthetics

The action of cisatracurium is potentiated by isoflurane, sevoflurane, and enflurane (24).

References

1. Belmont MR, Lien CA, Quessy S, Abou-Donia MM, Abalos A, Eppich L, Savarese JJ. The clinical neuromuscular pharmacology of 51W89 in patients receiving nitrous oxide/opioid/barbiturate anesthesia. Anesthesiology 1995;82(5):1139–45.
2. Lien CA, Schmith VD, Belmont MR, Abalos A, Kisor DF, Savarese JJ. Pharmacokinetics of cisatracurium in patients receiving nitrous oxide/opioid/barbiturate anesthesia. Anesthesiology 1996;84(2):300–8.
3. Lepage JY, Malinovsky JM, Malinge M, Lechevalier T, Dupuch C, Cozian A, Pinaud M, Souron R. Pharmacodynamic dose-response and safety study of cisatracurium (51W89) in adult surgical patients during N_2O-O_2-opioid anesthesia. Anesth Analg 1996;83(4):823–9.
4. Welch RM, Brown A, Ravitch J, Dahl R. The in vitro degradation of cisatracurium, the R, cis-R'-isomer of atracurium, in human and rat plasma. Clin Pharmacol Ther 1995;58(2):132–42.
5. Fisher DM, Canfell PC, Fahey MR, Rosen JI, Rupp SM, Sheiner LB, Miller RD. Elimination of atracurium in humans: contribution of Hofmann elimination and ester hydrolysis versus organ-based elimination. Anesthesiology 1986;65(1):6–12.
6. Kisor DF, Schmith VD, Wargin WA, Lien CA, Ornstein E, Cook DR. Importance of the organ-independent elimination of cisatracurium. Anesth Analg 1996;83(5):1065–71.
7. Tsui D, Graham GG, Torda TA. The pharmacokinetics of atracurium isomers in vitro and in humans. Anesthesiology 1987;67(5):722–8.
8. Lien CA, Belmont MR, Abalos A, Eppich L, Quessy S, Abou-Donia MM, Savarese JJ. The cardiovascular effects and histamine-releasing properties of 51W89 in patients

receiving nitrous oxide/opioid/barbiturate anesthesia. Anesthesiology 1995;82(5):1131–8.

9. Doenicke A, Soukup J, Hoernecke R, Moss J. The lack of histamine release with cisatracurium: a double-blind comparison with vecuronium. Anesth Analg 1997;84(3):623–8.

10. Doenicke AW, Czeslick E, Moss J, Hoernecke R. Onset time, endotracheal intubating conditions, and plasma histamine after cisatracurium and vecuronium administration. Anesth Analg 1998;87(2):434–8.

11. Schramm WM, Jesenko R, Bartunek A, Gilly H. Effects of cisatracurium on cerebral and cardiovascular hemodynamics in patients with severe brain injury. Acta Anaesthesiol Scand 1997;41(10):1319–23.

12. Schramm WM, Papousek A, Michalek-Sauberer A, Czech T, Illievich U. The cerebral and cardiovascular effects of cisatracurium and atracurium in neurosurgical patients. Anesth Analg 1998;86(1):123–7.

13. Reich DL, Mulier J, Viby-Mogensen J, Konstadt SN, van Aken HK, Jensen FS, DePerio M, Buckley SG. Comparison of the cardiovascular effects of cisatracurium and vecuronium in patients with coronary artery disease. Can J Anaesth 1998;45(8):794–7.

14. Searle NR, Thomson I, Dupont C, Cannon JE, Roy M, Rosenbloom M, Gagnon L, Carrier M. A two-center study evaluating the hemodynamic and pharmacodynamic effects of cisatracurium and vecuronium in patients undergoing coronary artery bypass surgery. J Cardiothorac Vasc Anesth 1999;13(1):20–5.

15. Fodale V, Pratico C, Girlanda P, Baradello A, Lucanto T, Rodolico C, Nicolosi C, Rovere V, Santamaria LB, Dattola R. Acute motor axonal polyneuropathy after a cisatracurium infusion and concomitant corticosteroid therapy. Br J Anaesth 2004;92:289–93.

16. Davis NA, Rodgers JE, Gonzalez ER, Fowler AA. Prolonged weakness after cisatracurium infusion: a case report. Crit Care Med 1998;26:1290–2.

17. Clendenen SR, Harper JV, Wharen RE Jr, Guarderas JC. Anaphylactic reaction after cisatracurium. Anesthesiology 1997;87(3):690–2.

18. Toh KW, Deacock SJ, Fawcett WJ. Severe anaphylactic reaction to cisatracurium. Anesth Analg 1999;88(2):462–4.

19. Iannuzzi E, Iannuzzi M, Pedicini MS, Cirillo V, Chiefari M, Sacerdoti G. Anaphylactic reaction after cisatracurium administration. Eur J Anaesthesiol 2002;19(9):691–3.

20. Sorooshian SS, Stafford MA, Eastwood NB, Boyd AH, Hull CJ, Wright PM. Pharmacokinetics and pharmacodynamics of cisatracurium in young and elderly adult patients. Anesthesiology 1996;84(5):1083–91.

21. Boyd AH, Eastwood NB, Parker CJ, Hunter JM. Pharmacodynamics of the 1R cis-1′R cis isomer of atracurium (51W89) in health and chronic renal failure. Br J Anaesth 1995;74(4):400–4.

22. Tullock W, Scott V, Smith DA, Phillips L. Cook DR. Kinetics/dynamics of 51W89 in liver transplant patients and in healthy patients. Anesthesiology 1994;81:A1076.

23. De Wolf AM, Freeman JA, Scott VL, Tullock W, Smith DA, Kisor DF, Kerls S, Cook DR. Pharmacokinetics and pharmacodynamics of cisatracurium in patients with end-stage liver disease undergoing liver transplantation Br J Anaesth 1996; 76(5):624–8.

24. Wulf H, Kahl M, Ledowski T. Augmentation of the neuromuscular blocking effects of cisatracurium during desflurane, sevoflurane, isoflurane or total i.v. anaesthesia Br J Anaesth 1998;80(3):308–12.

Decamethonium

General Information

Decamethonium, a depolarizing neuromuscular blocker, is little used nowadays. A dose of 3 mg provides adequate relaxation for intra-abdominal surgery for about 15 minutes, supplements being required at intervals of 10–30 minutes. It is not as rapid in onset of action as suxamethonium. It is not hydrolysed by plasma cholinesterase, but is eliminated by the kidneys (1).

Tachyphylaxis occurs and a phase II block develops readily (2). In high doses, muscarinic actions can be seen and histamine release can occur.

Organs and Systems

Cardiovascular

Cardiovascular effects are less frequent than with suxamethonium; a reduction in heart rate sometimes occurs after a second dose.

Nervous system

Fasciculation occurs, with similar consequences to those described with suxamethonium.

Myotonia has been precipitated by decamethonium in patients with myotonia congenita and dystrophia myotonica (3).

Susceptibility Factors

Decamethonium depends on renal excretion for the termination of its effects and is therefore contraindicated in renal insufficiency (1).

The action of decamethonium is prolonged by hypothermia (4).

Drug–Drug Interactions

Hexafluorenium and decamethonium are antagonistic. Potentiation of decamethonium block has been reported with ketamine, and can occur with neostigmine.

References

1. Prescott LF. Mechanisms of renal excretion of drugs (with special reference to drugs used by anaesthetists). Br J Anaesth 1972;44(3):246–51.

2. Hughes R, Al-Azawi S, Payne JP. Tachyphylaxis after repeated dosage of decamethonium in anaesthetized man. Br J Clin Pharmacol 1982;13(3):355–9.

3. Orndahl G, Stenberg K. Myotonic human musculature: stimulation with depolarizing agents. Mechanical registration of the effects of succinyldicholine, succinylmonocholine and decamethonium. Acta Med Scand 1962;172(Suppl 389):3–29.

4. England AJ, Wu X, Richards KM, Redai I, Feldman SA. The influence of cold on the recovery of three neuromuscular blocking agents in man. Anaesthesia 1996;51(3):236–40.

Fazadinium

General Information

Originally claimed, from animal experiments, to be of rapid onset, short duration, and free from important adverse effects, this non-depolarizing relaxant has been found to be less satisfactory in man. The usual doses are 0.5–0.75 mg/kg, although 1 mg/kg is sometimes advocated for fast intubation (within 1–2 minutes). The duration of action is similar in man to that of D-tubocurarine and pancuronium. Excretion is primarily in the urine (50–80%, mostly in the first 6 hours), although a biliary route has also been suggested. Metabolism occurs, probably to a minor extent, 1–3% being detected in the urine as inactive metabolites.

Organs and Systems

Cardiovascular

Cardiovascular effects account for the relative unpopularity of fazadinium. It has some ganglion-blocking activity (1) and blocks cardiac muscarinic receptors in the therapeutic dose range (2). Its vagolytic potency is about the same as that of gallamine. Fazadinium, like pancuronium, also blocks the reuptake of noradrenaline into sympathetic nerve endings. These actions explain its major cardiac adverse effect, namely significant tachycardia (3), which occurs even with small doses and is persistent. It is dose-related (4), the increase in heart rate varying between 30 and 100%, and is associated with a rise in cardiac output and falls in stroke volume and peripheral resistance. Hypertension or hypotension can occur (5,6). If fazadinium is used injudiciously, extreme and dangerous cardiovascular changes can ensue (7).

Immunologic

Histamine release from fazadinium is very uncommon, but hypotension associated with an urticarial rash and two cases of severe bronchospasm and cardiac arrest (in patients who had also received thiopental) have been reported (8) as probably being due to fazadinium.

Immunological investigations combined with positive intradermal tests have been used to confirm fazadinium as the causative agent in a severe reaction (9).

Second-Generation Effects

Fetotoxicity

Placental transfer occurs and, though there may be some fetal uptake, Apgar scores did not appear to be affected (10,11).

References

1. Hughes R, Chapple DJ. Effects on non-depolarizing neuromuscular blocking agents on peripheral autonomic mechanisms in cats. Br J Anaesth 1976;48(2):59–68.
2. Marshall IG. The ganglion blocking and vagolytic actions of three short-acting neuromuscular blocking drugs in the cat. J Pharm Pharmacol 1973;25(7):530–6.
3. Hughes R, Payne JP, Sugai N. Studies on fazadinium bromide (AH 8165): a new non-depolarizing neuromuscular blocking agent. Can Anaesth Soc J 1976;23(1):36–47.
4. Schuh FT. Clinical neuromuscular pharmacology of AH 8165 D, an azobis-arylimidazo-pyridinium-compound. Anaesthesist 1975;24(4):151–6.
5. Lyons SM, Clarke RS, Young HS. A clinical comparison of AH8165 and pancuronium as muscle relaxants in patients undergoing cardiac surgery. Br J Anaesth 1975;47(6):725–9.
6. Lienhart A, Tauvent A, Guggiari M. Effets hemodynamiques des curares. [Hemodynamic effects of curares.]. In: Curares et Curarisation 1. Paris: Librairie Arnette, 1979:384.
7. Pinaud M, Arnould F, Souron R, Nicolas F. Influence of cardiac rhythm on the haemodynamic effects of fazadinium in patients with heart failure. Br J Anaesth 1983;55(6):507–12.
8. Alexander JP. Adverse reactions following fazadinium–thiopentone induction. Anaesthesia 1979;34(7):661–5.
9. Baldassare M, Mastroianni A. Su un grave caso di shock da bromuro di fazadinio. [On a severe case of shock caused by fazadinium bromide.] Acta Anaesthesiol Ital 1983;34:91.
10. Bertrand JC, Duvaldestin P, Henzel D, Desmonts JM. Quantitative assessment of placental transfer of fazadinium in obstetric anaesthesia. Acta Anaesthesiol Scand 1980;24(2):135–7.
11. Rainaldi MP, Busi T, Melloni C, Boschi S. Pharmacokinetics and placental transmission of fazadinium in elective caesarean sections. Acta Anaesthesiol Scand 1984;28(2):222–5.

Gallamine triethiodide

General Information

Gallamine is a non-depolarizing muscle relaxant. For intubation about 2 mg/kg (some authors say 3–4 mg/kg) are necessary, and the duration of effect is then similar to the usual intubating doses of D-tubocurarine or pancuronium. A dose of 1–1.5 mg/kg is usually sufficient to produce apnea and adequate abdominal relaxation. Such doses are said to be short-acting (20 minutes) but can provide clinical relaxation (75% or more depression of twitch height) for some 30–40 minutes. Individual variation is considerable, and complete spontaneous reversal of blockade is relatively slow.

Organs and Systems

Cardiovascular

Tachycardia invariably accompanies the use of gallamine. It is seen after doses as low as 20 mg and reaches a maximum at around 100 mg in adults (1). It is often extreme, rates above 120 per minute being not uncommon. The increase in heart rate outlasts the neuromuscular blocking effect (1). Usual clinical doses also result in a slight increase in mean arterial pressure, a slight fall in systemic vascular resistance, and a marked rise in cardiac index (2,3). These cardiovascular effects are principally accounted for by the strong vagolytic action of gallamine, the cardiac muscarinic receptors being almost as sensitive to its blocking action as the acetylcholine receptors of the neuromuscular junction (4). Blockade of noradrenaline reuptake and an increased release of noradrenaline from cardiac adrenergic nerve endings (5,6) may contribute, although an inotropic effect in man is disputed (7). Ganglion-blocking activity is slight and is not seen in the usual dose range. The possible mechanisms have been reviewed (8–10). Gallamine should therefore not be used when tachycardia has to be avoided.

Immunologic

Histamine release may be associated with the use of gallamine more often than was previously believed, according to several studies involving large numbers of patients (11–14). There have been several reports of reactions involving skin flushing, bronchospasm, or cardiovascular collapse possibly due to gallamine, including anaphylactoid reactions to small precurarizing doses (15,16).

Second-Generation Effects

Fetotoxicity

Placental transfer has been variously reported, usually only small amounts being detected in the umbilical blood, with no clinically obvious effects on the newborn (17).

Susceptibility Factors

Renal disease

Gallamine does not undergo biotransformation and depends entirely on glomerular filtration for its excretion (17). In renal insufficiency the neuromuscular blockade that it causes is considerably prolonged and gallamine is contraindicated.

Drug–Drug Interactions

Azathioprine

Azathioprine reduces sensitivity to gallamine in experimental animals, possibly as a result of phosphodiesterase inhibition, increasing transmitter release (SEDA-4, 87) (18), (SEDA-13, 104).

References

1. Eisele JH, Marta JA, Davis HS. Quantitative aspects of the chronotropic and neuromuscular effects of gallamine in anesthetized man. Anesthesiology 1971;35(6):630–3.
2. Stoelting RK. Hemodynamic effects of gallamine during halothane–nitrous oxide anesthesia. Anesthesiology 1973;39(6):645–7.
3. Kennedy BR, Farman JV. Cardiovascular effects of gallamine triethiodide in man. Br J Anaesth 1968;40(10):773–80.
4. Riker WF Jr, Wescoe WC. The pharmacology of Flaxedil, with observations on certain analogues. Ann NY Acad Sci 1951;54(3):373–94.
5. Brown BR Jr, Crout JR. The sympathomimetic effect of gallamine on the heart. J Pharmacol Exp Ther 1970;172(2):266–73.
6. Vercruysse P, Bossuyt P, Hanegreefs G, Verbeuren TJ, Vanhoutte PM. Gallamine and pancuronium inhibit pre- and postjunctional muscarine receptors in canine saphenous veins. J Pharmacol Exp Ther 1979;209(2):225–30.
7. Reitan JA, Fraser AI, Eisele JH. Lack of cardiac inotropic effects of gallamine in anesthetized man. Anesth Analg 1973;52(6):974–9.
8. Marshall IG. Pharmacological effects of neuromuscular blocking agents: interaction with cholinoceptors other than nicotinic receptors of the neuromuscular junction. Anest Rianim 1986;27:19.
9. Bowman WC. Non-relaxant properties of neuromuscular blocking drugs. Br J Anaesth 1982;54(2):147–60.
10. Bowman WC. Pharmacology of Neuromuscular Function. 2nd ed. London/Boston/Singapore/Sydney/Toronto/ Wellington: Wright;. 1990.
11. Hatton F, Tiret L, Maujol L, N'Doye P, Vourc'h G, Desmonts JM, Otteni JC, Scherpereel P. Enquête épidémiologique sur les anesthésies. [INSERM. Epidemiological survey of anesthesia. Initial results.] Ann Fr Anesth Réanim 1983;2(5):331–86.
12. Fisher MM, Munro I. Life-threatening anaphylactoid reactions to muscle relaxants. Anesth Analg 1983;62(6):559–64.
13. Laxenaire MC, Moneret-Vautrin DA, Vervloet D. The French experience of anaphylactoid reactions. Int Anesthesiol Clin 1985;23(3):145–60.
14. Galletly DC, Treuren BC. Anaphylactoid reactions during anaesthesia. Seven years' experience of intradermal testing. Anaesthesia 1985;40(4):329–33.
15. Harrison GR, Thompson ID. Adverse reaction to methohexitone and gallamine. Anaesthesia 1981;36(1):40–4.
16. Harrison JF, Bird AG. Anaphylaxis to precurarising doses of gallamine triethiodide. Anaesthesia 1986;41(6):600–4.
17. Ramzan MI, Somogyi AA, Walker JS, Shanks CA, Triggs EJ. Clinical pharmacokinetics of the non-depolarising muscle relaxants. Clin Pharmacokinet 1981;6(1):25–60.
18. Dretchen KL, Morgenroth VH 3rd, Standaert FG, Walts LF. Azathioprine: effects on neuromuscular transmission. Anesthesiology 1976;45(6):604–9.

Metocurine

General Information

Metocurine is a non-depolarizing neuromuscular blocker, a synthetic derivative of D-tubocurarine. No metabolites have been detected and it depends almost entirely on renal function for its excretion; 40–50% of the drug is excreted in the urine and about 2% (possibly more) in the bile in 24 hours (1). It is about twice as potent as D-tubocurarine and a quarter as potent as pancuronium, measured during narcotic/nitrous oxide anesthesia. It has similar onset and duration of action and speed of recovery to D-tubocurarine and pancuronium (2).

The dose of metocurine for intubation is 0.3 mg/kg and adequate abdominal relaxation is achieved with 0.1–0.2 mg/kg in most patients. As with all neuromuscular blocking agents, there is great individual variation in response, and if it is desired to give minimal doses, monitoring of the neuromuscular response is advisable. Volatile anesthetics and prior suxamethonium would be expected to reduce dosage requirements, but clinical reports are lacking. Patients with burns require 2–3 times higher doses of metocurine (3) and this phenomenon can persist (in lessening degree) for 1 year or more (4).

Organs and Systems

Cardiovascular

Metocurine has significantly less ganglion-blocking activity than D-tubocurarine (5) and much less of a tendency to provoke histamine release (6,7). It does not block cardiac muscarinic receptors at neuromuscular blocking doses (8). Cardiovascular stability is therefore to be expected (9). Slight tachycardia and fall in blood pressure have been reported in one-third of patients given larger doses (0.4 mg/kg) rapidly, probably as a result of histamine release, but no bronchospasm was seen (2).

Susceptibility Factors

Renal disease

Greatly prolonged duration of paralysis and a reduced rate of return of neuromuscular function can occur in renal insufficiency, because of a reduced plasma clearance and a prolonged half-life (10). Metocurine is not the relaxant of choice when renal function is poor.

Drug–Drug Interactions

Phenytoin

Resistance to metocurine is also described in patients taking long-term phenytoin (SEDA-10, 110) (11).

References

1. Meijer DK, Weitering JG, Vermeer GA, Scaf AH. Comparative pharmacokinetics of d-tubocurarine and metocurine in man. Anesthesiology 1979;51(5):402–7.
2. Savarese JJ, Ali HH, Antonio RP. The clinical pharmacology of metocurine: dimethyltubocurarine revisited. Anesthesiology 1977;47(3):277–84.
3. Martyn JA, Goudsouzian NG, Matteo RS, Liu LM, Szyfelbein SK, Kaplan RF. Metocurine requirements and plasma concentrations in burned paediatric patients. Br J Anaesth 1983;55(4):263–8.
4. Martyn JA, Matteo RS, Szyfelbein SK, Kaplan RF. Unprecedented resistance to neuromuscular blocking effects of metocurine with persistence after complete recovery in a burned patient. Anesth Analg 1982;61(7):614–7.
5. Hughes R, Chapple DJ. Effects on non-depolarizing neuromuscular blocking agents on peripheral autonomic mechanisms in cats. Br J Anaesth 1976;48(2):59–68.
6. McCullough LS, Stone WA, Delaunois AL, Reier CE, Hamelberg W. The effect of dimethyl tubocurarine iodide on cardiovascular parameters, postganglionic sympathetic

activity, and histamine release. Anesth Analg 1972;51(4):554–9.
7. Basta SJ, Savarese JJ, Ali HH, Moss J, Gionfriddo M. Histamine-releasing potencies of atracurium, dimethyl tubocurarine and tubocurarine. Br J Anaesth 1983;55(Suppl 1):S105–6.
8. Hughes R, Chapple DJ. Cardiovascular and neuromuscular effects of dimethyl tubocurarine in anaesthetized cats and rhesus monkeys. Br J Anaesth 1976;48(9):847–52.
9. Hughes R, Ingram GS, Payne JP. Studies on dimethyl tubocurarine in anaesthetized man. Br J Anaesth 1976;48(10):969–74.
10. Brotherton WP, Matteo RS. Pharmacokinetics and pharmacodynamics of metocurine in humans with and without renal failure. Anesthesiology 1981;55(3):273–6.
11. Ornstein E, Matteo RS, Young WL, Diaz J. Resistance to metocurine in patients receiving phenytoin. Anesthesiology 1984;61:A314.

Mivacurium chloride

General Information

Mivacurium chloride is a non-depolarizing muscle relaxant, a benzylisoquinolinium diester compound with a duration of approximately twice that of suxamethonium. In vitro (1), it is metabolized to a significant extent by plasma cholinesterase, and minimally by acetylcholinesterase. The rate of metabolism in vitro is directly related to plasma cholinesterase activity. In pooled human plasma the rate of hydrolysis of mivacurium was 70% that of suxamethonium. Its half-life is 5–10 minutes compared with 2–5 minutes for suxamethonium. The in vitro hydrolysis of mivacurium by purified human plasma cholinesterase occurs at 88% of the rate for suxamethonium (2). There was a poor correlation between the duration of action of bolus doses of mivacurium and the plasma cholinesterase activity in individual patients (2), a finding that has also been reported by others (3). However, the average infusion rate to maintain around 95% blockade in individual patients correlated significantly with the patients' plasma cholinesterase activities (4). While metabolites have been detected in both urine and bile, mivacurium seems to depend principally on ester hydrolysis for its plasma clearance, so that reduced activity of plasma cholinesterase is likely to result in a prolonged duration of action.

Organs and Systems

Cardiovascular

Benzylisoquinolinium compounds have a tendency to evoke histamine release, the main source of the cardiovascular changes seen with mivacurium. These have been reported as minimal up to and including twice the ED_{95} dose in several studies (3,5–7). At higher dosages (0.2 mg/kg and over) transient hypotension, often associated with facial flushing and lasting only some 2–5 minutes, which correlated significantly with increases in plasma histamine, has been described (5). Reducing the speed of injection to 30 or 60 seconds reduced the degree of hypotension to insignificant levels. Similar findings in 50% of patients given doses of 0.2 and 0.25 mg/kg have been described elsewhere (3). In yet another series, mean arterial pressure fell by more than 20% (24–61%) in seven of 15 patients given rapid bolus injections of 0.2–0.25 mg/kg (6). Pretreatment with oral antihistamines has been suggested as an additional option to reduce histamine-related adverse effects after administration of high-dose mivacurium (8).

In patients scheduled for coronary artery bypass grafting or valve replacement (7), significant hypotension was seen in two patients (out of 27 given higher doses), even when mivacurium was injected slowly (over 60 seconds); the mean arterial pressure fell by 24 and 50% after the injection of 0.2 and 0.25 mg/kg respectively. Beta-blockers, calcium channel blockers, and nitrates were not discontinued preoperatively in this study. The authors concluded that "doses larger than 0.15 mg/kg are probably unnecessary and may contribute to hemodynamic instability at least in cardiac patients."

Respiratory

Because of requests for a medico-legal consultation for bronchospasm, the Food and Drug Administration's MedWatch database has been queried to assess whether adverse events leading to bronchospasm or asthma occurred more often with mivacurium than with other muscle relaxants (9). Bronchospasm constituted 22% of the events with mivacurium, 14% with atracurium, 11% with vecuronium, 7.6% with rocuronium, and 2.0% with pancuronium. These figures emphasize the recommendation of the manufacturers that caution be taken when giving mivacurium to "patients with clinically significant cardiovascular disease and patients with any history suggesting a greater sensitivity to the release of histamine or related mediators".

Susceptibility Factors

Genetic factors

Prolonged neuromuscular blockade, up to several hours duration, has been reported in patients with abnormal plasma cholinesterase activity, who were either homozygous for the atypical gene or the silent gene or heterozygous for the atypical and the silent genes (10–13). This is a particular problem if mivacurium is used for ambulatory anesthesia, after which the patient is expected to return home, since facilities for postoperative ventilatory support may not be available. As patients with atypical cholinesterase are usually not detected by preoperative screening, it has been suggested that the patient's response to mivacurium should be tested by using a very low initial dose. However, complete paralysis for nearly 5 hours has recently been observed after a test dose of mivacurium 14 µg/kg in a patient with atypical serum cholinesterase as diagnosed by standard phenotyping

and DNA sequencing (14). The authors concluded that neuromuscular monitoring and facilities for long-term ventilation should always be available when mivacurium is used.

Renal disease

The duration of mivacurium-induced neuromuscular blockade was prolonged in patients with kidney disease (SEDA-17, 25) (15,16). These results are probably due to reduced plasma cholinesterase activity.

Hepatic disease

The duration of mivacurium-induced neuromuscular blockade was prolonged in patients with liver disease (SEDA-17, 25) (17). These results are probably due to reduced plasma cholinesterase activity.

Drug–Drug Interactions

Bambuterol

Bambuterol has been reported to alter the metabolism of mivacurium (18). Bambuterol has a dose-dependent inhibitory effect on plasma cholinesterase activity and prolongs the effects of suxamethonium. Bambuterol 10 mg was given to 28 patients 2 hours before an elective operation requiring general anesthesia. The patients given bambuterol had a 67–97% fall in plasma cholinesterase activity, leading to reduced clearance of mivacurium. This resulted in a shorter onset and a 3- to 4-fold prolongation of action of the neuromuscular blockade produced by standard doses of mivacurium.

General anesthetics

Inhalation anesthetics potentiate the neuromuscular blocking action of mivacurium, as with other non-depolarizing relaxants. With isoflurane (3) and enflurane (19) the ED_{95} is reduced by about 25% and the duration of action is somewhat prolonged, although the extent of this is not clear. Halothane has much less of an effect (20,21).

References

1. Cook DR, Stiller RL, Weakly JN, Chakravorti S, Brandom BW, Welch RM. In vitro metabolism of mivacurium chloride (BW B1090U) and succinylcholine. Anesth Analg 1989;68(4):452–6.
2. Savarese JJ, Ali HH, Basta SJ, Embree PB, Scott RP, Sunder N, Weakly JN, Wastila WB, el-Sayad HA. The clinical neuromuscular pharmacology of mivacurium chloride (BW B1090U). A short-acting nondepolarizing ester neuromuscular blocking drug. Anesthesiology 1988;68(5):723–32.
3. Choi WW, Mehta MP, Murray DJ, Sokoll MD, Forbes RB, Gergis SD, Abou-Donia M, Kirchner J. Neuromuscular and cardiovascular effects of mivacurium chloride in surgical patients receiving nitrous oxide–narcotic or nitrous oxide–isoflurane anaesthesia. Can J Anaesth 1989;36(6):641–50.
4. Ali HH, Savarese JJ, Embree PB, Basta SJ, Stout RG, Bottros LH, Weakly JN. Clinical pharmacology of mivacurium chloride (BW B1090U) infusion: comparison with vecuronium and atracurium. Br J Anaesth 1988;61(5):541–6.

5. Savarese JJ, Ali HH, Basta SJ, Scott RP, Embree PB, Wastila WB, Abou-Donia MM, Gelb C. The cardiovascular effects of mivacurium chloride (BW B1090U) in patients receiving nitrous oxide-opiate-barbiturate anesthesia. Anesthesiology 1989;70(3):386–94.

6. Caldwell JE, Heier T, Kitts JB, Lynam DP, Fahey MR, Miller RD. Comparison of the neuromuscular block induced by mivacurium, suxamethonium or atracurium during nitrous oxide–fentanyl anaesthesia. Br J Anaesth 1989;63(4):393–9.

7. Stoops CM, Curtis CA, Kovach DA, McCammon RL, Stoelting RK, Warren TM, Miller D, Bopp SK, Jugovic DJ, Abou-Donia MM. Hemodynamic effects of mivacurium chloride administered to patients during oxygen–sufentanil anesthesia for coronary artery bypass grafting or valve replacement. Anesth Analg 1989;68(3):333–9.

8. Doenicke A, Moss J, Lorenz W, Mayer M, Rau J, Jedrzejewski A, Ostwald P. Effect of oral antihistamine premedication on mivacurium-induced histamine release and side effects. Br J Anaesth 1996;77(3):421–3.

9. Bishop MJ, JT OD, Salemi JR. Mivacurium and bronchospasm. Anesth Analg 2003;97:484–5.

10. Ostergaard D, Jensen FS, Jensen E, Skovgaard LT, Viby-Mogensen J. Mivacurium-induced neuromuscular blockade in patients with atypical plasma cholinesterase. Acta Anaesthesiol Scand 1993;37(3):314–8.

11. Petersen RS, Bailey PL, Kalameghan R, Ashwood ER. Prolonged neuromuscular block after mivacurium. Anesth Analg 1993;76(1):194–6.

12. Goudsouzian NG, d'Hollander AA, Viby-Mogensen J. Prolonged neuromuscular block from mivacurium in two patients with cholinesterase deficiency. Anesth Analg 1993;77(1):183–5.

13. Maddineni VR, Mirakhur RK. Prolonged neuromuscular block following mivacurium. Anesthesiology 1993;78(6):1181–4.

14. Vanlinthout LE, Bartels CF, Lockridge O, Callens K, Booij LH. Prolonged paralysis after a test dose of mivacurium in a patient with atypical serum cholinesterase. Anesth Analg 1998;87(5):1199–202.

15. Blobner M, Jelen-Esselborn S, Schneider G, Mann R, Kling M, Luppa P, Schneck HJ, Kochs E. Effect of renal function on neuromuscular block induced by continuous infusion of mivacurium. Br J Anaesth 1995;74(4):452–4.

16. Head-Rapson AG, Devlin JC, Parker CJ, Hunter JM. Pharmacokinetics and pharmacodynamics of the three isomers of mivacurium in health, in end-stage renal failure and in patients with impaired renal function. Br J Anaesth 1995;75(1):31–6.

17. Head-Rapson AG, Devlin JC, Parker CJ, Hunter JM. Pharmacokinetics of the three isomers of mivacurium and pharmacodynamics of the chiral mixture in hepatic cirrhosis. Br J Anaesth 1994;73(5):613–8.

18. Ostergaard D, Rasmussen SN, Viby-Mogensen J, Pedersen NA, Boysen R. The influence of drug-induced low plasma cholinesterase activity on the pharmacokinetics and pharmacodynamics of mivacurium. Anesthesiology 2000;92(6):1581–7.

19. Caldwell JE, Kitts JB, Heier T, Fahey MR, Lynam DP, Miller RD. The dose-response relationship of mivacurium chloride in humans during nitrous oxide-fentanyl or nitrous oxide-enflurane anesthesia. Anesthesiology 1989;70(1):31–5.

20. Brandom BW, Sarner JB, Woelfel SK, Dong ML, Horn MC, Borland LM, Cook DR, Foster VJ, McNulty BF, Weakly JN. Mivacurium infusion requirements in pediatric surgical patients during nitrous oxide–halothane and during nitrous oxide–narcotic anesthesia. Anesth Analg 1990;71(1):16–22.

21. From RP, Pearson KS, Choi WW, Abou-Donia M, Sokoll MD. Neuromuscular and cardiovascular effects of mivacurium chloride (BW B1090U) during nitrous oxide-fentanyl–thiopentone and nitrous oxide–halothane anaesthesia. Br J Anaesth 1990;64(2):193–8.

Pancuronium bromide

General Information

Pancuronium bromide is a non-depolarizing muscle relaxant (1) with two quaternary ammonium groups on a steroid (androstane) skeleton. It is about 5–7 times as potent as D-tubocurarine. Protein binding occurs to both albumins and globulins, probably only to a relatively slight extent (10–20%), although reports vary from 10 to 90%. In contrast to most other non-depolarizing relaxants, pancuronium is metabolized at about 10–20%. Deacetylation in the liver probably accounts for the greater part of this biotransformation. The major metabolites are 3-monohydroxypancuronium, 17-monohydroxypancuronium, and (3,17)-dihydroxypancuronium; they are active pharmacologically, 3-monohydroxypancuronium being half as potent and the other two having 2% of the potency of pancuronium. About 40–50% of a dose is normally excreted in the urine and 5–10% in the bile over 24 hours as pancuronium plus its metabolites.

Pancuronium is reported to inhibit plasma cholinesterase (2) and this may be partly why the action of suxamethonium, given after a small dose of pancuronium, is prolonged. It also weakly inhibits acetylcholinesterase.

For tracheal intubation the usual dose is 0.1 mg/kg. When given after suxamethonium, 0.05 mg/kg is sufficient for good abdominal relaxation. Further doses of about one-quarter to one-third of the initial dose are given at intervals of 30–40 minutes to maintain relaxation. Reversal is easily achieved with neostigmine, provided there is some spontaneous return of neuromuscular transmission beforehand. If the evoked twitch height is less than 10% of the control value, there can be difficulty in reversing the blockade; this applies to all non-depolarizing relaxants, except perhaps vecuronium and atracurium.

The onset time for complete neuromuscular blockade is similar to that of D-tubocurarine and other non-depolarizing agents, namely 2–4 minutes. However, this is to some extent dose-dependent, and because of the relative lack of cardiovascular effects and histamine release, pancuronium can safely be given in higher dosages, thus producing good intubation conditions within 2 minutes. The dose of D-tubocurarine required to achieve similar conditions in 2 minutes would result in hypotension. As with D-tubocurarine, repeated doses can lead to accumulation and prolonged blockade.

In burned patients resistance to the neuromuscular blocking action of pancuronium may be encountered (3), as with other non-depolarizing relaxants.

Patients in whom pancuronium bromide is of value (4) include:

- patients with hypoxemia resisting mechanical ventilation and so cardiovascularly unstable that the use of sedatives is precluded;
- patients with bronchospasm unresponsive to conventional therapy;
- patients with severe tetanus or poisoning when muscle spasm prohibits adequate ventilation;
- patients with status epilepticus unable to maintain their own ventilation;
- shivering patients in whom metabolic demands for oxygen should be reduced;
- patients requiring tracheal intubation in whom suxamethonium is contraindicated.

Organs and Systems

Cardiovascular

Cardiovascular adverse effects are minimal with pancuronium. Ganglion blockade does not occur. Slight dose-dependent rises in heart rate, blood pressure, and cardiac output are common (5), but are often masked by the actions of other co-administered agents, such as fentanyl or halothane, which cause bradycardia or hypotension. These adverse effects of pancuronium are thus often beneficial and can be deliberately harnessed. Several mechanisms contribute: vagal blockade via selective blockade of cardiac muscarinic receptors (6), release of noradrenaline from adrenergic nerve endings (7), increased blood catecholamine concentrations (8), inhibition of neuronal catecholamine reuptake (9–11), and direct effects on myocardial contractility (12). These have been reviewed (13–15).

Occasionally nodal rhythm, atrioventricular dissociation, and tachydysrhythmias (such as ventricular extra beats or even bigeminy) develop, but these usually occur in association with halothane.

Supraventricular tachycardia has been reported after 8 mg pancuronium in a patient taking aminophylline (800 mg/day) (16).

Nodal rhythm can occur after injection of pancuronium. This dysrhythmia and bradycardia appear to be more common when neostigmine (plus atropine) is given for reversal of pancuronium-induced neuromuscular blockade than for reversal of D-tubocurarine or alcuronium (17); cholinesterase inhibition by pancuronium may contribute to the bradycardia in these circumstances.

Respiratory

Histamine release and bronchospasm are relatively rare with pancuronium but have been reported (SEDA-12, 117) (18–21).

Nervous system

Accidental injection into the cerebrospinal fluid of 4 mg of pancuronium resulted in generalized hypotonia,

weakness, and hypoventilation (SEDA-15, 126) (22). Neostigmine given intravenously led to prompt recovery.

Sensory systems

Neonates with congenital diaphragmatic hernia often develop respiratory failure. To facilitate mechanical ventilation, neuromuscular blocking agents may be used. Sensorineural hearing loss can occur in survivors, with a reported incidence of up to 60%. It has been associated with the use of pancuronium. In a historical cohort study of 37 survivors of congenital diaphragmatic hernia, children with hearing loss had received significantly higher doses of pancuronium during respiratory failure than children without hearing loss (23). In addition, the cumulative dose of pancuronium correlated with the intensity of hearing loss in decibels. There were no differences with regard to oxygenation and ventilation parameters or to the cumulative dose of aminoglycosides, vancomycin, or furosemide, but children with hearing loss had received a higher cumulative dose of etacrynic acid. The authors admitted that the retrospective study design and the small sample size demanded cautious interpretation of their observations. For the time being, this report is not reason enough to avoid pancuronium if neuromuscular blockade is required. However, it should be remembered that the risk of severe neuromuscular disturbances associated with long-term administration of neuromuscular blocking agents militates against the routine use of these drugs in patients in intensive care, both children and adults. If muscle relaxants are given in this setting for more than a few hours, their effect should be monitored by a peripheral nerve stimulator to avoid overdose and drug accumulation. This may prove technically difficult in neonates.

Liver

Significant hyperbilirubinemia has been reported to occur more frequently in critically ill neonates given pancuronium than in a control group (24). The hyperbilirubinemia increased in the 4 days after withdrawal of pancuronium, whereas during the administration period the hyperbilirubinemia was less in the pancuronium group.

Body temperature

Malignant hyperthermia, possibly triggered by pancuronium, has been described (25), although pancuronium is generally considered to be safe in patients who are susceptible to the syndrome (26).

Second-Generation Effects

Fetotoxicity

There is placental transfer of pancuronium, but no untoward effects have been reported in neonates.

In a comparison of the onset and duration of paralysis produced by 0.2 mg/kg pancuronium ($n = 8$) or pipecuronium ($n = 8$) injected into the thighs of fetuses at 30–38 weeks gestational age, tachycardia occurred in four out of eight fetuses given pancuronium, and there was loss of beat-to-beat variability in two. No such changes were observed in any of the eight fetuses given pipecuronium (27).

Susceptibility Factors

Renal disease

Pancuronium appears to depend more on renal function for its elimination than D-tubocurarine does. Its action is, in most cases, significantly prolonged in renal insufficiency (28); in particular, spontaneous recovery is slow and adequate reversal of the block with neostigmine takes much longer than is generally expected (29). The response to pancuronium is much more unpredictable in renal insufficiency, with great interindividual variation in duration of blockade. Occasionally resistance to neuromuscular blockade with pancuronium is encountered (SEDA-13, 103) (28,30). This may be because of an increase in the volume of distribution. High plasma and tissue concentrations of 3-monohydroxypancuronium, sufficient to produce significant neuromuscular blockade, have also been measured in anuria (31). Monitoring of neuromuscular function is required in patients with appreciable renal dysfunction.

Hepatic disease

In hepatic disease, pancuronium seems to be more problematic than D-tubocurarine. Patients with cirrhosis have a prolonged half-life, a reduced clearance, and a markedly increased apparent volume of distribution (32). This is likely to result in the need for larger initial doses for adequate relaxation and prolongation of recovery of neuromuscular function.

Cholestasis can prolong the action of pancuronium, reducing its plasma clearance by 50%. This may be a result of raised bile salts, reducing the hepatic uptake of pancuronium (which is an important factor contributing to the total plasma clearance in normal patients) (SEDA-6, 130).

In patients undergoing liver transplantation, the dosage requirements for pancuronium and vecuronium by intravenous infusion were reduced by 57 and 50% respectively during the anhepatic phase (SEDA-17, 153), whereas atracurium requirements were not altered by exclusion of the liver from the circulation.

Other features of the patient

As with all muscle relaxants, abnormal reactions can occur in patients with neuromuscular diseases. In addition, muscle fibrillation has been reported, possibly due to pancuronium, in a patient with metachromatic leukodystrophy (33).

Pancuronium is relatively contraindicated, particularly in combination with halothane, in patients who may have raised catecholamine concentrations, or who are receiving drugs with sympathomimetic effects. Severe hypertension together with tachycardia can occur when pancuronium is given to a patient with a pheochromocytoma (34,35). Caution should also be exercised in patients with thyrotoxicosis and with valvular stenosis, coronary artery insufficiency (36), or other conditions in which a tachycardia is hazardous.

Drug–Drug Interactions

Aminophylline

Aminophylline facilitates neuromuscular transmission, perhaps by increasing neurotransmitter release, through raising cyclic AMP concentrations at the neuromuscular junction via phosphodiesterase inhibition (37). This would account for the antagonism of pancuronium-induced blockade that has been reported in the presence of very high serum concentrations of theophylline (38).

Anticonvulsants

The long-term use of phenytoin has been associated with increased pancuronium requirements during neurosurgical operations (39), although the opposite effect might be expected from the quinine-like membrane-stabilizing activity of phenytoin.

Azathioprine

Azathioprine reduces sensitivity to pancuronium in experimental animals, possibly as a result of phosphodiesterase inhibition, increasing transmitter release (SEDA-4, 87) (40), (SEDA-13, 104).

Carbamazepine

Resistance to pancuronium, with a considerable shortening of recovery time, has been seen in patients taking long-term carbamazepine (SEDA-12, 118) (41); there was an inverse correlation between the daily dose and the recovery time.

Ciclosporin

Ciclosporin can cause considerable prolongation of the neuromuscular paralysis induced by pancuronium (42) in one patient (and also in another given vecuronium). Reversal required both neostigmine and edrophonium. Subsequently, recurarization occurred (SEDA-14, 116). Contributing factors could have been the solvent Cremophor EL in the ciclosporin formulation (Sandimmun) and minor renal dysfunction.

Corticosteroids

Corticosteroids have been reported to antagonize neuromuscular blockade due to pancuronium (43,44). In vitro studies in rats have shown a direct facilitating action of prednisolone on neuromuscular transmission (45), so that one would expect some antagonism of non-depolarizing relaxants in general.

Furosemide

Furosemide (1 mg/kg) shortened the recovery time from pancuronium blockade in neurosurgical patients with normal renal function (46). Phosphodiesterase inhibition and increased pancuronium excretion were suggested as possible explanations.

General anesthetics

Halothane anesthesia increases the risks of tachydysrhythmias when pancuronium is used (47).

Pancuronium lowers the MAC for halothane by 25% (48), although this has been disputed (SEDA-15, 124) (49).

Glyceryl trinitrate

Experiments in cats have demonstrated a significant prolongation and potentiation of the neuromuscular blockade induced by pancuronium during glyceryl trinitrate infusion (1 mg/kg/minute) started before the muscle relaxant was given. No prolongation was seen if suxamethonium, D-tubocurarine, or gallamine were used instead of pancuronium. Neostigmine reversal of the pancuronium block was not affected and neither was the plasma clearance of pancuronium changed over the 2 hours after the injection (50,51). The cause of this phenomenon, and whether it is applicable to humans, remains to be elucidated. However, more recent experiments (also in cats), using only moderate doses of pancuronium (and vecuronium), have failed to elicit any potentiation by glyceryl trinitrate (52).

Lithium carbonate

Prolonged neuromuscular blockade has been reported in patients taking long-term lithium given pancuronium (53). In animal experiments, lithium prolonged neuromuscular block due to pancuronium, suxamethonium, and decamethonium, but not that due to D-tubocurarine and gallamine (54); on the other hand, lithium was reported to have no or minimal effects on the blockade produced by pancuronium or D-tubocurarine (55). The mechanism of this interaction is not known, although possible mechanisms have been discussed (54). Caution, and monitoring are advisable.

Tricyclic antidepressants

The use of both halothane and pancuronium in patients taking tricyclic antidepressant has been reported as resulting in severe tachydysrhythmias. Experiments in dogs have shown that this combination can produce ventricular fibrillation and cardiac arrest (56). Enflurane also resulted in tachycardias in dogs given both imipramine and pancuronium acutely, but not when the imipramine was given chronically for 15 days beforehand. Pancuronium should not be used in patients taking tricyclic antidepressants.

Interference with Diagnostic Tests

Radiography

Complete relaxation in artificially ventilated neonates has resulted in apparent "gasless abdomens" on radiography and confusion in diagnosis. On discontinuation of paralysis, the normal appearance of gas-filled bowel was restored (57).

References

1. Roizen MF, Feeley TW. Pancuronium bromide. Ann Intern Med 1978;88(1):64–8.
2. Stovner J, Oftedal N, Holmboe J. The inhibition of cholinesterases by pancuronium. Br J Anaesth 1975;47(9):949–54.
3. Yamashita M, Shiga T, Matsuki A, Oyama T. Unusual resistance to pancuronium in severely burned patients: case reports. Can Anaesth Soc J 1982;29(6):630–1.
4. Speight TM, Avery GS. Pancuronium bromide: a review of its pharmacological properties and clinical application. Drugs 1972;4(3):163–226.
5. Coleman AJ, Downing JW, Leary WP, Moyes DG, Styles M. The immediate cardiovascular effects of pancuronium, alcuronium and tubocurarine in man. Anaesthesia 1972;27(4):415–22.
6. Saxena PR, Bonta IL. Mechanism of selective cardiac vagolytic action of pancuronium bromide. Specific blockade of cardiac muscarinic receptors. Eur J Pharmacol 1970;11(3):332–41.
7. Domenech JS, Garcia RC, Sastain JM, Loyola AQ, Oroz JS. Pancuronium bromide: an indirect sympathomimetic agent. Br J Anaesth 1976;48(12):1143–8.
8. Cardan E, Nana A, Domokos M. Blood catecholamine changes after pancuronium bromide administration. Xth Congress of the Scandinavian Society of Anesthesiologists. Lund 1971;57:.
9. Quintana A. Effect of pancuronium bromide on the adrenergic reactivity of the isolated rat vas deferens. Eur J Pharmacol 1977;46(3):275–7.
10. Docherty JR, McGrath JC. Potentiation of cardiac sympathetic nerve responses in vivo by pancuronium bromide. Br J Pharmacol 1977;61(3):P472–3.
11. Docherty JR, McGrath JC. Sympathomimetic effects of pancuronium bromide on the cardiovascular system of the pithed rat: a comparison with the effects of drugs blocking the neuronal uptake of noradrenaline. Br J Pharmacol 1978;64(4):589–99.
12. Seed RF, Chamberlain JH. Myocardial stimulation by pancuronium bromide. Br J Anaesth 1977;49(5):401–7.
13. Bowman WC. Pharmacology of Neuromuscular Function. 2nd ed.. London/Boston/Singapore/Sydney/Toronto/Wellington: Wright;. 1990.
14. Bowman WC. Non-relaxant properties of neuromuscular blocking drugs. Br J Anaesth 1982;54(2):147–60.
15. Marshall IG. Pharmacological effects of neuromuscular blocking agents: interaction with cholinoceptors other than nicotinic receptors of the neuromuscular junction. Anest Rianim 1986;27:19.
16. Belani KG, Anderson WW, Buckley JJ. Adverse drug interaction involving pancuronium and aminophylline. Anesth Analg 1982;61(5):473–4.
17. Heinonen J, Takkunen O. Bradycardia during antagonism of pancuronium-induced neuromuscular block. Br J Anaesth 1977;49(11):1109–15.

18. Heath ML. Bronchospasm in an asthmatic patient following pancuronium. Anaesthesia 1973;28(4):437–40.

19. Buckland RW, Avery AF. Histamine release following pancuronium. A case report. Br J Anaesth 1973;45(5):518–21.

20. Mishima S, Yamamura T. Anaphylactoid reaction to pancuronium. Anesth Analg 1984;63(9):865–6.

21. Bonnet MC, Julia JM, Chardon P, Kienlen J, du Cailar J. Àpropos d'un cas d'anaphylaxie au pancuronium. [Apropos a case of anaphylaxis caused by pancuronium.] Cah Anesthesiol 1986;34(3):253–5.

22. Peduto VA, Gungui P, Di Martino MR, Napoleone M. Accidental subarachnoid injection of pancuronium. Anesth Analg 1989;69(4):516–7.

23. Cheung PY, Tyebkhan JM, Peliowski A, Ainsworth W, Robertson CM. Prolonged use of pancuronium bromide and sensorineural hearing loss in childhood survivors of congenital diaphragmatic hernia. J Pediatr 1999;135(2 Pt 1):233–9.

24. Freeman J, Lesko SM, Mitchell AA, Epstein MF, Shapiro S. Hyperbilirubinemia following exposure to pancuronium bromide in newborns. Dev Pharmacol Ther 1990;14(4):209–15.

25. Waterman PM, Albin MS, Smith RB. Malignant hyperthermia: a case report. Anesth Analg 1980;59(3):220–1.

26. Gronert GA. Malignant hyperthermia. Anesthesiology 1980;53(5):395–423.

27. Fan SZ, Susetio L, Tsai MC. Neuromuscular blockade of the fetus with pancuronium or pipecuronium for intra-uterine procedures. Anaesthesia 1994;49(4):284–6.

28. Somogyi AA, Shanks CA, Triggs EJ. The effect of renal failure on the disposition and neuromuscular blocking action of pancuronium bromide. Eur J Clin Pharmacol 1977;12(1):23–9.

29. Bevan DR, Archer D, Donati F, Ferguson A, Higgs BD. Antagonism of pancuronium in renal failure: no recurarization. Br J Anaesth 1982;54(1):63–8.

30. Gramstad L. Atracurium, vecuronium and pancuronium in end-stage renal failure. Dose-response properties and interactions with azathioprine. Br J Anaesth 1987;59(8):995–1003.

31. Vandenbrom RH, Wierda JM. Pancuronium bromide in the intensive care unit: a case of overdose. Anesthesiology 1988;69(6):996–7.

32. Duvaldestin P, Agoston S, Henzel D, Kersten UW, Desmonts JM. Pancuronium pharmacokinetics in patients with liver cirrhosis. Br J Anaesth 1978;50(11):1131–6.

33. Quader MA, Healy TE. Muscle fibrillation following thiopentone and pancuronium bromide. An association with metachromatic leucodystrophy. Anaesthesia 1977;32(7):644–6.

34. Hirano S, Ueki O, Misaki T, Hisazumi H, Hamatani K, Matsubara F, Miwa U. Severe hypertension and tachycardia associated with pancuronium bromide in a patient with asymptomatic pheochromocytoma. Hinyokika Kiyo 1984;30(5):709–13.

35. Jones RM, Hill AB. Severe hypertension associated with pancuronium in a patient with a phaeochromocytoma. Can Anaesth Soc J 1981;28(4):394–6.

36. Thomson IR, Putnins CL. Adverse effects of pancuronium during high-dose fentanyl anesthesia for coronary artery bypass grafting. Anesthesiology 1985;62(6):708–13.

37. Ono K, Nagano O, Ohta Y, Kosaka F. Neuromuscular effects of respiratory and metabolic acid–base changes in vitro with and without nondepolarizing muscle relaxants. Anesthesiology 1990;73(4):710–6.

38. Doll DC, Rosenberg H. Antagonism of neuromuscular blockage by theophylline. Anesth Analg 1979;58(2):139–40.

39. Chen J, Kim YD, Dubois M, et al. The increased requirement of pancuronium in neurosurgical patients receiving dilantin chronically. Anesthesiology 1983;59:A288.

40. Dretchen KL, Morgenroth VH 3rd, Standaert FG, Walts LF. Azathioprine: effects on neuromuscular transmission. Anesthesiology 1976;45(6):604–9.

41. Roth S, Ebrahim ZY. Resistance to pancuronium in patients receiving carbamazepine. Anesthesiology 1987;66(5):691–3.

42. Crosby E, Robblee JA. Cyclosporine-pancuronium interaction in a patient with a renal allograft. Can J Anaesth 1988;35(3 Pt 1):300–2.

43. Meyers EF. Partial recovery from pancuronium neuromuscular blockade following hydrocortisone administration. Anesthesiology 1977;46(2):148–50.

44. Laflin MJ. Interaction of pancuronium and corticosteroids. Anesthesiology 1977;47(5):471–2.

45. Wilson RW, Ward MD, Johns TR. Corticosteroids: a direct effect at the neuromuscular junction. Neurology 1974;24(11):1091–5.

46. Azar I, Cottrell J, Gupta B, Turndorf H. Furosemide facilitates recovery of evoked twitch response after pancuronium. Anesth Analg 1980;59(1):55–7.

47. Stirt JA, Sullivan SF. Aminophylline. Anesth Analg 1981;60(8):587–602.

48. Forbes AR, Cohen NH, Eger EI 2nd. Pancuronium reduces halothane requirement in man. Anesth Analg 1979;58(6):497–9.

49. Fahey MR, Sessler DI, Cannon JE, Brady K, Stoen R, Miller RD. Atracurium, vecuronium, and pancuronium do not alter the minimum alveolar concentration of halothane in humans. Anesthesiology 1989;71(1):53–6.

50. Glisson SN, El-Etr AA, Lim R. Prolongation of pancuronium-induced neuromuscular blockade by intravenous infusion of nitroglycerin. Anesthesiology 1979;51(1):47–9.

51. Glisson SN, Sanchez MM, El-Etr AA, Lim RA. Nitroglycerin and the neuromuscular blockade produced by gallamine, succinylcholine, D-tubocurarine, and pancuronium. Anesth Analg 1980;59(2):117–22.

52. Schwarz S, Agoston S, Houwertjes MC. Does intravenous infusion of nitroglycerin potentiate pancuronium- and vecuronium-induced neuromuscular blockade? Anesth Analg 1986;65(2):156–60.

53. Borden H, Clarke MT, Katz H. The use of pancuronium bromide in patients receiving lithium carbonate. Can Anaesth Soc J 1974;21(1):79–82.

54. Hill GE, Wong KC, Hodges MR. Lithium carbonate and neuromuscular blocking agents. Anesthesiology 1977;46(2):122–6.

55. Waud BE, Farrell L, Waud DR. Lithium and neuromuscular transmission. Anesth Analg 1982;61(5):399–402.

56. Edwards RP, Miller RD, Roizen MF, Ham J, Way WL, Lake CR, Roderick L. Cardiac responses to imipramine and pancuronium during anesthesia with halothane or enflurane. Anesthesiology 1979;50(5):421–5.

57. Siegle RL. Neonatal gasless abdomen: another cause. Am J Roentgenol 1979;133(3):522–3.

Pipecuronium bromide

General Information

Pipecuronium bromide is a bisquaternary steroid analogue of pancuronium. In vitro pipecuronium reversibly inhibits both human red cell acetylcholinesterase and human plasma cholinesterase to an extent that might have clinical implications (1). Its potency is similar to that of pancuronium and its onset and duration are also approximately the same. Accumulation can occur (2), and maintenance doses should be one-quarter to one-sixth of the initial dose to achieve a similar effect, depending on the anesthetic technique used.

From animal investigations hepatic uptake appears to be a factor in the drug's total plasma clearance, but renal excretion seems to be the main route of elimination. Ligation of renal pedicles in dogs (3) resulted in reduced elimination of pipecuronium, with a four-fold increase in mean residence time and a four-fold increase in hepatobiliary elimination, which did not compensate for the loss of urinary excretion. In humans, about 40% of pipecuronium is excreted unchanged in the urine together with another 15% as 3-hydroxypipecuronium in 24 hours (4). The half-life is around 135–160 minutes.

Organs and Systems

Cardiovascular

No histamine release has been reported with pipecuronium, and vagolytic or sympathomimetic effects are not seen in the usual dose range. Rarely, significant hypotension has been reported (2), but this was transient and occurred during an unstable phase of anesthesia. Bradycardia has also been seen (2) but is usually mild (5), and probably due to the vagotonic effects of co-administered drugs, as is seen with vecuronium and atracurium (that is a minor disadvantage of the relaxant's lack of vagolytic or sympathomimetic effects). Usually, no significant changes in heart rate or blood pressure are seen (6–8), even with doses up to three times the ED_{95} (9,10). Cardiovascular stability has also been reported in cardiac patients (11), including patients in ASA classes II and III about to undergo coronary artery bypass grafting who received doses up to 0.15 mg/kg (12) and those who received high-dose fentanyl anesthesia (13). The absence of tachycardia in these high-risk cardiac patients, in whom any increase in myocardial oxygen demand is unwanted, was considered an advantage of pipecuronium.

Susceptibility Factors

Renal disease

As expected, renal dysfunction is associated with an increase in volume of distribution, a decrease in plasma clearance (1.6 versus 2.4 ml/kg/minute), and an increase in half-life (263 versus 137 minutes) compared with patients with normal renal function (14). In the latter study there was no statistically significant prolongation of the mean duration of action of pipecuronium, but there was a much greater variation in those with renal insufficiency, with 25% recovery times (after 0.07 mg/kg) of 30–267 minutes (controls 55–198 minutes). These patients were also undergoing renal transplantation and most of the replacement kidneys would be expected to have some function and some glomerular excretion of pipecuronium. Prolongation of pipecuronium blockade should be expected in patients with renal insufficiency.

Drug–Drug Interactions

Barbiturates

Thiobutobarbital prolongs the duration of action of pipecuronium in dogs (15), but no interaction with barbiturates has been reported in man.

General anesthetics

In patients who have been exposed to volatile anesthetic agents for 30 minutes or so there is an increase in potency of pipecuronium to such an extent that doses can be reduced by about one-third with isoflurane (16) or enflurane (10) compared with those required for balanced anesthesia. Halothane appears to be associated with relatively minor changes in potency (16). When the same doses of pipecuronium are given, the duration of blockade is significantly longer during isoflurane anesthesia than during neuroleptanesthesia (17); halothane is also associated with a prolonged action but to a lesser extent.

References

1. Simon G, Biro K, Karpati E, Tuba Z. The effect of the steroid muscle relaxant pipecurium bromide on the acetylcholinesterase activity of red blood cells in vitro. Arzneimittelforschung 1980;30(2a):360–3.
2. Wittek L, Gecsenyi M, Barna B, Hargitay Z, Adorjan K. Report on clinical test of pipecurium bromide. Arzneimittelforschung 1980;30(2a):379–83.
3. Khuenl-Brady KS, Sharma M, Chung K, Miller RD, Agoston S, Caldwell JE. Pharmacokinetics and disposition of pipecuronium bromide in dogs with and without ligated renal pedicles. Anesthesiology 1989;71(6):919–22.
4. Wierda JM, Karliczek GF, Vandenbrom RH, Pinto I, Kersten-Kleef UW, Meijer DK, Agoston S. Pharmacokinetics and cardiovascular dynamics of pipecuronium during coronary artery surgery. Can J Anaesth 1990;37(2):183–91.
5. Boros M, Szenohradszky J, Marosi G, Toth I. Comparative clinical study of pipecurium bromide and pancuronium bromide. Arzneimittelforschung 1980;30(2a):389–93.
6. Alant O, Darvas K, Pulay I, Weltner J, Bihari I. First clinical experience with a new neuromuscular blocker pipecurium bromide. Arzneimittelforschung 1980;30(2a):374–9.
7. Bunjatjan AA, Miheev VI. Clinical experience with a new steroid muscle relaxant: pipecurium bromide. Arzneimittelforschung 1980;30(2a):383–5.
8. Newton DE, Richardson FJ, Agoston S. Preliminary studies in man with pipecurium bromide (Arduan), a new steroid neuromuscular blocking agent. Br J Anaesth 1982;54:P789.
9. Larijani GE, Bartkowski RR, Azad SS, Seltzer JL, Weinberger MJ, Beach CA, Goldberg ME. Clinical pharmacology of pipecuronium bromide. Anesth Analg 1989;68(6):734–9.
10. Foldes FF, Nagashima H, Nguyen HD, Duncalf D, Goldiner PL. Neuromuscular and cardiovascular effects of pipecuronium. Can J Anaesth 1990;37(5):549–55.
11. Barankay A. Circulatory effects of pipecurium bromide during anaesthesia of patients with severe valvular and ischaemic heart diseases. Arzneimittelforschung 1980;30(2a):386–9.

12. Tassonyi E, Neidhart P, Pittet JF, Morel DR, Gemperle M. Cardiovascular effects of pipecuronium and pancuronium in patients undergoing coronary artery bypass grafting. Anesthesiology 1988;69(5):793–6.
13. Stanley JC, Carson IW, Gibson FM, McMurray TJ, Elliott P, Lyons SM, Mirakhur RK. Comparison of the haemodynamic effects of pipecuronium and pancuronium during fentanyl anaesthesia. Acta Anaesthesiol Scand 1991;35(3):262–6.
14. Caldwell JE, Canfell PC, Castagnoli KP, Lynam DP, Fahey MR, Fisher DM, Miller RD. The influence of renal failure on the pharmacokinetics and duration of action of pipecuronium bromide in patients anesthetized with halothane and nitrous oxide. Anesthesiology 1989;70(1):7–12.
15. Pulay I, Alant O, Darvas K, Weltner J, Zeteny Z. Respiration paralysing and circulatory effects of a new non-depolarizing relaxant, pipecurium bromide, in anaesthetized dogs. Arzneimittelforschung 1980;30(2a):358–60.
16. Pittet JF, Tassonyi E, Morel DR, Gemperle G, Richter M, Rouge JC. Pipecuronium-induced neuromuscular blockade during nitrous oxide–fentanyl, isoflurane, and halothane anesthesia in adults and children. Anesthesiology 1989;71(2):210–3.
17. Wierda JM, Richardson FJ, Agoston S. Dose-response relation and time course of action of pipecuronium bromide in humans anesthetized with nitrous oxide and isoflurane, halothane, or droperidol and fentanyl. Anesth Analg 1989;68(3):208–13.

Rapacuronium

General Information

Rapacuronium, an aminosteroid non-depolarizing neuromuscular blocking agent with a rapid onset and a comparatively short duration of action (1,2), was withdrawn from the US market in March 2001 and subsequently worldwide. The manufacturers informed the FDA in an open letter about postmarketing reports of severe bronchospasm and some deaths of unknown origin associated with rapacuronium. The severity of the incidents recently reported to the manufacturers was impressive enough to cause fears about patient safety. This event highlights the need for continued surveillance, not only during clinical trials but also during the routine use of approved drugs.

Organs and Systems

Cardiovascular

A major adverse effect of rapacuronium is an increase in heart rate (3). Plasma histamine concentrations may increase after rapacuronium injection, but this was not correlated with changes in blood pressure or heart rate (4).

Respiratory

In a study of the effects of rapacuronium on respiratory function, performed while rapacuronium was still on the market in the USA, the authors observed statistically significant reductions in peak inspiratory flow rate, peak expiratory flow rate, and dynamic compliance, and increases in peak inflating pressure when rapacuronium 1.5 mg/kg was given under steady-state conditions to patients who were already anesthetized, intubated, and ventilated (5). In five of the 10 patients these changes amounted to more than 25% from baseline and were considered clinically relevant. As rapacuronium is no longer available this has no direct clinical impact. However, while discussing the mechanisms of rapacuronium-induced bronchospasm the authors speculated that differential effects of the drug on several subtypes of muscarinic acetylcholine receptors might be responsible. As raised histamine concentrations were not found in seven patients with rapacuronium-induced bronchospasm in another study (4), they reckoned that histamine release was an unlikely explanation. Referring to the observation that pipecuronium, another non-steroidal muscle relaxant, blocked pilocarpine-stimulated prejunctional M_2 receptors in vitro (6), they suggested that a similar effect might result in rapacuronium-induced bronchospasm. Prejunctional M_2 receptors are thought to have a role in negative feedback and inhibition of further acetylcholine release, thereby reducing smooth muscle relaxation. These aspects will need to be taken into account when new substances are considered for clinical use.

Second-Generation Effects

Pregnancy

Some controversy has been raised by the use of rapacuronium for rapid sequence induction in elective cesarean section (7). The authors reported that intubating conditions 60 seconds after rapacuronium 2.5 mg/kg were comparable with those after suxamethonium 1.5 mg. The percentage of the drug that crossed the placenta to the fetus was low (umbilical/maternal vein concentration ratio 0.088) compared with other non-depolarizing agents, and there were no adverse effects on the fetus. Others, however, would not use rapacuronium or other non-depolarizing agents for cesarean section, referring to the longer duration of action, which might be a problem in cases of failed intubation (8). Rapid sequence induction with thiopental plus suxamethonium is still standard for cesarean section. Rapacuronium should be considered for cesarean section only in patients in whom suxamethonium is contraindicated. In such cases, induction with propofol plus alfentanil without a neuromuscular blocking agent may be an alternative, which still awaits evaluation with regard to maternal and fetal safety.

Susceptibility Factors

Renal disease

Rapacuronium plasma clearance was reduced in patients with renal insufficiency, but this did not result in an increased duration of action (9).

Hepatic disease

Although not completely understood, hepatic uptake is assumed to be the reason for the short duration of action of rapacuronium. However, neither recovery time nor drug half-life after a single bolus of rapacuronium was prolonged in patients with liver cirrhosis compared with healthy controls (10).

References

1. Fleming NW, Chung F, Glass PS, Kitts JB, Kirkegaard-Nielsen H, Gronert GA, Chan V, Gan TJ, Cicutti N, Caldwell JE. Comparison of the intubation conditions provided by rapacuronium (ORG 9487) or succinylcholine in humans during anesthesia with fentanyl and propofol. Anesthesiology 1999;91(5):1311–7.
2. Sparr HJ, Mellinghoff H, Blobner M, Noldge-Schomburg G. Comparison of intubating conditions after rapacuronium (Org 9487) and succinylcholine following rapid sequence induction in adult patients. Br J Anaesth 1999;82(4):537–41.
3. Osmer C, Wulf K, Vogele C, Zickmann B, Hempelmann G. Cardiovascular effects of Org 9487 under isoflurane anaesthesia in man. Eur J Anaesthesiol 1998;15(5):585–9.
4. Levy JH, Pitts M, Thanopoulos A, Szlam F, Bastian R, Kim J. The effects of rapacuronium on histamine release and hemodynamics in adult patients undergoing general anesthesia. Anesth Analg 1999;89(2):290–5.
5. Tobias JD, Johnson JO, Sprague K, Johnson G. Effects of rapacuronium on respiratory function during general anesthesia: a comparison with cis-atracurium. Anesthesiology 2001;95(4):908–12.
6. Zappi L, Song P, Nicosia S, Nicosia F, Rehder K. Do pipecuronium and rocuronium affect human bronchial smooth muscle? Anesthesiology 1999;91(6):1616–21.
7. Abouleish EI, Abboud TK, Bikhazi G, Kenaan CA, Mroz L, Zhu J, Lee J, Abboud TS. Rapacuronium for modified rapid sequence induction in elective caesarean section: neuromuscular blocking effects and safety compared with succinylcholine, and placental transfer. Br J Anaesth 1999;83(6):862–7.
8. Young SJ, Kilpatrick A. Alternatives to succinylcholine at caesarean section. Br J Anaesth 2000;84(5):695–6.
9. Szenohradszky J, Caldwell JE, Wright PM, Brown R, Lau M, Luks AM, Fisher DM. Influence of renal failure on the pharmacokinetics and neuromuscular effects of a single dose of rapacuronium bromide. Anesthesiology 1999;90(1):24–35.
10. Duvaldestin P, Slavov V, Rebufat Y. Pharmacokinetics and pharmacodynamics of rapacuronium in patients with cirrhosis. Anesthesiology 1999;91(5):1305–10.

Rocuronium bromide

General Information

Rocuronium is a steroidal agent related chemically to vecuronium. It is less potent than vecuronium and has a quicker onset of action. The plasma clearance of rocuronium is primarily due to liver uptake and biliary excretion (1). About one-third of an injected dose is excreted unchanged in the urine (1). Good intubating conditions may be expected 90–120 seconds after the injection of 0.6 mg/kg rocuronium. Increasing the dose to 1 mg/kg will give acceptable intubating conditions at 60 seconds. There were no increases in plasma histamine concentrations with doses up to 1.2 mg/kg (2).

Organs and Systems

Cardiovascular

Rocuronium has virtually no cardiovascular adverse effects (2–4). Minor increases in heart rate can occur with higher doses owing to its mild vagolytic properties.

There are several reports of pain during injection of rocuronium (5,6). Eight of 10 patients complained of severe pain, one complained of moderate pain, and another reported an unpleasant sensation (5). This suggests that rocuronium will almost invariably cause pain. The mechanism of this phenomenon is not clear, but there appear to be some similarities to propofol injection pain. Several authors have suggested that rocuronium should not be given to awake patients (5,6). On the other hand, small doses of rocuronium have been used, with some success, to prevent fasciculations and myalgia after suxamethonium (7–10). With regard to the severity of injection pain, rocuronium pretreatment in awake patients does not seem advisable.

Immunologic

Several allergic reactions to rocuronium have been reported (11–20). Based on data from the UK, Australia, and France, it had been suggested that the incidence of such reactions after rocuronium administration parallels its frequency of use, as assessed by its market share, implying that rocuronium does not have unusual allergenic properties (15,21,22). In one hospital, the incidence of such reactions was 1 in 3000 (15) and in another 1 in 6000 (11). Also, the incidence of hypotension, tachycardia, or reduced oxygen saturation (which might suggest an anaphylactoid reaction) was relatively low after rocuronium administration compared with other muscle relaxants in a computerized analysis of 47 295 anesthetic records in one hospital (23).

However, the French Group on the Study of Perianesthetic Anaphylactoid Reactions (GERAP) has reported that the proportion of anaphylactoid reactions to rocuronium was similar to suxamethonium in relation to the individual market shares of these agents (22). There were 41 cases among 452 reported cases of anaphylaxis due to neuromuscular blocking agents that were attributed to rocuronium (24). This would make rocuronium look unfavorable, taking into account the fact that suxamethonium is believed to trigger anaphylactoid reactions more often than any non-depolarizing neuromuscular blocker. The authors assumed that their figures might have been partly due to anesthetists' paying more attention to the effects of drugs that had become available more recently, especially in cases of mild reactions. Reporting bias has also been offered as one possible explanation of 29 reports of anaphylaxis to rocuronium among 150 000 patients in Norway, in contrast to 8 cases among 800 000 patients in the other Scandinavian countries (25). This observation has prompted the Norwegian Medicines Agency to recommend that rocuronium be temporarily withdrawn from routine practice and that it be used for rapid-sequence induction only.

It is difficult to understand why such an increase in the number of reported cases should only be observed in France and Norway and not in other countries in which rocuronium is widely used. For the time being, it is not possible to decide whether anaphylactoid reactions are more common with rocuronium than with other non-depolarizing muscle relaxants. To get a clearer picture, a large longitudinal survey would be needed (26), which is unlikely to be performed, owing to the large number of cases that would be required. We shall probably have to rely on national surveys, like the French one cited above. International networking and pooling of data might be the way forward. All of this will depend on clinicians chasing every case of a suspected anaphylactoid reaction by immunological testing and reporting all confirmed cases to appropriate bodies.

The Norwegian Medicines Agency has recommended that rocuronium bromide should be withdrawn from routine practice, referring to 29 reported cases of anaphylaxis or anaphylactoid reactions among 150 000 administrations over 2.5 years. In response, and with regard to the paucity of reported cases of anaphylaxis to rocuronium in other Nordic countries, the statistical problems of surveying such rare adverse drug reactions have been highlighted (25).

One patient died after developing multiorgan failure due to a reaction to rocuronium (27).

- A 64-year-old obese man, scheduled for a hernia repair, had had previous episodes of venous thromboembolism, for which he was still taking an oral anticoagulant. Previous general anesthesia had been uneventful. General anesthesia was induced with sufentanil 15 µg and propofol 400 mg. He was given rocuronium 50 mg to facilitate endotracheal intubation, and shortly after developed bronchospasm, severe hypotension, tachycardia, and generalized erythema. He was resuscitated with adrenaline, hydrocortisone, and colloid infusion. However, his further course after admission to the intensive care unit was complicated by persistent hypotension, acute respiratory distress syndrome, acute renal insufficiency, disseminated intravascular coagulation, and pancreatitis, and he died 7 days after the incident. Blood samples drawn at 30 and 60 minutes after the initial presentation showed increased concentrations of histamine and tryptase. Specific IgE antibodies against quaternary ammonium groups were detected, with a positive radioimmunoassay inhibition by rocuronium.

Death caused by an anaphylactic reaction to a muscle relaxant seems to be rare, although mortality rates from intraoperative anaphylaxis in the range of 3.4–6% have been reported (28–31). The incidence of cardiac arrest was 4.9% among patients with anaphylactic reactions to muscle relaxants referred to the French GERAP centers for further testing, but these patients all survived (22).

Second-Generation Effects

Fetotoxicity

The maternofetal transfer or rocuronium, as indicated by a fetal/maternal plasma concentration ratio of 0.16, is between that of vecuronium and pancuronium (32). When rocuronium was used for cesarean section, no adverse effects on the fetus were observed (32). With regard to the duration of rocuronium-induced paralysis and the relatively high incidence of failed intubations in obstetric patients, however, it was agreed that rocuronium should be considered for rapid-sequence intubation for cesarean section only if suxamethonium is contraindicated (33–35).

Susceptibility Factors

Age

In elderly patients, because of reduced hepatic elimination, the duration of action of rocuronium can be prolonged (36,37).

Renal disease

Despite the predominantly biliary elimination of rocuronium, reduced clearance and a prolonged half-life have been reported in patients with chronic renal insufficiency requiring hemodialysis (38,39); however, the duration of action was not longer than in healthy controls (38).

Hepatic disease

The duration of action of rocuronium was significantly prolonged in patients with liver cirrhosis, which might be explained either by a larger central volume of distribution or by a lower plasma clearance (40,41).

Drug–Drug Interactions

Anticonvulsant drugs

The duration of action of rocuronium can be reduced during long-term therapy with anticonvulsants (42). In one study the mean times to recovery of twitch height to 25% of baseline after rocuronium 0.6 mg/kg were 21 minutes in patients taking either carbamazepine or phenytoin versus 45 minutes in controls (43). It was suggested that the dose of rocuronium should be increased in patients taking antiepileptic drugs.

General anesthetics

The neuromuscular blocking effects of rocuronium are potentiated by halothane, enflurane, and isoflurane (44–46).

References

1. Wierda JM, Kleef UW, Lambalk LM, Kloppenburg WD, Agoston S. The pharmacodynamics and pharmacokinetics of Org 9426, a new non-depolarizing neuromuscular blocking agent, in patients anaesthetized with nitrous oxide, halothane and fentanyl. Can J Anaesth 1991;38(4 Pt 1): 430–5.

2. Levy JH, Davis GK, Duggan J, Szlam F. Determination of the hemodynamics and histamine release of rocuronium (Org 9426) when administered in increased doses under N_2O/O_2– sufentanil anesthesia. Anesth Analg 1994;78(2): 318–21.

3. McCoy EP, Maddineni VR, Elliott P, Mirakhur RK, Carson IW, Cooper RA. Haemodynamic effects of rocuronium during fentanyl anaesthesia: comparison with vecuronium. Can J Anaesth 1993;40(8):703–8.

4. Hudson ME, Rothfield KP, Tullock WC, Firestone LL. Haemodynamic effects of rocuronium bromide in adult cardiac surgical patients. Can J Anaesth 1998;45(2):139–43.

5. Borgeat A, Kwiatkowski D. Spontaneous movements associated with rocuronium: is pain on injection the cause? Br J Anaesth 1997;79(3):382–3.

6. Steegers MA, Robertson EN. Pain on injection of rocuronium bromide. Anesth Analg 1996;83(1):203.

7. Demers-Pelletier J, Drolet P, Girard M, Donati F. Comparison of rocuronium and d-tubocurarine for prevention of succinylcholine-induced fasciculations and myalgia. Can J Anaesth 1997;44(11):1144–7.

8. Findlay GP, Spittal MJ. Rocuronium pretreatment reduces suxamethonium-induced myalgia: comparison with vecuronium. Br J Anaesth 1996;76(4):526–9.

9. Motamed C, Choquette R, Donati F. Rocuronium prevents succinylcholine-induced fasciculations. Can J Anaesth 1997;44(12):1262–8.

10. Tsui BC, Reid S, Gupta S, Kearney R, Mayson T, Finucane B. A rapid precurarization technique using rocuronium. Can J Anaesth 1998;45(5 Pt 1):397–401.

11. Allen SJ, Gallagher A, Paxton LD. Anaphylaxis to rocuronium. Anaesthesia 2000;55(12):1223–4.

12. Barthelet Y, Ryckwaert Y, Plasse C, Bonnet-Boyer MC, d'Athis F. Accidents anaphylactiques graves après administration de rocuronium. [Severe anaphylactic reactions after administration of rocuronium.] Ann Fr Anesth Reanim 1999;18(8):896–900.

13. Donnelly T. Anaphylaxis to rocuronium. Br J Anaesth 2000;84(5):696.

14. Heier T, Guttormsen AB. Anaphylactic reactions during induction of anaesthesia using rocuronium for muscle relaxation: a report including 3 cases. Acta Anaesthesiol Scand 2000;44(7):775–81.

15. Neal SM, Manthri PR, Gadiyar V, Wildsmith JA. Histaminoid reactions associated with rocuronium. Br J Anaesth 2000;84(1):108–11.

16. Matthey P, Wang P, Finegan BA, Donnelly M. Rocuronium anaphylaxis and multiple neuromuscular blocking drug sensitivities. Can J Anaesth 2000;47(9):890–3.

17. Yee R, Fernandez JA. Anaphylactic reaction to rocuronium bromide. Anaesth Intensive Care 1996;24(5):601–4.

18. Kierzek G, Audibert J, Pourriat JL. Anaphylaxis after rocuronium. Eur J Anaesthesiol 2003;20(2):169–70.

19. Thomas R, Wood M. Anaphylaxis to rocuronium. Anaesthesia 2003;58(2):196.

20. Joseph P, Benoit Y, Gressier M, Blanc P, Lehot JJ. Accident anaphylactique après administration de rocuronium: intérêt du bilan primaire pour le diagnostic précoce. [Anaphylaxis after rocuronium: advantage of blood tests for early diagnosis.] Ann Fr Anesth Reanim 2002;21(3):221–3.

21. Rose M, Fisher M. Rocuronium: high risk for anaphylaxis? Br J Anaesth 2001;86(5):678–82.

22. Laxenaire MC, Mertes PM. Groupe d'Etudes des Réactions Anaphylactoides Peranesthésiques. Anaphyl-axis during anaesthesia. Results of a two-year survey in France Br J Anaesth 2001;87(4):549–58.

23. Booij LH, Houweling PJ. Rocuronium: high risk for anaphylaxis? Br J Anaesth 2001;87(5):805–6.

24. Laxenaire MC. Epidemiologie des réactions anaphylactoides peranesthesiques. Quatrieme enquete multicentrique (juillet 1994–decembre 1996). Le Groupe d'Etudes des Réactions Anaphylactoides Peranésthesiques. [Epidemiology of anesthetic anaphylactoid reactions. Fourth multicenter survey (July 1994–December 1996).] Ann Fr Anesth Reanim 1999;18(7):796–809.

25. Laake JH, Rottingen JA. Rocuronium and anaphylaxis — a statistical challenge. Acta Anaesthesiol Scand 2001;45(10): 1196–203.

26. Fisher M, Baldo BA. Anaphylaxis during anaesthesia: current aspects of diagnosis and prevention. Eur J Anaesthesiol 1994;11(4):263–84.

27. Baillard C, Korinek AM, Galanton V, Le Manach Y, Larmignat P, Cupa M, Samama CM. Anaphylaxis to rocuronium. Br J Anaesth 2002;88(4):600–2.

28. Fisher MM, More DG. The epidemiology and clinical features of anaphylactic reactions in anaesthesia. Anaesth Intensive Care 1981;9(3):226–34.

29. Hatton F, Tiret L, Maujol L, N'Doye P, Vourc'h G, Desmonts JM, Otteni JC, Scherpereel P. Enquête épidémiologique sur les anesthesies. [INSERM. Epidemiological survey of anesthesia. Initial results.] Ann Fr Anesth Reanim 1983;2(5):331–86.

30. Currie M, Webb RK, Williamson JA, Russell WJ, Mackay P. The Australian Incident Monitoring Study. Clinical anaphylaxis: an analysis of 2000 incident reports. Anaesth Intensive Care 1993;21(5):621–5.

31. Mitsuhata H, Matsumoto S, Hasegawa J. [The epidemiology and clinical features of anaphylactic and anaphylactoid reactions in the perioperative period in Japan.]Masui 1992;41(10):1664–9.

32. Abouleish E, Abboud T, Lechevalier T, Zhu J, Chalian A, Alford K. Rocuronium (Org 9426) for caesarean section. Br J Anaesth 1994;73(3):336–41.

33. Abouleish E, Abboud T. Rocuronium for caesarean section. Br J Anaesth 1995;74:347–8.

34. McSwiney M, Edwards C, Wilkins A. Rocuronium for caesarean section. Br J Anaesth 1995;74(3):348.

35. Priestley GS, Swales HA, Gaylard DG. Rocuronium for caesarean section. Br J Anaesth 1995;74(3):348.

36. Bevan DR, Fiset P, Balendran P, Law-Min JC, Ratcliffe A, Donati F. Pharmacodynamic behaviour of rocuronium in the elderly. Can J Anaesth 1993;40(2):127–32.

37. Matteo RS, Ornstein E, Schwartz AE, Ostapkovich N, Stone JG. Pharmacokinetics and pharmacodynamics of rocuronium (Org 9426) in elderly surgical patients. Anesth Analg 1993;77(6):1193–7.

38. Cooper RA, Maddineni VR, Mirakhur RK, Wierda JM, Brady M, Fitzpatrick KT. Time course of neuromuscular effects and pharmacokinetics of rocuronium bromide (Org 9426) during isoflurane anaesthesia in patients with and without renal failure. Br J Anaesth 1993;71(2):222–6.

39. Szenohradszky J, Fisher DM, Segredo V, Caldwell JE, Bragg P, Sharma ML, Gruenke LD, Miller RD. Pharmaco-kinetics of rocuronium bromide (ORG 9426) in patients with normal renal function or patients undergoing cadaver renal transplantation Anesthesiology 1992;77(5):899–904.

40. Khalil M, D'Honneur G, Duvaldestin P, Slavov V, De Hys C, Gomeni R. Pharmacokinetics and pharmacodynamics of rocuronium in patients with cirrhosis. Anesthesiology 1994;80(6):1241–7.

41. van Miert MM, Eastwood NB, Boyd AH, Parker CJ, Hunter JM. The pharmacokinetics and pharmacodynamics

of rocuronium in patients with hepatic cirrhosis. Br J Clin Pharmacol 1997;44(2):139–44.

42. Loan PB, Connolly FM, Mirakhur RK, Kumar N, Farling P. Neuromuscular effects of rocuronium in patients receiving beta-adrenoreceptor blocking, calcium entry blocking and anticonvulsant drugs. Br J Anaesth 1997;78(1):90–1.

43. Koenig HM, Hoffman WE. The effect of anticonvulsant therapy on two doses of rocuronium-induced neuromuscular blockade. J Neurosurg Anesthesiol 1999;11(2):86–9.

44. Oris B, Crul JF, Vandermeersch E, Van Aken H, Van Egmond J, Sabbe MB. Muscle paralysis by rocuronium during halothane, enflurane, isoflurane, and total intravenous anesthesia. Anesth Analg 1993;77(3):570–3.

45. Olkkola KT, Tammisto T. Quantifying the interaction of rocuronium (Org 9426) with etomidate, fentanyl, midazolam, propofol, thiopental, and isoflurane using closed-loop feedback control of rocuronium infusion. Anesth Analg 1994;78(4):691–6.

46. Shanks CA, Fragen RJ, Ling D. Continuous intravenous infusion of rocuronium (ORG 9426) in patients receiving balanced, enflurane, or isoflurane anesthesia. Anesthesiology 1993;78(4):649–51.

Suxamethonium

General Information

Suxamethonium consists of two acetylcholine molecules linked together. Initially, it acts like acetylcholine by depolarizing the motor end-plate. However, unlike acetylcholine, which on dissociation from the receptor is immediately destroyed by acetylcholinesterase present in the neuromuscular junction, suxamethonium is hydrolysed by a (pseudo)cholinesterase present in the plasma but not at the neuromuscular junction. Most of an injected dose of suxamethonium is normally destroyed before it reaches the neuromuscular junction. If the activity of plasma cholinesterase in a particular patient is reduced, more of the suxamethonium reaches the neuromuscular junction and its action is proportionately prolonged. The molecules of suxamethonium that reach the acetylcholine receptor sites interact repeatedly with them, producing prolonged depolarization of the motor end-plate, which becomes surrounded by an electrically inactive zone. The end-result is flaccid paralysis. The action of suxamethonium is terminated by diffusion away from the neuromuscular junction. Hydrolysis results in choline and succinylmonocholine, which has a very weak competitive blocking action and is further slowly hydrolysed by plasma cholinesterase to choline and succinic acid.

About 10% of an intravenous dose of suxamethonium is excreted unchanged in the urine with a half-life of 1–2 minutes (1). The half-life is prolonged in patients with pseudocholinesterase deficiency or an abnormal pseudocholinesterase.

The usual adult dose of suxamethonium chloride is 0.5–1.5 mg/kg, which provides clinical relaxation for some 4–9 minutes. However, the normal response is highly variable and relaxation for up to 15 minutes can result from normal doses. Suxamethonium iodide has about two-thirds the potency of the chloride.

General adverse effects

Suxamethonium has several unwanted and potentially dangerous adverse effects. Generalized muscle fasciculations are associated, to a varying degree, with muscle pain, an acute rise in serum potassium, which under certain conditions can result in dysrhythmias and cardiac arrest, raised intraocular and intragastric pressures, and rhabdomyolysis and myoglobinuria with a rare risk of renal insufficiency. Bradycardia and junctional rhythms are relatively common. Normal doses can cause prolonged paralysis (on rare occasions for several hours) in patients with congenital or acquired plasma cholinesterase abnormality or deficiency.

Anaphylactoid reactions have been documented, and signs suggestive of histamine release are not uncommon. These are mostly mild such as flushing of the skin. Occasionally bronchospasm and/or hypotension can lead to circulatory arrest. Suxamethonium is the relaxant most commonly associated with the syndrome of malignant hyperthermia.

Tumor-inducing effects have not been reported.

Tachyphylaxis and resistance

Tachyphylaxis to the neuromuscular blocking effects of suxamethonium is associated with repeated doses. Prolonged exposure of the neuromuscular junction to suxamethonium (resulting from repeated bolus injections or during an infusion of the drug, or as a consequence of delayed hydrolysis subsequent to genetic or acquired plasma cholinesterase deficiency) is accompanied by the development of a phase II block, with non-depolarizing characteristics and a variably prolonged recovery. This depends on both the dose and the duration of exposure to suxamethonium. A cumulative dose of 3–4 mg/kg and an exposure time of 20–30 minutes can be sufficient during halothane anesthesia (2). However, there is wide variation between patients (3), and monitoring of neuromuscular transmission (train-of-four or post-tetanic count) is advisable with cumulative doses greater than 3 mg/kg.

Resistance to suxamethonium has been seen in von Recklinghausen's disease (4) and nemaline myopathy (5).

Organs and Systems

Cardiovascular

Bradycardia and other dysrhythmias are common (80% in some series) and occur after the first and subsequent injections of suxamethonium in infants and children. In adults, these effects are seen more commonly after second or later injections, particularly when the interval between the doses is 2–5 minutes. However, it has been suggested that bradycardia and asystole may now be more frequently seen than previously in adults after a single injection of suxamethonium, as a result of the increased use of fentanyl or the omission of atropine beforehand (6). Nodal rhythm and wandering pacemaker are frequent. The bradycardia is sometimes extreme (asystolic periods of 15–30 seconds duration have been reported). Usually these minor dysrhythmias revert to normal after a few minutes. Halothane can prolong their presence. The incidence of bradycardic asystole is not known, as atropine (the effective therapy) is usually quickly given.

Over the years cardiac arrest in apparently healthy children has occurred unexpectedly, most cases having been attributed to suxamethonium-induced hyperkalemia in patients with previously undetected myopathies (7–17). Several children have died of this complication. A diagnosis of Duchenne dystrophy or another unspecified progressive myopathy was made in 80% of the patients reported to the American Malignant Hyperthermia Registry who were subsequently tested for myopathies (18). Pointing out that hyperkalemia was detected in 72% of the patients from whom blood samples were taken, the authors suggested that calcium, sodium bicarbonate, hyperventilation, and glucose and insulin should be considered for the treatment of anesthesia-related cardiac arrest in children. This is certainly good advice. Standard resuscitative efforts in such cases are often ineffective, as severe hyperkalemia prevents the restoration of a stable cardiac rhythm. It should be stressed that resuscitative efforts should not be stopped until hyperkalemia has been aggressively treated. Excessive doses of adrenaline, calcium, sodium bicarbonate, and glucose/insulin may be required. Peritoneal dialysis (19), hemodialysis (20), and cardiopulmonary bypass (21) have been used successfully to treat suxamethonium-induced hyperkalemic cardiac arrest.

Regarding the risk of this rare but life-threatening complication in children with undetected myopathy or muscular dystrophy, it has been suggested that the routine use of suxamethonium in pediatric anesthesia be abandoned. It should be reserved for emergency intubation or when immediate securing of the airway is necessary.

Tachycardia and a rise in blood pressure are occasionally seen. Other supraventricular and ventricular dysrhythmias are much less common. Ventricular fibrillation associated with suxamethonium is usually the result of hyperkalemia, but has also been reported in hypercalcemia (22) and is often seen in the course of malignant hyperthermia. Atropine, especially when given intravenously just before suxamethonium, is the most effective agent for the prevention of dysrhythmias. Hexafluorenium, D-tubocurarine, pancuronium, and other non-depolarizer blockers have also been reported as being effective in prevention. Severe hypotension can occur in patients with anaphylactoid reactions.

On theoretical grounds, suxamethonium, being akin to acetylcholine, should produce effects not only at the neuromuscular junction, but also at autonomic ganglia, at muscarinic receptors, and at postganglionic parasympathetic receptors. However, these other types of cholinoceptors are not so sensitive to its action. Nevertheless, stimulation of sympathetic ganglia has been invoked as being possibly responsible for the tachycardia and rise in blood pressure that sometimes occur transiently after its use. Likewise, stimulation of parasympathetic ganglia or direct stimulation of cardiac muscarinic receptors may be responsible for bradycardia. Differences in resting sympathetic and vagal tone have been said to account for the more frequent occurrence of tachycardia in "vagotonic" adults and bradycardia in "sympathotonic" children. The transient mild rise in blood pressure is possibly the result of the initial fasciculation, inducing an increase in venous return, which may also reflexly result in a slowing of the heart rate. Stimulation of afferent receptors in the carotid sinus has also been claimed to cause reflex bradycardia. Small doses (20–25 mg) are said to convert nodal to sinus rhythm, and larger doses to depress the sinoatrial node and so to cause bradycardia and nodal rhythm. Fasciculation probably produces an increase in afferent discharge from muscle spindles, which may account for the reported arousal pattern on the electroencephalogram; this in turn is postulated as a cause of tachycardia and a rise in blood pressure.

It has been hypothesized that suxamethonium modulates noradrenaline release from postganglionic sympathetic nerve terminals by presynaptic nicotine (+) and muscarinic (−) receptors on these nerve terminals (23). The refractory period of these presynaptic nicotinic receptors is postulated as being longer than that of the muscarinic receptors, which results in a net muscarinic effect (bradycardia) after a second injection of suxamethonium within 4–5 minutes of the first. To explain the occurrence of bradycardia after an initial injection of suxamethonium in young children, it is postulated that sympathetic nerve terminals mature later, so that muscarinic (bradycardic) effects are unopposed by noradrenaline secretion in younger patients.

Some controversial correspondence has followed the report of four cases of fatal cardiac arrest among 150 patients who were given suxamethonium by paramedics in out-of-hospital emergencies (24). The authors suggested that this might militate against suxamethonium-facilitated endotracheal intubation in this setting. Others, however, have argued that there was no evidence for a causal role of suxamethonium in those cases (25). Patients with critical conditions, such as respiratory failure requiring endotracheal intubation, may have a cardiac arrest without being given suxamethonium. Furthermore, undetected esophageal intubation was considered to be an alternative explanation of cardiac arrest. Indeed, when endotracheal intubation is attempted in these often dramatic and stressful circumstances by health-care providers who have no routine experience in this, there may be a high rate of esophageal intubation. In one study 18 of 108 patients who had been intubated by paramedics were found to have the tube in their esophagus (26). So the role of suxamethonium in the above report is questionable. On the other hand, suxamethonium is part of the protocol for emergency intubation in many centers worldwide and suxamethonium-associated cardiac arrest, apart from anecdotal instances, has not been reported to be a relevant problem (27). Suxamethonium may increase the success rate of emergency intubations while reducing the incidence of traumatic intubations (28). Therefore, rapid-sequence intubation with an induction agent such as etomidate and suxamethonium is probably still the technique of choice for airway management in emergencies. Whoever uses this technique must be aware of contraindications to suxamethonium and must have frequent practice in endotracheal intubation.

Respiratory

Apnea of variable duration results from muscle paralysis. The return of spontaneous respiration is normally rapid, but it may be delayed if phase II block develops. This will only be of consequence if it is not detected and spontaneous respiration is permitted before it is adequate. Exacerbation of muscle weakness in Duchenne muscular dystrophy after injection of suxamethonium can lead to delayed respiratory failure postoperatively (29).

Bronchospasm is a feature of about one-third of anaphylactoid reactions to suxamethonium and laryngeal edema can also occur, producing intubation problems (30) or respiratory distress and cyanosis after extubation (31).

Nervous system

An arousal pattern can occur on the electroencephalogram, possibly as a result of increased afferent traffic from muscle spindles. This has been speculated as the cause of perioperative dreaming in children in whom an intermittent-suxamethonium technique has been used during light anesthesia (SEDA-13, 102) (32). Suxamethonium must be used with caution in neurological disease and is better avoided altogether when there is a risk of a dangerous rise in serum potassium. A transient rise in intracranial pressure has been observed after injection of suxamethonium, probably as a result of increased cerebral blood volume (33,34). This might be regarded as noxious in patients with intracranial lesions. However, when suxamethonium was given to patients with markedly raised intracranial pressure who received artificial ventilation on the intensive care unit, no adverse effects were observed (35).

Patients with severe head injuries require endotracheal intubation and controlled ventilation. Rapid-sequence intubation using an intravenous anesthetic plus suxamethonium is the standard technique for this, as the patient may have a full stomach. However, suxamethonium has been suggested by some to have a negative effect by causing increased intracranial pressure. The literature on this has been reviewed (36). The authors found only two studies that specifically addressed the effects of suxamethonium on intracranial pressure in patients with head injuries (35,37). In both studies suxamethonium was given to patients who were already being ventilated in the intensive care unit. There were no adverse effects of suxamethonium on intracranial pressure or cerebral perfusion pressure. However, when suxamethonium was given to lightly anesthetized patients undergoing resection of intracranial tumors, there were significant increases in intracranial pressure (38,39). These could be prevented by pretreatment with a small dose of a non-depolarizing muscle relaxant (39). The importance of an adequate level of anesthesia for intubating patients at risk of intracranial hypertension should be stressed. A lightly anesthetized patient will have large increases in intracranial pressure during intubation, no matter which muscle relaxant is used, because of a stress response that includes venous vasoconstriction and a massive increase in central venous pressure, resulting in impaired venous outflow from the cranium and thereby increased intracranial blood volume.

Neuromuscular function

Muscle pain
Generalized postoperative muscle pain associated with suxamethonium is a common problem that became apparent immediately after its introduction in the early 1950s (40). The depolarization of the motor end-plate receptors produced by suxamethonium (either directly or via repetitive discharge generation by the motor nerve terminals) (41) results in generalized and desynchronized contraction of skeletal muscle fibers. These fasciculations result in aching muscle pain (in up to 90% of patients), most commonly in the neck, pectoral region, shoulders, and back. The pain is most often experienced the day after operation and is worse in ambulatory patients. It is more common in women than in men. On average, 50% of the patients who receive suxamethonium during induction of anesthesia will complain of postoperative myalgia, which normally lasts 2 to 3 days (42). Children, elderly patients, athletes, and pregnant women (43) complain less often. Africans also seem to be less susceptible (44).

Mechanism
The cause of the pain is unknown, although there are many hypotheses such as damage to muscle (45,46) resulting from asynchronous contractions of adjacent muscle fibers (47), irreversible damage to muscle spindles (48), potassium flux (49), lactic acid (50), serotonin (51), calcium influx-associated damage to muscle spindles (52), and prostaglandins (53,54). However, no correlation was found between pain and biochemical changes that were assumed to represent muscle cell damage (55,56). Subsequently, it was believed that generalized suxamethonium-induced fasciculation and asynchronous contraction of adjacent muscle fibers might result in damage to muscle fibers, causing pain (57). Fasciculation is thought to be mediated via presynaptic acetylcholine receptors (58). But the severity of fasciculation does not seem to correspond to the frequency or intensity of postoperative myalgia (59,60,61,62,63,64,65,66).

Serum potassium concentrations were higher in patients who developed myalgia (67) than in those who did not, but the implication of this is not clear.

Intracellular lactic acid accumulation has also been considered but never substantiated (68).

Some have suggested an inflammatory component (62,69,70,71). However, the authors of a recent study were unable to show any effect of dexamethasone or to establish a relation between myalgia and post-suxamethonium increases in serum interleukin-6 concentrations, and therefore suggested that there was no evidence of an inflammatory origin (72).

Prevention

Various preventive measures have been recommended, but none is effective in all cases. One reliable method is the injection of a small non-paralysing dose of a non-depolarizing neuromuscular blocker 2–3 minutes before the injection of suxamethonium (73–77) in preventing fasciculations, but the patient must be carefully observed, since an unexpected degree of paralysis occasionally ensues (SEDA-6, 130).

Other measures, much disputed, include the prior injection of diazepam (78,79), procaine or lidocaine (77), vitamin C, suxamethonium itself (10 mg), and aspirin (53,54).

The combined use of atracurium 0.05 mg/kg and lidocaine 1.5 mg/kg reduced the incidence of postoperative myalgia to 5% compared with 75% in controls (77). Thiopental, injected immediately beforehand, is also said to have some effect, as is giving the suxamethonium slowly.

Patients who received a high dose (3.5 mg/kg) of propofol for induction of anesthesia had a significantly lower incidence of myalgia (29%) than patients who were given either a standard dose of propofol 2 mg/kg (61%) or thiopental 5mg/kg (63%) (66). Continuous propofol administration had previously been shown to be effective in preventing myalgia (80), while studies using a single dose had produced conflicting results (81,82).

Various preventive interventions have been subjected to meta-analysis (83). Small doses of non-depolarizing neuromuscular blocking agents (precurarization), sodium channel blockers (local anesthetics such as lidocaine), and non-steroidal anti-inflammatory drugs were effective, with numbers-needed-to-treat (NNT$_B$) of 2.5–6. Precurarization, however, was associated with adverse effects such as blurred vision (NNT$_H$ = 3), diplopia (NNT$_H$ = 5), heavy eyelids (NNT$_H$ = 2), weakness (NNT$_H$ = 4), difficulty in breathing (NNT$_H$ = 26), difficulty in swallowing (NNT$_H$ = 7), and a lower voice (NNT$_H$ = 6). The authors concluded that precurarization should only be used cautiously. In response to this publication, a correspondent highlighted the fact that the incidence of these adverse effects was dose-related and that the published doses used for precurarization studies had increased significantly over the last 20 years (84). This correspondent, a well-known expert in the field, suggested that precurarization with a non-depolarizing blocking agent is both safe and effective, provided that the dose does not exceed 10% of the ED95. We agree with this, but should also like to endorse the following statement: "Clinicians should be aware of this risk when using precurarization. To maximize patients' safety, close monitoring for precurarization-related side effects is strongly recommended." (85). It should also be noted that the incidence of myalgia in this meta-analysis was still rather high despite precurarization, at 21–38%. Because of their methods, the authors could not assess the impact of combining different interventions. An incidence of 5% has been reported for the combined use of atracurium (0.05 mg/kg) and lidocaine (1.5 mg/kg) for pre-treatment followed by suxamethonium 1.5 mg/kg (86). Similarly, the combination of a small dose of d-tubocurarine with lidocaine 1.5 mg/kg was more effective than either drug alone (87). All this could be summarized in a protocol for rapid-sequence intubation of the airway:

1. Preoxygenate for at least 2 minutes.
2. Give a small dose (no more than $0.1 \times$ ED95) of a non-depolarizing muscle relaxant.
3. Give lidocaine 1.5 mg/kg 90 seconds after the non-depolarizing muscle relaxant.
4. Give an induction agent no later than 120 seconds after the non-depolarizing muscle relaxant, followed by suxamethonium 1.5 mg/kg.
5. Intubate no earlier than 50 seconds after suxamethonium.

Myotonic reactions

Rarely, on injecting suxamethonium, contracture, instead of the usual relaxation, of skeletal muscles ensues. In denervated muscles the postulated mechanism is direct activation of the contractile mechanism by suxamethonium because of the widespread chemosensitivity of the muscle fiber membranes.

Paradoxical contracture is most often associated with myotonia dystrophica and myotonia congenita. A myotonic reaction has also been reported in a patient with hyperkalemic periodic paralysis (88). Suxamethonium is therefore contraindicated in these conditions, even though normal responses are sometimes seen. Contracture has also been reported as a result of denervation in Pancoast's syndrome and after plexus injuries and, rarely, in patients with amyotrophic lateral sclerosis or multiple sclerosis (89–91).

Failure of relaxation and generalized muscular rigidity after suxamethonium is sometimes also seen in patients who develop the syndrome of malignant hyperthermia. Isolated masseter muscle rigidity can occur after the administration of suxamethonium, being reported particularly in children given both suxamethonium and halothane. Most experts define masseter muscle rigidity as a major increase in masseter muscle tone severe enough to make mouth opening impossible and to prevent laryngoscopy and endotracheal intubation. Referring to the high incidence of positive results with halothane-caffeine contracture testing, some believe that up to 50% of patients with masseter muscle rigidity are susceptible to malignant hyperthermia (92–95). Others are not convinced of such a high degree of correlation (96) and hold that divers other factors are responsible for the majority of cases (97–99). While severe masseter muscle rigidity is rare (100), smaller increases in jaw tension of about 60 seconds duration occur almost invariably after suxamethonium administration (101,102). Such increases in masseter muscle tone can be attenuated by using propofol as an induction agent and by precurarization, that is pretreatment with a small dose of a non-depolarizing muscle relaxant (102) This might be important during rapid sequence induction of anesthesia.

A hypothesis has been offered to explain muscle hyperexcitability in response to suxamethonium (103). Voltage clamp experiments on alpha subunits of human muscle sodium channels, heterologously expressed in HEK 293 cells, showed that succinic acid, a metabolite of suxamethonium, shifted steady-state activation in the direction of more negative membrane potentials. The EC_{50} for this effect was 0.39 mmol/l. This might lead to muscle hyperexcitability in vivo. Clearly, it is not currently possible to claim any direct clinical implications of this study, but two facts should be considered. After the administration of a routine dose of suxamethonium, blood concentrations of 0.17 mmol/l have been reported (104) Thus, equimolar concentrations of succinic acid are to be expected, given that cholinesterase activity is not impaired. Moreover, succinic acid is a citric acid cycle intermediate, ubiquitous in body tissues. In conditions of ischemia and hypoxia, tissue and serum concentrations of succinic acid increase up to 0.2 mmol/l (105,106). Thus, the administration of suxamethonium to a hypoxic patient may well lead to succinic acid concentrations that affect muscle sodium channel excitability in vitro.

Rhabdomyolysis
Myoglobinuria (107) and raised serum creatine kinase activity (46) have been reported after suxamethonium and appear to be evidence of muscle damage, probably resulting from fasciculation. Repeated bolus doses of suxamethonium result in higher plasma myoglobin concentrations (108) and creatine kinase activities (46). Myoglobinemia seems to be much more common in children than in adults (SEDA-10, 107) (SEDA-11, 121) (109) and is more marked when halothane is used (110). On occasion, myoglobinuria results in renal insufficiency (111–116).

There is an association between (latent) muscular dystrophy (usually of the Duchenne or Becker type) and the production of rhabdomyolysis by suxamethonium (112,113,117,118). Suxamethonium can cause excessive muscle damage in these patients, as manifested not only by severe myoglobinemia and raised serum creatine kinase activity but also by acute exacerbation of muscle weakness postoperatively (SEDA-11, 121) (7,29,112,119,120). Massive potassium release can result in hyperkalemic cardiac arrest. Such patients may also develop features suggestive of the syndrome of malignant hyperthermia (121,122). Suxamethonium should not be used in patients with Duchenne muscular dystrophy or who have a family history suspect for the condition.

Prolonged paralysis
Prolonged paralysis can result from idiosyncrasy, overdose, or reduced or abnormal plasma cholinesterase activity. There are geographical and racial differences in sensitivity to suxamethonium (SEDA-6, 129) (123,124); some of these differences arise from dietary and other environmental factors and others result from variations in plasma cholinesterase genotypes. Genotypically normal patients may be paralysed by a usual (1 mg/kg) dose of suxamethonium for as short a time as 2 minutes or (rarely) as long as 20 minutes, and the duration in general inversely reflects plasma cholinesterase activity (125).

Prolonged paralysis after suxamethonium has also been reported in von Recklinghausen's disease (126), but resistance to suxamethonium has also been seen (4).

Sensory systems

Shortly after the introduction of suxamethonium it was noted that it can increase intraocular pressure (127), an observation that has subsequently been confirmed in several other studies (128–142). The increase in intraocular pressure occurs promptly after intravenous injection of suxamethonium, peaks at 1–2 minutes, and returns to baseline after 6–10 minutes (130,137). The mean increase is about 4–8 mmHg, with a range of 5–15 mmHg.

Mechanism
Several mechanisms have been suggested to explain the effect of suxamethonium on intraocular pressure. One of the first ideas was to blame fasciculation and contraction of the extraocular muscles of the eye (143). However, a study in humans undergoing enucleation showed that suxamethonium produces an increase in intraocular pressure even after detachment of the extraocular muscles (144). So activity of the extraocular muscles may increase intraocular pressure, but there must be other factors. Observing that suxamethonium administration was almost invariably followed by retraction of the eyeball, some investigators suggested increased tone of intraorbital smooth muscles as a mechanism (145), but in fact there is very little intraorbital extraocular smooth muscle in humans. This idea has therefore not been widely accepted. There appears to be some effect of suxamethonium on the intraocular smooth muscles, as indicated by the observation that there is a rapid rise in anterior chamber thickness and a diminution of lens thickness after suxamethonium administration (146). These changes could be explained by a relaxing effect of suxamethonium on the ciliary muscle, which would in turn result in increased aqueous humor outflow resistance and a consequent increase in intraocular pressure (144). However, this mechanism would not be expected to produce pressure increases of the magnitude observed after suxamethonium injection. A vasodilatory effect on conjunctival vessels has been observed (147), and this has been interpreted as indirect evidence of choroidal vasodilatation (148). On the other hand, an increase in ocular blood flow has not been detected after suxamethonium administration but after subsequent endotracheal intubation (149). In conclusion, there is no satisfactory explanation for the suxamethonium-associated increase in intraocular pressure, but increased tone of extraocular muscles, increased aqueous humor outflow resistance, and increased choroidal blood volume are probably important elements.

Prevention
Many efforts have been made to find a technique to prevent the suxamethonium-associated increase in intraocular pressure. Some attenuation of the pressure response has been demonstrated with defasciculation doses of nondepolarizing muscle relaxants (150), but this could not be reproduced in subsequent studies (128–130,151). The same is true for self-taming, that is pretreatment with a small dose of suxamethonium (152,153). Other drugs that have been used with some effect are diazepam

(133,154,155), lidocaine (135,142,149,156,157), glyceryl trinitrate (158), nifedipine (159), and beta-blockers (160), but none of these completely prevented increases in intraocular pressure.

The most effective method of attenuating the intraocular pressure response to suxamethonium plus endotracheal intubation is to provide a deep level of anesthesia by using intravenous anesthetics and opiates (161–165). In 60 patients who received thiopental/suxamethonium, propofol/suxamethonium, or propofol/alfentanil/suxamethonium for anesthesia induction, the increase in intraocular pressure after suxamethonium plus endotracheal intubation was completely blocked by propofol plus alfentanil (165). Combining an intravenous anesthetic with a rapid-onset opioid, such as alfentanil, prevents increases in intraocular pressure (165). When the ultra-short-acting opioid remifentanil (1 microgram/kg) was given in combination with propofol (2 mg/kg) and suxamethonium (1 mg/kg) for endotracheal intubation during induction of anesthesia the highest intraocular pressure recorded was 18 mmHg, whereas peak values up to 35 mmHg occurred in the control group without remifentanil (166).

Implications for surgery

A particular problem is the clinical impact of a rise in intraocular pressure during operation in cases of penetrating eye injury, which is usually performed as an emergency, when it is often not clear whether the patient has eaten recently. While it is commonly accepted that anesthesia in these patients should be induced in a rapid-sequence technique, that is by giving an hypnotic and suxamethonium followed rapidly by endotracheal intubation, in order to reduce the risk of pulmonary aspiration of gastric contents, there is considerable controversy about what to do in the case of penetrating eye injuries. As suxamethonium provokes an increase in intraocular pressure in intact eyes, there is concern that its use could result in loss of intraocular contents and damage to the eye if the eyeball is opened. This, however, has not hitherto been observed, either in clinical studies or in animal experiments (167–169). Several experts regard suxamethonium as being appropriate for rapid-sequence intubation in patients with penetrating eye injuries (170–174).

Similarly, there are difficulties in strabismus surgery, which is commonly performed in children, with the goal of correcting the optical axes of the eyes by shortening certain extraocular muscles. The "forced duction test" can be used to differentiate between a paretic muscle and a restrictive force that prevents ocular movement. Suxamethonium, by increasing the tone of the extraocular muscles, can produce considerable alterations in the results of that test, sometimes lasting as long as 20 minutes (175). Suxamethonium should therefore be avoided in strabismus surgery. Furthermore, in a retrospective study there was an increased incidence of masseter muscle rigidity in patients with strabismus (176). A positive halothane-caffeine contracture test was subsequently found in 25% of the adults and 50% of the children in whom masseter rigidity had occurred (92–95). In line with that, there were more patients with strabismus in a group

of patients who had experienced an episode of malignant hyperthermia than in the general surgical population in the USA (177). Based on these observations, it has been assumed that patients with strabismus might have an increased risk of malignant hyperthermia (174,178), which has been regarded as another reason for avoiding suxamethonium in strabismus surgery (179). On the other hand, the incidence of strabismus was not different in two groups of patients, with or without a positive halothane–caffeine contracture test (180). In conclusion, there are some indirect clues to an increased risk of malignant hyperthermia in patients with strabismus, but for the time being there is not enough evidence to contraindicate suxamethonium. However, there are reasons for reserving its use for special circumstances, such as rapid-sequence induction in patients with an increased risk of pulmonary aspiration. First, the surgical procedure can be impaired by increased tone in the extraocular muscles. Secondly, patients with strabismus may have a higher risk of suxamethonium-associated masseter muscle rigidity. Thirdly, most patients with strabismus are children, in whom the suxamethonium is best avoided (SEDA-19, 139).

Electrolyte balance

An immediate rise in serum potassium occurs after the administration of suxamethonium. The rise is normally small, 0.5 mmol/l or less (4). However, in some cases it can be larger, and cases of cardiac arrest associated with hyperkalemia have been reported in critically ill patients after prolonged immobilization (181–189). Cardiac arrest also occurred in a patient with wound botulism (190).

- A 28-year-old previously healthy man was admitted with a 4-week history of progressive symmetrical muscle weakness that had started in his neck and descended to both arms and legs. He also complained of diplopia, dysphonia, and dysphagia. On the day of admission, he noted difficulty in breathing. He had a history of intermittent diamorphine abuse, and had been injecting "black tar" heroin subcutaneously for the past month. Several hours after admission he had to be intubated, and was given etomidate 20 mg plus suxamethonium 80 mg. Within 60 seconds he developed a wide complex tachycardia, which degenerated into ventricular fibrillation refractory to electrical countershock and standard resuscitative measures. His serum potassium concentration 10–12 minutes after the onset of cardiocirculatory arrest was 6.8 mmol/l, having been 4.7 mmol/l several hours before. Calcium chloride, sodium bicarbonate, and glucose/insulin were given, and 25 minutes after the arrest began the heart rhythm converted to sinus tachycardia. The electrocardiogram subsequently showed no structural abnormalities. A serological test taken on the day of admission was positive for botulinum toxin type A. He eventually survived without any residual deficits and was discharged from hospital after 63 days.

The authors suggested that suxamethonium should be avoided in patients with suspected botulism and in patients with muscle weakness of unknown origin. Wound botulism had been observed before in drug users who have injected black tar heroin (191). Botulinum toxin inhibits presynaptic acetylcholine release, resulting in muscle weakness. In animals chronic administration of botulinum toxin caused an increase in the number of postsynaptic acetylcholine receptors with distribution across the muscle surface (192) and postsynaptic acetylcholine receptors converted into the immature type with prolonged channel opening times (193). With huge numbers of muscle fibers altered in that way, suxamethonium may cause hyperkalemic cardiac arrest by producing massive potassium efflux.

One major concern for anesthetists is suxamethonium-associated hyperkalemia in apparently fit patients without obvious risk factors. Life-threatening hyperkalemia occurred in three Japanese women who underwent cesarean section (194).

- Cardiac arrest occurred in a 34-year-old woman who was given suxamethonium 120 mg. She had been immobilized and treated with high-dose magnesium sulfate and ritodrine for 5 weeks before the event because of preterm uterine contractions. Her preoperative creatine kinase activity was 4050 IU/l. After rapid-sequence induction of anesthesia and injection of suxamethonium she became cyanotic and pulseless and the electrocardiogram showed ventricular fibrillation. The serum potassium concentration after 25 minutes of cardiopulmonary resuscitation, which included the administration of adrenaline, sodium bicarbonate, and calcium chloride, was 5.7 mmol/l. During resuscitation vaginal vacuum delivery was performed. Finally, she was defibrillated successfully and made a full recovery.
- Two other patients had been immobilized and treated with magnesium and ritodrine for several weeks. Preoperative creatine kinase activities were 2120 IU/l and 630 IU/l. In both cases, serum potassium increased by 2.3 mmol/l within 2–3 minutes after suxamethonium injection (from 4.0 to 6.3 mmol/l and from 4.9 to 7.2 mmol/l). This was accompanied by tall peaked T waves and a short period of ventricular tachycardia in one case and by tall peaked T waves and widened QRS complexes in the other.

The authors suggested that the combined effects of immobilization and prolonged magnesium administration might have resulted in a denervation-like state of large groups of skeletal muscles. The drawback of that explanation is that an awake and healthy person will always move normally even when confined to bed. As long as muscle cells receive physiological stimulation via the neuromuscular junction in patients without muscle weakness, denervation-like changes should not occur to a significant extent. In addition, denervation alone is not known to be associated with an increase in plasma creatine kinase activity, a strong indicator of muscle cell damage, which was found in all the patients reported here. Unfortunately, the authors did not document creatine kinase activities or myoglobin concentrations after suxamethonium, which might have given some idea about additional suxamethonium-induced rhabdomyolysis.

It can be assumed that these three patients had some form of myopathy, either acquired during their previous course or pre-existing. It would have been interesting to know if they had any clinical symptoms, such as muscle pain or weakness. Pre-existing myopathy would be unlikely if plasma creatine kinase activities had been normal before. However, this information was not given in the paper. On the other hand, myopathy could have been acquired during the course of pregnancy and hospital treatment. Various drugs and toxins have been associated with myopathies (195). Hypermagnesemia can produce muscle weakness but magnesium sulfate has not so far been reported to cause myopathy. Therefore, the role of ritodrine in these cases should be questioned. This selective beta$_2$-adrenoceptor agonist has previously been linked to myopathic changes in a patient treated for preterm labor (196). In addition, glucocorticoid treatment, probably used to promote fetal lung development, might be a contributory factor. Long-term glucocorticoid treatment is associated with myopathic changes (195).

In the end, the exact mechanism of suxamethonium-associated hyperkalemia in these cases cannot be determined. Given the huge numbers of patients who receive suxamethonium during rapid-sequence induction of anesthesia for cesarean section, even after some time of treatment for preterm labor without adverse effects, it would be overzealous to call for a restricted use of suxamethonium in these patients. Rather, this report is in support of preoperative screening of plasma creatine kinase activity. Probably suxamethonium should not be used in patients with raised plasma creatine kinase activity. It is a good idea to check creatine kinase activity preoperatively in women due to undergo cesarean section after prolonged immobilization and pretreatment with magnesium sulfate and a beta$_2$-adrenoceptor agonist such as ritodrine.

Mechanism

The underlying mechanisms of and mortality from suxamethonium-associated hyperkalemic cardiac arrest have been reviewed (197). The rise in serum potassium probably results from repetitive opening of receptor-linked ion channels and suxamethonium-induced fasciculation, although it can occur in the absence of visible fasciculation. Muscle injury with excessive leakage of potassium is postulated as a cause of the hyperkalemia. Reuptake of potassium into muscle cells may also be hindered. It has been shown that denervation results in a spread of the normally small receptor area of the motor end-plate over the entire muscle fiber membrane, so that eventually the whole membrane surface is directly excitable by depolarizing agents such as acetylcholine or suxamethonium (198). The immature extrajunctional receptor-linked ion channels so formed remain open for a longer time than those at normal motor end-plates. Depolarization by suxamethonium thereby results in an excessive efflux of potassium from ion channels spread over the entire muscle fiber membrane and not just, as normally occurs, from the circumscribed motor end-plate region (199–201). Prolonged immobilization can also result in extrajunctional receptor spread (202) and a greater increase in serum potassium than usual after suxamethonium.

Rhabdomyolysis is also a mechanism for hyperkalemia, and it has been said that almost all reported cases of hyperkalemic cardiac arrest considered to have resulted from rhabdomyolysis occurred in children and adolescents with underlying muscular dystrophies (197). Hyperkalemia during rapid acute rhabdomyolysis is more likely to result in unsuccessful resuscitation than hyperkalemia due to the potassium efflux that results from upregulation of acetylcholine receptors.

Susceptibility factors
The rise in serum potassium can be prolonged (SEDA-11, 122) (203) and exaggerated (SEDA-10, 108) (204) in patients taking beta-blockers. In renal insufficiency the rise after suxamethonium is similar to that in healthy patients (205) and is only dangerous if the serum potassium is already high (above 5.5 mmol/l). However, several conditions can lead to a massive rise in serum potassium, resulting in ventricular fibrillation and cardiac arrest. These include burns (206,207), massive trauma (208,209), and neurological diseases or injuries, especially when denervation is a feature, such as spinal cord injury (210), hemiplegia, multiple sclerosis, or muscular dystrophy (211), peripheral nerve injuries (90,212) and polyneuropathy (213,214). Hyperkalemia has also been reported after suxamethonium in patients with tetanus (215), encephalitis (216), Parkinson's disease (SEDA-6, 129) (217), muscle wasting secondary to chronic arterial insufficiency (218), metastatic embryonal rhabdomyosarcoma (SEDA-14, 114) (219), ruptured cerebral aneurysms (SEDA-5, 134) (220), hyperparathyroidism (22), and in patients with severe and long-lasting sepsis (221,222).

There are times when patients are most susceptible to hyperkalemia. In patients with burns or trauma this is generally between 10 and 60 days after the injury, or longer if there is persistent infection and delayed healing. In neurological diseases or injuries the danger period is usually from 3 weeks to 6 months after onset. However, in some cases, such as patients with transverse spinal lesions and tetraplegia, dangerous hyperkalemia has been reported as early as 24–48 hours after the injury, and likewise severe potassium rises have been reported more than 6 months after injury or onset of disease, particularly in patients with progressive lesions (SEDA-6, 128) (211).

Extrajunctional spread of acetylcholine receptors and expression of the immature type of these receptors with prolonged channel opening times have been shown after burns, which may be why there can be massive potassium release after suxamethonium administration. As the increase in acetylcholine receptor density on the muscle surface takes some time to develop, there should be an interval after the accident during which suxamethonium can be safely given. However, the length of this interval is controversial. Referring to a lack of reports of hyperkalemic complications during the first week after the injury, it has been suggested that suxamethonium can be given safely during the first 6–7 days after major thermal injury (223). However, based on the results of animal experiments, suxamethonium might be safe for up to 48 hours after the injury only (223).

The use of suxamethonium in intensive care units has been critically reviewed (224). Several cases of hyperkalemic cardiac arrest after suxamethonium have occurred in intensive care patients (181,183–185,187,188). Of particular concern is the risk of hyperkalemic cardiac arrest when suxamethonium is given to critically ill patients after a period of immobilization (182). The exact mechanism is not known, but extrajunctional spread of acetylcholine receptors is believed to play a major role. It is strongly recommended that suxamethonium should not be given to patients who have been immobilized in the intensive care unit for more than a few days.

In yet another report of suxamethonium-induced fatal hyperkalemic cardiac arrest in an intensive care unit it was assumed that severe mucositis after cancer chemotherapy might have contributed to the hyperkalemic response (225).

- A 37-year-old woman with acute myelogenous leukemia was admitted to an intensive care unit (ICU) with mental status changes and progressive dyspnea due to pneumonia. Intubation was performed before ICU admission using a sedative without neuromuscular blockade. She had received chemotherapy with cytarabine, daunorubicin, and intrathecal methotrexate for brain metastases. After chemotherapy and before ICU admission her course was complicated by continuous neutropenic fevers and by painful mucositis causing dysphagia and bleeding. After 10 days of ventilator treatment in the ICU and treatment with ceftazidime, gentamicin, metronidazole, vancomycin, amphotericin, and aciclovir, her condition improved, allowing withdrawal of ventilator support and extubation. A few hours later, however, she gradually developed severe respiratory distress and required re-intubation. The serum potassium concentration before intubation was 4.3 mmol/l. For endotracheal intubation she received intravenous etomidate 14 mg and suxamethonium 100 mg. Immediately after intubation she developed a broad-complex tachycardia and her blood pressure could not be measured. Chest compression and advanced cardiac life support were started. Her serum potassium concentration was 13.1 mmol/l. Intravenous calcium chloride, sodium bicarbonate, and insulin/glucose were therefore given. The serum potassium fell to 6.5 mmol/l but rose to 7.4 mmol/l 15 minutes later, despite additional antihyperkalemic treatment. She finally died.

Despite this having been a case of suxamethonium-induced hyperkalemic cardiac arrest after several days of ventilator treatment on the intensive care unit, the authors did not believe that upregulation and extrajunctional spread of acetylcholine receptors were the underlying mechanisms. They implied that mobilization and daily physiotherapy would have both prevented these typical denervation-like changes and ruled out a neuromuscular disorder. Rather they suggested that severe generalized mucositis had resulted in a state that they compared to an "internal burns injury." However, these speculations were not substantiated by additional data. In particular, they gave no information on the presuxamethonium neuromuscular state of the patient. Some form of polyneuropathy and/or myopathy could have been present, and this was not ruled out by the fact that the patient could breathe spontaneously and sit in a chair. While it is true that severe mucositis represents a state of widespread cellular damage similar to severe burn injuries, it is not clear why this itself should result in hyperkalemia after suxamethonium. To our knowledge suxamethonium only has effects on excitable cells. Even in patients with severe thermal injuries, no case of hyperkalemia after suxamethonium has been reported within the first 48 hours after the accident, and suxamethonium-induced hyperkalemia in burned patients is believed to result from upregulation of acetylcholine receptors, owing to thermal damage of nerve fibers (structural denervation) and immobilization (functional denervation) (198). Apart from immobilization due to the severity of the illness it is very unlikely that mucositis should have similar effects. Mucositis itself should therefore not be regarded as a risk factor for suxamethonium-associated hyperkalemia.

In a survey of intensive care units in the UK, more than two-thirds of the respondents would have chosen suxamethonium in a clinical scenario requiring re-intubation in a patient with abdominal sepsis and weaning failure after 20 days of ICU stay (226). The authors concluded that there is a lack of appreciation of the dangers of suxamethonium in critically ill patients in intensive care units.

The use of suxamethonium in patients with renal insufficiency was controversial in the 1970s, after some cases of hyperkalemic cardiac arrest in such patients. As several studies did not show exaggerated potassium release, suxamethonium is now considered safe for patients with renal insufficiency, if preoperative hyperkalemia is excluded. The observation of some cases of postoperative hyperkalemia recently prompted a review of the literature (227). The authors found sufficient evidence to support the current consensus: suxamethonium can be used in patients with renal insufficiency, but it should not be given if there is pre-existing hyperkalemia; doses of suxamethonium should not be given repeatedly, as this can result in sinus bradycardia.

Suxamethonium is said to be contraindicated in patients with hyperkalemia (that is a serum potassium concentration over 5.5 mmol/l). This, however, has been questioned (228). In an analysis of their anesthetic database, the authors identified 38 patients with a preoperative serum potassium concentration over 5.5 mmol/l who subsequently received suxamethonium. In no case were dysrhythmias or any complications documented and there were no deaths. While they admitted that minor complications might not have found their way into the database, the authors felt that major problems caused by suxamethonium in these patients were unlikely. They suggested that the use of suxamethonium in patients with serum potassium concentrations above 5.5 mmol/l may be acceptable when other muscle relaxants have inappropriate profiles. As their analysis included only a few patients with serum potassium concentrations above 6.0 mmol/l they recommended the use of antihyperkalemic treatment before suxamethonium in these patients.

Prevention

It has been claimed that non-depolarizing drugs given before suxamethonium attenuate the rise in potassium, but this has been repeatedly shown to be unreliable. It seems advisable to avoid the use of suxamethonium completely in such patients. This subject has been extensively reviewed (229,230).

Gastrointestinal

Suxamethonium can increase intragastric pressure. This is probably a result of fasciculation of the abdominal muscles (231), although a vagal effect can also contribute. The rise is highly variable, ranging from zero to more than 85 cm H_2O according to many different investigations (232–235). The intragastric pressure at which the lower esophageal sphincter opens is also variable, with a mean of about 28 cm H_2O, depending partly on the angle between the esophagus and the cardia of the stomach (236,237). There is therefore a danger that the suxamethonium-induced rise in intragastric pressure may produce incompetence of the lower esophageal sphincter and result in regurgitation. This risk is likely to be increased in patients with hiatus hernia, gastric and intestinal dilatation, ascites, and intra-abdominal tumors. Pregnant patients are especially susceptible, as the tonus of the lower esophageal sphincter can also be reduced in pregnancy. It has been suggested, however, that suxamethonium causes, either by a direct action on the lower esophageal sphincter or indirectly through a pinch action of the diaphragm, increased resistance to opening of the lower esophagus, which counteracts the increased intragastric pressure (238). Attenuating fasciculation by giving small doses of non-depolarizing blockers reduces the rise in gastric pressure (231,234,239).

Urinary tract

In severe renal disease, suxamethonium should only be given if the serum potassium is below 5.5 mmol/l. The excretion of neostigmine and pyridostigmine can be impaired in renal insufficiency, and this has been reported to have resulted in prolongation of the action of suxamethonium given some hours later (240).

Myoglobinuria resulting from suxamethonium administration can cause acute renal insufficiency (111,112,241).

Musculoskeletal

The problem of suxamethonium-associated postoperative myalgia has been reviewed (242). Key statements are:

- there is no correlation between the severity of muscle fasciculation, changes in serum creatine phosphokinase or serum potassium, and postoperative myalgia;
- although not proven, mechanical muscle damage is still assumed to be an underlying mechanism;
- several classes of pretreatment drugs reduce the incidence and severity of myalgia; combining two agents may be the most useful method;
- so far, the lowest incidence of post-suxamethonium myalgia has been reported when a small dose of a

non-depolarizing neuromuscular blocking agent was given together with lidocaine as pretreatment.

In addition, there was a reduced incidence and intensity of post-suxamethonium myalgia when anesthesia had been maintained by propofol infusion compared with isoflurane (243).

Immunologic

From the results of intradermal injections, suxamethonium has only 1% of the histamine-releasing activity of D-tubocurarine (244). However, through the years there have been many reports of reactions, varying from flushing and urticaria to bronchospasm (245,246) and severe shock (247–250). That suxamethonium was responsible was suggested in some cases by the fact that the patients reacted on different occasions with raised plasma histamine and catecholamine concentrations (251–253). The association was confirmed in other cases by repeatedly injecting the drug, thereby producing bronchospasm several times in the course of the one anesthetic (254,255). Skin testing has also yielded confirmation, although this can be dangerous (248). Analysis of large series of patients (256–261) who have had severe anaphylactoid reactions during anesthesia, using more sophisticated laboratory and immunological investigations in addition to intradermal skin tests, suggests that suxamethonium may be much more commonly associated with such reactions than was previously believed. In 18 cases (262) cardiovascular collapse was the predominant feature in 72% and bronchospasm in 33%; cardiac arrest occurred in five patients. In addition, two reports (263,264) of anaphylactic reactions involving both thiopental and suxamethonium have raised the question of "aggregate"-induced reactions (263) occurring when drugs are given in such a way that they can interact in the injection system.

Body temperature

The syndrome of malignant hyperthermia can be triggered by suxamethonium. Mortality is more than 60% in untreated patients. This syndrome is reported as occurring once in every 15 000–150 000 anesthetics. It may be more common in the Japanese. However, there are also abortive forms of malignant hyperthermia, and many of the typical signs may be produced by other conditions, so that it is difficult to ascertain the precise incidence. Autosomal dominant inheritance, with reduced penetrance and variable expressivity, is the proposed genetic basis. The cause is unknown, but it is thought to be associated with a rise in free ionized myoplasmic calcium, possibly owing to a failure of the sarcoplasmic reticulum to bind calcium. As a result, aerobic and anaerobic metabolism are increased, resulting in the typical features of the syndrome. Halothane and suxamethonium are the most frequent triggers, although almost all of the inhalational anesthetic agents have been incriminated. While other muscle relaxants (pancuronium, D-tubocurarine) have been suggested as triggers in a few cases, and many other drugs used in anesthetized patients also, convincing

evidence is lacking. It has been suggested that stress plays a role in the development of malignant hyperthermia (265).

Dantrolene (266,267) is the agent of choice for treatment of malignant hyperthermia and greatly reduces the mortality to under 10% if given in time (268) together with general supportive measures. Dantrolene itself has adverse effects that are mostly minor in nature, such as nausea and vomiting, when it is used acutely. However, a report has suggested that it may have contributed to uterine atony, with resulting excessive hemorrhage when given prophylactically after a cesarean section (269), and muscle weakness associated with its oral prophylactic use in a patient with compromised respiratory function is reported to have exacerbated postoperative respiratory depression to such an extent that artificial ventilation was required (SEDA-14, 114) (270). The combination with calcium channel blockers, such as verapamil, may result in severe cardiovascular depression and hyperkalemia (SEDA-12, 113) (271,272), so that extreme care is required.

Second-Generation Effects

Pregnancy

Maternal doses of suxamethonium up to 200 mg have been reported as not resulting in detectable concentrations in neonates. Very large bolus doses (300–500 mg) have produced umbilical vein concentrations up to 2 micrograms/ml, but the neonates showed no adverse effects (273,274). Extreme reduction in plasma cholinesterase activity, either caused by organophosphorus poisoning (275) or genetically determined (SEDA-15, 123) (276,277), has resulted in weakness and respiratory depression in neonates after normal or small (275) maternal doses.

Susceptibility Factors

Genetic factors

Plasma cholinesterase deficiency can be hereditary or acquired. The hereditary form is believed to account for two-thirds of suxamethonium-sensitive patients. Genetically determined plasma cholinesterase variants hydrolyse suxamethonium much more slowly. About 96% of the population are homozygotes for the normal "typical" gene, one in 25 are heterozygotes ("typical"/ "atypical") and have a slightly prolonged (about 2–4 times normal) response to suxamethonium, and one in 2000–3000 are homozygotes for the "atypical" gene and have a markedly prolonged response (2–3 hours). The "silent" gene is much rarer and homozygotes (about 0.0006% of the population) have virtually no plasma cholinesterase activity; in them complete paralysis after suxamethonium lasts many hours.

Acquired plasma cholinesterase deficiency is clinically less important, since paralysis from suxamethonium seldom lasts for more than 20–30 minutes. However, this can be avoided by not using suxamethonium in patients known to be at risk. Clinically important prolongation of suxamethonium-paralysis is only to be expected, with the exception of some drug-induced effects, in patients with more than one cause for a reduction in pseudocholinesterase activity. In malnutrition and liver disease (278,279) the synthesis of plasma cholinesterase in the liver is reduced. Neonates have about 50% of normal adult plasma cholinesterase activity. In pregnancy there is a rapid fall in plasma cholinesterase activity of about 25% in the first trimester, which only returns to normal some 6–8 weeks postpartum (280–282). Occasionally much larger falls occur. The lowest average values have been reported during the first week of the puerperium (SEDA-5, 135) (283,284). Similar changes have been reported in gestational trophoblastic disease (hydatidiform mole) (285). Cancer is sometimes associated with lower plasma cholinesterase activity (SEDA-5, 136) (286). There is also a report of multiple esterase deficiencies in Hodgkin's disease (287). Plasma cholinesterase activity has also been reported to be reduced by up to 70–80% in patients with renal disease and burns. Plasmapheresis (SEDA-5, 135) (288,289) removes cholinesterase, along with other proteins, from the plasma.

Numerous drugs also reduce plasma cholinesterase synthesis or activity, for example estrogens, glucocorticoids, phenelzine, organophosphorus compounds (such as ecothiopate eye-drops, insecticides), carbamates (insecticides, bambuterol), cytotoxic drugs, metoclopramide, the ester-type local anesthetic drugs, and pancuronium. Anticholinesterases also prolong the action of suxamethonium. Several reviews are recommended for detailed information about plasma cholinesterase and its relevance in anesthetic practice (124,290–292).

Hepatic disease

In severe liver dysfunction the synthesis of plasma cholinesterase may be reduced to such an extent that the action of suxamethonium can be prolonged (SED-8, 282). This is usually not more than 2 or 3 times the normal duration.

Other features of the patient

Suxamethonium-induced fasciculation or increased muscle tone can be dangerous in patients with fractures or dislocations (especially vertebral, when the drug is relatively contraindicated), in patients with open-eye injuries or after the eyeball is opened surgically, when an increase in abdominal pressure must be avoided (pheochromocytoma, aortic aneurysm, full stomach, ileus), and in patients in whom a rise in arterial pressure may be catastrophic (cerebral aneurysm, raised intracranial pressure). Prolonged paralysis, occasionally lasting hours, is a risk if the patient is, or has been, taking certain drugs.

Pregnancy

In pregnancy the risk of regurgitation has to be weighed against the advantage of rapid intubation. The use of "precurarization" with small doses of non-depolarizing drugs may reduce the intensity of the fasciculation, but is by no means reliable. If possible, relaxation is better achieved by using a non-depolarizing agent alone.

Muscle disorders

Patients with muscle disorders (dystrophia myotonica, myotonia congenita, myasthenia gravis, and hyperkalemic periodic paralysis) tend to react unpredictably to suxamethonium. In myasthenia gravis, small doses of suxamethonium may be tried and the resulting effect monitored. In the other diseases listed non-depolarizers, cautiously used, are preferable. Cardiac arrest has been reported in patients with pseudohypertrophic muscular dystrophy (Duchenne type) and excessive muscle damage may be produced by suxamethonium in this condition.

Myasthenic syndromes

In myasthenia gravis responses to suxamethonium are unpredictable (293–296). Resistance has been reported and the development of a phase II block can occur more readily, occasionally leading to prolonged paralysis. The measures used to treat the condition, for example plasmapheresis or anticholinesterases, further complicate the picture. Patients with the Eaton–Lambert syndrome are very sensitive to all relaxants.

Asthma or allergic reactions

In patients with asthma or a history of previous allergy, suxamethonium should be used with caution, in view of its potential for causing allergic reactions and bronchospasm. When a patient or a relative has had a previous adverse reaction to an anesthetic, the possibilities of an atypical cholinesterase genotype or malignant hyperthermia should also be considered. Patients with certain musculoskeletal and developmental abnormalities, such as a tendency to joint dislocations, squint, ptosis, hernias, some forms of cryptorchidism, pectus excavatum, kyphosis, foot deformities, and myopathic features, and also those who have reacted to a previous injection of suxamethonium with generalized muscle rigidity or masseter spasm, may be more prone to malignant hyperthermia. Dantrolene should be available to every area where anesthetic agents are used.

Patients at risk of aspiration

The choice of muscle relaxants for rapid sequence induction of anesthesia in patients at risk of aspiration has been controversial for many years. Suxamethonium has been used for decades, because it has a fast onset and a short duration of action, although it can have severe adverse effects. Alternatives have been suggested, all of which have their own pros and cons, but suxamethonium has withstood the test of time and is still widely used. On this background, the use of rocuronium versus suxamethonium has been subjected to a Cochrane review, in which 40 studies addressing the issue were identified, 26 of which were combined for analysis (297). For rocuronium, the relative risk of excellent intubating conditions was 0.87 (95% CI = 0.81, 0.94) compared with suxamethonium. In a subgroup of patients who had been given propofol as an induction agent, there was no difference between rocuronium and suxamethonium. The reviewers concluded that overall suxamethonium creates excellent intubation conditions more reliably than rocuronium and should still be used as a first-line muscle relaxant for rapid sequence intubation. Rocuronium, when used with propofol, reliably created excellent intubation conditions and was consequently suggested as a second-line alternative to suxamethonium. In addition, some have suggested that intubating under deep anesthesia without a neuromuscular blocker is an acceptable third-line alternative if neither suxamethonium nor rocuronium is considered appropriate. To allow rapid-sequence intubation of the trachea without a muscle relaxant, adequate doses of propofol (2.0–2.5 mg/kg) or etomidate (0.3 mg/kg) and a fast-onset opioid, such as alfentanil (50 micrograms/kg) or remifentanil (4 micrograms/kg) are required (298–303).

Drug Administration

Drug dosage regimens

The short duration of action of suxamethonium is regarded as one of its big advantages over other muscle relaxants, as return of spontaneous ventilation can be expected within a few minutes in cases of failed intubation. Recently, the optimal dose in this respect has received some attention. In one study, a dose of 0.56 mg/kg was found to result in acceptable intubation conditions in 95% of the patients (304), while the authors of another paper reported that the duration of action shortened significantly when the dose was reduced to 0.6 mg/kg (305). However, as highlighted in an accompanying editorial (306), this does not apply to all patients, and even with such a low dose the duration of action was still as long as 11 minutes in some individuals. The reduced dose is not intrinsically safer but is associated with a higher incidence of unacceptable intubation conditions. Therefore, we agree with Donati, who concluded in his editorial that the traditional dose of 1 mg/kg is not a bad choice after all.

Drug–Drug Interactions

Alkylating agents

As suxamethonium is normally metabolized by plasma cholinesterase, only a small proportion of the injected dose reaches the neuromuscular junction. When plasma cholinesterase activity is significantly reduced a larger proportion of suxamethonium enters the neuromuscular junction, resulting in prolonged neuromuscular blockade. A variety of drugs and medical conditions are associated with this problem, and another example has recently been described (307).

- A 65-year-old man became severely depressed after his first dose of chemotherapy for non-Hodgkin lymphoma. He was given venlafaxine, olanzapine, and lithium, but his depression worsened and electroconvulsive therapy was started. After three uneventful treatment sessions he allowed chemotherapy to be restarted with cyclophosphamide, doxorubicin, vincristine, and prednisolone. After the fourth electroconvulsive

treatment, he had apnea for 45 minutes after thiopental 200 mg and suxamethonium 40 mg. Using a peripheral nerve stimulator, four equal twitch responses to train-of-four stimulation were observed after 30 minutes. He recovered fully. A blood sample taken during the episode showed a dibucaine number of 73 (reference range 76×83), a fluoride number of 53 (73×82), a K002/0683 number of 86 (110×115), and a plasma cholinesterase activity of 339 units/l (600×1400).

Referring to previous reports the authors suggested that cyclophosphamide-induced inhibition of plasma cholinesterase might have caused prolonged neuromuscular blockade after suxamethonium. Indeed, it has long been known that nitrogen mustards and related agents, such as cyclophosphamide, chlorambucil, triethylmelamine, and thiophosphoramide, can prolong the action of suxamethonium, which probably reduce plasma cholinesterase activity by alkylation of the enzyme (SED 14, 368). On the other hand, suxamethonium has been used in a patient taking cyclophosphamide without any evidence of prolonged action (308). If it is indicated, suxamethonium can be used in these patients, but neuromuscular transmission should be monitored.

Antidysrhythmic drugs

Quinidine potentiates not only non-depolarizing muscle relaxants but also depolarizing drugs (309).

Verapamil can potentiate the block produced by both types of neuromuscular blocking agent (310).

Beta-blockers can prolong and possibly exaggerate the rise in serum potassium resulting from the injection of suxamethonium (SEDA-10, 108) (SEDA-11, 122) (203,204).

Aprotinin (Trasylol)

Aprotinin (Trasylol) slightly reduces plasma cholinesterase activity and would only be expected to prolong the action of suxamethonium in combination with other factors. However, re-paralysis has been reported when this agent was used after operations during which suxamethonium had been given alone or in combination with normal doses of D-tubocurarine (311).

Atracurium dibesilate

Prior administration of suxamethonium potentiates the action of atracurium by about 30% (312).

Bambuterol

Bambuterol, a beta$_2$-adrenoceptor agonist that is used to relieve bronchospasm, approximately doubles the duration of action of suxamethonium (SEDA-14, 114) (313). Plasma cholinesterase activity was reduced significantly even 10–12.5 hours after a single dose of 30 mg had been given to patients. The interaction is due to the binding of carbamate groups to plasma cholinesterase.

Cardiac glycosides

Cardiac glycosides and suxamethonium can interact, resulting in an increased risk of dysrhythmias (314), perhaps through alterations in intracellular calcium (22). In

24 patients with ischemic heart disease taking digoxin who underwent abdominal surgery ventricular extra beats with bigemini or severe bradycardia were recorded in two patients and episodes of torsade de pointes occurred in two others during endotracheal intubation (315). The authors suggested that endotracheal intubation in digitalized patients should be performed without suxamethonium. However, considering the frequency with which digitalized patients receive suxamethonium and the paucity of reports of clinical problems, this interaction is probably of minor importance.

Chloroprocaine

Because it is hydrolysed by plasma cholinesterase, chloroprocaine may competitively enhance the action of suxamethonium (316).

Cocaine

Procaine and cocaine are esters that are hydrolysed by plasma cholinesterase and may therefore competitively enhance the action of suxamethonium (succinylcholine) (317). Chloroprocaine may have a similar action. Lidocaine also interacts, although the mechanism is not clear unless very high doses are used (318).

Cytotoxic and immunosuppressive drugs

Nitrogen mustard and related alkylating agents, such as cyclophosphamide, chlorambucil, triethylmelamine, and thiophosphoramide, prolong the action of suxamethonium (319,320). Plasma cholinesterase activity is reduced, possibly by alkylation of the enzyme. It has been suggested that azathioprine may potentiate suxamethonium by inhibition of phosphodiesterase activity (SEDA-4, 87) (321).

Donepezil

Donepezil acts primarily as a reversible inhibitor of acetylcholinesterase with a half-life of over 70 hours. Prolonged paralysis lasting several hours and requiring postoperative mechanical ventilation in the intensive care unit has been reported after the use of suxamethonium in a patient taking long-term donepezil (322).

- An 85-year-old woman with a history of mild Alzheimer's disease and hypertension underwent abdominal hysterectomy. Anesthesia was induced with suxamethonium 100 mg and 40 minutes later pancuronium 2 mg. After 2 hours, when surgery was finished, train-of-four stimulation elicited three twitches, and neostigmine 5 mg plus glycopyrrolate 1 mg was given to reverse neuromuscular block. She was subsequently able to follow commands and was breathing adequately; four twitches were observed during train-of-four stimulation. Several minutes after extubation she became apneic and had to be reintubated. Further neostigmine 1 mg was given, but neuromuscular block persisted without any response to peripheral nerve stimulation. In a blood sample taken 60 minutes after the second dose of neostigmine plasma cholinesterase activity was 2.1 (reference range 7.1–19) U/ml. The dibucaine

number was 45 (reference range 81–87)%, and the fluoride number was 84 (44–54)%.

The authors of this report subsequently tested the effect of donepezil on plasma cholinesterase activity in vitro. Supratherapeutic concentrations (0.02 mg/ml) reduced plasma cholinesterase activity to 53% of baseline. Dibucaine and fluoride numbers were not affected by neostigmine or donepezil. Others have shown previously that therapeutic doses of donepezil inhibit acetylcholinesterase by 64% (323). Prolonged paralysis in this case may have been due to the combined effects of atypical plasma cholinesterase and additional inhibition of plasma cholinesterase activity by donepezil. Unfortunately, preoperative plasma cholinesterase activity was not known and low cholinesterase activity was detected under the influence of neostigmine, which inhibits both plasma cholinesterase and acetylcholinesterase. Because a very high dose of neostigmine resulted in intensification rather than reversal of neuromuscular block, overdose of neostigmine may have caused paradoxical neuromuscular block (324). Hypothetically, paradoxical block is a combination of desensitization and open channel block (SED-13, 298). So the additional dose of neostigmine should have been omitted. In addition, an excess of acetylcholine at the end-plate might have been the result of combined inhibition of acetylcholinesterase by both donepezil and neostigmine. Until more is known, neostigmine and other cholinesterase inhibitors should be used with caution in patients taking donepezil.

- A 72-year-old woman with a symptomatic hiatus hernia, osteoarthritis, and Alzheimer's disease was taking fluoxetine 20 mg/day, donepezil hydrochloride 10 mg/day, nimesulide 12.5 mg/day, and omeprazole 20 mg/day (325). There still was no twitch response to peripheral nerve stimulation 20 minutes after rapid-sequence induction of anesthesia with propofol 2.5 mg/kg and suxamethonium 1 mg/kg. She then gradually developed a weak twitch response, and 50 minutes after induction of anesthesia four twitches with a fade were elicited by train-of-four stimulation. No additional medication was given and after the end of the procedure 10 minutes later she was extubated uneventfully. She refused further blood testing and so her plasma cholinesterase activity at that time is not known. However, her anesthetic notes from a previous operation did not reveal any problems with prolonged paralysis after suxamethonium.

It is not proven that donepezil was the cause of the prolonged duration of action of suxamethonium in this case. However, a case with some similarities has been reported before (322). In addition, there has been another report linking donepezil therapy to both prolonged duration of action of suxamethonium and reduced sensitivity to atracurium (326). Recovery of neuromuscular function should therefore be monitored when suxamethonium is given to patients taking donepezil. The withdrawal of donepezil 2–3 weeks before an operation cannot be supported, because this might have adverse effects on cognitive function. The issue has been highlighted in a recent letter, and the author concluded that "a brief prolongation of muscle relaxation is very rarely a problem (although its mismanagement may be)" (327).

Ecothiopate

Ecothiopate eye-drops, used in the treatment of glaucoma, prolong the action of suxamethonium considerably (328,329). Ecothiopate is a long-acting anticholinesterase that inhibits the activity of both acetylcholinesterase and plasma cholinesterase. Plasma cholinesterase activity may be reduced to 5% or less and on withdrawal requires 1–2 months for recovery to normal values (330,331). The prolonged anticholinesterase effect is due to conversion of the enzyme to its stable phosphoryl derivative. If a patient has used ecothiopate eye-drops in the previous 2 months or so, suxamethonium should not be given, unless normal plasma cholinesterase activity can be demonstrated. Various organophosphorus insecticides, such as parathion and malathion, may also result in prolonged paralysis after suxamethonium due to reduced free cholinesterase activity (275,332), produced in a similar manner to that in the case of ecothiopate.

Estrogens and estrogen-containing contraceptives

Estrogens and estrogen-containing contraceptives prolong the action of suxamethonium. Plasma cholinesterase activity is reduced, possibly by estrogenic inhibition of the hepatic synthesis of plasma cholinesterase, and its isozymes are modified (290,333,334). Diethylstilbestrol, included in this group, is reported to have caused paralysis for 3 hours in a patient with other aggravating factors (SEDA-4, 89) (335). One would, however, expect little prolongation of suxamethonium paralysis since the decrease in plasma cholinesterase activity (after contraceptives, at least) averages only about 20%. Prednisone, cortisol, and dexamethasone also reduce plasma cholinesterase activity to a mild or moderate degree (SEDA-15, 122) (336–338).

General anesthetics

When mixed in solution, thiopental will hydrolyse suxamethonium, owing to a pH effect. Ketamine may prolong the action of suxamethonium slightly (339,340); a phase II block might be prolonged more significantly (340), although there is no clinical experience reported. Decreased presynaptic acetylcholine synthesis or release has been postulated as the mechanism (341). In another study there was no significant shift in the dose–response curve for suxamethonium with ketamine (342). Inhalational agents potentiate muscle relaxants, which is of more clinical importance with regard to non-depolarizing agents. Tachyphylaxis and phase II block develop earlier and after smaller total doses of suxamethonium when volatile agents such as halothane, enflurane, or isoflurane (343,344) are used instead of balanced anesthesia. Halothane can increase the incidence of cardiac dysrhythmias, especially bradycardia and nodal rhythm, after suxamethonium. Atropine and glycopyrrolate, particularly when given intravenously just before, afford some protection (SEDA-5, 136) (345).

Isoflurane

Isoflurane in nitrous oxide inhibited suxamethonium-induced muscle fasciculation in children (346).

Lidocaine

Procaine and cocaine are esters that are hydrolysed by plasma cholinesterase and may therefore competitively enhance the action of suxamethonium (347). Chloroprocaine may have a similar action. Lidocaine also interacts, although the mechanism is not clear unless very high doses are used (348).

Lithium carbonate

Lithium carbonate delays the onset and prolongs the action of depolarizing relaxants (349,350). The principal mechanism of action is disputed. Factors suggested have been the development of dual block, reduced sensitivity of the end-plate for suxamethonium, diminished synthesis or release of acetylcholine, and plasma cholinesterase inhibition (350–352). The clinical importance is also disputed.

Local anesthetics

Procaine and cocaine are esters that are hydrolysed by plasma cholinesterase and can therefore competitively enhance the action of suxamethonium (353). Chloroprocaine may have a similar action. Lidocaine also interacts, although the mechanism is not clear unless very high doses are used (354).

Magnesium sulfate

Magnesium sulfate is used mostly in the treatment of toxemia of pregnancy. Serum magnesium concentrations may be raised and, as magnesium inhibits the release of acetylcholine and reduces the sensitivity of the postjunctional membrane, the action of non-depolarizing agents will be prolonged. It is not so clear, however, why the action of suxamethonium is also prolonged (355–358). Suxamethonium-induced fasciculation are reportedly prevented (SEDA-5, 135) (359). It has been suggested that the administration of intravenous magnesium sulfate should be stopped 20–30 minutes before muscle relaxants are given. Monitoring with a nerve stimulator is advisable.

Metoclopramide

Metoclopramide inhibits the activity of plasma cholinesterase and can prolong the action of suxamethonium (SEDA-14, 115) (360–362).

Neostigmine

Neostigmine inhibits both plasma cholinesterase and acetylcholinesterase, so that if any suxamethonium is still circulating, its action will be prolonged (by about a factor of two). This may present problems when neostigmine is administered to antagonize phase II block (363) (in which hypothetical desensitization block and open channel block elements may also be intensified) or shortly after suxamethonium is given. In renal insufficiency both neostigmine and pyridostigmine can cause prolongation (by 1–2 hours) of the action of suxamethonium given several hours after renal transplant operations.

Non-depolarizing muscle relaxants

Non-depolarizing muscle relaxants and suxamethonium are mutually antagonistic. These agents are often given in small non-paralysing doses before suxamethonium to reduce fasciculation and other adverse effects. Gallamine is slightly more effective than D-tubocurarine, and both are more effective than pancuronium. This precurarization tends to prolong the onset of action of (probably by direct antagonism) and to shorten (D-tubocurarine) or lengthen (pancuronium) its duration of action (364). The latter effect may well be due to inhibition of plasma cholinesterase by pancuronium. When compared with pancuronium, pretreatment with either atracurium or vecuronium was associated with a significantly shorter time to 90% twitch recovery after a standard dose of suxamethonium (365). When non-depolarizing agents are given after suxamethonium, even more than 30 minutes later, their action is considerably potentiated and prolonged (117,366,367). This effect (and also the production of a phase II block when suxamethonium is used alone in high or frequently repeated doses) may be the result of inhibition of transmitter release through a pre-junctional action of suxamethonium (368). Suxamethonium given some time after a paralysing dose of a non-depolarizing agent (for example for peritoneal closure) produces varying effects depending on the depth of residual curarization and on the dosage of suxamethonium (SEDA-21, 141) (369–371). As it is uncertain what type of block results, this practice cannot be recommended, although few problems with subsequent reversal have been reported.

Phenelzine

Phenelzine, a monoamine oxidase inhibitor, has been reported to cause significant prolongation of suxamethonium paralysis due to depressed plasma cholinesterase levels (to about 10% of normal). Recovery of plasma cholinesterase activity took 2 weeks (372).

Procaine

Procaine is hydrolysed by plasma cholinesterase and may therefore competitively enhance the action of suxamethonium (316).

Tacrine (tetrahydroaminoacridine) and hexafluorenium

Tacrine (tetrahydroaminoacridine) and hexafluorenium, used sometimes to potentiate and prolong the action of suxamethonium (373,374), inhibit plasma cholinesterase. Hexafluorenium also inhibits acetylcholinesterase and has a weak neuromuscular blocking action of the non-depolarizing type; a phase II block develops fairly rapidly when repeated injections of even small doses (0.2–0.3 mg/kg) of suxamethonium are given in combination with hexafluorenium (375). Fasciculation is reportedly reduced and hyperkalemia prevented (376), as is the increase in intraocular pressure (377), when hexafluorenium is given before suxamethonium. Because of a lack of consistency of successful results from various investigators, this method is not recommended for patients who are especially at risk from hyperkalemia or increased intraocular pressure. Simultaneous injection of hexafluorenium and suxamethonium can cause severe bronchospasm.

Trimetaphan

Trimetaphan can double the duration of suxamethonium block (378–380). The mechanism is not clear, but may be a competitive effect at the neuromuscular junction. Blockade of end-plate ionic channels has also been suggested (381).

References

1. Dal Santo G. Kinetics of distribution of radioactive labeled muscle relaxants. 3. Investigations with ^{14}C-succinyldicholine and ^{14}C-succinylmonocholine during controlled conditions. Anesthesiology 1968;29(3):435–43.
2. DeCook TH, Goudsouzian NG. Tachyphylaxis and phase II block development during infusion of succinylcholine in children. Anesth Analg 1980;59(9):639–43.
3. Ramsey FM, Lebowitz PW, Savarese JJ, Ali HH. Clinical characteristics of long-term succinylcholine neuromuscular blockade during balanced anesthesia. Anesth Analg 1980;59(2):110–6.
4. Baraka A. Myasthenic response to muscle relaxants in von Recklinghausen's disease. Br J Anaesth 1974;46(9):701–3.
5. Heard SO, Kaplan RF. Neuromuscular blockade in a patient with nemaline myopathy. Anesthesiology 1983;59(6):588–90.
6. Sorensen M, Engbaek J, Viby-Mogensen J, Guldager H, Molke Jensen F. Bradycardia and cardiac asystole following a single injection of suxamethonium. Acta Anaesthesiol Scand 1984;28(2):232–5.
7. Linter SP, Thomas PR, Withington PS, Hall MG. Suxamethonium associated hypertonicity and cardiac arrest in unsuspected pseudohypertrophic muscular dystrophy. Br J Anaesth 1982;54(12):1331–2.
8. Genever EE. Suxamethonium-induced cardiac arrest in unsuspected pseudohypertrophic muscular dystrophy. Case report. Br J Anaesth 1971;43(10):984–6.
9. Henderson WA. Succinylcholine-induced cardiac arrest in unsuspected Duchenne muscular dystrophy. Can Anaesth Soc J 1984;31(4):444–6.
10. Solares G, Herranz JL, Sanz MD. Suxamethonium-induced cardiac arrest as an initial manifestation of Duchenne muscular dystrophy. Br J Anaesth 1986;58(5):576.
11. Sullivan M, Thompson WK, Hill GD. Succinylcholine-induced cardiac arrest in children with undiagnosed myopathy. Can J Anaesth 1994;41(6):497–501.
12. Bush GH. Suxamethonium-associated hypertonicity and cardiac arrest in unsuspected pseudohypertrophic muscular dystrophy. Br J Anaesth 1983;55(9):923.
13. Schaer H, Steinmann B, Jerusalem S, Maier C. Rhabdomyolysis induced by anaesthesia with intraoperative cardiac arrest. Br J Anaesth 1977;49(5):495–9.
14. Seay AR, Ziter FA, Thompson JA. Cardiac arrest during induction of anesthesia in Duchenne muscular dystrophy. J Pediatr 1978;93(1):88–90.
15. Parker SF, Bailey A, Drake AF. Infant hyperkalemic arrest after succinylcholine. Anesth Analg 1995;80(1):206–7.
16. Schulte-Sasse U, Eberlein HJ, Schmucker I, Underwood D, Wolbert R. Sollte die verwendung von succinylcholin in der kinderanästhesie neu uberdacht werden?. [Should the use of

succinylcholine in pediatric anesthesia be re-evaluated?.] Anaesthesiol Reanim 1993;18(1):13–9.

17. Farrell PT. Anaesthesia-induced rhabdomyolysis causing cardiac arrest: case report and review of anaesthesia and the dystrophinopathies. Anaesth Intensive Care 1994; 22(5):597–601.

18. Larach MG, Rosenberg H, Gronert GA, Allen GC. Hyperkalemic cardiac arrest during anesthesia in infants and children with occult myopathies. Clin Pediatr (Phila) 1997;36(1):9–16.

19. Jackson MA, Lodwick R, Hutchinson SG. Hyperkalaemic cardiac arrest successfully treated with peritoneal dialysis. BMJ 1996;312(7041):1289–90.

20. Lin JL, Huang CC. Successful initiation of hemodialysis during cardiopulmonary resuscitation due to lethal hyperkalemia. Crit Care Med 1990;18(3):342–3.

21. Lee G, Antognini JF, Gronert GA. Complete recovery after prolonged resuscitation and cardiopulmonary bypass for hyperkalemic cardiac arrest. Anesth Analg 1994;79(1):172–4.

22. Smith RB, Petruscak J. Succinylcholine, digitalis, and hypercalcemia: a case report. Anesth Analg 1972;51(2):202–5.

23. Nigrovic V. Succinylcholine, cholinoceptors and catecholamines: proposed mechanism of early adverse haemodynamic reactions. Can Anaesth Soc J 1984;31(4):382–94.

24. Pace SA, Fuller FP. Out-of-hospital succinylcholine-assisted endotracheal intubation by paramedics. Ann Emerg Med 2000;35(6):568–72.

25. Menegazzi JJ, Wayne MA. Succinylcholine-assisted endotracheal intubation by paramedics. Ann Emerg Med 2001;37(3):360–1.

26. Katz SH, Falk JL. Misplaced endotracheal tubes by paramedics in an urban emergency medical services system. Ann Emerg Med 2001;37(1):32–7.

27. Zink BJ, Snyder HS, Raccio-Robak N. Lack of a hyperkalemic response in emergency department patients receiving succinylcholine. Acad Emerg Med 1995;2(11):974–8.

28. Dronen SC, Merigian KS, Hedges JR, Hoekstra JW, Borron SW. A comparison of blind nasotracheal and succinylcholine-assisted intubation in the poisoned patient. Ann Emerg Med 1987;16(6):650–2.

29. Smith CL, Bush GH. Anaesthesia and progressive muscular dystrophy. Br J Anaesth 1985;57(11):1113–8.

30. Ravindran RS, Klemm JE. Anaphylaxis to succinylcholine in a patient allergic to penicillin. Anesth Analg 1980;59(12):944–5.

31. Cohen S, Liu KH, Marx GF. Upper airway edema — an anaphylactoid reaction to succinylcholine? Anesthesiology 1982;56(6):467–8.

32. O'Sullivan EP, Childs D, Bush GH. Peri-operative dreaming in paediatric patients who receive suxamethonium. Anaesthesia 1988;43(2):104–6.

33. Halldin M, Wahlin A. Effect of succinylcholine on the intraspinal fluid pressure. Acta Anaesthesiol Scand 1959; 3:155–61.

34. Marsh ML, Dunlop BJ, Shapiro HM, Gagnon RL, Rockoff MA. Succinylcholine-intracranial pressure effects in neurosurgical patients. Anesth Analg 1980;59:550–1.

35. Kovarik WD, Mayberg TS, Lam AM, Mathisen TL, Winn HR. Succinylcholine does not change intracranial pressure, cerebral blood flow velocity, or the electroencephalogram in patients with neurologic injury. Anesth Analg 1994;78(3):469–73.

36. Clancy M, Halford S, Walls R, Murphy M. In patients with head injuries who undergo rapid sequence intubation using succinylcholine, does pretreatment with a competitive neuromuscular blocking agent improve outcome? A literature review. Emerg Med J 2001;18(5):373–5.

37. Brown MM, Parr MJ, Manara AR. The effect of suxamethonium on intracranial pressure and cerebral perfusion pressure in patients with severe head injuries following blunt trauma. Eur J Anaesthesiol 1996;13(5):474–7.

38. Minton MD, Grosslight K, Stirt JA, Bedford RF. Increases in intracranial pressure from succinylcholine: prevention by prior nondepolarizing blockade. Anesthesiology 1986;65(2):165–9.

39. Stirt JA, Grosslight KR, Bedford RF, Vollmer D. "Defasciculation" with metocurine prevents succinylcholine-induced increases in intracranial pressure. Anesthesiology 1987;67(1):50–3.

40. Churchill-Davidson HC. Suxamethonium (succinylcholine) chloride and muscle pains. Br Med J 1954;4853:74–5.

41. Standaert FG, Adams JE. The actions of succinylcholine on the mammalian motor nerve terminal. J Pharmacol Exp Ther 1965;149:113–23.

42. Wong SF, Chung F. Succinylcholine-associated postoperative myalgia. Anaesthesia 2000;55:144–52.

43. Thind GS, Bryson TH. Single dose suxamethonium and muscle pain in pregnancy. Br J Anaesth 1983;55(8):743–5.

44. Coxon JD. Muscle pain after suxamethonium. Br Anaesth 1962;34:750.

45. Paton WD. The effects of muscle relaxants other than muscular relaxation. Anesthesiology 1959;20(4):453–63.

46. Tammisto T, Airaksinen M. Increase of creatine kinase activity in serum as sign of muscular injury caused by intermittently administred suxamethonium during halothane anaesthesia. Br J Anaesth 1966;38(7):510–5.

47. Waters DJ, Mapleson WW. Suxamethonium pains: hypothesis and observation. Anaesthesia 1971;26(2):127–41.

48. Rack PM, Westbury DR. The effects of suxamethonium and acetylcholine on the behaviour of cat muscle spindles during dynamics stretching, and during fusimotor stimulation. J Physiol 1966;186(3):698–713.

49. Mayrhofer O. Die Wirksamheit von d-Tubocurarin zur Verhütung der Muskelschmerzen nach Succinylcholin. [The efficacy of d-tubocurarine in the prevention of muscle pain after succinylcholine.] Anaesthesist 1959;8:313.

50. Konig W. Über Beschwerden nach Anwendung von Succinylcholin. Anaesthesist 1956;5:50.

51. Kaniaris P, Galanopoulou T, Varonos D. Effects of succinylcholine on plasma 5-HT levels. Anesth Analg 1973;52(3):425–7.

52. Collier CB. Suxamethonium pains and early electrolyte changes. Anaesthesia 1978;33(5):454–61.

53. Naguib M, Farag H, Magbagbeola JA. Effect of pre-treatment with lysine acetyl salicylate on suxamethonium-induced myalgia. Br J Anaesth 1987;59(5):606–10.

54. McLoughlin C, Nesbitt GA, Howe JP. Suxamethonium induced myalgia and the effect of pre-operative administration of oral aspirin. A comparison with a standard treatment and an untreated group. Anaesthesia 1988;43(7):565–7.

55. Laurence AS. Myalgia and biochemical changes following intermittent suxamethonium administration. Effects of alcuronium, lignocaine, midazolam and suxamethonium pretreatments on serum myoglobin, creatinine kinase and myalgia. Anaesthesia 1987;42:503–10.

56. McLoughlin C, Elliott P, McCarthy G, Mirakhur RK. Muscle pains and biochemical changes following suxamethonium administration after six pretreatment regimens. Anaesthesia 1992;47:202–6.

57. Waters DJ, Mapleson WW. Suxamethonium pains: hypothesis and observation. Anaesthesia 1971;26:127–41.

58. Bowman WC. Prejunctional and postjunctional cholinoceptors at the neuromuscular junction. Anesth Analg 1980;59:935–43.

59. Ferres CJ, Mirakhur RK, Craig HJ, Browne ES, Clarke RS. Pretreatment with vecuronium as a prophylactic against post-suxamethonium muscle pain. Br J Anaesth 1983;55:735–41.

60. O'Sullivan EWilliams N, Calvey T. Differential effects of neuromuscular blocking agents on suxamethonium-induced fasciculations and myalgia. Br J Anaesth 1988;60:367–71.

61. Lee TL, Aw TC. Prevention of succinylcholine-induced myalgia with lidocaine pretreatment. J Anesth 1991;5:239–46.

62. Leeson-Payne CG, Nicoll JM, Hobbs GJ. Use of ketorolac in the prevention of suxamethonium myalgia. Br J Anaesth 1994;73:788–90.

63. Nigrovic V, Wierda JM. Post-succinylcholine muscle pain and smoking. Can J Anaesth 1994;41:453–4.

64. Findlay GP, Spittal MJ. Rocuronium pretreatment reduces suxamethonium-induced myalgia: comparison with vecuronium. Br J Anaesth 1996;76:526–9.

65. Harvey SC, Roland P, Bailey MK, Tomlin MK, Williams A. A randomized, double-blind comparison of rocuronium, d-tubocurarine, and "mini-dose" succinylcholine for preventing succinylcholine-induced muscle fasciculations. Anesth Analg 1998;87:719–22.

66. Kararmaz A, Kaya S, Turhanoglu S, Ozyilmaz MA. Effects of high-dose propofol on succinylcholine-induced fasciculations and myalgia. Acta Anaesthesiol Scand 2003;47:180–4.

67. Collier CB. Suxamethonium pains and early electrolyte changes. Anaesthesia 1978;33:454–61.

68. König W. Über Beschwerden nach Anwendung von Succinylcholin. Anaesthesist 1956;5:50.

69. Naguib M, Farag H, Magbagbeola JA. Effect of pre-treatment with lysine acetyl salicylate on suxamethonium-induced myalgia. Br J Anaesth 1987;59:606–10.

70. McLoughlin C, Nesbitt GA, Howe JP. Suxamethonium induced myalgia and the effect of pre-operative administration of oral aspirin. A comparison with a standard treatment and an untreated group. Anaesthesia 1988;43:565–7.

71. Kahraman S, Ercan S, Aypar U, Erdem K. Effect of preoperative i.m. administration of diclofenac on suxamethonium-induced myalgia Br J Anaesth 1993;71:238–41.

72. Schreiber JU, Mencke T, Biedler A, Furst O, Kleinschmidt S, Buchinger H, Fuchs-Buder T. Postoperative myalgia after succinylcholine: no evidence for an inflammatory origin. Anesth Analg 2003;96:1640–4.

73. Cullen DJ. The effect of pretreatment with nondepolarizing muscle relaxants on the neuromuscular blocking action of succinylcholine. Anesthesiology 1971;35(6):572–8.

74. Jansen EC, Hansen PH. Objective measurement of succinylcholine-induced fasciculations and the effect of pretreatment with pancuronium or gallamine. Anesthesiology 1979;51(2):159–60.

75. Blitt CD, Carlson GL, Rolling GD, Hameroff SR, Otto CW. A comparative evaluation of pretreatment with nondepolarizing neuromuscular blockers prior to the administration of succinylcholine. Anesthesiology 1981;55(6):687–9.

76. Erkola O, Salmenpera A, Kuoppamaki R. Five nondepolarizing muscle relaxants in precurarization Acta Anaesthesiol Scand 1983;27(6):427–32.

77. Raman SK, San WM. Fasciculations, myalgia and biochemical changes following succinylcholine with atracurium and lidocaine pretreatment. Can J Anaesth 1997;44(5 Pt 1):498–502.

78. Fahmy NR, Malek NS, Lappas DG. Diazepam prevents some adverse effects of succinylcholine. Clin Pharmacol Ther 1979;26(3):395–8.

79. Manchikanti L. Diazepam does not prevent succinylcholine-induced fasciculations and myalgia. A comparative evaluation of the effect of diazepam and d-tubocurarine pretreatments. Acta Anaesthesiol Scand 1984;28(5):523–8.

80. Manataki AD, Arnaoutoglou HM, Tefa LK, Glatzounis GK, Papadopoulos GS. Continuous propofol administration for suxamethonium-induced postoperative myalgia. Anaesthesia 1999;54:419–22.

81. Maddineni VR, Mirakhur RK, Cooper AR. Myalgia and biochemical changes following suxamethonium after induction of anaesthesia with thiopentone or propofol. Anaesthesia 1993;48:626–8.

82. McClymont C. A comparison of the effect of propofol or thiopentone on the incidence and severity of suxamethonium-induced myalgia. Anaesth Intensive Care 1994;22:147–9.

83. Schreiber JU, Lysakowski C, Fuchs-Buder T, Tramer MR. Prevention of succinylcholine-induced fasciculation and myalgia: a meta-analysis of randomized trials. Anesthesiology 2005;103:877–84.

84. Donati F. Dose inflation when using precurarization. Anesthesiology 2006;105:222–3.

85. Schreiber J, Fuchs-Buder T, Lysakowski C, Tramer M. Dose inflation when using precurarization: authors' reply. Anesthesiology 2006;105:223.

86. Raman SK, San WM. Fasciculations, myalgia and biochemical changes following succinylcholine with atracurium and lidocaine pretreatment. Can J Anaesth 1997;44:498–502.

87. Melnick B, Chalasani J, Uy NT, Phitayakorn P, Mallett SV, Rudy TE. Decreasing post-succinylcholine myalgia in outpatients. Can J Anaesth 1987;34:238–41.

88. Flewellen EH, Bodensteiner JB. Anesthetic experience in a patient with hyperkalemic periodic paralysis. Anesthesiol Rev 1980;7:44.

89. Brim VD. Denervation supersensitivity: the response to depolarizing muscle relaxants. Br J Anaesth 1973;45(2):222–6.

90. Kelly EP. A rise in serum potassium after suxamethonium following brachial plexus injury. Anaesthesia 1982;37(6):694–5.

91. Orndahl G, Stenberg K. Myotonic human musculature: stimulation with depolarizing agents. Mechanical registration of the effects of succinyldicholine, succinylmonocholine and decamethonium. Acta Med Scand 1962;172(Suppl 389):3–29.

92. Allen GC, Rosenberg H. Malignant hyperthermia susceptibility in adult patients with masseter muscle rigidity. Can J Anaesth 1990;37(1):31–5.

93. Flewellen EH, Nelson TE. Halothane-succinylcholine induced masseter spasm: indicative of malignant hyperthermia susceptibility? Anesth Analg 1984;63(7):693–7.

94. O'Flynn RP, Shutack JG, Rosenberg H, Fletcher JE. Masseter muscle rigidity and malignant hyperthermia susceptibility in pediatric patients. An update on management and diagnosis. Anesthesiology 1994;80(6):1228–33.

95. Rosenberg H, Fletcher JE. Masseter muscle rigidity and malignant hyperthermia susceptibility. Anesth Analg 1986;65(2):161–4.

96. Gronert GA. Management of patients in whom trismus occurs following succinylcholine. Anesthesiology 1988;68(4):653–5.

97. Van der Spek AF, Fang WB, Ashton-Miller JA, Stohler CS, Carlson DS, Schork MA. The effects of succinylcholine on mouth opening. Anesthesiology 1987;67(4):459–65.

98. Meakin G, Walker RW, Dearlove OR. Myotonic and neuromuscular blocking effects of increased doses of suxamethonium in infants and children. Br J Anaesth 1990;65(6):816–8.

99. Littleford JA, Patel LR, Bose D, Cameron CB, McKillop C. Masseter muscle spasm in children:

implications of continuing the triggering anesthetic. Anesth Analg 1991;72(2):151–60.

100. Lazzell VA, Carr AS, Lerman J, Burrows FA, Creighton RE. The incidence of masseter muscle rigidity after succinylcholine in infants and children. Can J Anaesth 1994;41(6):475–9.

101. Leary NP, Ellis FR. Masseteric muscle spasm as a normal response to suxamethonium. Br J Anaesth 1990;64(4):488–92.

102. Ummenhofer WC, Kindler C, Tschaler G, Hampl KF, Drewe J, Urwyler A. Propofol reduces succinylcholine induced increase of masseter muscle tone. Can J Anaesth 1998;45(5 Pt 1):417–23.

103. Jenkins JG. Masseter muscle rigidity after vecuronium. Eur J Anaesthesiol 1999;16(2):137–9.

104. Polta TA, Hanisch EC Jr, Nasser JG, Ramsborg GC, Roelofs RI. Masseter spasm after pancuronium. Anesth Analg 1980;59(7):509–11.

105. Albrecht A, Wedel DJ, Gronert GA. Masseter muscle rigidity and nondepolarizing neuromuscular blocking agents. Mayo Clin Proc 1997;72(4):329–32.

106. Cheung PY, Tyebkhan JM, Peliowski A, Ainsworth W, Robertson CM. Prolonged use of pancuronium bromide and sensorineural hearing loss in childhood survivors of congenital diaphragmatic hernia. J Pediatr 1999;135(2 Pt 1):233–9.

107. Airaksinen MM, Tammisto T. Myoglobinuria after intermittent administration of succinylcholine during halothane anesthesia. Clin Pharmacol Ther 1966;7(5):583–7.

108. Plotz J, Braun J. Serummyoglobin nach Wiederholungsgaben von Succinylcholin und der Einfluss von Dantrolen. [Serum myoglobin following intermittent administration of succinylcholine and the effect of dantrolene. Clinical studies of children in halothane anesthesia.] Anaesthesist 1985;34(10): 513–5.

109. Plotz J. Nebenwirkungen von Succinylcholin auf die Skelettmuskulatur in Halothannarkose bei Kindern: Prophylaxe mit Diallylnortoxiferin, 'self-taming' und Dantrolen. Therapiewoche 1984;34:3168.

110. Harrington JF, Ford DJ, Striker TW. Myoglobinemia after succinylcholine in children undergoing halothane and non-halothane anesthesia. Anesthesiology 1984;61:A431.

111. Hool GJ, Lawrence PJ, Sivaneswaran N. Acute rhabdomyolytic renal failure due to suxamethonium. Anaesth Intensive Care 1984;12(4):360–4.

112. McKishnie JD, Muir JM, Girvan DP. Anaesthesia-induced rhabdomyolysis—a case report. Can Anaesth Soc J 1983;30(3 Pt 1):295–8.

113. Pedrozzi NE, Ramelli GP, Tomasetti R, Nobile-Buetti L, Bianchetti MG. Rhabdomyolysis and anesthesia: a report of two cases and review of the literature. Pediatr Neurol 1996;15(3):254–7.

114. Bhave CG, Gadre KC, Gharpure BS. Myoglobinuria following the use of succinylcholine. J Postgrad Med 1993;39(3):157–9.

115. Gokhale YA, Marathe P, Patil RD, Prasar S, Kamble P, Hase NK, Agrawal MB, Deshmukh SN, Menon PS. Rhabdomyolysis and acute renal failure following a single dose of succinylcholine. J Assoc Physicians India 1991;39(12):968–70.

116. Lee SC, Abe T, Sato T. Rhabdomyolysis and acute renal failure following use of succinylcholine and enflurane: report of a case. J Oral Maxillofac Surg 1987;45(9): 789–92.

117. Ryan JF, Kagen LJ, Hyman AI. Myoglobinemia after a single dose of succinylcholine. N Engl J Med 1971; 285(15):824–7.

118. Gibbs JM. A case of rhabdomyolysis associated with suxamethonium. Anaesth Intensive Care 1978;6(2):141–5.

119. Miyamoto K, Sasaki M, Okudo T, et al. Four cases suspected of malignant hyperthermia induced by halothane and succinylcholine. Hiroshima J Anesth 1983;18:157.

120. Lewandowski KB. Strabismus as a possible sign of subclinical muscular dystrophy predisposing to rhabdomyolysis and myoglobinuria: a study of an affected family. Can Anaesth Soc J 1982;29(4):372–6.

121. Larsen UT, Juhl B, Hein-Sorensen O, de Fine Olivarius B. Complications during anaesthesia in patients with Duchenne's muscular dystrophy (a retrospective study). Can J Anaesth 1989;36(4):418–22.

122. Wang JM, Stanley TH. Duchenne muscular dystrophy and malignant hyperthermia—two case reports. Can Anaesth Soc J 1986;33(4):492–7.

123. Steegmuller H. On the geographical distribution of pseudocholinesterase variants. Humangenetik 1975;26(3): 167–85.

124. Pantuck EJ, Pantuck CB. Cholinesterases and anticholinesterases. In: Katz RL, editor. Muscle Relaxants. Amsterdam: Excerpta Medica, 1975:155.

125. Viby-Mogensen J. Correlation of succinylcholine duration of action with plasma cholinesterase activity in subjects with the genotypically normal enzyme. Anesthesiology 1980;53(6):517–20.

126. Yamashita M, Matsuki A, Oyama T. Anaesthetic considerations on von Recklinghausen's disease (multiple neurofibromatosis). Abnormal response to muscle relaxants. Anaesthesist 1977;26(6):317–8.

127. Hofmann H, Holzer H. Die Wirkung von Muskelrelaxanzien auf den intraokularen Druck. [Effect of muscle relaxants on the intraocular pressure.] Klin Monatsbl Augenheilkd 1953;123(1):1–16.

128. Bowen DJ, McGrand JC, Palmer RJ. Intraocular pressures after suxamethonium and endotracheal intubation in patients pretreated with pancuronium. Br J Anaesth 1976;48(12):1201–5.

129. Bowen DJ, McGrand JC, Hamilton AG. Intraocular pressure after suxamethonium and endotracheal intubation. The effect of pre-treatment with tubocurarine or gallamine. Anaesthesia 1978;33(6):518–22.

130. Cook JH. The effect of suxamethonium on intraocular pressure. Anaesthesia 1981;36(4):359–65.

131. Craythorne NW, Rottenstein HS, Dripps RD. The effect of succinylcholine on intraocular pressure in adults, infants and children during general anesthesia. Anesthesiology 1960;21:59–63.

132. Dear GD, Hammerton M, Hatch DJ, Taylor D. Anaesthesia and intra-ocular pressure in young children. A study of three different techniques of anaesthesia. Anaesthesia 1987;42(3):259–65.

133. Feneck RO, Cook JH. Failure of diazepam to prevent the suxamethonium-induced rise in intra-ocular pressure. Anaesthesia 1983;38(2):120–7.

134. Goldsmith E. An evaluation of succinylcholine and gallamine as muscle relaxants in relation to intraocular tension. Anesth Analg 1967;46(5):557–61.

135. Grover VK, Lata K, Sharma S, Kaushik S, Gupta A. Efficacy of lignocaine in the suppression of the intra-ocular pressure response to suxamethonium and tracheal intubation. Anaesthesia 1989;44(1):22–5.

136. Lincoff HA, Ellis CH, DeVoe AG, DeBeer EJ, Impastato DJ, Berg S, Orkin L, Magda H. The effect of succinylcholine on the intraocular pressure. Am J Ophthalmol 1955;40(4):501–10.

137. Pandey K, Badola RP, Kumar S. Time course of intraocular hypertension produced by suxamethonium. Br J Anaesth 1972;44(2):191–6.

138. Robertson GS, Gibson PF. Suxamethonium and intraocular pressure. Anaesthesia 1968;23(3):342–9.

139. Sarmany BJ. Über die Wirkung von verschiedenen Narkotica auf den intraoculären Druck. [On the effect of various narcotics on intraocular pressure.] Anaesthesist 1967;16(10):296–8.

140. Schwartz H, DeRoetth A. Effect of succinylcholine on intraocular pressure in human. Anesthesiology 1958; 19:112–3.

141. Taylor TH, Mulcahy M, Nightingale DA. Suxamethonium chloride in intraocular surgery. Br J Anaesth 1968; 40(2):113–8.

142. Warner LO, Bremer DL, Davidson PJ, Rogers GL, Beach TP. Effects of lidocaine, succinylcholine, and tracheal intubation on intraocular pressure in children anesthetized with halothane–nitrous oxide. Anesth Analg 1989;69(5):687–90.

143. Kornblueth W, Jampolsky A, Tamler E, Marg E. Contraction of the oculorotary muscles and intraocular pressure. A tonographic and electromyographic study of the effect of edrophonium chloride (Tensilon) and succinylcholine (Anectine) on the intraocular pressure. Am J Ophthalmol 1960;49:1381–7.

144. Kelly RE, Dinner M, Turner LS, Haik B, Abramson DH, Daines P. Succinylcholine increases intraocular pressure in the human eye with the extraocular muscles detached. Anesthesiology 1993;79(5):948–52.

145. Bjork A, Halldin M, Wahlin A. Enophthalmus elicited by succinylcholine; some observations on the effect of succinylcholine and noradrenaline on the intraorbital muscles studied on man experimental animals. Acta Anaesthesiol Scand 1957;1(1–2):41–53.

146. Abramson DH. Anterior chamber and lens thickness changes induced by succinylcholine. Arch Ophthalmol 1971;86(6):643–7.

147. Halldin M, Wahlin A, Koch T. Observations of the conjunctival vessels under the influence of succinylcholine with intravenous anaesthesia. Acta Anaesthesiol Scand 1959;3:163–71.

148. Adams AK, Barnett KC. Anaesthesia and intraocular pressure. Anaesthesia 1966;21(2):202–10.

149. Robinson R, White M, McCann P, Magner J, Eustace P. Effect of anaesthesia on intraocular blood flow. Br J Ophthalmol 1991;75(2):92–3.

150. Miller RD, Way WL, Hickey RF. Inhibition of succinylcholine-induced increased intraocular pressure by non-depolarizing muscle relaxants. Anesthesiology 1968;29(1):123–6.

151. Meyers EF, Krupin T, Johnson M, Zink H. Failure of nondepolarizing neuromuscular blockers to inhibit succinylcholine-induced increased intraocular pressure, a controlled study. Anesthesiology 1978;48(2):149–51.

152. Verma RS. "Self-taming" of succinylcholine-induced fasciculations and intraocular pressure. Anesthesiology 1979;50(3):245–7.

153. Meyers EF, Singer P, Otto A. A controlled study of the effect of succinylcholine self-taming on intraocular pressure. Anesthesiology 1980;53(1):72–4.

154. Cunningham AJ, Albert O, Cameron J, Watson AG. The effect of intravenous diazepam on rise of intraocular pressure following succinylcholine. Can Anaesth Soc J 1981; 28(6):591–6.

155. Fjeldborg P, Hecht PS, Busted N, Nissen AB. The effect of diazepam pretreatment on the succinylcholine-induced rise in intraocular pressure. Acta Anaesthesiol Scand 1985;29(4):415–7.

156. Mahajan RP, Grover VK, Munjal VP, Singh H. Double-blind comparison of lidocaine, tubocurarine and diazepam pretreatment in modifying intraocular pressure increases. Can J Anaesth 1987;34(1):41–5.

157. Murphy DF, Eustace P, Unwin A, Magner JB. Intravenous lignocaine pretreatment to prevent intraocular pressure rise following suxamethonium and tracheal intubation. Br J Ophthalmol 1986;70(8):596–8.

158. Mahajan RP, Grover VK, Sharma SL, Singh H. Intranasal nitroglycerin and intraocular pressure during general anesthesia. Anesth Analg 1988;67(7):631–6.

159. Indu B, Batra YK, Puri GD, Singh H. Nifedipine attenuates the intraocular pressure response to intubation following succinylcholine. Can J Anaesth 1989;36(3 Pt 1):269–72.

160. Grover VK, Kakkar RK, Grewal S, Sharma S, Gupta A. Efficacy of topical timolol to prevent intraocular pressor response to suxamethonium and tracheal intubation. J Anaesth Clin Pharmacol 1996;12:107–11.

161. Edmondson L, Lindsay SL, Lanigan LP, Woods M, Chew HE. Intra-ocular pressure changes during rapid sequence induction of anaesthesia. A comparison between thiopentone and suxamethonium and thiopentone and atracurium. Anaesthesia 1988;43(12):1005–10.

162. Mirakhur RK, Shepherd WF, Darrah WC. Propofol or thiopentone: effects on intraocular pressure associated with induction of anaesthesia and tracheal intubation (facilitated with suxamethonium). Br J Anaesth 1987; 59(4):431–6.

163. Polarz H, Bohrer H, Fleischer F, Huster T, Bauer H, Wolfrum J. Effects of thiopentone/suxamethonium on intraocular pressure after pretreatment with alfentanil. Eur J Clin Pharmacol 1992;43(3):311–3.

164. Sweeney J, Underhill S, Dowd T, Mostafa SM. Modification by fentanyl and alfentanil of the intraocular pressure response to suxamethonium and tracheal intubation. Br J Anaesth 1989;63(6):688–91.

165. Zimmerman AA, Funk KJ, Tidwell JL. Propofol and alfentanil prevent the increase in intraocular pressure caused by succinylcholine and endotracheal intubation during a rapid sequence induction of anesthesia. Anesth Analg 1996;83(4):814–7.

166. Alexander R, Hill R, Lipham WJ, Weatherwax KJ, el-Moalem HE. Remifentanil prevents an increase in intraocular pressure after succinylcholine and tracheal intubation. Br J Anaesth 1998;81(4):606–7.

167. Donlon JV. Succinylcholine and open eye injury. Anesthesiology 1986;64:525–6.

168. Wang ML, Seiff SR, Drasner K. A comparison of visual outcome in open-globe repair: succinylcholine with D-tubocurarine vs nondepolarizing agents. Ophthalmic Surg 1992;23(11):746–51.

169. Moreno RJ, Kloess P, Carlson DW. Effect of succinylcholine on the intraocular contents of open globes. Ophthalmology 1991;98(5):636–8.

170. Cunningham AJ, Barry P. Intraocular pressure—physiology and implications for anaesthetic management. Can Anaesth Soc J 1986;33(2):195–208.

171. Donlon JV. Anesthesia and eye, ear, nose, and throat surgery. In: Miller RD, editor. Anesthesia. 4th ed.. New York: Churchill Livingstone, 1994:2175–96.

172. Hunter JM. Anaesthetic drugs and the eye. In: Mostafa SM, editor. Anaesthesia for Ophthalmic Surgery. Oxford: Oxford University Press, 1991:32–44.

173. McGoldrick KE. The open globe: is an alternative to succinylcholine necessary? J Clin Anesth 1993;5(1):1–4.

174. McGoldrick KE. Anesthesia and the eye. In: Barash PG, Cullen BF, Stoelting RK, editors. Clinical Anesthesia. 3rd ed.. Philadelphia: Lippincott-Raven, 1996:911–28.

175. France NK, France TD, Woodburn JD Jr, Burbank DP. Succinylcholine alteration of the forced duction test. Ophthalmology 1980;87(12):1282–7.

176. Carroll JB. Increased incidence of masseter spasm in children with strabismus anesthetized with halothane and succinylcholine. Anesthesiology 1987;67(4):559–61.

177. Strazis KP, Fox AW. Malignant hyperthermia: a review of published cases. Anesth Analg 1993;77(2):297–304.

178. Dodd MJ, Phattiyakul P, Silpasuvan S. Suspected malignant hyperthermia in a strabismus patient. A case report. Arch Ophthalmol 1981;99(7):1247–50.

179. Schwartz N, Eisenkraft JB, Raab EL. Masseter muscle spasm, succinylcholine, and strabismus surgery. Anesthesiology 1988;69(4):635–6.

180. Ranklev E, Henriksson KG, Fletcher R, Germundsson K, Oldfors A, Kalimo H. Clinical and muscle biopsy findings in malignant hyperthermia susceptibility. Acta Neurol Scand 1986;74(6):452–9.

181. Berkahn JM, Sleigh JW. Hyperkalaemic cardiac arrest following succinylcholine in a longterm intensive care patient. Anaesth Intensive Care 1997;25(5):588–9.

182. Biccard BM, Grant IS, Wright DJ, Nimmo SR, Hughes M. Suxamethonium and critical illness polyneuropathy. Anaesth Intensive Care 1998;26(5):590–1.

183. Dornan RI, Royston D. Suxamethonium-related hyperkalaemic cardiac arrest in intensive care. Anaesthesia 1995;50(11):1006.

184. Hansen D. Suxamethonium-induced cardiac arrest and death following 5 days of immobilization. Eur J. Anaesthesiol 1998;15(2):240–1.

185. Hemming AE, Charlton S, Kelly P. Hyperkalaemia, cardiac arrest, suxamethonium and intensive care. Anaesthesia 1990;45(11):990–1.

186. Horton WA, Fergusson NV. Hyperkalaemia and cardiac arrest after the use of suxamethonium in intensive care. Anaesthesia 1988;43(10):890–1.

187. Lee YM, Fountain SW. Suxamethonium and cardiac arrest. Singapore Med J 1997;38(7):300–1.

188. Markewitz BA, Elstad MR. Succinylcholine-induced hyperkalemia following prolonged pharmacologic neuromuscular blockade. Chest 1997;111(1):248–50.

189. Matthews JM. Succinylcholine-induced hyperkalemia and rhabdomyolysis in a patient with necrotizing pancreatitis. Anesth Analg 2000;91(6):1552–4.

190. Chakravarty EF, Kirsch CM, Jensen WA, Kagawa FT. Cardiac arrest due to succinylcholine-induced hyperkalemia in a patient with wound botulism. J Clin Anesth 2000;12(1):80–2.

191. Passaro DJ, Werner SB, McGee J, Mac Kenzie WR, Vugia DJ. Wound botulism associated with black tar heroin among injecting drug users. JAMA 1998;279(11):859–63.

192. Simpson LL. The effects of acute and chronic botulinum toxin treatment on receptor number, receptor distribution and tissue sensitivity in rat diaphragm. J Pharmacol Exp Ther 1977;200(2):343–51.

193. Koltgen D, Ceballos-Baumann AO, Franke C. Botulinum toxin converts muscle acetylcholine receptors from adult to embryonic type. Muscle Nerve 1994;17(7):779–84.

194. Sato K, Nishiwaki K, Kuno N, Kumagai K, Kitamura H, Yano K, Okamoto S, Ishikawa K, Shimada Y. Unexpected hyperkalemia following succinylcholine administration in prolonged immobilized parturients treated with magnesium and ritodrine. Anesthesiology 2000;93(6):1539–41.

195. Pascuzzi RM. Drugs and toxins associated with myopathies. Curr Opin Rheumatol 1998;10(6):511–20.

196. Sholl JS, Hughey MJ, Hirschmann RA. Myotonic muscular dystrophy associated with ritodrine tocolysis. Am J Obstet Gynecol 1985;151(1):83–6.

197. Gronert GA. Cardiac arrest after succinylcholine: mortality greater with rhabdomyolysis than receptor upregulation. Anesthesiology 2001;94(3):523–9.

198. Martyn JA, White DA, Gronert GA, Jaffe RS, Ward JM. Up-and-down regulation of skeletal muscle acetylcholine receptors. Effects on neuromuscular blockers. Anesthesiology 1992;76(5):822–43.

199. Axelsson J, Thesleff S. A study of supersensitivity in denervated mammalian skeletal muscle. J Physiol 1959;147(1):178–93.

200. Kendig JJ, Bunker JP, Endow S. Succinylcholine-induced hyperkalemia: effects of succinylcholine on resting potentials and electrolyte distributions in normal and denervated muscle. Anesthesiology 1972;36(2):132–7.

201. Gronert GA, Lambert EH, Theye RA. The response of denervated skeletal muscle to succinylcholine. Anesthesiology 1973;39(1):13–22.

202. Fischbach GD, Robbins N. Effect of chronic disuse of rat soleus neuromuscular junctions on postsynaptic membrane. J Neurophysiol 1971;34(4):562–9.

203. O'Brien DJ, Moriarty DC, Hope CE. The effect of pre-existing beta blockade on potassium flux in patients receiving succinylcholine. Can Anaesth Soc J 1986;3:S89.

204. McCammon RL, Stoelting RK. Exaggerated increase in serum potassium following succinylcholine in dogs with beta blockade. Anesthesiology 1984;61(6):723–5.

205. Koide M, Waud BE. Serum potassium concentrations after succinylcholine in patients with renal failure. Anesthesiology 1972;36(2):142–5.

206. Schaner PJ, Brown RL, Kirksey TD, Gunther RC, Ritchey CR, Gronert GA. Succinylcholine-induced hyperkalemia in burned patients. 1. Anesth Analg 1969;48(5):764–70.

207. Tolmie JD, Joyce TH, Mitchell GD. Succinylcholine danger in the burned patient. Anesthesiology 1967;28(2):467–70.

208. Mazze RI, Escue HM, Houston JB. Hyperkalemia and cardiovascular collapse following administration of succinylcholine to the traumatized patient. Anesthesiology 1969;31(6):540–7.

209. Birch AA Jr, Mitchell GD, Playford GA, Lang CA. Changes in serum potassium response to succinylcholine following trauma. JAMA 1969;210(3):490–3.

210. Stone WA, Beach TP, Hamelberg W. Succinylcholine — danger in the spinal-cord-injured patient. Anesthesiology 1970;32(2):168–9.

211. Cooperman LH. Succinylcholine-induced hyperkalemia in neuromuscular disease. JAMA 1970;213(11):1867–71.

212. Tobey RE, Jacobsen PM, Kahle CT, Clubb RJ, Dean MA. The serum potassium response to muscle relaxants in neural injury. Anesthesiology 1972;37(3):332–7.

213. Beach TP, Stone WA, Hamelberg W. Circulatory collapse following succinylcholine: report of a patient with diffuse lower motor neuron disease. Anesth Analg 1971;50(3):431–7.

214. Fergusson RJ, Wright DJ, Willey RF, Crompton GK, Grant IW. Suxamethonium is dangerous in polyneuropathy. BMJ (Clin Res Ed) 1981;282(6260):298–9.

215. Roth F, Wuthrich H. The clinical importance of hyperkalaemia following suxamethonium administration. Br J Anaesth 1969;41(4):311–6.

216. Cowgill DB, Mostello LA, Shapiro HM. Encephalitis and a hyperkalemic response to succinycholine. Anesthesiology 1974;40(4):409–11.

217. Gravlee GP. Succinylcholine-induced hyperkalemia in a patient with Parkinson's disease. Anesth Analg 1980;59(6):444–6.

218. Rao TL, Shanmugam M. Succinylcholine administration — another contraindication? Anesth Analg 1979;58(1):61–2.

219. Krikken-Hogenberk LG, de Jong JR, Bovill JG. Succinylcholine-induced hyperkalemia in a patient with metastatic rhabdomyosarcoma. Anesthesiology 1989;70(3):553–5.

220. Iwatsuki N, Kuroda N, Amaha K, Iwatsuki K. Succinylcholine-induced hyperkalemia in patients with ruptured cerebral aneurysms. Anesthesiology 1980;53(1):64–7.

221. Kohlschutter B, Baur H, Roth F. Suxamethonium-induced hyperkalaemia in patients with severe intra-abdominal infections. Br J Anaesth 1976;48(6):557–62.

222. Khan TZ, Khan RM. Changes in serum potassium following succinylcholine in patients with infections. Anesth Analg 1983;62(3):327–31.

223. Gronert GA. Succinylcholine hyperkalemia after burns. Anesthesiology 1999;91(1):320–2.

224. Booij LH. Is succinylcholine appropriate or obsolete in the intensive care unit? Crit Care 2001;5(5):245–6.

225. Al-Khafaji AH, Dewhirst WE, Cornell CJ Jr, Quill TJ. Succinylcholine-induced hyperkalemia in a patient with mucositis secondary to chemotherapy. Crit Care Med 2001;29(6):1274–6.

226. Soliman IE, Park TS, Berkelhamer MC. Transient paralysis after intrathecal bolus of baclofen for the treatment of post-selective dorsal rhizotomy pain in children. Anesth Analg 1999;89(5):1233–5.

227. Yaksh TL. A drug has to do what a drug has to do. Anesth Analg 1999;89(5):1075–7.

228. Schow AJ, Lubarsky DA, Olson RP, Gan TJ. Can succinylcholine be used safely in hyperkalemic patients? Anesth Analg 2002;95(1):119–22.

229. Gronert GA, Theye RA. Pathophysiology of hyperkalemia induced by succinylcholine. Anesthesiology 1975;43(1):89–99.

230. Yentis SM. Suxamethonium and hyperkalaemia. Anaesth Intensive Care 1990;18(1):92–101.

231. Muravchick S, Burkett L, Gold MI. Succinylcholine-induce fasciculations and intragastric pressure during induction of anesthesia. Anesthesiology 1981;55(2):180–3.

232. Salem MR, Wong AY, Lin YH. The effect of suxamethonium on the intragastric pressure in infants and children. Br J Anaesth 1972;44(2):166–70.

233. Roe RB. The effect of suxamethonium on intragastric pressure. Anaesthesia 1962;17:179–81.

234. Miller RD, Way WL. Inhibition of succinylcholine-induced increased intragastric pressure by nondepolarizing muscle relaxants and lidocaine. Anesthesiology 1971;34(2):185–8.

235. La Cour D. Rise in intragastric pressure caused by suxamethonium fasciculations. Acta Anaesthesiol Scand 1969;13(4):255–61.

236. Marchand P. The gastro-oesophageal sphincter and the mechanism of regurgitation. Br J Surg 1955;42(175):504–13.

237. Greenan J. The cardio-oesophageal junction. Br J Anaesth 1961;33:432–9.

238. Smith G, Dalling R, Williams TI. Gastro-oesophageal pressure gradient changes produced by induction of anaesthesia and suxamethonium. Br J Anaesth 1978;50(11):1137–43.

239. La Cour D. Prevention of rise in intragastric pressure due to suxamethonium fasciculations by prior dose of D-tubocurarine. Acta Anaesthesiol Scand 1970;14(1):5–15.

240. Bishop MJ, Hornbein TF. Prolonged effect of succinylcholine after neostigmine and pyridostigmine administration in patients with renal failure. Anesthesiology 1983;58(4):384–6.

241. Bennike KA, Jarnum S. Myoglobinuria with acute renal failure possibly induced by suxamethonium. A case report. Br J Anaesth 1964;36:730–6.

242. Wong SF, Chung F. Succinylcholine-associated postoperative myalgia. Anaesthesia 2000;55(2):144–52.

243. Manataki AD, Arnaoutoglou HM, Tefa LK, Glatzounis GK, Papadopoulos GS. Continuous propofol administration for suxamethonium-induced postoperative myalgia. Anaesthesia 1999;54(5):419–22.

244. Bourne JG, Collier HO, Somers GF. Succinylcholine (succinoylcholine), muscle-relaxant of short action. Lancet 1952;1(25):1225–9.

245. Smith NL. Histamine release by suxamethonium. Anaesthesia 1957;12(3):293–8.

246. Bele-Binda N, Valeri F. A case of bronchospasm induced by succinylcholine. Can Anaesth Soc J 1971;18(1):116–9.

247. Redderson C, Perkins HM, Adler WH, Gravenstein JS. Systemic reaction to succinylcholine: a case report. Anesth Analg 1971;50(1):49–52.

248. Sitarz L. Anaphylactic shock following injection of suxamethonium. Anaesth Resusc Intensive Ther 1974;2(1):83–6.

249. Mandappa JM, Chandrasekhara PM, Nelvigi RG. Anaphylaxis to suxamethonium. Two case reports. Br J Anaesth 1975;47(4):523–5.

250. James OF, Aseervatham SD, Fortunaso B, Clancy R. Anaphylactoid reaction to suxamethonium. Anaesth Intensive Care 1979;7(3):288.

251. Kepes ER, Haimovici H. Allergic reaction to succinylcholine. JAMA 1959;171:548–9.

252. Jerums G, Whittingham S, Wilson P. Anaphylaxis to suxamethonium. A case report. Br J Anaesth 1967;39(1):73–7.

253. Moss J, Fahmy NR, Sunder N, Beaven MA. Hormonal and hemodynamic profile of an anaphylactic reaction in man. Circulation 1981;63(1):210–3.

254. Fellini AA, Bernstein RL, Zauder HL. Bronchospasm due to suxamethonium; report of a case. Br J Anaesth 1963;35:657–9.

255. Katz AM, Mulligan PG. Bronchospasm induced by suxamethonium. A case report. Br J Anaesth 1972;44(10):1097–9.

256. Fisher MM, Munro I. Life-threatening anaphylactoid reactions to muscle relaxants. Anesth Analg 1983;62(6):559–64.

257. Laxenaire MC, Moneret-Vautrin DA, Vervloet D, Alazia M, Francois G. Accidents anaphylactoïdes graves peranesthésiques. [Severe peranesthetic anaphylactic accident.] Ann Fr Anesth Reanim 1985;4(1):30–46.

258. Laxenaire MC, Moneret-Vautrin DA, Vervloet D. The French experience of anaphylactoid reactions. Int Anesthesiol Clin 1985;23(3):145–60.

259. Galletly DC, Treuren BC. Anaphylactoid reactions during anaesthesia. Seven years' experience of intradermal testing. Anaesthesia 1985;40(4):329–33.

260. Youngman PR, Taylor KM, Wilson JD. Anaphylactoid reactions to neuromuscular blocking agents: a commonly undiagnosed condition? Lancet 1983;2(8350):597–9.

261. Vuitton D, Neidhardt-Audion M, Girardin P, Racadot E, Geissmann C, Laurent R, Barale F. Caractéristiques épidemiologiques de 21 accidents anaphylactoïdes peranesthésiques observés dans une population de 12,855 sujets opérés. [Epidemiologic characteristics of 21 peranesthetic anaphylactoid accidents observed in a population of 12,855 surgically treated patients.] Ann Fr Anesth Reanim 1985;4(2):167–72.

262. Laxenaire MC, Moneret-Vautrin DA, Boileau S. Choc anaphylactique au suxaméthonium: à propos de 18 cas. [Anaphylactic shock induced by suxamethonium.] Ann Fr Anesth Reanim 1982;1(1):29–36.

263. Wright PJ, Shortland JR, Stevens JD, Parsons MA, Watkins J. Fatal haemopathological consequences of general anaesthesia. Br J Anaesth 1989;62(1):104–7.

264. Moneret-Vautrin DA, Widmer S, Gueant JL, Kamel L, Laxenaire MC, Mouton C, Gerard H. Simultaneous anaphylaxis to thiopentone and a neuromuscular blocker: a study of two cases. Br J Anaesth 1990;64(6):743–5.

265. Gronert GA, Thompson RL, Onofrio BM. Human malignant hyperthermia: awake episodes and correction by dantrolene. Anesth Analg 1980;59(5):377–8.

266. Britt BA. Dantrolene. Can Anaesth Soc J 1984;31(1):61–75.

267. Ward A, Chaffman MO, Sorkin EM. Dantrolene. A review of its pharmacodynamic and pharmacokinetic properties and therapeutic use in malignant hyperthermia, the neuroleptic malignant syndrome and an update of its use in muscle spasticity. Drugs 1986;32(2):130–68.

268. Kolb ME, Horne ML, Martz R. Dantrolene in human malignant hyperthermia. Anesthesiology 1982;56(4):254–62.

269. Weingarten AE, Korsh JI, Neuman GG, Stern SB. Postpartum uterine atony after intravenous dantrolene. Anesth Analg 1987;66(3):269–70.

270. Hara Y, Kato A, Horikawa H, Kato Y, Ichiyanagi K. [Postoperative respiratory depression thought to be due to oral dantrolene pretreatment in a malignant hyperthermia-susceptible patient.]Masui 1988;37(4):483–7.

271. Saltzman LS, Kates RA, Corke BC, Norfleet EA, Heath KR. Hyperkalemia and cardiovascular collapse after verapamil and dantrolene administration in swine. Anesth Analg 1984;63(5):473–8.

272. Rubin AS, Zablocki AD. Hyperkalemia, verapamil, and dantrolene. Anesthesiology 1987;66(2):246–9.

273. Moya F, Kvisselgaard N. The placental transmission of succinylcholine. Anesthesiology 1961;22:1–6.

274. Kvisselgaard N, Moya F. Investigation of placental thresholds to succinylcholine. Anesthesiology 1961;22:7–10.

275. Weis OF, Muller FO, Lyell H, Badenhorst CH, van Niekerk P. Materno-fetal cholinesterase inhibitor poisoning. Anesth Analg 1983;62(2):233–5.

276. Hoefnagel D, Harris NA, Kim TH. Transient respiratory depression of the newborn. Its occurrence after succinylcholine administration to the mother. Am J Dis Child 1979;133(8):825–6.

277. Cherala SR, Eddie DN, Sechzer PH. Placental transfer of succinylcholine causing transient respiratory depression in the newborn. Anaesth Intensive Care 1989;17(2):202–4.

278. Hodges RJ, Harkness J. Suxamethonium sensitivity in health and disease; a clinical evaluation of pseudo-cholinesterase levels. BMJ 1954;4878:18–22.

279. Birch JH, Foldes FF, Rendell-Baker L. Causes and prevention of prolonged apnea with succinylcholine. Curr Res Anesth Analg 1956;35(6):609–33.

280. Shnider SM. Serum chlonesterase activity during pregnancy, labor and the puerperium. Anesthesiology 1965;26:335–9.

281. Robertson GS. Serum cholinesterase deficiency. II. Pregnancy. Br J Anaesth 1966;38(5):361–9.

282. Hazel B, Monier D. Human serum cholinesterase: variations during pregnancy and post-partum. Can Anaesth Soc J 1971;18(3):272–7.

283. Evans RT, Wroe JM. Plasma cholinesterase changes during pregnancy. Their interpretation as a cause of suxamethonium-induced apnoea. Anaesthesia 1980;35(7):651–4.

284. Robson N, Robertson I, Whittaker M. Plasma cholinesterase changes during the puerperium. Anaesthesia 1986;41(3):243–9.

285. Davies JM, Carmichael D, Dymond C. Plasma cholinesterase and trophoblastic disease. Gestational trophoblastic disease and reduced activity of plasma cholinesterase. Anaesthesia 1983;38(11):1071–4.

286. Kaniaris P, Fassoulaki A, Liarmakopoulou K, Dermitzakis E. Serum cholinesterase levels in patients with cancer. Anesth Analg 1979;58(2):82–4.

287. Goertz B, Spieckermann B, Leven B, et al. Succinylunverträglichkeit mit achtwöchiger Atemlähmung. Intensivmedizin 1977;14:88.

288. Evans RT, MacDonald R, Robinson A. Suxamethonium apnoea associated with plasmaphoresis. Anaesthesia 1980;35(2):198–201.

289. Paterson JL, Walsh ES, Hall GM. Progressive depletion of plasma cholinesterase during daily plasma exchange. BMJ 1979;2(6190):580.

290. Whittaker M. Plasma cholinesterase variants and the anaesthetist. Anaesthesia 1980;35(2):174–97.

291. Jensen FS, Viby-Mogensen J, Ostergaard D. Significance of plasma cholinesterase for the anaesthetist. Curr Anaesth Crit Care 1991;2:232.

292. Davis L, Britten JJ, Morgan M. Cholinesterase. Its significance in anaesthetic practice. Anaesthesia 1997;52(3):244–60.

293. Foldes FF. Myasthenia gravis. In: Katz RL, editor. Muscle Relaxants. Amsterdam: Excerpta Medica, 1975:345.

294. Azar I. The response of patients with neuromuscular disorders to muscle relaxants: a review. Anesthesiology 1984;61(2):173–87.

295. Martz DG, Schreibman DL, Matjasko MJ. Neurological diseases. In: Katz RL, Benumof JL, Kadis LB, editors. Anesthesia and Uncommon Diseases. 3rd ed.. Philadelphia: W.B. Saunders, 1990:560.

296. Miller JD, Lee C. Muscle diseases. In: Katz RL, Benumof JL, Kadis LB, editors. Anesthesia and Uncommon Diseases. 3rd ed.. Philadelphia: W.B. Saunders, 1990:590.

297. Perry J, Lee J, Wells G. Rocuronium versus succinylcholine for rapid sequence induction intubation (Cochrane Review). In: The Cochrane Library. Oxford: Update Software, 2003:1.

298. Beck GN, Masterson GR, Richards J, Bunting P. Comparison of intubation following propofol and alfentanil with intubation following thiopentone and suxamethonium. Anaesthesia 1993;48(10):876–80.

299. Scheller MS, Zornow MH, Saidman LJ. Tracheal intubation without the use of muscle relaxants: a technique using propofol and varying doses of alfentanil. Anesth Analg 1992;75(5):788–93.

300. Wong AK, Teoh GS. Intubation without muscle relaxant: an alternative technique for rapid tracheal intubation. Anaesth Intensive Care 1996;24(2):224–30.

301. Stevens JB, Vescovo MV, Harris KC, Walker SC, Hickey R. Tracheal intubation using alfentanil and no muscle relaxant: is the choice of hypnotic important? Anesth Analg 1997;84(6):1222–6.

302. Klemola UM, Mennander S, Saarnivaara L. Tracheal intubation without the use of muscle relaxants: remifentanil or alfentanil in combination with propofol. Acta Anaesthesiol Scand 2000;44(4):465–9.

303. Erhan E, Ugur G, Alper I, Gunusen I, Ozyar B. Tracheal intubation without muscle relaxants: remifentanil or alfentanil in combination with propofol. Eur J Anaesthesiol 2003;20(1):37–43.

304. Naguib M, Samarkandi A, Riad W, Alharby SW. Optimal dose of succinylcholine revisited. Anesthesiology 2003;99:1045–9.

305. Kopman AF, Zhaku B, Lai KS. The "intubating dose" of succinylcholine: the effect of decreasing doses on recovery time. Anesthesiology 2003;99:1050–4.

306. Donati F. The right dose of succinylcholine. Anesthesiology 2003;99:1037–8.

307. Norris JC. Prolonged succinylcholine apnoea resulting from acquired deficiency of plasma cholinesterase. Anaesthesia 2003;58:1137.

308. Dillman JB. Safe use of succinylcholine during repeated anesthetics in a patient treated with cyclophosphamide. Anesth Analg 1987;66:351–3.

309. Miller RD, Way WL, Katzung BG. The potentiation of neuromuscular blocking agents by quinidine. Anesthesiology 1967;28(6):1036–41.

310. Durant NN, Nguyen N, Katz RL. Potentiation of neuromuscular blockade by verapamil. Anesthesiology 1984; 60(4):298–303.

311. Chasapakis G, Dimas C. Possible interaction between muscle relaxants and the kallikrein-trypsin inactivator "Trasylol". Report of three cases. Br J Anaesth 1966;38(10):838–9.

312. Fisher DM, Caldwell JE, Sharma M, Wiren JE. The influence of bambuterol (carbamylated terbutaline) on the duration of action of succinylcholine-induced paralysis in humans. Anesthesiology 1988;69(5):757–9.

313. Avery GS. Check-list to potential clinically important interactions. Drugs 1973;5(3):187–211.

314. Blanloeil Y, Pinaud M, Nicolas F. Arythmies per-operatoires chez le coronarien digitalise. Vingt-quatre cas. [Perioperative cardiac arrhythmias in digitalized patients with ischemic heart disease.] Anesth Analg (Paris) 1980; 37(11–12):669–74.

315. Zsigmond EK, Robins G. The effect of a series of anti-cancer drugs on plasma cholinesterase activity. Can Anaesth Soc J 1972;19(1):75–82.

316. Gurman GM. Prolonged apnea after succinylcholine in a case treated with cytostatics for cancer. Anesth Analg 1972;51(5):761–5.

317. Dretchen KL, Morgenroth VH 3rd, Standaert FG, Walts LF. Azathioprine: effects on neuromuscular transmission. Anesthesiology 1976;45(6):604–9.

318. Sprung J, Castellani WJ, Srinivasan V, Udayashankar S. The effects of donepezil and neostigmine in a patient with unusual pseudocholinesterase activity. Anesth Analg 1998;87(5):1203–5.

319. Friedhoff LT, Rogers SL. Correlation between the clinical efficacy of donepezil HCl (E2020) and red-blood cell (RBC) acetylcholinesterase (ACHE) inhibition in patients with Alzheimer's disease. Clin Pharmacol Ther 1997;61:177.

320. Bevan DR, Donati F, Kopman AF. Reversal of neuromuscular blockade. Anesthesiology 1992;77(4):785–805.

321. Crowe S, Collins L. Suxamethonium and donepezil: a cause of prolonged paralysis. Anesthesiology 2003;98(2):574–5.

322. Sanchez Morillo J, Demartini Ferrari A, Roca de Togores Lopez A. Interacción entre donepezilo y bloqueantes musculares en la enfermedad de Alzheimer. [Interaction of donepezil and muscular blockers in Alzheimer's disease.] Rev Esp Anestesiol Reanim 2003;50(2):97–100.

323. Heath ML. Donepezil and succinylcholine. Anaesthesia 2003;58(2):202.

324. Gesztes T. Prolonged apnoea after suxamethonium injection associated with eye drops containing an anticholinesterase agent. Br J Anaesth 1966;38(5):408–9.

325. Pantuck EJ. Ecothiopate iodide eye drops and prolonged response to suxamethonium. Br J Anaesth 1966;38(5):406–7.

326. Deroetth A Jr, Dettbarn WD, Rosenberg P, Wilensky JG, Wong A. Effect of phospholine iodide on blood cholinesterase levels of normal and glaucoma subjects. Am J Ophthalmol 1965;59:586–92.

327. McGavi DD. Depressed levels of serum-pseudocholinesterase with ecothiophate–iodide eyedrops. Lancet 1965; 19:272–3.

328. Barnes JM, Davies DR. Blood cholinesterase levels in workers exposed to organo-phosphorus insecticides. BMJ 1951;4735:816–9.

329. Robertson GS. Serum protein and cholinesterase changes in association with contraceptive pills. Lancet 1967;1(7484):232–5.

330. Whittaker M, Charlier AR, Ramaswamy S. Changes in plasma cholinesterase isoenzymes due to oral contraceptives. J Reprod Fertil 1971;26(3):373–5.

331. Archer TL, Janowsky EC. Plasma pseudocholinesterase deficiency associated with diethylstilbestrol therapy. Anesth Analg 1978;57(6):726–32.

332. Foldes FF, Arai T, Gentsch HH, Zarday Z. The influence of glucocorticoids on plasma cholinesterase. Proc Soc Exp Biol Med 1974;146(3):918–20.

333. Verjee ZH, Behal R, Ayim EM. Effect of glucocorticoids on liver and blood cholinesterases. Clin Chim Acta 1977; 81(1):41–6.

334. Bradamante V, Kunec-Vajic E, Lisic M, Dobric I, Beus I. Plasma cholinesterase activity in patients during therapy with dexamethasone or prednisone. Eur J Clin Pharmacol 1989;36(3):253–7.

335. Bovill JG, Coppel DL, Dundee JW, Moore J. Current status of ketamine anaesthesia. Lancet 1971;1(7712):1285–8.

336. Tsai SK, Lee CM, Tran B. Ketamine enhances phase I and phase II neuromuscular block of succinylcholine. Can J Anaesth 1989;36(2):120–3.

337. Amaki Y, Nagashima H, Radnay PA, Foldes FF. Ketamine interaction with neuromuscular blocking agents in the phrenic nerve-hemidiaphragm preparation of the rat. Anesth Analg 1978;57(2):238–43.

338. Johnston RR, Miller RD, Way WL. The interaction of ketamine with D-tubocurarine, pancuronium, and succinylcholine in man. Anesth Analg 1974;53(4):496–501.

339. Hilgenberg JC, Stoelting RK. Characteristics of succinylcholine-produced phase II neuromuscular block during enflurane, halothane, and fentanyl anesthesia. Anesth Analg 1981;60(4):192–6.

340. Donati F, Bevan DR. Long-term succinylcholine infusion during isoflurane anesthesia. Anesthesiology 1983;58(1):6–10.

341. Cozanitis DA, Dundee JW, Khan MM. Comparative study of atropine and glycopyrrolate on suxamethonium-induced changes in cardiac rate and rhythm. Br J Anaesth 1980;52(3):291–3.

342. Hill GE, Wong KC, Hodges MR. Potentiation of succinylcholine neuromuscular blockade by lithium carbonate. Anesthesiology 1976;44(5):439–42.

343. Hill GE, Wong KC, Hodges MR. Lithium carbonate and neuromuscular blocking agents. Anesthesiology 1977; 46(2):122–6.

344. Schou M. Possible mechanisms of action of lithium salts: approaches and perspectives. Biochem Soc Trans 1973;1:81.

345. Whittaker M, Spencer R. Plasma cholinesterase variants in patients having lithium therapy. Clin Chim Acta 1977;75(3):421–5.

346. Matsuo S, Rao DB, Chaudry I, Foldes FF. Interaction of muscle relaxants and local anesthetics at the neuromuscular junction. Anesth Analg 1978;57(5):580–7.

347. Usubiaga JE, Wikinski JA, Morales RL, Usubiaga LE. Interaction of intravenously administered procaine, lidocaine and succinylcholine in anesthetized subjects. Anesth Analg 1967;46(1):39–45.

348. Morris R, Ciesecke A. Potentiation of muscle relaxants by magnesium sulfate therapy in toxemia in pregnancy. South Med J 1968;61:25.

349. Skaredoff MN, Roaf ER, Datta S. Hypermagnesaemia and anaesthetic management. Can Anaesth Soc J 1982;29(1):35–41.

350. Ghoneim MM, Long JP. The interaction between magnesium and other neuromuscular blocking agents. Anesthesiology 1970;32(1):23–7.

351. Giesecke AH Jr, Morris RE, Dalton MD, Stephen CR. Of magnesium, muscle relaxants, toxemic parturients, and cats. Anesth Analg 1968;47(6):689–95.

352. De Vore JS, Asrani R. Magnesium sulfate prevents succinylcholine-induced fasciculations in toxemic parturients. Anesthesiology 1980;52(1):76–7.

353. Kambam JR, Parris WC, Franks JJ, Sastry BV. The inhibitory effect of metoclopramide on plasma cholinesterase activity. Anesth Analg 1988;67:S107.

354. Kao YJ, Turner DR. Prolongation of succinylcholine block by metoclopramide. Anesthesiology 1989;70(6):905–8.

355. Kao YJ, Tellez J, Turner DR. Dose-dependent effect of metoclopramide on cholinesterases and suxamethonium metabolism. Br J Anaesth 1990;65(2):220–4.

356. Gissen AJ, Katz RL, Karis JH, Papper EM. Neuromuscular block in man during prolonged arterial infusion with succinylcholine. Anesthesiology 1966;27(3):242–9.

357. Ivankovich AD, Sidell N, Cairoli VJ, Dietz AA, Albrecht RF. Dual action of pancuronium on succinylcholine block. Can Anaesth Soc J 1977;24(2):228–42.

358. Ebeling BJ, Keienburg T, Hausmann D, Apffelstaedt C. Das Wirkungsprofil von Succinylcholin nach Präcurarisierung mit Atracurium, Vecuronium oder Pancuronium. [Profile of the effect of succinylcholine after pre-curarization with atracurium, vecuronium or pancuronium.] Anästhesiol Intensivmed Notfallmed Schmerzther 1996;31(5):304–8.

359. d'Hollander AA, Agoston S, De Ville A, Cuvelier F. Clinical and pharmacological actions of a bolus injection of suxamethonium: two phenomena of distinct duration. Br J Anaesth 1983;55(2):131–4.

360. Katz RL. Modification of the action of pancuronium by succinylcholine and halothane. Anesthesiology 1971;35(6):602–6.

361. Bowman WC. Non-relaxant properties of neuromuscular blocking drugs. Br J Anaesth 1982;54(2):147–60.

362. Walts LF, Dillon JB. Clinical studies of the interaction between D-tubocurarine and succinylcholine. Anesthesiology 1969;31(1):35–8.

363. Scott RP, Norman J. Effect of suxamethonium given during recovery from atracurium. Br J Anaesth 1988;61(3):292–6.

364. Kim KS, Na DJ, Chon SU. Interactions between suxamethonium and mivacurium or atracurium. Br J Anaesth 1996;77(5):612–6.

365. Bodley PO, Halwax K, Potts L. Low serum pseudocholinesterase levels complicating treatment with phenelzine. BMJ 1969;3(669):510–2.

366. Foldes FF, Hillmer NR, Molloy RE, Monte AP. Potentiation of the neuromuscular effect of succinylcholine by hexafluorenium. Anesthesiology 1960;21:50–8.

367. Gordh T, Wahlin A. Potentiation of the neuromuscular effect of succinylcholine by tetrahydro-amino-acridine. Acta Anaesthesiol Scand 1961;5:55–61.

368. Walts LF, DeAngelis J, Dillon JB. Clinical studies of the interaction of hexafluorenium and succinylcholine in man. Anesthesiology 1970;33(5):503–7.

369. Radnay PA, El-Gaweet ES, Novakovic M, Badola R, Cizmar S, Duncalf D. Prevention of succinylcholine

370. Katz RL, Eakins KE, Lord CO. The effects of hexafluorenium in preventing the increase in intraocular pressure produced by succinylcholine. Anesthesiology 1968;29(1):70–8.

371. Tewfik GI. Trimetaphan; its effect on the pseudo-cholinesterase level of man. Anaesthesia 1957;12(3):326–9.

372. Sklar GS, Lanks KW. Effects of trimethaphan and sodium nitroprusside on hydrolysis of succinylcholine in vitro. Anesthesiology 1977;47(1):31–3.

373. Poulton TJ, James FM 3rd, Lockridge O. Prolonged apnea following trimethaphan and succinylcholine. Anesthesiology 1979;50(1):54–6.

374. Nakamura K, Hatano Y, Mori K. The site of action of trimethaphan-induced neuromuscular blockade in isolated rat and frog muscle. Acta Anaesthesiol Scand 1988;32(2):125–30.

375 Matsuo S, Rao DB, Chaudry I, Foldes FF. Interaction of muscle relaxants and local anesthetics at the neuromuscular junction. Anesth Analg 1978;57(5):580–7.

376 Usubiaga JE, Wikinski JA, Morales RL, Usubiaga LE. Interaction of intravenously administered procaine, lidocaine and succinylcholine in anesthetized subjects. Anesth Analg 1967;46(1):39–45.

377 Matsuo S, Rao DB, Chaudry I, Foldes FF. Interaction of muscle relaxants and local anesthetics at the neuromuscular junction. Anesth Analg 1978;57(5):580–7.

378 Matsuo S, Rao DB, Chaudry I, Foldes FF. Interaction of muscle relaxants and local anesthetics at the neuromuscular junction. Anesth Analg 1978;57(5):580–7.

379 Usubiaga JE, Wikinski JA, Morales RL, Usubiaga LE. Interaction of intravenously administered procaine, lidocaine and succinylcholine in anesthetized subjects. Anesth Analg 1967;46(1):39–45.

380 Stirt JA, Katz RL, Murray AL, Schehl DL, Lee C. Modification of atracurium blockade by halothane and by suxamethonium. A review of clinical experience. Br J Anaesth 1983;55(Suppl 1):S71–5.

381 Randell T, Yli-Hankala A, Lindgren L. Isoflurane inhibits muscle fasciculations caused by succinylcholine in children. Acta Anaesthesiol Scand 1993;37(3):262–4.

induced hyperkalemia by neuroleptanesthesia and hexafluorenium in anephric patients. Anaesthesist 1981;30(7):334–7.

Tubocurarine

General Information

D-Tubocurarine is the standard non-depolarizing neuromuscular blocking agent against which all others of the group are compared. The molecule has one quaternary and one tertiary nitrogen, the latter being protonated at body pH, making it a bisquaternary entity. Its main action at the neuromuscular junction is to block the access of acetylcholine to the receptor recognition sites competitively; it may also block some ion channels, but only to a small extent and at very high concentrations.

Blockade of neuromuscular transmission by D-tubocurarine is easily reversed (if twitch height has recovered to at least 10%) by anticholinesterases. Sensitivity to D-tubocurarine and other non-depolarizing relaxants is highly variable, even in apparently healthy patients, so that the small doses given for precurarization can lead to appreciable paralysis (1–3). More commonly, residual blockade can be detected postoperatively (4,5), long after the expected recovery of neuromuscular transmission.

About 40–50% of a normal dose of D-tubocurarine is bound to plasma proteins, mostly gammaglobulins (about 25%). This binding is highly variable, giving a variable amount of non-bound drug available for neuromuscular blockade. Metabolism does not occur. Tubocurarine is eliminated principally via glomerular filtration (about 40–60% in 24 hours), but has an alternative pathway for excretion in the bile (normally only about 12% in 24 hours). The initial dose for healthy patients is 0.2–0.5 mg/kg, dependent on the anesthetic agents used and whether suxamethonium is given beforehand or not. Maintenance doses are about one-third of the initial dose and are required at approximately 30–40-minute intervals. Accumulation can occur and is more likely if large doses are given too frequently or if excretion is impaired. Smaller doses should be given if the patient has received D-tubocurarine within the previous 24 hours.

General adverse effects

A fall in blood pressure occurs almost always with D-tubocurarine. It is often mild, but may be marked, particularly if a large dose is given rapidly or if the patient is hypovolemic, or has a diminished cardiac reserve or capacity for vasoconstriction (as is not infrequently the case in old age, in diabetes, and in other diseases with sympathetic neuropathy), and is potentiated by other anesthetic agents such as halothane. Myasthenic patients or patients with other neuromuscular pathology are markedly sensitive to non-depolarizing relaxants.

Histamine-mediated reactions are common, leading to local wheal-and-flare effects near the injection site, frequent hypotension (mostly about a 20% fall), and occasionally bronchospasm.

Malignant hyperthermia has also been reported after D-tubocurarine.

Tumor-inducing effects have not been reported.

Drug resistance

Patients with burns require more D-tubocurarine (and higher plasma concentrations) for the same degree of blockade compared with non-burned patients (6). The mechanism is not known, but it appears not to be altered pharmacokinetics (7). The resistance to non-depolarizing neuromuscular blocking agents (SEDA-8, 136) appears to be influenced by the size of the body surface area burned and by the time which has elapsed since the injury (see Atracurium). In extensive burns dose requirements are increased approximately by a factor of 2–3.

Patients with upper motor neuron lesions such as hemiplegia (8–11) and possibly multiple sclerosis (SEDA-13, 105) (12) can be resistant to various non-depolarizing blockers. Lower motor neuron injury has so far only been reported to produce this phenomenon in rats (13) and dogs. Affected muscles in these conditions are paralysed to a lesser degree than unaffected muscles, and this

has to be taken into account when siting the electrodes for monitoring a block and in assessing recovery therefrom. The mechanism is probably a quantitative and/or qualitative change in acetylcholine receptors. Resistance is seen too in patients taking certain drugs such as phenytoin, carbamazepine, and, disputedly, azathioprine.

In liver disease, increased amounts of D-tubocurarine may be required. In the past it has been suggested that this could be due to reduced synthesis of acetylcholinesterase, or to increased concentrations of gammaglobulins binding the relaxant (14), although this is disputed (15). Similar kinetic mechanisms to those suggested for pancuronium may be involved, but there are no studies on D-tubocurarine. In primary liver cancer in children, resistance to D-tubocurarine (and alcuronium) has been reported (SEDA-13, 104) (16).

Hyperkalemia tends to reduce the neuromuscular blocking effects of tubocurarine.

Organs and Systems

Cardiovascular

D-Tubocurarine commonly causes a fall in blood pressure, associated with a slight tachycardia and a reduction in total peripheral resistance; cardiac output is not affected. The frequency of hypotension is reported as being 20–90%. This wide range probably reflects the methods of measurement, the anesthetic agents used, and the general condition of the patients in the various studies, as well as the criteria for diagnosing hypotension. The magnitude of the fall in blood pressure is generally about 20%, and it occurs within 5 minutes of injection. Histamine release is considered to be the principal cause (17), but blockade of autonomic ganglia may also contribute. It has been suggested that prostacycline, released by histamine acting on H_1 receptors, is the final mediator; intravenous administration of aspirin or an H_1 receptor antagonist beforehand affords some protection (SEDA-15, 126) (18). Ganglion blockade may also contribute, particularly if high doses are used (19). Reduction in venous return secondary to muscle relaxation and alterations in intrathoracic and intra-abdominal pressures may also play a role. The fall in blood pressure can be greatly exaggerated in hypovolemic patients, in the elderly, and in others with reduced sympathetic tone. Tubocurarine should be used very cautiously in such patients or another relaxant should be chosen. Concurrent administration of agents known to cause circulatory depression aggravates the problem. The higher the halothane concentration, for example, the greater the fall in blood pressure after D-tubocurarine (20). Since the degree of hypotension seems to be linked to dose (17) and the rate of injection (21), it seems reasonable to use the smallest dose that produces adequate relaxation (under 0.5 mg/kg) and to inject it slowly (over at least 180 seconds) (SEDA-7, 141).

Respiratory

Tubocurarine can cause apnea. The muscles involved in protecting and maintaining the airway are more sensitive to D-tubocurarine than the muscles of ventilation (22,23) so that aspiration and airway obstruction are possible in the partially curarized patient at a time when spontaneous ventilation is adequate. Airway obstruction in the presence of vigorous respiratory efforts can eventually (and is rarely reported to) lead to negative pressure pulmonary edema (24,25). Hypoventilation can occur after doses as low as 1.5 mg in exceptionally sensitive patients. Postoperative hypoventilation, or apnea, is a danger in patients given certain antibiotics and antidysrhythmic drugs before or after apparently successful spontaneous reversal or antagonism of a non-depolarizing block.

Potentiation of undetected residual curarization can also occur postoperatively from respiratory acidosis.

Histamine release, common with D-tubocurarine, can cause bronchospasm. Tubocurarine is relatively contraindicated in asthmatic patients and in those with an allergic tendency.

Nervous system

Minute amounts of D-tubocurarine have been detected in cerebrospinal fluid (26). Although convulsions have been produced in animals by injection into the cerebrospinal fluid, and it has been suggested that exceptionally large doses can cause depression of medullary centers, there is insufficient information to draw any conclusions.

Pancuronium is reported to lower the MAC for halothane, but whether this is a central or peripheral action is not known.

Gastrointestinal

The motility of the gut may be reduced by tubocurarine, as a result of ganglion blockade.

Body temperature

Tubocurarine has been implicated as a trigger of malignant hyperthermia, particularly in combination with halothane (27), although doubts have been expressed (28). Increased muscular tone is not a feature with D-tubocurarine.

Second-Generation Effects

Pregnancy

Placental transfer of D-tubocurarine occurs (as with all relaxants) and low concentrations of the drug have been detected in umbilical blood. Under normal circumstances no untoward effects have been reported in neonates.

Paralysis occurred in a 28-week fetus, whose mother received D-tubocurarine for status epilepticus, and joint deformities possibly resulting from 4 weeks' maternal curarization during the first trimester have been reported (29).

Experiments in chick embryos have shown that D-tubocurarine can cause retardation of bone growth (30) and that malformations can be produced by in utero curarization (31). Long-term curarization during pregnancy is undesirable.

Susceptibility Factors

Genetic factors

Individual responses to these compounds differ (32–34). Racial differences and environmental factors can influence the response to relaxants and hence the extent of problems due to excessive activity. Patients in the USA reportedly require less D-tubocurarine than in the UK, and the West Indians need more. Difference in cholinesterase activities, perhaps brought about by more organophosphorus insecticides being used in one country than in another, or differences in protein-binding as a result of dietary factors, are possible explanations (35). Vecuronium has been reported to be approximately 30% more potent in Montreal than in Paris (36).

Age

In the elderly extreme falls in blood pressure can occur with D-tubocurarine (37).

Renal disease

In renal insufficiency the action of D-tubocurarine is increased (38) and prolonged (39).

The half-life in the complete absence of renal function is increased by 70% or more. The reduced ability of plasma proteins to bind the drug (40), if this indeed occurs, will result in a greater proportion of unbound D-tubocurarine and therefore increased potency.

Increased biliary excretion of D-tubocurarine occurs in renal insufficiency and compensates to a varying degree for reduced renal excretion (41). The slower rate of biliary (as opposed to renal) excretion will result in sharply increasing prolongation of neuromuscular blockade if large single doses are used or if multiple doses are given (42). A single small dose will result in little or no prolongation of effect, since redistribution will be mainly responsible for termination of the drug's effect. It has been suggested for several other non-depolarizing relaxants that the initial dose produces less effect in renal insufficiency (SEDA-13, 103).

The problem of accumulation may be marked in intensive care situations, where D-tubocurarine is used to maintain long-term paralysis (42). These patients may also have impaired renal and hepatic function, with protein and electrolyte imbalance. The timing of repeat injections of D-tubocurarine (and, indeed, all relaxant drugs) in such cases should be guided by monitoring of neuromuscular function (by response to single twitch, train-of-four, or tetanic stimulation, which is more sensitive but painful), or clinically by observing the return of muscle tone.

Other features of the patient

In hypovolemic patients, in patients with impaired sympathetic autonomic activity, and in patients operated on in the anti-Trendelenburg position, extreme falls in blood pressure can occur with D-tubocurarine. Hypotension is aggravated by the use of halothane in particular, and by other drugs that produce circulatory depression. In such cases, and in patients with hypertension, coronary artery disease, and arteriosclerosis, D-tubocurarine is better avoided.

Asthmatic and atopic individuals are at special risk from D-tubocurarine's histamine-releasing potential, and severe bronchospasm can result (43).

Greatly increased sensitivity occurs in myasthenia (44) and may even be seen in "premyasthenic" patients with no overt symptoms (45). Increased sensitivity has also been reported in amyotrophic lateral sclerosis (46), von Recklinghausen's disease (47), and ocular muscular dystrophy (48). Patients with Duchenne muscular dystrophy have prolonged block in the regional curare test (49), but other investigators have disputed whether an altered response to non-depolarizing relaxants occurs in this condition.

Patients with thyrotoxic myopathy, as with all forms of myopathy, are exceedingly sensitive to all non-depolarizing agents.

Drug–Drug Interactions

Antidysrhythmic drugs

Class I antidysrhythmic drugs, such as procainamide, lidocaine, propranolol, diphenylhydantoin (50), quinidine (51), and lidocaine (52) have all been claimed to enhance neuromuscular blockade by D-tubocurarine and other non-depolarizing agents. Bretylium (53) and disopyramide (54) are also reported to have their neuromuscular blocking activities potentiated by low concentrations of D-tubocurarine in animal experiments; neostigmine failed to reverse disopyramide-induced blockade (SEDA-13, 102) (55). The greatest hazard from these agents is that they can cause "recurarization" when given postoperatively. With bretylium this can occur several hours after its administration, as a result of its slow kinetics (53). Effects in man have still to be documented for bretylium, but "recurarization" 15 minutes after adequate reversal of vecuronium blockade with neostigmine has been described in a patient given disopyramide intravenously (SEDA-14, 116) (56).

Aprotinin

Reparalysis has been reported when aprotinin was used after operations during which suxamethonium had been given alone or in combination with normal doses of D-tubocurarine (57).

Atracurium dibesilate

Small doses of D-tubocurarine (0.05 or 0.1 mg/kg) administered 3 minutes before atracurium potentiated its action synergistically (SEDA-12, 117) (70).

Azathioprine

Azathioprine reduces sensitivity to D-tubocurarine in experimental animals, possibly as a result of phosphodiesterase inhibition, increasing transmitter release (SEDA-4, 87) (58), (SEDA-13, 104).

Calcium channel blockers

Calcium channel blockers, such as verapamil and nifedipine, can potentiate neuromuscular blocking agents (59,60) and it has been suggested that in long-term use they can accumulate in muscle and make block-reversal difficult (61).

Corticosteroids

There have been several contradictory reports of possible interactions of tubocurarine with corticosteroids. In general, it seems that the long-term use of steroids can reduce sensitivity to non-depolarizing neuromuscular blocking agents, while acute administration can cause potentiation (62). Long-term steroid treatment may be associated with the development of a myasthenic syndrome in some patients, who will therefore be very sensitive to neuromuscular blocking agents.

Diuretics

Furosemide (40–80 mg) has been reported to enhance and prolong D-tubocurarine-induced block in anephric patients (63). In animals low doses potentiated D-tubocurarine (and suxamethonium) probably via presynaptic effects, while high doses (1–40 mg/kg in cats) reversed the neuromuscular actions of these relaxants (64). The effects of high doses were similar to those of theophylline, and phosphodiesterase inhibition leading to increased acetylcholine release was postulated as a possible mechanism for the antagonism.

Potassium and magnesium loss as a result of the use of diuretics can affect non-depolarizing relaxants.

Doxapram

Doxapram, used as a respiratory stimulant, increased partial D-tubocurarine and pancuronium neuromuscular blockade when used in high concentrations in rats (SEDA-14, 113) (65). There have been no reports in man so far.

Ganglion-blocking agents

Trimetaphan and hexamethonium can potentiate D-tubocurarine-induced block, but clinical reports clearly showing this are lacking. Tubocurarine will increase their hypotensive effect. Neostigmine could theoretically facilitate the postulated end-plate ion channel block of trimetaphan (SEDA-13, 102) (66), which would complicate reversal of neuromuscular block.

Local anesthetics

Local anesthetics have diverse effects on the neuromuscular junction. In very large doses they produce paralysis on their own. When the recommended doses are used for local anesthesia, systemic absorption is small and interaction with relaxants is not to be expected. However, large doses injected intravascularly (accidentally, or therapeutically for dysrhythmias) can potentiate relaxants of both types (67,68).

Magnesium sulfate

Magnesium inhibits the release of acetylcholine and reduces the sensitivity of the postjunctional membrane. Thus, magnesium sulfate can cause neuromuscular transmission failure and enhance the effect of D-tubocurarine and other non-depolarizing neuromuscular blocking drugs (69). Not only have potentiation and prolongation of D-tubocurarine block been reported, but also respiratory depression when magnesium sulfate was given an hour after reversal of the relaxant. Presumably the muscle weakness resulted from potentiation of residual curarization. Whether the effects are additive or synergistic is disputed. Muscle relaxants must be used with caution and in reduced dosage in patients receiving magnesium sulfate. Reversal of the block may be difficult.

References

1. Rao TL, Jacobs HK. Pulmonary function following "pretreatment" dose of pancuronium in volunteers. Anesth Analg 1980;59(9):659–61.
2. Mayrhofer O. Die Wirksamheit von d-Tubocurarin zur Verhütung der Muskelschmerzen nach Succinylcholin. [The efficacy of d-tubocurarine in the prevention of muscle pains after succinylcholine.] Anaesthesist 1959;8:313.
3. Musich J, Walts LF. Pulmonary aspiration after a priming dose of vecuronium. Anesthesiology 1986;64(4):517–9.
4. Viby-Mogensen J, Jorgensen BC, Ording H. Residual curarization in the recovery room. Anesthesiology 1979;50(6):539–41.
5. Lennmarken C, Lofstrom JB. Partial curarization in the postoperative period. Acta Anaesthesiol Scand 1984;28(3):260–2.
6. Martyn JA, Szyfelbein SK, Ali HH, Matteo RS, Savarese JJ. Increased d-tubocurarine requirement following major thermal injury. Anesthesiology 1980;52(4):352–5.
7. Martyn JA, Matteo RS, Greenblatt DJ, Lebowitz PW, Savarese JJ. Pharmacokinetics of d-tubocurarine in patients with thermal injury. Anesth Analg 1982;61(3):241–6.
8. Shayevitz JR, Matteo RS. Decreased sensitivity to metocurine in patients with upper motoneuron disease. Anesth Analg 1985;64(8):767–72.
9. Moorthy SS, Hilgenberg JC. Resistance to non-depolarizing muscle relaxants in paretic upper extremities of patients with residual hemiplegia. Anesth Analg 1980;59(8):624–7.
10. Graham DH. Monitoring neuromuscular block may be unreliable in patients with upper-motor-neuron lesions. Anesthesiology 1980;52(1):74–5.
11. Laycock JR, Smith CE, Donati F, Bevan DR. Sensitivity of the adductor pollicis and diaphragm muscles to atracurium in a hemiplegic patient. Anesthesiology 1987;67(5):851–3.
12. Brett RS, Schmidt JH, Gage JS, Schartel SA, Poppers PJ. Measurement of acetylcholine receptor concentration in skeletal muscle from a patient with multiple sclerosis and resistance to atracurium. Anesthesiology 1987;66(6):837–9.
13. Hogue CW Jr, Itani MS, Martyn JA. Resistance to d-tubocurarine in lower motor neuron injury is related to increased acetylcholine receptors at the neuromuscular junction. Anesthesiology 1990;73(4):703–9.
14. Stovner J, Theodorsen L, Bjelke E. Sensitivity to tubocurarine and alcuronium with special reference to plasma protein pattern. Br J Anaesth 1971;43(4):385–91.
15. Duvaldestin P. Common disease states affecting the action of neuromuscular blocking drugs. In: Agoston S, Bowman WC, editors. Monographs in Anaesthesiology 19. Amsterdam: Elsevier Science Publishers BV, 1990:253.
16. Brown TC, Gregory M, Bell B, Campbell PC. Liver tumours and muscle relaxants. Electromyographic studies in children. Anaesthesia 1987;42(12):1284–6.
17. Moss J, Rosow CE, Savarese JJ, Philbin DM, Kniffen KJ. Role of histamine in the hypotensive action of d-tubocurarine in humans. Anesthesiology 1981;55(1):19–25.
18. Hatano Y, Arai T, Noda J, Komatsu K, Shinkura R, Nakajima Y, Sawada M, Mori K. Contribution of prostacyclin to D-tubocurarine-induced hypotension in humans. Anesthesiology 1990;72(1):28–32.
19. Marshall IG. Pharmacological effects of neuromuscular blocking agents: interaction with cholinoceptors other than nicotinic receptors of the neuromuscular junction. Anest Rianim 1986;27:19.
20. Munger WL, Miller RD, Stevens WC. The dependence of a d-tubocurarine-induced hypotension on alveolar concentration of halothane, dose of d-tubocurarine, and nitrous oxide. Anesthesiology 1974;40(5):442–8.
21. Stoelting RK, McCammon RL, Hilgenberg JC. Changes in blood pressure with varying rates of administration of d-tubocurarine. Anesth Analg 1980;59(9):697–9.
22. Pavlin EG, Holle RH. Schoene RB. Recovery of airway protection compared with ventilation in humans after paralysis with curare. Anesthesiology 1989;70(3):381–5.
23. Knill RL. D-tubocurarine and upper airway obstruction: a historical perspective. Anesthesiology 1989;71(3):480–1.
24. Warner LO, Martino JD, Davidson PJ, Beach TP. Negative pressure pulmonary oedema: a potential hazard of muscle relaxants in awake infants. Can J Anaesth 1990;37(5):580–3.
25. Brown RE. Negative pressure pulmonary edema. In: Berry FA, editor. Anesthetic Management of Difficult and Routine Pediatric Patients. New York: Churchill Livingstone, 1986:169.
26. Matteo RS, Pua EK, Khambatta HJ, Spector S. Cerebrospinal fluid levels of d-tubocurarine in man. Anesthesiology 1977;46(6):396–9.
27. Britt BA, Webb GE, LeDuc C. Malignant hyperthermia induced by curare. Can Anaesth Soc J 1974;21(4):371–5.
28. Gronert GA. Malignant hyperthermia. Anesthesiology 1980;53(5):395–423.
29. Older PO, Harris JM. Placental transfer of tubocurarine. Case report. Br J Anaesth 1968;40(6):459–63.
30. Ahmed W. The effect of relaxant drugs on the growth and development of bone and cartilage in the chick embryo. Ain Shams Med J 1970;21:679.
31. Drachman DB, Coulombre AJ. Experimental clubfoot and arthrogryposis multiplex congenita. Lancet 1962;2:523–6.
32. Azar I. The response of patients with neuromuscular disorders to muscle relaxants: a review. Anesthesiology 1984;61(2):173–87.
33. Martz DG, Schreibman DL, Matjasko MJ. Neurological diseases. In: Katz RL, Benumof JL, Kadis LB, editors. Anesthesia and Uncommon Diseases. 3rd ed.. Philadelphia: W.B. Saunders, 1990:560.
34. Miller JD, Lee C. Muscle diseases. In: Katz RL, Benumof JL, Kadis LB, editors. Anesthesia and Uncommon Diseases. 3rd ed.. Philadelphia: W.B. Saunders, 1990:590.
35. Stovner J. Clinical use of relaxants in Europe. In: Katz RL, editor. Muscle Relaxants. Amsterdam: Excerpta Medica, 1975:268.
36. Fiset P, Donati F, Balendran P, Meistelman C, Lira E, Bevan DR. Vecuronium is more potent in Montreal than in Paris. Can J Anaesth 1991;38(6):717–21.
37. McCullough LS, Reier CE, Delaunois AL, Gardier RW, Hamelberg W. The effects of d-tubocurarine on

spontaneous postganglionic sympathetic activity and histamine release. Anesthesiology 1970;33(3):328–34.

38. Orko R, Heino A, Rosenberg PH, Alanen T. Dose-response of tubocurarine in patients with and without renal failure. Acta Anaesthesiol Scand 1984;28(4):452–6.

39. Miller RD, Matteo RS, Benet LZ, Sohn YJ. The pharmacokinetics of d-tubocurarine in man with and without renal failure. J Pharmacol Exp Ther 1977;202(1):1–7.

40. Miller RD, Eger EI 2nd. Early and late relative potencies of pancuronium and d-tubocurarine in man. Anesthesiology 1976;44(4):297–300.

41. Cohen EN, Brewer HW, Smith D. The metabolism and elimination of d-tubocurarine-H3. Anesthesiology 1967;28(2):309–17.

42. Riordan DD, Gilbertson AA. Prolonged curarization in a patient with renal failure. Case report. Br J Anaesth 1971;43(5):506–8.

43. Yeung ML, Ng LY, Koo AW. Severe bronchospasm in an asthmatic patient following alcuronium and D-tubocurarine. Anaesth Intensive Care 1979;7(1):62–4.

44. Foldes FF. Myasthenia gravis. In: Katz RL, editor. Muscle Relaxants. Amsterdam: Excerpta Medica, 1975:345.

45. Enoki T, Naito Y, Hirokawa Y, Nomura R, Hatano Y, Mori K. Marked sensitivity to pancuronium in a patient without clinical manifestations of myasthenia gravis. Anesth Analg 1989;69(6):840–2.

46. Rosenbaum KJ, Neigh JL, Strobel GE. Sensitivity to nondepolarizing muscle relaxants in amyotrophic lateral sclerosis: report of two cases. Anesthesiology 1971;35(6):638–41.

47. Baraka A. Myasthenic response to muscle relaxants in von Recklinghausen's disease. Br J Anaesth 1974;46(9):701–3.

48. Robertson JA. Ocular muscular dystrophy. A cause of curare sensitivity. Anaesthesia 1984;39(3):251–3.

49. Brown JC, Charlton JE. Study of sensitivity to curare in certain neurological disorders using a regional technique. J Neurol Neurosurg Psychiatry 1975;38(1):34–45.

50. Harrah MD, Way WL, Katzung BG. The interaction of d-tubocurarine with antiarrhythmic drugs. Anesthesiology 1970;33(4):406–10.

51. Miller RD, Way WL, Katzung BG. The potentiation of neuromuscular blocking agents by quinidine. Anesthesiology 1967;28(6):1036–41.

52. Katz RL, Gissen AJ. Effects of intravenous and intra-arterial procaine and lidocaine on neuromuscular transmission in man. Acta Anaesthesiol Scand Suppl 1969;36:103–13.

53. Welch GW, Waud BE. Effect of bretylium on neuromuscular transmission. Anesth Analg 1982;61(5):442–4.

54. Healy TE, O'Shea M, Massey J. Disopyramide and neuromuscular transmission. Br J Anaesth 1981;53(5):495–8.

55. Jones SV, Marshall IG. Non-competitive effects of disopyramide at the neuromuscular junction: evidence for endplate ion channel block. Br J Anaesth 1987;59(6):776–83.

56. Baurain M, Barvais L, d'Hollander A, Hennart D. Impairment of the antagonism of vecuronium-induced paralysis and intra-operative disopyramide administration. Anaesthesia 1989;44(1):34–6.

57. Chasapakis G, Dimas C. Possible interaction between muscle relaxants and the kallikrein-trypsin inactivator "Trasylol". Report of three cases. Br J Anaesth 1966;38(10):838–9.

58. Dretchen KL, Morgenroth VH 3rd, Standaert FG, Walts LF. Azathioprine: effects on neuromuscular transmission. Anesthesiology 1976;45(6):604–9.

59. Durant NN, Nguyen N, Katz RL. Potentiation of neuromuscular blockade by verapamil. Anesthesiology 1984;60(4):298–303.

60. Jones RM, Cashman JN, Casson WR, Broadbent MP. Verapamil potentiation of neuromuscular blockade: failure of reversal with neostigmine but prompt reversal with edrophonium. Anesth Analg 1985;64(10):1021–5.

61. Bikhazi GB, Leung I, Flores C, Mikati HM, Foldes FF. Potentiation of neuromuscular blocking agents by calcium channel blockers in rats. Anesth Analg 1988;67(1):1–8.

62. Maestrone E. Interaction of neuromuscular blocking agents in surgical patients. In: Agoston S, Bowman WC, editors. Monographs in Anaesthesiology 19. Amsterdam: Elsevier Science Publishers BV, 1990:199.

63. Miller RD, Sohn YJ, Matteo RS. Enhancement of d-tuborcurarine neuromuscular blockade by diuretics in man. Anesthesiology 1976;45(4):442–5.

64. Scappaticci KA, Ham JA, Sohn YJ, Miller RD, Dretchen KL. Effects of furosemide on the neuromuscular junction. Anesthesiology 1982;57(5):381–8.

65. Pollard BJ, Randall NP, Pleuvry BJ. Doxapram and the neuromuscular junction. Br J Anaesth 1989;62(6):664–8.

66. Nakamura K, Hatano Y, Mori K. The site of action of trimethaphan-induced neuromuscular blockade in isolated rat and frog muscle. Acta Anaesthesiol Scand 1988;32(2):125–30.

67. Matsuo S, Rao DB, Chaudry I, Foldes FF. Interaction of muscle relaxants and local anesthetics at the neuromuscular junction. Anesth Analg 1978;57(5):580–7.

68. Telivuo L, Katz RL. The effects of modern intravenous local analgesics on respiration during partial neuromuscular block in man. Anaesthesia 1970;25(1):30–5.

69. Giesecke AH Jr, Morris RE, Dalton MD, Stephen CR. Of magnesium, muscle relaxants, toxemic parturients, and cats. Anesth Analg 1968;47(6):689–95.

70. Gerber HR, Romppainen J, Schwinn W. Potentiation of atracurium by pancuronium and D-tubocurarine. Can Anaesth Soc J 1986;33(5):563–70.

Vecuronium bromide

General Information

Vecuronium is a monoquaternary analogue of pancuronium, with a similar speed of onset, a duration of action of 15–30 minutes, rapid spontaneous recovery, and virtually no cumulative effects (1). Being monoquaternary, it is more lipophilic than pancuronium. About 30% is bound to plasma proteins. It is deacetylated in the liver, the principal metabolite being 3-desacetylvecuronium, which is believed to have about 50% of the neuromuscular blocking potency of the parent drug in man; small amounts of 17-desacetylvecuronium and 3,17-didesacetylvecuronium are also formed. In balanced anesthesia vecuronium is slightly more potent than pancuronium, but during halothane anesthesia it has been reported to be 1.4 times as potent as the latter. Suitable doses during balanced anesthesia are similar to those for pancuronium; potentiation by volatile agents (2) allows these doses to be reduced, after equilibration has occurred between the volatile agent and the tissues, by 25 or 45% when halothane or enflurane are used (3,4). In another study, after 1 hour of constant 90% neuromuscular blockade under nitrous oxide (60%), isoflurane (1.2% end-tidal), or enflurane (1.2% end-tidal) anesthesia the vecuronium infusion requirements were reduced by as much as 70% (compared with the nitrous oxide/fentanyl group) (SEDA-13, 105) (5).

In animals, histamine release, cholinesterase inhibition, and autonomic effects are minimal and occur only at concentrations of vecuronium considerably greater than those required for neuromuscular block (6–9). Interactions with antimicrobial drugs, analgesics, and anesthetic agents were similar to those known for other non-depolarizing relaxants, apart from a possible potentiating effect by metronidazole (6). These animal findings have been confirmed in man by the relative paucity of reported adverse effects. In man, the intradermal injection of vecuronium produces a considerably smaller local histamine reaction than d-tubocurarine, metocurine, pancuronium, or atracurium do (10,11) and plasma histamine is not raised in the clinical dose range (12,13). Nevertheless, minor skin reactions have been reported (14,15), as well as hypotension (16) and severe anaphylactoid reactions with circulatory collapse (17,18) and bronchospasm (19,20). Cross-sensitivity with pancuronium may occur (SEDA-10, 111).

Organs and Systems

Cardiovascular

The expected cardiovascular stability of vecuronium has been confirmed in man (2,21–23). Even doses as large as 0.28 mg/kg in patients undergoing coronary artery bypass grafting produced negligible effects (24). Bradycardia is the only cardiovascular adverse effect reported, and this is seen in association with opioids such as fentanyl (25) and sufentanil (SEDA-11, 125) (26) or other drugs that are themselves capable of producing bradycardia. The lack of vagolytic and sympathomimetic activity of vecuronium means that it does not counteract the bradycardia or the hypotensive effects of other drugs or surgical manipulations. It is an ideal relaxant for patients with pheochromocytoma (27).

Musculoskeletal

Masseter muscle rigidity is a rare but potentially dangerous adverse effect of suxamethonium and can prevent successful airway management. Furthermore, it can be the first sign of malignant hyperthermia and rhabdomyolysis. Non-depolarizing neuromuscular blocking agents are thought to be safe with regard to masseter muscle rigidity. However, masseter muscle rigidity not associated with the use of suxamethonium can also complicate airway management (28).

- A 42-year-old woman had anesthesia induced with propofol 200 mg, vecuronium 8 mg, and mask ventilation with oxygen, nitrous oxide, and 2% isoflurane. Laryngoscopy proved impossible because of spasm of the masseter muscles, and the airway was secured by

blind nasal intubation. There was no evidence of rigidity of other muscle groups. Body temperature and end-tidal carbon dioxide concentration remained in the reference ranges. Masseter muscle rigidity persisted throughout the operation and resolved during recovery from anesthesia after neostigmine 2.5 mg had been given.

The authors suggested that in this case the phenomenon had been caused by vecuronium. Masseter muscle rigidity persisted during anesthesia and resolved during recovery from anesthesia after neostigmine had been given and isoflurane inhalation had been stopped. If vecuronium caused muscle rigidity in this case it was probably not mediated by effects on acetylcholine receptors, but rather by an interaction of vecuronium with ion channels (sodium, potassium, and/or calcium), but it is hard to imagine how this effect could have been antagonized by a cholinesterase inhibitor. It therefore seems likely that the masseter muscle rigidity was rather caused by isoflurane, which would explain why the symptoms improved after withdrawal of isoflurane. There have been previous reports of masseter muscle rigidity associated with non-depolarizing neuromuscular blocking agents (SEDA-21, 144) (29,30). The mechanism is unclear. One wonders how muscle specimens from these patients might react to exposure to an inhalational anesthetic during in vitro contracture testing. Regarding the link between masseter muscle rigidity and malignant hyperthermia, muscle biopsy would not be inappropriate in patients who have masseter muscle rigidity severe enough to prevent mouth opening and conventional orotracheal intubation.

Second-Generation Effects

Fetotoxicity

There is placental transfer of vecuronium, but no effects have been detected in the newborn (the feto-maternal concentration ratio is about 10% less than for pancuronium (31). Postpartum, vecuronium has been reported to have an appreciably longer duration of action (SEDA-13, 105) (32,33) when given in a dose of 0.1 mg/kg.

Susceptibility Factors

Age

Spontaneous recovery of neuromuscular function after a bolus dose of vecuronium (0.1 mg/kg) was significantly prolonged in elderly patients compared with younger adults (SEDA-17, 153). The elimination half-life was significantly prolonged (125 versus 78 minutes) and the plasma clearance reduced (2.5 versus 5.6 ml/kg/minute) in the elderly versus the younger patients.

Renal disease

About 25–30% of an injected dose of vecuronium is excreted in the urine in normal patients, mostly as unchanged drug. Renal dysfunction has been reported as having no significant effect on the duration of action of vecuronium (SEDA-11, 125) (34–36). Nevertheless, slight resistance to the neuromuscular blocking effect of an initial dose (ED_{50} increased by 20%) and a small reduction (of 23%) in infusion requirements to maintain a 90% block after 1 hour of relaxation have been described in end-stage renal insufficiency (SEDA-13, 103) (37). These findings are in line with those for other non-depolarizing agents, with the exception of atracurium; the changes, however, are minor compared with the older relaxants, as is to be expected from the kinetics of vecuronium. There is a slight tendency for the action of vecuronium to be prolonged in renal insufficiency, and monitoring of neuromuscular transmission is advisable if several doses are to be given.

Hepatic disease

In liver disease (cirrhosis and cholestasis), the plasma clearance of vecuronium is reduced, its half-life is increased, and its duration of action is prolonged (SEDA-10, 112) (38,39). Rapid uptake in the liver appears to be an important factor in its plasma clearance and in determining its relatively short duration of action; it is estimated that about 40% of the injected drug is excreted via the bile (40). Prolongation of the action of large single doses and accumulation after repeated doses are therefore to be expected in liver disease.

Drug–Drug Interactions

Azathioprine

In humans with renal insufficiency, azathioprine 3 mg/kg produced a negligible and transient reduction in neuromuscular blockade maintained by infusion of vecuronium (37).

Carbamazepine

Resistance to vecuronium has been described in patients taking carbamazepine (41).

Ciclosporin

Ciclosporin can cause considerable prolongation of the neuromuscular paralysis induced by vecuronium (42), causing difficulties with reversal (SEDA-14, 116) (43). Potentiation of vecuronium in cats has also been described (SEDA-12, 188) (44).

Disopyramide

Disopyramide has also been associated with impairment of neostigmine antagonism of vecuronium-induced neuromuscular blockade (45).

- A 63-year-old man was given vecuronium 70 µg/kg followed by increments of 20 µg/kg, and three intravenous doses of disopyramide 10 mg for supraventricular extra beats, followed by an infusion of 25 mg/hour. Paralysis was reversed using atropine 0.75 mg and neostigmine 2.5 mg. The twitch height returned to normal and the train-of-four was above 85%, but the responses to

tetanic stimulation at 100 and 50 Hz remained severely depressed (10 and 45% respectively). The plasma concentration of disopyramide was 5.1 µg/ml.

Metronidazole

Metronidazole can potentiate the effects of non-depolarizing muscle relaxants (49).

Serum concentrations of metronidazole rose during concomitant administration of ciprofloxacin and metronidazole (50). The authors speculated that the mechanism was inhibition of cytochrome P_{450} by ciprofloxacin.

Phenytoin

Acute administration of phenytoin (10 mg/kg intravenously) has been reported to enhance slightly, but statistically significantly, steady blockade maintained by an infusion of vecuronium (SEDA-15, 124) (46). This is in contrast to reports of resistance to non-depolarizing neuromuscular blocking agents, including vecuronium, associated with long-term phenytoin (SEDA-13, 104) (47).

Testosterone

Testosterone enanthate, given over 10 years to produce virilization, has been claimed to have been responsible for a case of marked resistance to vecuronium (SEDA-14, 116) (48).

References

1. Miller RD, Rupp SM, Fisher DM, Cronnelly R, Fahey MR, Sohn YJ. Clinical pharmacology of vecuronium and atracurium. Anesthesiology 1984;61(4):444–53.
2. Mirakhur RK, Ferres CJ, Clarke RS, Bali IM, Dundee JW. Clinical evaluation of Org NC 45. Br J Anaesth 1983;55(2):119–24.
3. Foldes FF, Bencini A, Newton D. Influence of halothane and enflurane on the neuromuscular effects of ORG NC 45 in man. Br J Anaesth 1980;52(Suppl 1):S64–5.
4. Ording H, Viby-Mogensen J. Dose response curves for Org NC 45 and pancuronium. Acta Anaesthesiol Scand 1981;25(Suppl 72):73.
5. Cannon JE, Fahey MR, Castagnoli KP, Furuta T, Canfell PC, Sharma M, Miller RD. Continuous infusion of vecuronium: the effect of anesthetic agents. Anesthesiology 1987;67(4):503–6.
6. McIndewar IC, Marshall RJ. Interactions between the neuromuscular blocking drug Org NC 45 and some anaesthetic, analgesic and antimicrobial agents. Br J Anaesth 1981;53(8):785–92.
7. Son SL, Waud BE, Waud DR. A comparison of the neuromuscular blocking and vagolytic effects of ORG NC45 and pancuronium. Anesthesiology 1981;55(1):12–8.
8. Durant NN, Marshall IG, Savage DS, Nelson DJ, Sleigh T, Carlyle IC. The neuromuscular and autonomic blocking activities of pancuronium, Org NC 45, and other pancuronium analogues, in the cat. J Pharm Pharmacol 1979;31(12):831–6.
9. Marshall RJ, McGrath JC, Miller RD, Docherty JR, Lamar JC. Comparison of the cardiovascular actions of ORG NC 45 with those produced by other non-depolarizing neuromuscular blocking agents in experimental animals. Br J Anaesth 1980;52(Suppl 1):S21–32.

10. Booij LH, Krieg N, Crul JF. Intradermal histamine releasing effect caused by Org-NC 45. A comparison with pancuronium, metocurine and d-tubocurarine Acta Anaesthesiol Scand 1980;24(5):393–4.

11. Robertson EN, Booij LH, Fragen RJ, Crul JF. Intradermal histamine release by 3 muscle relaxants. Acta Anaesthesiol Scand 1983;27(3):203–5.

12. Basta SJ, Savarese JJ, Ali HH, et al. Vecuronium does not alter serum histamine within the clinical dose range. Anesthesiology 1983;59:A273.

13. Goudsouzian NG, Young ET, Moss J, Liu LM. Histamine release during the administration of atracurium or vecuronium in children. Br J Anaesth 1986;58(11):1229–33.

14. Clayton DG, Watkins J. Histamine release with vecuronium. Anaesthesia 1984;39(11):1143–4.

15. Spence AG, Barnetson RS. Reaction to vecuronium bromide. Lancet 1985;1(8435):979–80.

16. Lavery GG, Hewitt AJ, Kenny NT. Possible histamine release after vecuronium. Anaesthesia 1985;40(4):389–90.

17. Thacker MA, Boon von Ochssee D. Anaphylactoid reaction to vecuronium. Anaesth Intensive Care 1988;16(1):129–30.

18. Treuren BC, Buckley DH. Anaphylactoid reaction to vecuronium. Br J Anaesth 1990;64(1):125–6.

19. Conil C, Bornet JL, Jean-Noel M, Conil JM, Brouchet A. Choc anaphylactique au pancuronium et au vécuronium. [Anaphylactic shock caused by pancuronium and vecuronium.] Ann Fr Anesth Reanim 1985;4(2):241–3.

20. Holt AW, Vedig AE. Anaphylaxis following vecuronium. Anaesth Intensive Care 1988;16(3):378–9.

21. Barnes PK, Smith GB, White WD, Tennant R. Comparison of the effects of Org NC 45 and pancuronium bromide on heart rate and arterial pressure in anaesthetized man. Br J Anaesth 1982;54(4):435–9.

22. Gregoretti SM, Sohn YJ, Sia RL. Heart rate and blood pressure changes after ORG NC45 (vecuronium) and pancuronium during halothane and enflurane anesthesia. Anesthesiology 1982;56(5):392–5.

23. Lienhart A, Desnault H, Guggiari M, et al. Vecuronium bromide: dose response curve and haemodynamic effects in anaesthetized man. In: Agoston S, editor. Clinical Experiences with Norcuron. Amsterdam: Excerpta Medica, 1982:46.

24. Morris RB, Cahalan MK, Miller RD, Wilkinson PL, Quasha AL, Robinson SL. The cardiovascular effects of vecuronium (ORG NC45) and pancuronium in patients undergoing coronary artery bypass grafting. Anesthesiology 1983;58(5):438–40.

25. Salmenpera M, Peltola K, Takkunen O, Heinonen J. Cardiovascular effects of pancuronium and vecuronium during high-dose fentanyl anesthesia. Anesth Analg 1983;62(12):1059–64.

26. Starr NJ, Sethna DH, Estafanous FG. Bradycardia and asystole following the rapid administration of sufentanil with vecuronium. Anesthesiology 1986;64(4):521–3.

27. Gencarelli PJ, Roizen MF, Miller RD, Joyce J, Hunt TK, Tyrrell JB. ORG NC45 (Norcuron) and pheochromocytoma: a report of three cases. Anesthesiology 1981;55(6):690–3.

28. Jenkins JG. Masseter muscle rigidity after vecuronium. Eur J Anaesthesiol 1999;16(2):137–9.

29. Polta TA, Hanisch EC Jr, Nasser JG, Ramsborg GC, Roelofs RI. Masseter spasm after pancuronium. Anesth Analg 1980;59(7):509–11.

30. Albrecht A, Wedel DJ, Gronert GA. Masseter muscle rigidity and nondepolarizing neuromuscular blocking agents. Mayo Clin Proc 1997;72(4):329–32.

31. Demetriou M, Depoix JP, Diakite B, Fromentin M, Duvaldestin P. Placental transfer of org nc 45 in women undergoing Caesarean section. Br J Anaesth 1982;54(6):643–5.

32. Hawkins JL, Adenwala J, Camp C, Joyce TH 3rd. The effect of H2-receptor antagonist premedication on the duration of vecuronium-induced neuromuscular blockade in postpartum patients. Anesthesiology 1989;71(2):175–7.

33. Camp CE, Tessem J, Adenwala J, Joyce TH 3rd. Vecuronium and prolonged neuromuscular blockade in postpartum patients. Anesthesiology 1987;67(6):1006–8.

34. Fahey MR, Morris RB, Miller RD, Nguyen TL, Upton RA. Pharmacokinetics of Org NC45 (Norcuron) in patients with and without renal failure. Br J Anaesth 1981;53(10):1049–53.

35. Bencini AF, Scaf AH, Sohn YJ, Meistelman C, Lienhart A, Kersten UW, Schwarz S, Agoston S. Disposition and urinary excretion of vecuronium bromide in anesthetized patients with normal renal function or renal failure. Anesth Analg 1986;65(3):245–51.

36. Bevan DR, Donati F, Gyasi H, Williams A. Vecuronium in renal failure. Can Anaesth Soc J 1984;31(5):491–6.

37. Gramstad L. Atracurium, vecuronium and pancuronium in end-stage renal failure. Dose-response properties and interactions with azathioprine. Br J Anaesth 1987;59(8):995–1003.

38. Lebrault C, Berger JL, D'Hollander AA, Gomeni R, Henzel D, Duvaldestin P. Pharmacokinetics and pharmacodynamics of vecuronium (ORG NC 45) in patients with cirrhosis. Anesthesiology 1985;62(5):601–5.

39. Lebrault C, Duvaldestin P, Henzel D, Chauvin M, Guesnon P. Pharmacokinetics and pharmacodynamics of vecuronium in patients with cholestasis. Br J Anaesth 1986;58(9):983–7.

40. Bencini AF, Scaf AH, Sohn YJ, Kersten-Kleef UW, Agoston S. Hepatobiliary disposition of vecuronium bromide in man. Br J Anaesth 1986;58(9):988–95.

41. Ebrahim Z, Bulkley R, Roth S. Carbamazepine therapy and neuromuscular blockade with atracurium and vecuronium. Anesth Analg 1988;67:555.

42. Crosby E, Robblee JA. Cyclosporine–pancuronium interaction in a patient with a renal allograft. Can J Anaesth 1988;35(3 Pt 1):300–2.

43. Wood GG. Cyclosporine-vecuronium interaction. Can J Anaesth 1989;36(3 Pt 1):358.

44. Gramstad L, Gjerlow JA, Hysing ES, Rugstad HE. Interaction of cyclosporin and its solvent, Cremophor, with atracurium and vecuronium. Studies in the cat. Br J Anaesth 1986;58(10):1149–55.

45. Baurain M, Barvais L, d'Hollander A, Hennart D. Impairment of the antagonism of vecuronium-induced paralysis and intra-operative disopyramide administration. Anaesthesia 1989;44(1):34–6.

46. Gray HS, Slater RM, Pollard BJ. The effect of acutely administered phenytoin on vecuronium-induced neuromuscular blockade. Anaesthesia 1989;44(5):379–81.

47. Ornstein E, Matteo RS, Schwartz AE, Silverberg PA, Young WL, Diaz J. The effect of phenytoin on the magnitude and duration of neuromuscular block following atracurium or vecuronium. Anesthesiology 1987;67(2):191–6.

48. Reddy P, Guzman A, Robalino J, Shevde K. Resistance to muscle relaxants in a patient receiving prolonged testosterone therapy. Anesthesiology 1989;70(5):871–3.

49. McIndewar IC, Marshall RJ. Interactions between the neuromuscular blocking drug Org NC 45 and some anaesthetic, analgesic and antimicrobial agents. Br J Anaesth 1981;53(8):785–92.

50. Cooke CE, Sklar GE, Nappi JM. Possible pharmacokinetic interaction with quinidine: ciprofloxacin or metronidazole? Ann Pharmacother 1996;30(4):364–6.

MUSCLE RELAXANTS

Baclofen

General Information

Baclofen is a chlorophenyl derivative of gamma-aminobutyric acid (GABA), a naturally occurring inhibitory neurotransmitter in the brain and spinal cord. It is of proven therapeutic value in reducing the severity of flexor or extensor spasms resulting from spinal cord injury or disease. The recommended oral dose is 5 mg tds, which can be carefully increased; however, the total daily dose should not exceed 80 mg (20 mg qds). It is also used for the treatment of intractable hiccups, especially in patients with uremia.

The most commonly reported adverse effects are drowsiness, dizziness, fatigue, confusion, hypotension, and nausea.

The adverse effects of baclofen in the treatment of gastroesophageal reflux have been reviewed (1). The most common adverse effects were *somnolence, dizziness, nausea, vomiting*, and *seizures*. In 16 patients with non-acid duodenogastroesophageal reflux (or duodenal reflux) baclofen improved reflux and symptoms (2). The dose of baclofen was 5 mg tds, increasing by 5 mg every fourth day to a dose of 20 mg tds. Four patients reported adverse effects of nausea or drowsiness.

Organs and Systems

Nervous system

Altered consciousness is a major adverse effect of baclofen, because of its GABA-mimetic effects. While this reflects global nervous system depression, other adverse effects, such as seizures and dyskinesias, are probably better explained by selective effects on different brain areas. A case of akinetic mutism associated with baclofen might be an example of this (3).

- A 76-year-old man with a history of cognitive decline of unknown origin had severe contractures with increasing pain in his legs. He was given baclofen 10 mg tds, and 2 days later had difficulty following commands. Another 2 days later he could not speak and would not follow commands, although he was alert with his eyes open. He had no spontaneous movements, but would withdraw to painful stimuli. The electroencephalogram showed intermittent, bilateral, symmetrical, sharp waves. Computed tomography and laboratory tests showed no specific abnormalities. Baclofen was withdrawn and he improved over the next 4 days, after which there was no difference to his prebaclofen condition.

The authors explained that akinetic mutism occurs when bilateral frontal lobe or diencephalic–mesencephalic dysfunction interrupts the limbic circuitry. As symptoms were observed immediately after the start of treatment and resolved completely after withdrawal, the condition was probably caused by baclofen. It is not known why baclofen in this case impaired neuronal activity specifically in these areas. The authors found only one previous report describing the case of a 57-year-old woman with end-stage renal insufficiency, who developed akinetic mutism after a single dose of baclofen (4). In this case, the symptoms resolved after dialysis. Therefore, adverse effects of baclofen should be suspected if neuropsychiatric symptoms occur after baclofen treatment has been started. Electroencephalography and computerized tomography may be necessary to exclude other causes.

Because the systemic effects of baclofen can cause a reduced level of consciousness, intrathecal administration via a catheter is widely used to avoid systemic effects. However, because a continuous infusion is required, implantable pumps containing a very concentrated solution of baclofen are used to avoid frequent refills. Inadvertent subarachnoid bolus administration of a concentrated solution will produce cranial spread of baclofen within the CSF, resulting in cerebral effects. This is most likely to occur when a new catheter or pump is implanted or during surgical revision of a catheter or implantable pump in cases of malfunction. A report of coma after implantation of a baclofen pump in five out of nine consecutive children illustrates this (5). The authors suggested that these children should be monitored in the recovery room for 5 hours postoperatively, in order to cover both the peak effect of any baclofen bolus and the additive effects of other perioperative CNS suppressants, such as opioids, benzodiazepines, or sedative antiemetics. In another report of transient coma after perioperative intrathecal bolus administration it was shown that the management of this complication can require admission to an intensive care unit (6).

Impairment of speech, memory, and mental acuity, associated with an abnormal electroencephalogram, has been described in a young patient taking normal doses (20 mg bd); gradual withdrawal restored the patient and electroencephalogram to normal (SEDA-12, 119) (7). Abnormal electroencephalographic changes have also been reported in a patient with deteriorating multiple sclerosis who developed encephalopathy 48 hours after starting baclofen in low dosage (10 mg tds), but this patient also had renal impairment; withdrawal led to reversal of symptoms in this case (8).

Epilepsy, progressing to status epilepticus, has been ascribed to baclofen (80 mg/day); the fits stopped on gradual withdrawal of the baclofen (9). In contrast to other reports, this patient had no history of seizures.

Concern has been raised that baclofen might be associated with new-onset seizures in children (10). Among 35 children with cerebral palsy aged 1–10 years, five developed new-onset seizures within 1–2.5 months after baclofen was started or the dose was increased (dosage range 0.36–1.5 mg/kg/day). While the authors admitted that young children with cerebral palsy have a significant risk of developing seizures independent of other factors, they still felt that there might be an association with baclofen. Indeed, studies in animals have suggested that baclofen may have proconvulsive properties (11), and three clinical papers have linked baclofen to convulsions. In one of these, two patients with tonic-clonic seizures among 14 adolescents with baclofen intoxication were described (12). There were also cases of seizures in three adults with traumatic brain injury who were treated with intrathecal baclofen and in a patient with multiple sclerosis (13,14). We conclude that baclofen has some proconvulsive properties, which rarely result in clinically important effects. In most of the reported cases baclofen was continued with concomitant antiepileptic medication.

An elderly patient with a 4-year history of Alzheimer's disease developed chorea 2 weeks after starting a trial of baclofen (SEDA-16, 23). The dosage had been gradually increased to 15 mg tds. The chorea resolved within 24 hours after the baclofen was withdrawn. The authors suggested that the chorea might have resulted from the combination of the GABA-agonist drug and deficient cholinergic function in Alzheimer's disease.

A case of aseptic meningitis after intrathecal administration of baclofen has been reported but, as viral causes could not be ruled out, the causative role of baclofen was unclear (15).

Psychological, psychiatric

Euphoria or depression can occur, and mania has been reported in a patient with schizophrenia (16).

Gastrointestinal

A possible effect of intrathecal baclofen on intestinal motility has been proposed (17). Triggered by two cases of paralytic ileus in patients receiving continuous intrathecal baclofen, the authors reviewed the case notes of 14 patients and summed the days without bowel movements before and after intrathecal baclofen therapy. Intestinal function deteriorated in 10 patients, was unchanged in one, and improved in three. They therefore advised that intestinal activity should be closely observed in patients receiving intrathecal baclofen. However, they felt that treatment could be continued, even in particularly sensitive patients, if prokinetic, laxative, or eubiotic drugs were used to promote peristaltic function.

Liver

Rarely, deterioration in liver function tests (increases in aspartate transaminase and alkaline phosphatase) can occur (SEDA-6, 132).

Musculoskeletal

With regard to its effects on spinal GABA receptors, intrathecal baclofen has been compared with intrathecal fentanyl for postoperative pain treatment in six children (mean age 4.2 years) with cerebral palsy undergoing bilateral dorsal rhizotomy (18). Both intrathecal baclofen and intrathecal fentanyl reduced postoperative pain. However, three of five children had severe muscle weakness after intrathecal baclofen 1–1.5 µg/kg, which prompted the authors to discontinue their study. An accompanying editorial dealt with the possible mechanisms of action of spinal GABA agonists on postoperative pain, suggesting that the effects on sensory processing probably cannot be separated from the changes in motor function (19). Therefore, this report of muscle weakness should not prompt us to close the file on intrathecal baclofen for pain treatment. More experience is needed and different dose regimens should be tested.

Sexual function

Intrathecal baclofen caused a reduction in erection rigidity and duration in eight of nine men. When ejaculation was possible before the start of baclofen treatment it disappeared or was more difficult to obtain during treatment. These effects resolved after withdrawal of baclofen (20).

Body temperature

Febrile reactions after intrathecal baclofen stopped a patient from receiving this treatment for spinal spasticity (21).

- A 33-year-old woman with spasticity caused by a myelopathy after numerous operations on her spine received a single bolus dose of baclofen 50 µg via a lumbar puncture, which resulted in complete resolution of her spasticity for almost 24 hours. However, her temperature increased to 39.0°C within 2 hours after the injection, and she had flu-like symptoms. Influenza was assumed to be the most likely explanation, as a child in her house had influenza at that time. Subsequently, an intrathecal catheter was placed and a baclofen pump implanted. However, her temperature rose again after baclofen administration had been started and the pump was halted. Subsequently, several attempts were made to restart the infusion, followed each time by spikes of fever. In the end, continuous intrathecal baclofen therapy had to be abandoned, and the fever did not recur. Several investigations to identify other causes of fever were mostly negative. However, based on bilateral hilar adenopathy on the chest X-ray and increased concentrations of angiotensin-converting enzyme, sarcoidosis was suspected.

The authors claimed that this was the first report of this problem. Referring to the observation that baclofen injection into the cerebral ventricles can produce fever in rats (22), they assumed that rostral spread of baclofen could have initiated a thermoregulatory response via the chemotrigger zone in the third ventricle. They suggested that a percutaneous subarachnoid catheter could facilitate the decision to either proceed with or abort surgical catheter or pump implantation when baclofen is associated with fever.

Long-Term Effects

Drug tolerance

Tolerance to intrathecal baclofen developed in three of 23 patients with spinal spasticity (23).

Drug withdrawal

Like many other agents that act at the GABA receptor, abrupt termination of long-term administration of baclofen can result in withdrawal symptoms, even after intrathecal administration (24,25). Patients can present with different symptoms, not all of which would be considered classical of drug withdrawal.

Clinical presentation

Common presenting features are muscular hyperactivity, hyperthermia, metabolic derangements, and rhabdomyolysis when baclofen therapy is abruptly discontinued, and several deaths have occurred (26). Clinicians should be suspicious of baclofen withdrawal if patients taking baclofen present with fever, muscle cramps, and hypotension. A case of brain death due to baclofen withdrawal with severe hypotension and hyperthermia up to 43°C has underscored the need for immediate and aggressive treatment (27).

Sudden withdrawal can cause hallucinations and grand mal convulsions or worsening of pre-existing epilepsy (SED-9, 206) (28,29).

There is a similarity between baclofen withdrawal and the neuroleptic malignant syndrome.

- A 36-year-old man with paraplegia after a spinal cord injury became disoriented (30). He had marked rigidity in both arms and legs, he was sweating and pyrexial (38°C), and his heart rate was 112/minute. His serum creatine kinase was raised at 2668 U/l and rose to 2982 U/l on day 3. At that time, baclofen was restarted. Within 3 days he was fully oriented. Over 2 weeks his creatine kinase activity gradually fell to normal and his temperature settled. It turned out that he had neglected to take any medication for several days before admission.

The authors believed that symptoms in this case resembled the neuroleptic malignant syndrome, based on the combination of muscle rigidity, pyrexia, signs of autonomic disturbance, and altered consciousness. They did not think that the raised serum creatine kinase activity was associated with rhabdomyolysis, stating that there was no evidence from urinalysis to suggest this. Unfortunately, they did not specify whether there was myoglobin in the urine or not. Creatine kinase activities up to 40 000 U/l have been noted during baclofen withdrawal (31), compared with which creatine kinase activity in this case was much lower, suggesting only moderate muscle damage. One might assume that muscle damage after baclofen withdrawal correlates with the duration and intensity of muscular hyperactivity. In addition, prolonged muscular hyperactivity may be expected to be followed by an increase in both body temperature and heart rate, owing to hypermetabolism and sympathetic activation. Sweating will result from sympathetic activation and a thermoregulatory response to hyperthermia and is not necessarily an autonomic disturbance. Disorientation is also an expected symptom of baclofen withdrawal. In conclusion, this patient's combination of symptoms could have been explained by baclofen withdrawal alone. Assuming that disturbances in central dopaminergic systems could have been involved, as in neuroleptic malignant syndrome, is speculative.

This is not the first report of similarities between the neuroleptic malignant syndrome and baclofen withdrawal (25,27,31). In addition, hyperthermia seems to be common in baclofen withdrawal (27).

- A 14-year-old child receiving continuous intrathecal baclofen treatment developed a fever of up to 40°C and painful muscle spasms, attributed to baclofen withdrawal due to failure of the intrathecal catheter. The symptoms resolved promptly after reintroduction of intrathecal baclofen (32).

If intrathecal baclofen has to be interrupted or cannot be restarted immediately, enteral baclofen should be given. However, finding the appropriate dose for this can be difficult and close observation of the patient is required, as illustrated in the following report (33).

- A 34-year-old man who was receiving continuous intrathecal baclofen (700 micrograms/day) for muscle spasticity after a spinal cord injury developed a fever, and infection of the implanted baclofen pump was suspected. The device was removed and he was given replacement therapy with oral baclofen (40 mg tds). He developed a tremor 12 hours after pump removal and his heart rate increased to 120/minute. Another 12 hours later he was somnolent, agitated, and confused, and had visual hallucinations. His blood pressure rose to 198/108 mmHg and his temperature to 40°C. This was followed by atrial fibrillation with a ventricular rate of 170/minute. The dose of oral baclofen was increased to 80 mg tds and he was given intravenous lorazepam 6–8 mg every 4 hours. During the following 24 hours his blood pressure, pulse, and temperature normalized and he recovered fully.

Management

Baclofen should always be withdrawn gradually. If a patient stops taking baclofen, a blood sample for baclofen serum concentration measurement should be taken if possible, to confirm the diagnosis post hoc if hyperthermia occurs. If a patient taking long-term baclofen presents with similar symptoms, baclofen withdrawal should be considered. If this is not effective and the patient deteriorates, with hyperthermia, increasing creatine kinase activity, and metabolic sequelae, dantrolene can be given.

Dantrolene is life-saving in malignant hyperthermia associated with volatile anesthetics and suxamethonium and is also the drug of choice for the treatment of neuroleptic malignant syndrome. Dantrolene has therefore been suggested as an additional therapeutic option in baclofen withdrawal (25), but there is only limited experience (31). In one case of baclofen withdrawal, dantrolene was given with success (31).

It should be stressed that baclofen withdrawal is a potentially fatal emergency. Because of the risk of rhabdomyolysis, disseminated intravascular coagulation, acute renal insufficiency, and other organ complications, patients should be transferred to the intensive care unit and given parenteral baclofen.

Since it has been hypothesized that the baclofen withdrawal syndrome might have similarities with the serotonin syndrome caused by overdose of serotonin reuptake inhibitors or amphetamines, the serotonin receptor antagonist cyproheptadine has been used in combination with oral baclofen and a benzodiazepine in four patients with baclofen withdrawal syndrome after continuous intrathecal baclofen therapy (34). The authors claimed that their patients improved significantly when cyproheptadine was given. Body temperature fell by at least 1.5°C and heart rate fell from 120–140/minute to under 100/minute. Muscular tone and myoclonus improved. Two patients also reported that itching was less intense. All this was felt to be temporarily related to the repeated administration of cyproheptadine. The authors concluded that cyproheptadine was a useful adjunct for the treatment of baclofen withdrawal syndrome. However, one of their patients suffered severe brain damage during withdrawal and subsequently died of pulmonary complications. This illustrates that early intensive care is required.

Second-Generation Effects

Fetotoxicity

Convulsions have been attributed to withdrawal of baclofen after in utero exposure (35).

- A 7-day-old baby was admitted to hospital with generalized convulsions, which did not respond to phenobarbital, phenytoin, clonazepam, lidocaine, or pyridoxine. A variety of investigations all gave negative results. Electroencephalography 4 days later showed prolonged episodes of epileptic activity. At that time baclofen withdrawal was suspected, as the paraplegic mother had been taking baclofen 20 mg tds throughout pregnancy. The baby was given baclofen 0.25 mg/kg qds and 30 minutes after the first dose the convulsions stopped. The baclofen was then slowly withdrawn over 2 weeks. An MRI scan of the brain on day 17 suggested a hypoxic ischemic insult in the perinatal period, which was considered to have been secondary to convulsions.

As convincingly presented by the authors, baclofen withdrawal was the most likely explanation for the convulsions. In discussing the possible mechanisms of the delayed onset of convulsions the authors assumed that a secondary increase in baclofen serum concentration due to redistribution might have prevented earlier onset of the withdrawal symptoms. This is of course speculative; nothing is known about baclofen pharmacokinetics in neonates. On the other hand, the authors stated that the mother had noted some abnormal movements starting on the second day postpartum, which might have represented the first signs of withdrawal. The half-life of baclofen in adults is 3–6 hours, and adults usually become symptomatic 24–72 hours after baclofen is reduced or withdrawn (27). In conclusion, baclofen withdrawal should be suspected if postnatal convulsions occur after intrauterine exposure. The first priority in such a case is to rule out other causes, such as infections, electrolyte disturbances, and intracranial pathology, and to prevent secondary brain damage due to prolonged convulsions.

Baclofen should probably be considered at an early stage, as it might be the most effective anticonvulsant in such cases.

Susceptibility Factors

Renal disease

As 70% of baclofen is excreted unchanged in the urine (36), accumulation and overdosage of baclofen can occur in patients with end-stage renal disease. Confusion, drowsiness, and coma after standard doses have been reported (37). In addition, abdominal pain was a common adverse effect of baclofen in patients with severe renal insufficiency (38). Toxic reactions characterized by a psychotic syndrome and myoclonus have also been reported (39). Patients with severely impaired renal function typically present with altered consciousness after very small doses of baclofen (38). Symptoms of overdose may resolve after hemodialysis (37,38).

- An 82-year-old man with left ventricular dysfunction and gout had worsening renal function (40). He was taking lisinopril, furosemide, naproxen, allopurinol, and baclofen 20 mg tds. As no reason could be found for the use of baclofen the dose was halved and then stopped 10 days later. The next day he had visual hallucinations, confusion, and agitation, and required sedation with diazepam. He was afebrile, with normal inflammatory markers, and a CT scan of the brain showed only cerebral atrophy. Baclofen was reintroduced, with complete resolution of neuropsychiatric symptoms within 48 hours.

Epilepsy

Generally, patients with a history of seizures, convulsive disorders, or psychiatric disturbances, and also elderly patients with cerebrovascular disease, should be regarded as patients at risk of developing the more serious side effects (SED-9, 206).

Baclofen is used to treat spasticity in children with cerebral palsy. These children often have epilepsy as well. The effect of baclofen on the frequency of seizures may therefore be relevant. It has been suggested that baclofen may increase seizure frequency and have proconvulsive properties (SEDA-27, 141) (41,42,43). In the largest study so far, the seizure frequency in 150 children with cerebral palsy before and after the institution of intrathecal baclofen therapy was recorded (44). The prevalence of epilepsy before the intervention was 60/150 (40%). Eight of those 60 children had a reduced seizure frequency after intrathecal baclofen was started; in four of those eight no more seizures occurred and antiepileptic treatment was withdrawn. On the other hand, two of 60 children had an increased frequency of seizures. In addition, one child developed new-onset seizures after intrathecal baclofen was started. The authors concluded that baclofen does not aggravate seizure activity in epileptic patients. Indeed, their results support the use of intrathecal baclofen to treat spasticity in patients with cerebral palsy and seizures. To what extent this can be extrapolated to other conditions, for example in patients with spasticity after trauma, who might also have post-traumatic epilepsy, is currently not clear.

Drug Administration

Drug administration route

Intrathecal baclofen is becoming increasingly popular for the treatment of severe spasticity in an attempt to reduce the incidence and severity of systemic adverse effects. However, hypotonia, respiratory depression, and coma can occur. Severe arterial hypotension also has been observed in two of 23 patients (16). Occasionally, nervous system suppression can be severe enough to require mechanical ventilation. Adverse effects have been seen not only with high doses (2000 micrograms/day produced flaccid quadriplegia with total areflexia) (SEDA-12, 119) (45), but also after a single bolus dose of 80 micrograms in a patient known to be very sensitive to the action of baclofen (SEDA-15, 128) (46).

Drugs injected directly into the cerebrospinal fluid have a tendency to produce unpredictable effects, their spread being influenced not only by the volume administered, but also by the concentration of the drug, its specific gravity in relation to that of cerebrospinal fluid, the positioning of the patient (head-up or head-down), and on the speed of injection of bolus doses. Truncal muscle spasms can also increase the spread of drug within the cerebrospinal fluid. All these parameters need to be taken into consideration. Standardization is required as a first step. Rapid bolus injection in particular can produce unexpectedly severe adverse effects.

Drug overdose

Overdose, which may be absolute or relative (due to impaired renal excretion or in elderly patients who develop adverse effects at lower dosages), leads to severe hypotonia, mental confusion and somnolence, respiratory depression, and eventually apnea, bradycardia, cardiac conduction abnormalities, hypotension, and coma.

Seizures have been reported in cases of baclofen overdose (47). In a review of cases presenting to an Australian toxicology service there were 23 cases in which baclofen intoxication was involved (48). In eight of these, baclofen was the only agent involved, and seizures occurred in four. Therefore, although it is a potent nervous system depressant, baclofen can have proconvulsive effects, especially in overdose. Other symptoms associated with overdose were miosis or mydriasis, depressed level of consciousness or coma, absent or depressed reflexes, hypertension, and bradycardia or tachycardia.

It is possible that during recovery the picture may be complicated by an acute withdrawal syndrome, with agitation, psychosis, tremor and dystonic movements, convulsions, and hallucinations (SEDA-11, 126) (49–53).

Physostigmine is rapidly effective in reversing not only the respiratory depression but also the coma and hypotonia seen in cases of intrathecal baclofen overdosage

(SEDA-15, 128) (46). The doses recommended for physostigmine salicylate are 1–2 mg intravenously over 5–10 minutes, which may have to be repeated after 30–40 minutes, as the action of physostigmine is fairly short. However, physostigmine may be ineffective when large doses of baclofen are involved (54), and it also has adverse effects of its own, so that the above dosage guidelines should not be exceeded. In particular, bradycardia and cardiac conduction defects can be worsened (cardiac arrest has been reported in connection with baclofen) and it should not be used in these circumstances, respiratory support and symptomatic treatment being recommended (55).

Phaclofen is a more specific baclofen antagonist (56), but more research is required to ascertain if it can be safely used in the treatment of baclofen overdose.

Drug–Drug Interactions

Tricyclic antidepressants

Tricyclic antidepressants can potentiate the muscle relaxant effects of baclofen, resulting in severe hypotonic weakness (57); the combination has also been incriminated in the causation of short-term memory impairment (SEDA-11, 127) (58).

References

1. Cappell MS. Clinical presentation, diagnosis and management of gastroesophageal reflux disease. Med Clin N Am 2005;89:243–91.
2. Koek GH, Sifrim D, Lerut T, Janssens J, Tack J. Effect of the GABA$_B$ agonist baclofen in patients with symptoms and duodeno-gastro-oesophageal reflux refractory to proton pump inhibitors. Gut 2003;52:1397–402.
3. Rubin DI, So EL. Reversible akinetic mutism possibly induced by baclofen. Pharmacotherapy 1999;19(4):468–70.
4. Parmar MS. Akinetic mutism after baclofen. Ann Intern Med 1991;115(6):499–500.
5. Anderson KJ, Farmer JP, Brown K. Reversible coma in children after improper baclofen pump insertion. Paediatr Anaesth 2002;12(5):454–60.
6. Lyew MA, Mondy C, Eagle S, Chernich SE. Hemodynamic instability and delayed emergence from general anesthesia associated with inadvertent intrathecal baclofen overdose. Anesthesiology 2003;98(1):265–8.
7. Wainapel SF, Lee L, Riley TL. Reversible electroencephalogram changes associated with administration of baclofen in a quadriplegic patient: case report. Paraplegia 1986;24(2):123–6.
8. Hormes JT, Benarroch EE, Rodriguez M, Klass DW. Periodic sharp waves in baclofen-induced encephalopathy. Arch Neurol 1988;45(7):814–5.
9. Rush JM, Gibberd FB. Baclofen-induced epilepsy. J R Soc Med 1990;83(2):115–6.
10. Hansel DE, Hansel CR, Shindle MK, Reinhardt EM, Madden L, Levey EB, Johnston MV, Hoon AH, Jr. Oral baclofen in cerebral palsy: possible seizure potentiation? Pediatr Neurol 2003;29:203–6.
11. Burgard EC, Sarvey JM. Long-lasting potentiation and epileptiform activity produced by GABA$_B$ receptor activation

in the dentate gyrus of rat hippocampal slice. J Neurosci 1991;11:1198–209.

12. Perry HE, Wright RO, Shannon MW, Woolf AD. Baclofen overdose: drug experimentation in a group of adolescents. Pediatrics 1998;101:1045–8.

13. Kofler M, Kronenberg MF, Rifici C, Saltuari L, Bauer G. Epileptic seizures associated with intrathecal baclofen application. Neurology 1994;44:25–7.

14. Zak R, Solomon G, Petito F, Labar D. Baclofen-induced generalized nonconvulsive status epilepticus. Ann Neurol 1994;36:113–4.

15. Naveira FA, Speight KL, Rauck RL, Carpenter RL. Meningitis after injection of intrathecal baclofen. Anesth Analg 1996;82(6):1297–9.

16. Wolf ME, Almy G, Toll M, Mosnaim AD. Mania associated with the use of baclofen. Biol Psychiatry 1982;17(6):757–9.

17. Kofler M, Matzak H, Saltuari L. The impact of intrathecal baclofen on gastrointestinal function. Brain Inj 2002;16(9): 825–36.

18. Soliman IE, Park TS, Berkelhamer MC. Transient paralysis after intrathecal bolus of baclofen for the treatment of post-selective dorsal rhizotomy pain in children. Anesth Analg 1999;89(5):1233–5.

19. Yaksh TL. A drug has to do what a drug has to do. Anesth Analg 1999;89(5):1075–7.

20. Denys P, Mane M, Azouvi P, Chartier-Kastler E, Thiebaut JB, Bussel B. Side effects of chronic intrathecal baclofen on erection and ejaculation in patients with spinal cord lesions. Arch Phys Med Rehabil 1998;79(5):494–6.

21. Wu SS, Dolan KA, Michael Ferrante F. Febrile reaction to subarachnoid baclofen administration. Anesthesiology 2002;96(5):1270–2.

22. Zarrindast MR, Oveissi Y. GABA$_A$ and GABA$_B$ receptor sites involvement in rat thermoregulation. Gen Pharmacol 1988;19(2):223–6.

23. Abel NA, Smith RA. Intrathecal baclofen for treatment of intractable spinal spasticity. Arch Phys Med Rehabil 1994;75(1):54–8.

24. Sampathkumar P, Scanlon PD, Plevak DJ. Baclofen withdrawal presenting as multiorgan system failure. Anesth Analg 1998;87(3):562–3.

25. Reeves RK, Stolp-Smith KA, Christopherson MW. Hyperthermia, rhabdomyolysis, and disseminated intravascular coagulation associated with baclofen pump catheter failure. Arch Phys Med Rehabil 1998;79(3):353–6.

26. Coffey RJ, Edgar TS, Francisco GE, Graziani V, Meythaler JM, Ridgely PM, Sadiq SA, Turner MS. Abrupt withdrawal from intrathecal baclofen: recognition and management of a potentially life-threatening syndrome. Arch Phys Med Rehabil 2002;83(6):735–41.

27. Green LB, Nelson VS. Death after acute withdrawal of intrathecal baclofen: case report and literature review. Arch Phys Med Rehabil 1999;80(12):1600–4.

28. Lees AJ, Clarke CRA, Harrison MJ. Hallucinations after sudden withdrawal of baclofen. Lancet 1977;2(8027):44–5.

29. Fromm GH, Terrence CF, Chattha AS, Glass JD. Baclofen in trigeminal neuralgia: its effect on the spinal trigeminal nucleus: a pilot study. Arch Neurol 1980;37(12):768–71.

30. Turner MR, Gainsborough N. Neuroleptic malignant-like syndrome after abrupt withdrawal of baclofen. J Psychopharmacol 2001;15(1):61–3.

31. Khorasani A, Peruzzi WT. Dantrolene treatment for abrupt intrathecal baclofen withdrawal. Anesth Analg 1995;80(5): 1054–6.

32. Alden TD, Lytle RA, Park TS, Noetzel MJ, Ojemann JG. Intrathecal baclofen withdrawal: a case report and review of the literature. Childs Nerv Syst 2002;18(9–10):522–5.

33. Greenberg MI, Hendrickson RG. Baclofen withdrawal following removal of an intrathecal baclofen pump despite oral baclofen replacement. J Toxicol Clin Toxicol 2003; 41(1):83–5.

34. Meythaler JM, Roper JF, Brunner RC. Cyproheptadine for intrathecal baclofen withdrawal. Arch Phys Med Rehabil 2003;84(5):638–42.

35. Ratnayaka BD, Dhaliwal H, Watkin S. Drug points. Neonatal convulsions after withdrawal of baclofen. BMJ 2001;323(7304):85.

36. Faigle JW, Keberle H, Degen PH. Chemistry and pharmacokinetics of baclofen. In: Feldman RG, Young RR, Koella WP, editors. Spasticity: Disordered Motor Control. Chicago: Year Book, 1980:461–75.

37. Peces R, Navascues RA, Baltar J, Laures AS, Alvarez-Grande J. Baclofen neurotoxicity in chronic haemodialysis patients with hiccups. Nephrol Dial Transplant 1998;13(7): 1896–7.

38. Chen KS, Bullard MJ, Chien YY, Lee SY. Baclofen toxicity in patients with severely impaired renal function. Ann Pharmacother 1997;31(11):1315–20.

39. Seyfert S, Kraft D, Wagner K. Baclofen-Dosis bei Haemodialyse und Niereninsuffizienz. [Baclofen toxicity during intermittent renal dialysis.] Nervenarzt 1981;52(10): 616–7.

40. O'Rourke F, Steinberg R, Ghosh P, Khan S. Withdrawal of baclofen may cause acute confusion in elderly patients. BMJ 2001;323(7317):870.

41. Hansel DE, Hansel CR, Shindle MK, Reinhardt EM, Madden L, Levey EB, Johnston MV, Hoon AH Jr. Oral baclofen in cerebral palsy: possible seizure potentiation? Pediatr Neurol 2003;29:203–6.

42. Kofler M, Kronenberg MF, Rifici C, Saltuari L, Bauer G. Epileptic seizures associated with intrathecal baclofen application. Neurology 1994;44:25–7.

43. Zak R, Solomon G, Petito F, Labar D. Baclofen-induced generalized nonconvulsive status epilepticus. Ann Neurol 1994;36:113–4.

44. Buonaguro V, Scelsa B, Curci D, Monforte S, Iuorno T, Motta F. Epilepsy and intrathecal baclofen therapy in children with cerebral palsy. Pediatr Neurol 2005;33:110–3.

45. Romijn JA, van Lieshout JJ, Velis DN. Reversible coma due to intrathecal baclofen. Lancet 1986;2(8508):696.

46. Muller-Schwefe G, Penn RD. Physostigmine in the treatment of intrathecal baclofen overdose. Report of three cases. J Neurosurg 1989;71(2):273–5.

47. Perry HE, Wright RO, Shannon MW, Woolf AD. Baclofen overdose: drug experimentation in a group of adolescents. Pediatrics 1998;101:1045–8.

48. Leung NY, Whyte IM, Isbister GK. Baclofen overdose: defining the spectrum of toxicity. Emerg Med Australas 2006;18:77–82.

49. Wimmer C. Über Lioresal- (Baclofen-) Intoxikationen— Ein kasuistischer Beitrag. Dtsch Gesundheitsw 1982; 37:1500.

50. May CR. Baclofen overdose. Ann Emerg Med 1983; 12(3):171–3.

51. White WB. Aggravated CNS depression with urinary retention secondary to baclofen administration. Arch Intern Med 1985;145(9):1717–8.

52. Nugent S, Katz MD, Little TE. Baclofen overdose with cardiac conduction abnormalities: case report and review of the literature. J Toxicol Clin Toxicol 1986;24(4):321–8.

53. Perry HE, Wright RO, Shannon MW, Woolf AD. Baclofen overdose: drug experimentation in a group of adolescents. Pediatrics 1998;101(6):1045–8.

54. Saltuari L, Baumgartner H, Kofler M, Schmutzhard E, Russegger L, Aichner F, Gerstenbrand F. Failure of physostigmine in treatment of acute severe intrathecal baclofen intoxication. N Engl J Med 1990;322(21):1533–4.
55. Penn RD, Kroin JS. Failure of physostigmine in treatment of acute severe intrathecal baclofen intoxication. N Engl J Med 1990;322:1533.
56. Kerr DI, Ong J, Prager RH, Gynther BD, Curtis DR. Phaclofen: a peripheral and central baclofen antagonist. Brain Res 1987;405(1):150–4.
57. Silverglat MJ. Baclofen and tricyclic antidepressants: possible interaction. JAMA 1981;246(15):1659.
58. Sandyk R, Gillman MA. Baclofen-induced memory impairment. Clin Neuropharmacol 1985;8(3):294–5.

Botulinum toxins

General Information

Botulinum toxins A and B, which are produced by the bacterium *Clostridium botulinum*, are used for the treatment of facial rhytides (for example, lateral orbital wrinkles, lower eyelid wrinkles, and labial lines), by producing weakness or paralysis of the associated muscles, and in the treatment of hyperhidrosis. The toxin binds with high affinity to peripheral cholinergic nerve endings, such as those at the neuromuscular junction and in the autonomic nervous system, preventing the release of the neurotransmitter acetylcholine (1). This action at the neuromuscular junction can cause weakness and even paralysis of the muscles supplied by the affected nerves. Sprouting of the terminal nerves eventually results in re-innervation of the muscles and return of function. Doses are measured in mouse units (MU), 1 MU being the LD_{50} in Swiss–Webster mice.

Botulinum toxin is used in the treatment of excessive muscle contraction disorders (dystonias), such as strabismus, blepharospasm, focal dystonias, and spasticity. One of its uses is in the removal of facial wrinkles by paralysing mimic muscles. It can reduce sweat production by blocking cholinergic innervation of eccrine sweat glands.

Fortunately, adverse effects and undesirable sequelae after injection are temporary. Several extensive reviews have covered these complications and their management (2,3,4).

Observational studies

For blepharospasm, injections of about 12.5–25 MU are made into the periocular muscles of each eye. When so used, adverse effects are seen in 20–50% of treatments. They consist of mild ptosis, increased or reduced tear function, diplopia, and ectropion. These effects are transient, most lasting about 2 weeks, and generally well tolerated. Occasionally ptosis is so severe as to be inconvenient for the patient. The blepharospasm is relieved for 2–4 months. Systemic effects have not been reported (5).

In the treatment of spastic torticollis there is a tendency to use larger doses (up to 1000 MU) injected into the neck muscles, and weakness of the pharyngeal muscles, resulting in dysphagia and paralysis of the vocal cords, has been reported. Difficulty in swallowing and deepening of the voice were found in up to 30% of cases in one series, resolving after 2–3 weeks (6). In one case there was severe dysphagia 2 days after an injection, with unilateral vocal cord paralysis a week later; swallowing was normal again after 6 weeks (7). The possibility of appreciable effects from this neurotoxin at more distant neuromuscular junctions and the development of antibodies are potential dangers here.

Treatment of spasmodic torticollis with botulinum toxin has been reviewed retrospectively in 107 patients (SEDA-17, 45). It was efficacious in 93% but adverse effects occurred in 84%. Initially, 500 MU were injected into each muscle, but the incidence of adverse effects led to a reduction in dosage, 200–500 MU being injected depending on the muscle used and on neck thickness. The median dose per treatment was 1000 (range 200–1600) MU on the first visit and 800 MU subsequently. Dysphagia occurred after 44% of the treatments. This was severe in 2% of treatments, allowing only sips of fluid and necessitating hospitalization for two patients because of dehydration. Two patients developed stridor, two had substantial weight loss, and one developed pneumonia as a result of aspiration. According to the authors, the risk of dysphagia is 40% if a sternomastoid is injected and 25% if it is not. The risks of moderate or severe dysphagia are 7% and under 1% respectively. The authors estimated that there is a 3% chance of antibody production with reduced responsiveness during the first 15 months of treatment. They recommended antibody testing for patients who have initial but not subsequent improvement after repeated injections of botulinum toxin. The problem of immunological resistance to the effects of botulinum toxin associated with repeat injections has been reviewed elsewhere (8).

The long-term effectiveness of high-dose botulinum toxin (200 MU per axilla) has been evaluated in an open study in patients with axillary hyperhidrosis unresponsive to previous therapies (9). In 34 patients follow-up was for at least 12 months. Four relapsed within 12 months and two relapsed after 16 and 19 months. Mild pain and a burning sensation, sometimes lasting up to 1 hour after injection, were the most frequent adverse effects. No compensatory hyperhidrosis at other body sites was reported.

In a review of all adverse events after therapeutic and cosmetic use reported to the FDA during the 13.5 years since botulinum A toxin was first licensed, there were 1437 reports—406 after therapeutic use (217 serious and 189 non-serious) and 1031 after cosmetic use (36 serious and 995 non-serious) (10). The adverse events occurred predominantly in women, median age 50 years. Over a single year the proportion of reports classified as serious was 33-fold higher for therapeutic than for cosmetic cases. The 217 serious adverse events reported in therapeutic cases included all 28 reported deaths; six deaths were attributed to *respiratory arrest*, five to *myocardial infarction*, three to *strokes*, two to *pulmonary embolism*, two to *pneumonia*, five to other causes, and five to unknown causes. Of the 36 serious events after cosmetic use of botulinum toxin, 30 were included as possible complications in the FDA-approved label; the other six may not have been related to the drug. *Seizures* were reported in 17 patients; 15 of these had either a history of seizures or a condition that increase their risk of seizures (for example a history of cerebral infarction). Other serious adverse events included dysphagia (n = 26), muscle weakness (11), allergic reactions (13), flu-like syndromes (10), injection site trauma (9), dysrhythmias (9), and myocardial infarction (6). Among the 995 cosmetic cases associated with non-serious events, the most common were lack of effect (63%), injection site reactions (19%), and ptosis (11%).

While this review revealed very interesting information about the adverse effects of botulinum toxin, it did not allow the incidence of such effects to be estimated. The survey covered 1989–2003, but the cosmetic use of botulinum toxin was only approved by the FDA in 2002. On the other hand, the estimated number of cosmetic uses over those 2 years in the USA was impressive (1 123 510 injections in 2002 and 2 891 390 injections in 2003) (11). Of course, botulinum toxin was also used for cosmetic purposes, even before FDA approval.

Adverse events have been studied in 327 patients (202 women, 125 men) who received 1043 injections of botulinum A toxin for cervical dystonia (n = 58), blepharospasm (n = 31), hemifacial spasm (n = 39), spasticity due to cerebral palsy (n = 96), chronic anal fissure (n = 96), or esophageal achalasia (n = 7) (12). The following adverse events were observed in those with cervical dystonias: dysphagia (27% of patients and 7% of sessions), weakness of the neck muscles (6.7% and 1.3%), pain during swallowing (5.1% and 1%), and a flu-like syndrome (3.4%, 0.7%); the dysphagia appeared 8.2 days after injection and lasted 15 days on average. In patients with blepharospasm there were unilateral ptosis (22%, 6.3%), bilateral ptosis (3%, 1.9%), and hematomas (3%, 0.6%), and in hemifacial spasm excessive weakness resulting in asymmetry of the face, either mild (28% and 20%) or moderate (46% and 27%). In spasticity due to cerebral palsy there was excessive weakness of the legs, which lasted 14 days on average (6.2% and 1.9%), pain (5.2% and 1.6%), and a flu-like syndrome (4.1% and 1.3%). In chronic anal fissure there were mild incontinence of flatus and feces (9% and 5%), hematomas (5%), a flu-like syndrome (3%), inflammation of external anal varices (2%), and epididymitis (1%). In esophageal achalasia, chest pain in six patients (on the day of injection and for 2–4 days) and esophageal reflux in two (4–8 weeks after the injection, lasting 2–3 weeks). The adverse effects were transient, mostly local, and completely reversible.

Placebo-controlled studies

In a multicenter, randomized, placebo-controlled trial in 145 patients with axillary hyperhidrosis, refractory to treatment with topical aluminium chloride, both 100 and 200 MU of botulinum toxin reduced sweat production by about 80% (13). After 24 weeks, sweat production in the treated axillae was about 45% of baseline. Temporary adverse events during the first 14 weeks included headache, soreness of the muscles of the shoulder girdle, axillary itching, and increased facial sweating.

A multicenter, double-blind, randomized, placebo-controlled study in 320 patients with untreated hyperhidrosis showed a more than 50% reduction in sweat production at 4 and 16 weeks after treatment respectively in 94 and 82% of patients treated with botulinum toxin (50 MU per axilla) and in 36 and 21% of placebo-treated patients (14). The major treatment-related adverse effect was an increase in sweating in non-axillary sites after treatment. Open treatment with botulinum toxin A was offered to patients in whom sweat production was at least 50% of baseline values (15). Of 207 study subjects, 39% had one treatment, 45% had two treatments and 15% had three treatments. Response rates 4 weeks after treatment were 96, 91, and 83% after the first, second, and third treatments respectively. In one of 207 patients there was possible transient seroconversion from negative to positive for neutralizing antibodies to botulinum toxin, and subsequent treatment with botulinum toxin resulted in complete disappearance of axillary sweating 7 days after injection.

Systematic reviews

In a review of four publications reporting adverse events after local injection of botulinum toxin into the lower urinary tract the reported adverse effects included generalized muscle weakness, arm weakness, hyposthenia with reduced supralesional muscle force, vision disturbances, and fever (16). All the adverse effects were self-limiting and lasted 2 weeks to 2 months after injection.

Organs and Systems

Nervous system

Five cases of severe headache refractory to oral analgesics have been reported in patients treated with 10–38 MU of botulinum toxin for glabella frown lines (n = 4) and in a patient treated with 120 MU for palmar hyperhidrosis (17). The headache lasted for 8 days to 4 weeks, did not respond to oral prednisolone, and in some patients was accompanied by photophobia, ear tenderness, or nasal congestion. Two patients had had a similar headache after a previous treatment with botulinum toxin and in another patient a similar headache occurred after the next treatment. None of the patients had a history of severe headaches.

In a double-blind, randomized, placebo-controlled trial in 60 patients with lateral epicondylitis a single injection of botulinum toxin type A significantly reduced pain (18). However, there was mild paresis of the fingers at 4 weeks in four patients who received botulinum and in none of those who received placebo; 10 patients who received botulinum and six who received placebo had weak finger extension on the same side as the injection.

Sensory systems

Parasympathetic dysfunction of the visual system occurred in three patients after injection of botulinum toxin type B at remote sites (19).

Neuromuscular function

Muscle weakness after botulinum toxin injection is usually due to local spread of the agent. Asymptomatic systemic effects have been detected in patients with cervical dystonia after repeated botulinum toxin injections, when muscle biopsies from the vastus lateralis muscle were examined (20). However, generalized neuromuscular symptoms are rare. Patients with a reduced margin of safety with regard to neuromuscular transmission might be considered prone to systemic effects, but even in patients with myasthenia gravis symptoms distal from the injection site have been reported only occasionally (21). However, generalized muscle weakness can occur if higher doses of botulinum toxin are used, and a recent report has illustrated that this may happen in patients after many uneventful treatment sessions (22). Electrophysiological findings in these patients were suggestive of mild botulism, with doses of botulinum toxin of 600–900 units. Two similar cases had been reported previously (21). Therefore, constant long-term monitoring of patients is recommended, even if they have been receiving injections for many years without adverse effects.

Generalized muscular weakness associated with signs of systemic cholinergic autonomic impairment has been reported.

- A 25-year-old woman was treated with botulinum toxin for hyperhidrosis of the axillae and hands in one session with a total amount of 1400 MU. Six days later she complained of diffuse weakness, diplopia, mild bilateral ptosis, severe weakness in the fingers, and reduced lacrimation, salivary production, and sweating (23). She recovered completely within 2 months.

Permanent extraocular muscle damage has been reported (24).

- A 70-year-old man had increasing difficulty in maintaining binocular vision while reading. There was imbalance of his extraocular muscle activity. Botulinum toxin 2.5 MU was therefore injected into the left inferior rectus muscle under electromyography control using a 27-gauge needle. At the next visit 1 month later he complained of diplopia in all directions of gaze, in keeping with a left inferior rectus muscle palsy. Over the next 10 months there was no improvement. Magnetic resonance imaging then showed atrophy of the left inferior rectus muscle. Inferior transposition of the medial and lateral recti muscles was performed, which produced satisfactory alignment.

Botulinum-induced atrophy of extraocular muscles of the eye cannot be excluded in this case. This mechanism is supported by the observation that botulinum toxin can cause histological changes in the extraocular muscles in adult monkeys (25). The authors of the present report also suggested that intramuscular hematoma or direct damage to the nerve to the muscle may have been responsible. So far, permanent extraocular muscle damage after botulinum toxin injection seems to be rare. If additional cases are reported, patients should be informed about this possible complication before treatment.

Skin

An unusual case of a generalized rash starting 30 hours after an injection of botulinum toxin A to treat blepharospasm has been reported (26).

A man who received botulinum A toxin injections every 3 months for 18 months for left-sided oromandibular dystonia developed left-sided madarosis and facial alopecia (27).

Musculoskeletal

Myofascial mecrosis has been attributed to botulinum toxin (28)

- A 36-year-old woman with multiple sclerosis was given electromyographically guided botulinum toxin (total dose 400 IU) into the medial hamstrings and adductor muscles in both legs. Two months she presented with a foul-smelling, painless, necrotic lesion measuring 2–3 cm in diameter in the groin skin crease overlying the adductor compartment of both thighs with no surrounding erythema. A large amount of foul-smelling pus, necrosed skin, and underlying adductor muscles was debrided. No organisms were grown.

The authors suggested that the necrosis might have been linked to excessive paralysis caused by the toxin, but they could not explain the underlying mechanism. Previous reports of botulinum-induced local paralysis did not mention necrosis. Previously, muscle fiber necrosis has only been noted in animal experiments (29). If excessive paralysis of the adductor muscles was the precipitating event, the patient should have noticed a significant change in muscle tone, but that was not mentioned. Also, negative cultures do not rule out infectious causes. Despite these uncertainties, the authors concluded that all patients who receive injections of botulinum toxin should be warned of this effect. For the time being we do not think there is enough evidence to back up this conclusion. This case report does not justify the assumption that extensive myofascial necrosis is a direct adverse effect of botulinum toxin. However, patients who receive deep intramuscular injections still need to be warned of infectious complications, which include abscess formation and soft tissue infections.

Immunologic

In a long-term study of 45 patients (mean age 69 years, 32 women) who had received injection of botulinum toxin repeatedly for at least 12 years (mean 16 years), there were 20 adverse events in 16 patients after their initial visit and 11 adverse events in 10 patients at their most recent injection visit (30). In four of 22 non-responsive patients *blocking antibodies* were confirmed by the mouse protection assay. Of the antibody-negative patients, 16 again became responsive after dosage adjustments and two remained non-responders.

Long-term effects

Drug tolerance

Secondary non-responsiveness can occur in patients who are given repeated injections of botulinum toxin type A, especially for focal dystonias and spasticity. Botulinum toxin type B has been used as an alternative but has been disappointing. Of 36 patients with cervical dystonia resistant to type A toxin, only 13 had a reasonable response to type B; the other 23 patients had either no response or a poor response, or had unacceptable adverse effects and stopped treatment (31). A few patients with blepharospasm, hemifacial spasm, or foot dystonia also had disappointing responses. Of 20 patients with spasticity, seven had some response to type B without unacceptable adverse effects.

Resistance to botulinum toxin type B has also been described in those with and without prior resistance to botulinum toxin type A (32). Of 24 patients with cervical dystonias treated with botulinum toxin type B for up to 64 months, mean treatment dose 14 828 (range 2500–28 000) units, eight became secondarily resistant, and four were primary non-responders, possibly because of the severity and nature of their disease.

Susceptibility Factors

Neuromuscular disorders

Patients with diseases that affect the neuromuscular junction, such as myasthenia gravis or Lambert–Eaton syndrome can develop systemic muscle weakness (33), even with low doses of botulinum toxin; they should therefore not be treated with botulinum toxin.

- An 80-year-old woman had severe difficulty in swallowing and flaccid paralysis of her cervical muscles starting 4 days after the periocular injection of botulinum toxin 120 MU for blepharospasm (21). She also developed bilateral facial nerve paralysis and slurred speech and could not fully close her eyes. Barium swallow and fluoroscopy showed signs of aspiration. The serum concentration of antiacetylcholine receptor antibodies was 6.9 units (reference range 0–0.7 units). Mestinone and prednisone improved her symptoms. She had been treated with botulinum toxin on 18 occasions over the previous 13 years without any untoward effects.

While the exact cause of muscle weakness was unclear, this case argues against the use of botulinum toxin in patients with myasthenic syndromes. When the margin of safety is reduced with regard to neuromuscular transmission, botulinum toxin can result in increased morbidity or even mortality. Generalized muscle weakness after botulinum toxin has also been reported in patients with other neuromuscular disorders (34). In addition, it should be remembered that both dysphagia and muscle weakness can occur after botulinum toxin injection, even in patients who do not suffer from generalized neuromuscular disorders (35).

Patients with mitochondrial cytopathies seem to be hypersensitive to the effects of botulinum toxin and have an increased risk of adverse reactions, as has been reported in two siblings with mitochondrial myopathy (36).

- A 30-year-old man with complex II and III deficiency of the mitochondrial respiratory chain had unspecified intellectual and movement disorders going back to infancy, was wheelchair bound, and could only speak single words or simple phrases, but had good comprehension and memory and normal sphincter function. He received two injections of botulinum toxin, (Dysport 120 mU in each parotid gland for excessive drooling and 100 mU into the right tibialis anterior muscle and 200 mU into the right tibialis posterior muscle for right foot inturning). There were no adverse effects. About 2 months later he received Dysport 120 mU into each parotid gland and 60 mU into each submandibular gland, 300 mU into the right tibialis anterior muscle, and 100 mU into the right tibialis posterior muscle. Ten days later he developed swallowing difficulties which resolved within 2 months.
- The second patient was the first patient's 32-year-old sister, who had a very similar clinical picture. She received Dysport 120 mU into each parotid gland, and 50 mU into each submandibular gland. She developed fluctuating dysphagia, which lasted 2 months.

The authors quoted one previous report of remote symptoms after botulinum toxin in a patient with mitochondrial myopathy (37). They suggested that neuromuscular junction defects might have resulted in the exacerbated response to botulinum toxin and concluded that botulinum toxin should be avoided in patients with mitochondrial cytopathies.

Generalized weakness has been reported after botulinum toxin treatment in a patient with amyotrophic lateral sclerosis (34).

Drug Administration

Drug formulations

Pain due to injection of botulinum toxin has been reported to be less severe with botulinum toxin reconstituted in preservative-containing saline 0.9% (benzyl alcohol 0.9% w/v) than with botulinum toxin reconstituted in preservative-free saline 0.9% in patients with glabella-frown lines (38).

Drug–Drug Interactions

Neuromuscular blocking drugs

As botulinum toxin inhibits acetylcholine release it can interfere with neuromuscular blocking agents (39). It has been suggested that each dose of botulinum toxin may have two effects: first, a direct increase in sensitivity to neuromuscular blocking agents; second, compensatory synaptic remodeling resulting in reduced sensitivity (39). Thus, the effects of neuromuscular blocking agents on neuromuscular transmission cannot be predicted in patients receiving botulinum toxin.

Management of Adverse Drug Reactions

Prevention of the adverse effects of botulinum toxin has been reviewed (40). The correct injection technique is essential, since most unwanted effects are caused by incorrect technique. The most common adverse effects are pain and hematoma. In the periocular region, lid and brow ptosis are important. Pain and bruising can also occur in the upper and lower face and at extrafacial sites. The most important methods of avoiding most unwanted adverse effects are the proper techniques of dilution, storage, and injection, and careful exclusion of patients with contraindications. Pain and bruising can be prevented by cooling the skin before and after injection. Upper lid ptosis can be partly corrected using apraclonidine or phenylephrine eye-drops.

Apraclonidine, an α_2 adrenoceptor agonist that causes Muller's muscles to contract, quickly raising the upper eyelid by 1–3 mm, has been used to treat ptosis secondary to the use of botulinum toxin (41).

References

1. Hambleton P. Clostridium botulinum toxins: a general review of involvement in disease, structure, mode of action and preparation for clinical use. J Neurol 1992;239(1):16–20.
2. Carruthers A, Carruthers J. Botulinum toxin type A. J Am Acad Dermatol 2005;53:284–90.
3. Vartanian AJ, Dayan SH. Complications of botulinum toxin A use in facial rejuvenation. Facial Plast Surg Clin North Am 2005;13:1–10.
4. Wollina U, Konrad H. Managing adverse events associated with botulinum toxin type A. A focus on cosmetic procedures. Am J Clin Dermatol 2005;6:141–50.
5. Cohen DA, Savino PJ, Stern MB, Hurtig HI. Botulinum injection therapy for blepharospasm: a review and report of 75 patients. Clin Neuropharmacol 1986;9(5):415–29.
6. Stell R, Coleman R, Thompson P, Marsden CD. Botulinum toxin treatment of spasmodic torticollis. BMJ 1988;297(6648):616.
7. Koay CE, Alun-Jones T. Pharyngeal paralysis due to botulinum toxin injection. J Laryngol Otol 1989;103(7):698–9.
8. Borodic G, Johnson E, Goodnough M, Schantz E. Botulinum toxin therapy, immunologic resistance, and problems with available materials. Neurology 1996;46(1):26–9.
9. Wollina U, Karamfilov T, Konrad H. High-dose botulinum toxin type A therapy for axillary hyperhidrosis markedly prolongs the relapse-free interval. J Am Acad Dermatol 2002;46(4):536–40.
10. Coté TR, Mohan AK, Polder JA, Walton MK, Braun MM. Botulinum toxin type A injections: adverse events reported to the US Food and Drug Administration in therapeutic and cosmetic cases. J Am Acad Dermatol 2005;53:407–15.
11. American Society of Plastic Surgeons. 2000/2001/2002/2003 National Plastic Surgery Statistics. Available at http://www.plasticsurgery.org/media/statistics/2003Statistics.cfm, accessed October 2007.
12. Slawek J, Madalinski MH, Maciag-Tymecka I, Duzynski W. (Frequency of side effects after botulinum toxin A injections in neurology, rehabilitation and gastroenterology.) Pol Merkur Lekarski 2005;18(105):298–302.
13. Heckmann M, Ceballos-Baumann AO, Plewig GHyperhidrosis Study Group. Botulinum toxin A for axillary hyperhidrosis (excessive sweating). N Engl J Med 2001;344(7):488–93.
14. Naumann M, Lowe NJ. Botulinum toxin type A in treatment of bilateral primary axillary hyperhidrosis: randomised, parallel group, double blind, placebo controlled trial. BMJ 2001;323(7313):596–9.
15. Naumann M, Lowe NJ, Kumar CR, Hamm HHyperhidrosis Clinical Investigators Group. Botulinum toxin type a is a safe and effective treatment for axillary hyperhidrosis over 16 months: a prospective study. Arch Dermatol 2003;139(6):731–6.
16. De Laet K, Wyndaele JJ. Adverse events after botulinum A toxin injection for neurogenic voiding disorders. Spinal Cord 2005;43(7):397–9.
17. Alam M, Arndt KA, Dover JS. Severe, intractable headache after injection with botulinum A exotoxin: report of 5 cases. J Am Acad Dermatol 2002;46(1):62–5.
18. Wong SM, Hui AC, Tong PY, Poon DW, Yu E, Wong LK. Treatment of lateral epicondylitis with botulinum toxin: a randomized, double-blind, placebo-controlled trial. Ann Intern Med 2005;143(11):793–7.
19. Dubow J, Kim A, Leikin J, Cumpston K, Bryant S, Rezak M. Visual system side effects caused by parasympathetic dysfunction after botulinum toxin type B injections. Mov Disord 2005;20(7):877–80.
20. Ansved T, Odergren T, Borg K. Muscle fiber atrophy in leg muscles after botulinum toxin type A treatment of cervical dystonia. Neurology 1997;48(5):1440–2.
21. Borodic G. Myasthenic crisis after botulinum toxin. Lancet 1998;352(9143):1832.
22. Bhatia KP, Munchau A, Thompson PD, Houser M, Chauhan VS, Hutchinson M, Shapira AH, Marsden CD. Generalised muscular weakness after botulinum toxin injections for dystonia: a report of three cases. J Neurol Neurosurg Psychiatry 1999;67(1):90–3.
23. Tugnoli V, Eleopra R, Quatrale R, Capone JG, Sensi M, Gastaldo E. Botulism-like syndrome after botulinum toxin type A injections for focal hyperhidrosis. Br J Dermatol 2002;147(4):808–9.
24. Mohan M, Tow S, Fleck BW, Lee JP. Permanent extraocular muscle damage following botulinum toxin injection. Br J Ophthalmol 1999;83(11):1309–10.
25. Spencer RF, McNeer KW. Botulinum toxin paralysis of adult monkey extraocular muscle. Structural alterations in orbital, singly innervated muscle fibers. Arch Ophthalmol 1987;105(12):1703–11.
26. Mezaki T, Sakai R. Botulinum toxin and skin reaction. Mov Disord 2005;20:770.
27. Kowing D. Madarosis and facial alopecia presumed secondary to botulinum a toxin injections. Optom Vis Sci 2005;82(7):579–82.
28. Agaba AE, Mahmoud S, Esmail H, Sutton J, Bertalot JC, Jibani MM. Extensive myofascial necrosis: a delayed complication of botulinum toxin therapy. Eur J Intern Med 2005;16(8):603–5.
29. Kim HS, Hwang JH, Jeong ST, Lee YT, Lee PK, Suh YL, Shim JS. Effect of muscle activity and botulinum toxin dilution volume on muscle paralysis. Dev Med Child Neurol 2003;45:200–6.
30. Mejia NI, Vuong KD, Jankovic J. Long-term botulinum toxin efficacy, safety, and immunogenicity. Mov Disord 2005;20(5):592–7.

31. Barnes MP, Best D, Kidd L, Roberts B, Stark S, Weeks P, Whitaker J. The use of botulinum toxin type-B in the treatment of patients who have become unresponsive to botulinum toxin type-A—initial experiences. Eur J Neurol 2005;12(12):947–55.
32. Berman B, Seeberger L, Kumar R. Long-term safety, efficacy, dosing, and development of resistance with botulinum toxin type B in cervical dystonia. Mov Disord 2005;20(2):233–7.
33. Barohn RJ, Jackson CE, Rogers SJ, Ridings LW, McVey AL. Prolonged paralysis due to nondepolarizing neuromuscular blocking agents and corticosteroids. Muscle Nerve 1994;17(6):647–54.
34. Mezaki T, Kaji R, Kohara N, Kimura J. Development of general weakness in a patient with amyotrophic lateral sclerosis after focal botulinum toxin injection. Neurology 1996;46(3):845–6.
35. Bakheit AM, Ward CD, McLellan DL. Generalised botulism-like syndrome after intramuscular injections of botulinum toxin type A: a report of two cases. J Neurol Neurosurg Psychiatry 1997;62(2):198.
36. Gioltzoglou T, Cordivari C, Lee PJ, Hanna MG, Lees AJ. Problems with botulinum toxin treatment in mitochondrial cytopathy: case report and review of the literature. J Neurol Neurosurg Psychiatry 2005;76(11):1594–6.
37. Muller-Vahl KR, Kolbe H, Egensperger R, Dengler R. Mitochondriopathy, blepharospasm, and treatment with botulinum toxin. Muscle Nerve 2000;23:647–8.
38. Alam M, Dover JS, Arndt KA. Pain associated with injection of botulinum A exotoxin reconstituted using isotonic sodium chloride with and without preservative: a double-blind, randomized controlled trial. Arch Dermatol 2002;138(4):510–4.
39. Fiacchino F, Grandi L, Soliveri P, Carella F, Bricchi M. Sensitivity to vecuronium after botulinum toxin administration. J Neurosurg Anesthesiol 1997;9(2):149–53.
40. Wollina U, Konrad H. Managing adverse events associated with botulinum toxin type A: a focus on cosmetic procedures. Am J Clin Dermatol 2005;6(3):141–50.
41. Scheinfeld N. The use of apraclonidine eyedrops to treat ptosis after the administration of botulinum toxin to the upper face. Dermatol Online J 2005;11(1):9.

Carisoprodol

General Information

Carisoprodol is a precursor of meprobamate, an oral anxiolytic with similarities to benzodiazepines. The spasmolytic effect of carisoprodol is thought to be due to interruption of neuronal communication within the reticular formation and spinal cord. Major adverse effects are sedation and drowsiness.

Organs and Systems

Nervous system

In 104 cases carisoprodol and its metabolite meprobamate were detected in the blood of car drivers who were either involved in accidents or arrested for impaired driving (1). In many of these cases, either alcohol or other nervous system depressants were also found. In 21 cases carisoprodol/meprobamate were the only drugs detected. Symptoms and reported driving behavior were similar in all cases. Impairment of driving ability appeared to be possible at any concentration of these two drugs. However, the most severe driving impairment and most overt symptoms of intoxication were noted when the combined concentration of carisoprodol and meprobamate exceeded 10 mg/l.

The potential effect of carisoprodol abuse on the ability to drive has been addressed in a retrospective analysis (2). Among 140 000 blood samples from drivers stopped by the police, carisoprodol and its metabolite meprobamate were the only substances found in 62 cases. Drivers with psychomotor impairment had higher plasma carisoprodol concentrations than those not impaired. There was no conclusive relation between driving impairment and plasma meprobamate concentration, which led the authors to suggest that carisoprodol itself in supratherapeutic concentration had an effect on the ability to drive, independent from the effect of its metabolite. In an earlier study, the most severe driving impairment and most overt symptoms of intoxication were noted when the combined concentration of carisoprodol and meprobamate exceeded 10 mg/l (3).

Long-Term Effects

Drug dependence

Because of its relation to benzodiazepines, dependence on carisoprodol can be a problem. Among patients who had taken carisoprodol for 3 months or more, up to 40% had used it in amounts larger than prescribed, and up to 30% had used it for an effect other than that for which it was prescribed (4). A significant percentage of physicians were unaware of the potential of carisoprodol for abuse and of its metabolism to meprobamate. Patients with carisoprodol withdrawal can present with agitation, restlessness, hallucinations, seizures, anorexia, and vomiting.

Drug Administration

Drug overdose

Symptoms of carisoprodol intoxication include agitation, impaired consciousness, myoclonus, generalized muscle spasms, shivering, tremor, tachycardia, and hypertension, not all of which can easily be explained by nervous system depression via a $GABA_A$ receptor-mediated mechanism of action. Based on an analysis of four cases of carisoprodol intoxication, the serotonin syndrome has been offered as an alternative explanation (5). This would have implications for the treatment of carisoprodol overdose, and there have been reports of the successful use of antiserotonergic drugs in this context. The authors admitted that the symptoms and signs of the serotonin syndrome are rather unspecific and could have been caused by other mechanisms. Therefore, their interesting hypothesis should be regarded with caution.

Carisoprodol overdose is reportedly rarely fatal. However, a review of the deaths examined at the Jefferson County Medical Examiner Office from 1986 to 1997 revealed 24 cases of carisoprodol overdosage (6). In all 24 cases other co-intoxicants were involved. Since the mechanism of death was respiratory depression in 82% of the cases, the authors suggested that carisoprodol had contributed to the fatal outcome. Carisoprodol overdosage should be regarded as potentially fatal if other respiratory depressants add to its effect.

Carisoprodol intoxication can also be associated with symptoms of nervous system overactivity rather than depression. Agitation and myoclonic movement disorders have been observed (7).

As carisoprodol and its metabolite meprobamate are GABA receptor agonists, the use of the benzodiazepine receptor antagonist flumazenil might be considered in some cases of carisoprodol toxicity (8).

- A 51-year-old woman took 87 tablets of carisoprodol (350 mg each) over 13 days and developed lethargy and abnormal speech. She was confused and her Glasgow Coma Score was 9/15. Her pupils were small and reactive. Two boluses of naloxone 2 mg were administered with no effect. After flumazenil 0.2 mg she became more alert but was still mildly somnolent. After a second dose of flumazenil 0.2 mg all signs of intoxication were reversed within 2 minutes. Her blood concentrations at admission were 7.4 µg/ml for carisoprodol and 30.7 µg/ml for meprobamate.

This suggests that flumazenil may be an effective therapeutic option if carisoprodol intoxication results in nervous system depression. However, carisoprodol overdose can also produce myoclonic movements or agitation (4), in which case it is questionable if flumazenil should be used.

References

1. Logan BK, Case GA, Gordon AM. Carisoprodol, meprobamate, and driving impairment. J Forensic Sci 2000;45(3): 619–623.
2. Bramness JG, Skurtveit S, Morland J. Impairment due to intake of carisoprodol. Drug Alcohol Depend 2004;74:311–8.
3. Logan BK, Case GA, Gordon AM. Carisoprodol, meprobamate, and driving impairment. J Forensic Sci 2000;45:619–23.
4. Reeves RR, Carter OS, Pinkofsky HB, Struve FA, Bennett DM. Carisoprodol (Soma): abuse potential and physician unawareness. J Addict Dis 1999;18(2):51–6.
5. Bramness JG, Morland J, Sorlid HK, Rudberg N, Jacobsen D. Carisoprodol intoxications and serotonergic features. Clin Toxicol (Phila) 2005;43:39–45.
6. Davis GG, Alexander CB. A review of carisoprodol deaths in Jefferson County, Alabama. South Med J 1998;91(8): 726–30.
7. Roth BA, Vinson DR, Kim S. Carisoprodol-induced myoclonic encephalopathy. J Toxicol Clin Toxicol 1998; 36(6):609–12.
8. Roberge RJ, Lin E, Krenzelok EP. Flumazenil reversal of carisoprodol (Soma) intoxication. J Emerg Med 2000; 18(1):61–4.

Chlormezanone

General Information

Chlormezanone is a tranquillizer with central muscle relaxant effects. In reaction to some case reports of serious, sometimes fatal, cutaneous toxicity and after intervention by drug regulatory authorities in some European countries, all major manufacturers have stopped production of chlormezanone. It may still be available in combination products in some Asian countries.

For the most part chlormezanone causes only minor adverse effects, such as sedation, dizziness, nausea, and headache, which clear on stopping the drug.

Organs and Systems

Hematologic

Rarely, thombocytopenia can occur in a patient taking chlormezanone (1).

Liver

Rarely, cholestatic hepatitis can occur with chlormezanone.

- A 46-year-old woman with rheumatoid arthritis developed cholestatic liver disease while taking chlormezanone and paracetamol (2).
- Fulminant liver necrosis requiring liver transplantation occurred in a young pregnant woman who had taken chlormezanone 600 mg/day for 3 weeks (SEDA-17, 157).

Skin

Toxic epidermal necrolysis and Stevens–Johnson syndrome have been attributed to chlormezanone (3).

Drug–Drug Interactions

Paracetamol

The concomitant use of paracetamol may increase the chance of adverse effects, especially erythema and urticaria (4).

References

1. Finney RD, Apps J. Unreviewed reports: Trancopal (chlormezanone) and thrombocytopenia. BMJ (Clin Res Ed) 1985;290:1112.
2. Pomiersky C, Blaich E. Arzneimittelbedingte Hepatitis mit Cholestase nach Therapie mit Chlormezanon. [Drug-induced hepatitis with cholestasis following therapy with chlormezanone.] Z Gastroenterol 1985;23(12):684–6.
3. Roujeau JC, Kelly JP, Naldi L, Rzany B, Stern RS, Anderson T, Auquier A, Bastuji-Garin S, Correia O, Locati F, et al. Medication use and the risk of Stevens-Johnson syndrome or toxic epidermal necrolysis. N Engl J Med 1995;333(24):1600–7.
4. Verbov J. Fixed drug eruption due to a drug combination but not to its constituents. Dermatologica 1985;171(1):60–1.

Chlorzoxazone

General Information

Chlorzoxazone is a centrally acting benzoxazole derivative with a weak muscle relaxing effect (1). It is usually used in combination with paracetamol for the treatment of painful muscle spasms. The usual dose is 500 mg tds. Drowsiness, weakness, dizziness, and gastrointestinal complaints are the most frequent unwanted effects.

Organs and Systems

Nervous system

A spasmodic torticollis-like syndrome, repeatedly evoked after the ingestion of chlorzoxazone, is an unusual adverse effect of the drug. Benzatropine mesilate 1 mg intravenously led to resolution of the symptoms within 10 minutes (2).

Liver

The most serious adverse effect of chlorzoxazone, which fortunately occurs only rarely, is hepatotoxicity.

In one case jaundice occurred and rechallenge with a single tablet of Parafon Forte (chlorzoxazone plus paracetamol) resulted in a dramatic reaction after 5 hours, with fever, chills, nausea, vomiting, and recurrence of icterus. Paracetamol on its own had no adverse effect in this case.

The authors reviewed some 23 other cases (SEDA-12, 119) (3).

References

1. Elenbaas JK. Centrally acting oral skeletal muscle relaxants. Am J Hosp Pharm 1980;37(10):1313–23.
2. Rosin MA. Chlorzoxazone-induced spasmotic torticollis. JAMA 1981;246(22):2575.
3. Powers BJ, Cattau EL Jr, Zimmerman HJ. Chlorzoxazone hepatotoxic reactions. An analysis of 21 identified or presumed cases. Arch Intern Med 1986;146(6):1183–6.

Cyclobenzaprine

General Information

Cyclobenzaprine is a centrally acting skeletal-muscle relaxant, claimed to be effective in providing relief of muscle spasm, pain and tenderness, and in reducing the limitations imposed thereby on normal daily activities. The recommended total oral daily dose is 10–30 mg (1). It is structurally similar to the tricyclic antidepressants and adverse effects similar to those seen with the tricyclic antidepressants are therefore to be expected.

The most common adverse effects of cyclobenzaprine are somnolence, dry mucous membranes, dizziness, and confusion. Less commonly, tachycardia, dysarthria, disorientation, and hallucinations have been reported (2).

Organs and Systems

Cardiovascular

Cyclobenzaprine can occasionally cause marked arteriolar spasm due to increased adrenergic tone, precipitating Raynaud's syndrome (SEDA-6, 132).

Psychological, psychiatric

Rarely, manic psychosis can be activated in patients with bipolar affective disorders (3).

First-onset paranoid psychosis has also been reported (4).

- A 36-year-old woman with no past psychiatric problems took 23 tablets of cyclobenzaprine (10 mg each) over 6 weeks to ease back pain resulting from a back injury. She developed insomnia, reduced appetite, poor concentration, irritability, disorganized thoughts, persecutory delusions, and auditory hallucinations. Cyclobenzaprine was withdrawn and a course of loxapine was started, leading to rapid and complete resolution of her agitation and psychotic symptoms within 72 hours. Loxapine was subsequently quickly withdrawn with no ill effects and she recovered fully.

The authors thought that this psychotic episode was related to cyclobenzaprine, in view of the temporal relation of the symptoms to the administration of cyclobenzaprine and their rapid resolution after withdrawal.

Drug Administration

Drug overdose

Common effects of cyclobenzaprine overdose were lethargy, agitation, sinus tachycardia, and both hypertension and hypotension (5).

References

1. Azoury FJ. Double-blind comparison of Parafon Forte and Flexeril in the treatment of acute musculoskeletal disorders. Curr Ther Res 1979;26:189.
2. Nibbelink DW, Strickland SC. Cyclobenzaprine (Flexeril) Report of a postmarketing surveillance program. Curr Ther Res 1980;28:894.
3. Beeber AR, Manring JM Jr. Psychosis following cyclobenzaprine use. J Clin Psychiatry 1983;44(4):151–2.
4. O'Neil BA, Knudson GA, Bhaskara SM. First episode psychosis following cyclobenzaprine use. Can J Psychiatry 2000;45(8):763–4.
5. Spiller HA, Winter ML, Mann KV, Borys DJ, Muir S, Krenzelok EP. Five-year multicenter retrospective review of cyclobenzaprine toxicity. J Emerg Med 1995;13(6):781–5.

Dantrolene

General Information

Dantrolene, a hydantoin derivative, is well established in clinical practice, being of greatest value for the reduction of clonus and involuntary muscle spasms (1,2). The recommended oral doses for the treatment of spastic conditions are 75–400 mg/day.

Dantrolene (1,2) is the agent of choice for treatment of malignant hyperthermia and greatly reduces the mortality to under 10% if given in time (3) together with general supportive measures.

Dantrolene differs from the centrally acting muscle relaxants in that its site of action is beyond the muscle cell membrane. It interferes with the excitation–contraction coupling mechanism of striated muscle, presumably by inhibition of calcium release from the sarcoplasmic reticulum.

The most common adverse reactions, seen in up to 75% of patients, are weakness, fatigue, drowsiness, and dizziness. Nausea, vomiting, and diarrhea or constipation are also common, but all these adverse reactions tend to disappear as treatment continues. In general, by adjusting the dose a satisfactory effect can be achieved with acceptable adverse effects.

Rare, but occasionally very serious, adverse effects include hepatotoxicity, respiratory depression, seizures, pleuropericardial reaction, and lymphocytic lymphoma (SEDA-5, 137).

Organs and Systems

Respiratory

Muscle weakness associated with the oral prophylactic use of dantrolene in a patient with compromised respiratory function is reported to have exacerbated postoperative respiratory depression to such an extent that artificial ventilation was required (SEDA-14, 114) (4).

Pleuropericardial reactions, with sterile effusions and eosinophilia, have also rarely been reported in patients taking 225–400 mg/day for 3 months to 4 years (5). There is no proof of a causal relation, but the chemically related nitrofurantoin has also been associated with pulmonary reactions. Patients taking dantrolene should be screened periodically.

Nervous system

Numbness of the hands and feet has been reported (6); long-term use of the structurally related phenytoin has been incriminated in causing polyneuropathy.

Exacerbation or precipitation of seizures has been reported in children with cerebral palsy taking long-term treatment with high doses of dantrolene (4–12 mg/kg) (7).

Sensory systems

Deafness occurred after 5 days' treatment with dantrolene 25 mg/day in a patient who was also taking long-term baclofen and diazepam (8). This may have been coincidental, but the authors suggested that dantrolene may have caused the effect by interfering with the release of calcium from the sarcoplasmic reticulum. It is therefore interesting that one hypothesis that explains the ototoxicity of aminoglycoside antibiotics involves disturbance of calcium ion binding and phosphorylation processes (SED-11, 549).

Hematologic

Fatal lymphocytic lymphoma has been described during high-dose dantrolene therapy (600 mg/day over 3 years) (9). Although the association was only circumstantial, another hydantoin derivative, phenytoin, is known to cause pseudolymphoma.

Liver

Hepatotoxicity from dantrolene consists mainly of minor liver function disturbances (in 1% of patients), with symptoms in 0.35–0.5% and fatal hepatitis in 0.3% (10,11). The risk of severe liver damage is greater with doses above 300–400 mg/day, with prolonged treatment (more than 60 days), in women and in patients older than 35 years.

Reproductive system

Dantrolene may have contributed to uterine atony, with resulting excessive hemorrhage when given prophylactically after a cesarean section (12).

Drug–Drug Interactions

Calcium channel blockers

The combination of dantrolene with calcium channel blockers, such as verapamil, can result in severe cardiovascular depression and hyperkalemia (SEDA-12, 113) (13,14), so that extreme care is required.

Dantrolene interacts with verapamil and with diltiazem, causing myocardial depression and cardiogenic shock (SEDA-16, 199).

Metoclopramide

The absorption of oral dantrolene can be significantly increased by metoclopramide (15). As the risk of hepatotoxicity has been related to the dosage of dantrolene, increased clinical surveillance is necessary to avoid toxicity of dantrolene during concurrent treatment with metoclopramide.

References

1. Britt BA. Dantrolene. Can Anaesth Soc J 1984;31(1):61–75.
2. Ward A, Chaffman MO, Sorkin EM. Dantrolene. A review of its pharmacodynamic and pharmacokinetic properties and therapeutic use in malignant hyperthermia, the neuroleptic malignant syndrome and an update of its use in muscle spasticity. Drugs 1986;32(2):130–68.
3. Kolb ME, Horne ML, Martz R. Dantrolene in human malignant hyperthermia. Anesthesiology 1982;56(4):254–62.
4. Hara Y, Kato A, Horikawa H, Kato Y, Ichiyanagi K. [Postoperative respiratory depression thought to be due to oral dantrolene pretreatment in a malignant hyperthermia-susceptible patient.]Masui 1988;37(4):483–7.
5. Petusevsky ML, Faling LJ, Rocklin RE, Snider GL, Merliss AD, Moses JM, Dorman SA. Pleuropericardial reaction to treatment with dantrolene. JAMA 1979; 242(25):2772–4.
6. Luisto M, Moller K, Nuutila A, Palo J. Dantrolene sodium in chronic spasticity of varying etiology. A double-blind study. Acta Neurol Scand 1982;65(4):355–62.
7. Denhoff E, Feldman S, Smith MG, Litchman H, Holden W. Treatment of spastic cerebral-palsied children with sodium dantrolene. Dev Med Child Neurol 1975;17(6):736–42.
8. Pace-Balzan A, Ramsden RT. Sudden bilateral sensorineural hearing loss during treatment with dantrolene sodium (Dantrium). J Laryngol Otol 1988;102(1):57–8.
9. Wan HH, Tucker JS. Dantrolene and lymphocytic lymphoma. Postgrad Med J 1980;56(654):261–2.
10. Utili R, Boitnott JK, Zimmerman HJ. Dantrolene-associated hepatic injury. Incidence and character. Gastroenterology 1977;72(4 Pt 1):610–6.
11. Pinder RM, Brogden RN, Speight TM, Avery GS. Dantrolene sodium: a review of its pharmacological properties and therapeutic efficacy in spasticity. Drugs 1977;13(1):3–23.
12. Weingarten AE, Korsh JI, Neuman GG, Stern SB. Postpartum uterine atony after intravenous dantrolene. Anesth Analg 1987;66(3):269–70.
13. Saltzman LS, Kates RA, Corke BC, Norfleet EA, Heath KR. Hyperkalemia and cardiovascular collapse after verapamil and dantrolene administration in swine. Anesth Analg 1984;63(5):473–8.
14. Rubin AS, Zablocki AD. Hyperkalemia, verapamil, and dantrolene. Anesthesiology 1987;66(2):246–9.
15. Gilman TM, Segal JL, Brunnemann SR. Metoclopramide increases the bioavailability of dantrolene in spinal cord injury. J Clin Pharmacol 1996;36(1):64–71.

Dioxium

General Information

Dioxium is obsolete. Accounts of its adverse effects will be found in earlier volumes in this series (SED-10, 213; SEDA-6, 131).

Doxacurium chloride

General Information

Doxacurium chloride is a long-acting non-depolarizing neuromuscular blocking agent. It is a bisquaternary benzylisoquinolinium derivative (a diester). It is subject to minimal hydrolysis by plasma cholinesterase (at about 6% of the rate of hydrolysis of suxamethonium when incubated with purified pooled human plasma cholinesterase) (1). Antagonism by edrophonium (1 mg/kg) was considered inadequate in one study, whereas no difficulties were experienced with neostigmine (0.05 mg/kg) (2).

Organs and Systems

Cardiovascular

No rise in plasma histamine concentration was found with bolus doses up to 0.08 mg/kg (1), but in one case there was transient hypotension 1 minute after a bolus dose of 0.05 mg/kg via a pulmonary artery cannula, with cutaneous flushing at 2 minutes, suggesting that histamine release can occur on occasion (3). There was no tachycardia or bronchospasm, but the mean arterial pressure fell from 88 to 40 mmHg and recovered with therapy within 3 minutes, by which time the skin flushing was fading.

In a study of 54 patients, plasma histamine concentrations increased by 200% following doxacurium in two patients, but there were no changes in heart rate or blood pressure (4). Indeed, cardiovascular stability has been reported in several studies (1,4) and only minor clinically insignificant changes have been seen with doses up to 0.08 mg/kg, even in cardiac patients (AHA classes III–IV) (5,6).

Bradycardia is occasionally seen (2), but this may be due to co-administration of vagotonic drugs with atracurium, vecuronium, and pipecuronium.

Susceptibility Factors

Renal disease

Renal excretion is the main route of elimination of doxacurium, and its duration of action would be expected to be prolonged in patients with renal dysfunction. There have been two reports of the use of doxacurium in patients with chronic renal insufficiency. In the first it was reported that the action of doxacurium (0.025 mg/kg bolus dose) was "markedly but not statistically prolonged"; the mean time to 25% recovery of the twitch height was 121 minutes in the group of patients with renal insufficiency as opposed to 67 minutes in the control group, with great interindividual variation in both groups (7). The second was a study of the pharmacokinetics and pharmacodynamics of doxacurium in patients undergoing cadaveric kidney or liver transplantation (8). The duration of action of doxacurium was more variable and greatly prolonged in patients with end-stage renal insufficiency, although once again the results were clinically but not statistically significant, because of the small numbers of patients and large variability. Plasma clearance was significantly slower and mean residence time significantly greater in the renal transplant group than in control patients. In the patients with liver disease there were no significant pharmacokinetic changes, but the duration of action of the low dose used (15 mg/kg) did tend to be somewhat prolonged.

References

1. Basta SJ, Savarese JJ, Ali HH, Embree PB, Schwartz AF, Rudd GD, Wastila WB. Clinical pharmacology of doxacurium chloride. A new long-acting nondepolarizing muscle relaxant. Anesthesiology 1988;69(4):478–86.
2. Scott RP, Norman J. Doxacurium chloride: a preliminary clinical trial. Br J Anaesth 1989;62(4):373–7.
3. Reich DL. Transient systemic arterial hypotension and cutaneous flushing in response to doxacurium chloride. Anesthesiology 1989;71(5):783–5.
4. Murray DJ, Mehta MP, Choi WW, Forbes RB, Sokoll MD, Gergis SD, Rudd GD, Abou-Donia MM. The neuromuscular blocking and cardiovascular effects of doxacurium chloride in patients receiving nitrous oxide narcotic anesthesia. Anesthesiology 1988;69(4):472–7.
5. Stoops CM, Curtis CA, Kovach DA, McCammon RL, Stoelting RK, Warren TM, Miller D, Abou-Donia MM. Hemodynamic effects of doxacurium chloride in patients receiving oxygen sufentanil anesthesia for coronary artery bypass grafting or valve replacement. Anesthesiology 1988;69(3):365–70.
6. Reich DL, Konstadt SN, Thys DM, Hillel Z, Raymond R, Kaplan JA. Effects of doxacurium chloride on biventricular cardiac function in patients with cardiac disease. Br J Anaesth 1989;63(6):675–81.
7. Cashman JN, Luke JJ, Jones RM. Neuromuscular block with doxacurium (BW A938U) in patients with normal or absent renal function. Br J Anaesth 1990;64(2):186–92.
8. Cook DR, Freeman JA, Lai AA, Robertson KA, Kang Y, Stiller RL, Aggarwal S, Abou-Donia MM, Welch RM. Pharmacokinetics and pharmacodynamics of doxacurium in normal patients and in those with hepatic or renal failure. Anesth Analg 1991;72(2):145–50.

Hexacarbacholine

General Information

Hexacarbacholine is obsolete. Accounts of its adverse effects will be found in earlier volumes in this series (SED-10, 213; SEDA-6, 131).

Tizanidine

General Information

Tizanidine is a centrally acting benzothiadiazol derivative with myotonolytic activity. Although its mechanism of action has not been fully clarified, facilitation of glycine-mediated transmission in the spinal cord may play an important role (1). A total daily dose of 15 mg (5 mg 3 times) is reported to be effective and well tolerated by most patients (2).

The documentation of adverse effects is still fragmentary. Tizanidine seems to be a relatively well tolerated and useful antispastic agent. The most frequently reported adverse effects include drowsiness, dry mouth, and muscle weakness (3). Occasionally, hypotension can occur; it is usually mild (4,5) but can be more severe in patients taking antihypertensive drugs (6–8), in whom tizanidine should be used with great caution. A small fall in heart rate has also been reported (9).

In an open study of tizanidine for neuropathic pain, several adverse effects were noted, such as dizziness, drowsiness, fatigue/weakness, dry mouth, gastrointestinal upset, and sleep difficulty (10).

Organs and Systems

Liver

In an open study of tizanidine for neuropathic pain, one patient developed abnormal liver function tests accompanied by nausea and vomiting, fatigue, confusion, weakness, and muscle aches (10). Within three weeks after withdrawal of tizanidine, the liver function tests returned to baseline and the symptoms resolved. Two other patients had transient asymptomatic rises in liver function tests, which returned to normal despite continuation of tizanidine. Transiently raised liver function tests during tizanidine treatment have occasionally been reported before (11–13).

Drug-drug interactions

Ciprofloxacin

Ciprofloxacin inhibits CYP1A2, which is involved in the metabolism of tizanidine. In healthy volunteers, ciprofloxacin 500 mg/day was given for 3 days followed by a single dose of tizanidine 4 mg (14). The peak plasma concentration was 1.2 ng/ml after placebo pre-treatment and 8.2 ng/ml after ciprofloxacin pre-treatment, a more than six-fold increase. The half-life of tizanidine was only slightly prolonged (1.8 hours after ciprofloxacin versus 1.5 hours after placebo). However, the AUC increased 10-fold. This was accompanied by low blood pressure, cognitive impairment, and drowsiness. The extent of these adverse effects correlated with the tizanidine plasma concentration.

Fluvoxamine

Fluvoxamine inhibits the metabolism of tizanidine, particularly by CYP1A2. In healthy volunteers who took fluvoxamine 100mg/day for 4 days, peak plasma concentrations of tizanidine after a single dose of 4 mg were 12 times higher than those observed previously in the same individuals without fluvoxamine (15). At the same time, the half-life increased from 1.5 to 4.3 hours. This was accompanied by a low arterial blood pressure, cognitive impairment, and drowsiness. The underlying mechanism seemed to be inhibition by fluvoxamine of tizanidine metabolism, by CYP1A2 in particular. There has also been a report of similar problems in clinical practice (16).

- A 70-year old woman had a stroke and developed pain and numbness in her leg. She was taking fluvoxamine 150 mg/day for depression. She was given tizanidine 3 mg/day and soon afterwards developed a dry mouth and anuria. This was accompanied by a fall in heart rate (to 56–60/minute) and body temperature (to 36.1–36.3°C). Tizanidine was withdrawn and her symptoms resolved immediately.

The authors subsequently surveyed the medical records of 913 patients looking for combined use of tizanidine and fluvoxamine. Of 23 patients who had taken these drugs simultaneously six had adverse effects: a low heart rate in six, dizziness in three, and a low body temperature, drowsiness, speech disorder, and hypotension in two. They recommended that the combination of tizanidine and fluvoxamine should be avoided.

References

1. Sayers AC, Burki HR, Eichenberger E. The pharmacology of 5-chloro-4-(2-imidazolin-2-yl-amino)-2,1,3-benzothiadiazole (DS 103-282), a novel myotonolytic agent. Arzneimittelforschung 1980;30(5):793–803.
2. Rinne UK. Tizanidine treatment of spasticity in multiple sclerosis and chronic myelopathy. Curr Ther Res 1980;28:827.
3. Hutchinson DR. Modified release tizanidine: a review. J Int Med Res 1989;17(6):565–73.
4. Fryda-Kaurimsky Z, Muller-Fassbender H. Tizanidine (DS 103-282) in the treatment of acute paravertebral muscle spasm: a controlled trial comparing tizanidine and diazepam. J Int Med Res 1981;9(6):501–5.
5. Goei HS, Whitehouse IJ. Acomparative trial of tizanidine and diazepam in the treatment of acute cervical muscle spasm. Clin Trials J 1982;19:20.
6. Hennies OL. A new skeletal muscle relaxant (DS 103-282) compared to diazepam in the treatment of muscle spasm of local origin. J Int Med Res 1981;9(1):62–8.
7. Hassan N, McLellan DL. Double-blind comparison of single doses of DS103-282, baclofen and placebo for suppression of spasticity. J Neurol Neurosurg Psychiatry 1980;43(12):1132–6.
8. Stien R, Nordal HJ, Oftedal SI, Slettebo M. The treatment of spasticity in multiple sclerosis: a double-blind clinical trial of a new anti-spastic drug tizanidine compared with baclofen. Acta Neurol Scand 1987;75(3):190–4.
9. Mathias CJ, Luckitt J, Desai P, Baker H, el Masri W, Frankel HL. Pharmacodynamics and pharmacokinetics of the oral antispastic agent tizanidine in patients with spinal cord injury. J Rehabil Res Dev 1989;26(4):9–16.
10. Semenchuk MR, Sherman S. Effectiveness of tizanidine in neuropathic pain: an open-label study. J Pain 2000;1(4):285–92.
11. de Graaf EM, Oosterveld M, Tjabbes T, Stricker BH. A case of tizanidine-induced hepatic injury. J Hepatol 1996;25(5):772–3.
12. Saper JR, Winner PK, Lake AE 3rd. An open-label dose-titration study of the efficacy and tolerability of tizanidine hydrochloride tablets in the prophylaxis of chronic daily headache. Headache 2001;41(4):357–68.
13. Lapierre Y, Bouchard S, Tansey C, Gendron D, Barkas WJ, Francis GS. Treatment of spasticity with tizanidine in multiple sclerosis. Can J Neurol Sci 1987;14(Suppl 3):513–7.
14. Granfors MT, Backman JT, Neuvonen M, Neuvonen PJ. Ciprofloxacin greatly increases concentrations and hypotensive effect of tizanidine by inhibiting its cytochrome P450 1A2-mediated presystemic metabolism. Clin Pharmacol Ther 2004;76:598–606.
15. Granfors MT, Backman JT, Neuvonen M, Ahonen J, Neuvonen PJ. Fluvoxamine drastically increases concentrations and effects of tizanidine: a potentially hazardous interaction. Clin Pharmacol Ther 2004;75:331–41.
16. Momo K, Doki K, Hosono H, Homma M, Kohda Y. Drug interaction of tizanidine and fluvoxamine. Clin Pharmacol Ther 2004;76:509–10.

Index of drug names

Printed and bound by CPI Group (UK) Ltd, Croydon, CR0 4YY

04/10/2024

01041143-0001